NURSING RESEARCH

Methods, Critical Appraisal, and Utilization

DATE DUE

Cat. No. 23-221

FIFTH EDITION

NURSING RESEARCH

Methods, Critical Appraisal, and Utilization

Geri LoBiondo-Wood, PhD, RN, FAAN
Associate Professor,
University of Texas Health Sciences Center,
School of Nursing,
Nursing Systems and Technology,
Houston, Texas

Judith Haber, PhD, APRN, CS, FAAN
Professor and Director,
Master's Program and Post-Master's Advanced Certificate Program,
Division of Nursing,
New York University,
New York, New York

With 57 illustrations

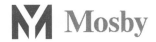

Mosby

St. Louis   London   Philadelphia   Sydney   Toronto

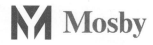

Vice-President and Publishing Director: Sally Schrefer
Executive Editor: Barbara Nelson Cullen
Managing Editor: Linda Caldwell
Developmental Editor: Eric Ham
Project Manager: Catherine Jackson
Production Editor: Jodi Everding
Designer: Amy Buxton

FIFTH EDITION
Copyright © 2002 by Mosby, Inc.

Previous editions copyrighted 1986, 1990, 1994, 1998

NOTICE
Pharmacology is an ever-changing field. Standard safety precautions must be followed, but as new research and clinical experience broaden our knowledge, changes in treatment and drug therapy may become necessary or appropriate. Readers are advised to check the most current product information provided by the manufacturer of each drug to be administered to verify the recommended dose, the method and duration of administration, and contraindications. It is the responsibility of the licensed prescriber, relying on experience and knowledge of the patient, to determine dosages and the best treatment for each individual patient. Neither the Publisher nor the editor assume any liability for any injury and/or damage to persons or property arising from this publication.

Mosby, Inc.
11830 Westline Industrial Drive
St. Louis, Missouri 63146

Printed in the United States of America.

International Standard Book Number 0-323-01287-6

01 02 03 04 05 CA/FF 9 8 7 6 5 4 3 2 1

Contributors

Ann Bello, MA, RN
Professor of Nursing,
Norwalk Community College,
Norwalk, Connecticut
Descriptive Data Analysis

Marlene Z. Cohen, PhD, RN
The John Dunn, Sr. Distinguished Professor in
  Oncology Nursing,
The University of Texas,
Houston Health Science Center, School of Nursing;
Director of Applied Nursing Research,
The University of Texas,
M.D. Anderson Cancer Center,
Houston, Texas
Introduction to Qualitative Research

Betty J. Craft, PhD, RN, CS
Associate Professor,
University of Nebraska Medical Center,
College of Nursing,
Omaha, Nebraska
Evaluating Quantitative Research

Margaret Grey, DrPH, RN, FAAN
Independence Foundation Professor of Nursing,
Associate Dean for Research Affairs,
Yale University School of Nursing,
New Haven, Connecticut
*Experimental and Quasiexperimental Designs; Data-
  Collection Methods; Inferential Data Analysis*

Judith Haber, PhD, APRN, CS, FAAN
Professor and Director,
Master's Program and Post-Master's Advanced
  Certificate Program,
Division of Nursing,
New York University,
New York, New York
*The Role of Research in Nursing; Critical Reading
  Strategies: Overview of the Research Process;
  Research Problems and Hypotheses; Sampling; Legal
  and Ethical Issues; Reliability and Validity*

Judith A. Heermann, PhD, RN
Associate Professor,
University of Nebraska Medical Center,
College of Nursing,
Omaha, Nebraska
Evaluating Quantitative Research

Barbara Krainovich-Miller, EdD, RN
Visiting Professor,
New York University,
School of Nursing,
New York, New York
*Critical Reading Strategies: Overview of the Research
  Process; Literature Review; Critical Thinking
  Challenges*

Patricia R. Liehr, PhD, RN
Associate Professor,
University of Texas Health Science Center—
  Houston,
School of Nursing,
Nursing Systems and Technology,
Houston, Texas
*Theoretical Framework; Qualitative Approaches to
  Research*

Geri LoBiondo-Wood PhD, RN, FAAN
Associate Professor,
University of Texas Health Science Center—
  Houston,
School of Nursing,
Nursing Systems and Technology,
Houston, Texas
*The Role of Research in Nursing; Critical Reading
  Strategies: Overview of the Research Process;
  Introduction to Quantitative Research;
  Nonexperimental Designs; Reliability and Validity;
  Analysis of Findings*

Marianne T. Marcus, EdD, RN, FAAN
Professor and Chairperson, Nursing Systems and
  Technology,
University of Texas Health Science Center—
  Houston,
School of Nursing,
Nursing Systems and Technology,
Houston, Texas
Qualitative Approaches to Research

Janet C. Meininger, PhD, RN, FAAN
Lee & Joseph D. Jamail Distinguished Professor,
University of Texas Health Science Center—
  Houston,
School of Nursing,
Nursing Systems and Technology,
Houston, Texas
Research Vignette

Merle H. Mishel, PhD, RN, FAAN
Kenan Professor of Nursing,
School of Nursing,
The University of North Carolina at Chapel Hill,
Chapel Hill, North Carolina
Research Vignette

Mary Naylor, PhD, RN, FAAN
Ralston Endowed Term Professor,
University of Pennsylvania School of Nursing,
Philadelphia, Pennsylvania
Research Vignette

Elizabeth Norman, PhD, RN, FAAN
Professor and Director, Doctoral Program,
Division of Nursing,
New York University,
New York, New York
Research Vignette

Mary Jane Smith, PhD, RN
Professor and Associate Dean for Graduate
  Academic Affairs,
West Virginia University School of Nursing,
Morgantown, West Virginia
Theoretical Framework

Helen J. Streubert Speziale, EdD, RN
Professor,
Nursing Department,
College Misericordia,
Dallas, Pennsylvania
Evaluating Qualitative Research

Susan Sullivan-Bolyai, DNSc, RN
Post-Doctoral Fellow,
Yale University,
School of Nursing,
New Haven, Connecticut
*Experimental and Quasiexperimental Designs; Data-
  Collection Methods; Inferential Data Analysis*

Marita Titler, PhD, RN, FAAN
Director of Research, Quality and Outcomes
  Management,
Department of Nursing Services and Patient Care,
University of Iowa Hospitals and Clinics,
Iowa City, Iowa
Use of Research in Practice

Foreword

A meaningful overview of the evolution of nursing research with excellent "real world" examples sets the stage for the fifth edition of *Nursing Research: Methods, Critical Appraisal, and Utilization* by LoBiondo-Wood and Haber. The authors tackle the enormously complex issues of how to incorporate the knowledge generated by research studies into care of patients, families, and communities, citing both successes and challenges for the twenty-first century. A combination of models for evidence-based practice, with practical illustrations, is particularly useful for students, clinicians, researchers, educators, and administrators who are committed to the value and importance of research and its application to practice. A rich overview of the strategies that have been developed and used provides an incentive for readers to absorb the content. A turbulent health care climate characterized by ever-present change brings an enormous challenge to the discipline. Use of research findings generated by means of sound theoretical and methodological methods can only strengthen the effectiveness of practice and, therefore, outcomes to which nursing is committed.

The wider community of the world is another focus of the fifth edition, and rightfully so. As the globe shrinks, technology expands, and health problems become world health problems, nursing must take its place in grappling with the enormous discrepancies between industrialized, developing, and third-world countries. The work by LoBiondo-Wood and Haber has proven its value as a superb contribution to international collaboration. Having had the opportunity to live and teach in highly diverse countries including Finland, Greece, Spain, India, and Thailand, I have found that *Nursing Research: Methods, Critical Appraisal, and Utilization* serves as an excellent resource for both faculties and students. Out of these international opportunities, I have developed a strong belief that appreciation of cultural differences is the only basis for meaningful research, educational, and clinical collaboration. Health care systems, political and economic structures, and—most importantly—the health of societies are enormously diverse. It follows that the purposes and foci of nursing research in different countries are widely discrepant. Thus global collaboration will be effective only to the extent that there is a commitment to fully understand differences between particular cultures and a desire to research the needs and find methods and solutions that will enable the nursing profession to transcend its differences by using research evidence as the worldwide foundation of clinical practice.

In this extremely timely work, LoBiondo-Wood and Haber address the urgent needs of quality, cost, and outcomes of care. The book is designed specifically to provide baccalaureate students with the essential knowledge and competency to evaluate critically the findings from studies pertaining to all three issues. The ability of "entry-level consumers" of research to critically evaluate their practice and participate in the research process may be a determining factor in nursing's survival as a profession.

Excellent examples of studies addressing populations central to the focus of twenty-first century health care delivery are provided. The list is extensive: the chronically ill, the aged, persons with AIDS, and vulnerable groups (e.g., the abused, single parents, children with life-threatening illnesses, and family caregivers). LoBiondo-Wood and Haber point out the importance of new information acquired by sound methodologies, which must be the cornerstone for testing theories and models of care relevant to the growing numbers in these populations. Both nurses with asssociate and/or baccalaureate degrees must be involved in the research process as the only legitimate route by which we learn about the specific needs of populations and design evidence-based care and evaluate its effectiveness by sound studies of outcomes. Further, the authors have provided another state-of-the-art guide to the literature review and an innovative new web-based instructor's manual. As computer technology becomes a part of every facet of care, it also provides an entree to the most current information for any discipline.

Finally, a major strength of the book is the infectious enthusiasm of the authors. The writing style invites the interest of the reader, and the content serves as a genuine inspiration for the intended audience.

Carol Noll Hoskins, PhD, RN, FAAN
Professor,
Division of Nursing,
School of Education,
New York University,
New York, New York

Preface

The foundation of the fifth edition of *Nursing Research: Methods, Critical Appraisal, and Utilization* continues to be the belief that nursing research is integral to all levels of nursing education and practice. Over the past 15 years since the first edition of this textbook, we have seen the depth and breadth of nursing research grow, with more nurses conducting and using research to shape clinical practice, education, administration, and public policy. Nurses are using research data to influence the nature and direction of health care delivery and document outcomes related to the quality and cost-effectiveness of patient care. As nurses continue to develop a unique body of nursing knowledge through research, decisions about clinical nursing practice will be increasingly research- and evidence-based.

As editors, we believe that all nurses need not only to understand the research process but also to know how to critically read, evaluate, and apply research findings in practice. We realize that understanding research is a challenge for every student, but believe that the challenge can be accomplished in a stimulating, lively, and learner-friendly manner.

Consistent with this perspective is the belief that nursing research must be an integral dimension of baccalaureate education, evident not only in the undergraduate nursing research course but also threaded throughout the curriculum. The research role of baccalaureate graduates calls for the skills of critical appraisal—that is, nurses should be competent research consumers.

Preparing students for this role involves developing their critical thinking and reading skills, thus enhancing their understanding of the research process, appreciation of the role of the critiquer, and ability to actually critique research. An undergraduate course in nursing research should develop this basic level of competence, which is an essential requirement if students are to engage in evidence-based clinical decision making and practice. This is in contrast to a graduate level research course in which the emphasis is on carrying out research, as well as understanding and appraising it.

The primary audience for this textbook remains undergraduate students who are learning the steps of the research process, as well as how to critique published research literature and use research findings to support evidence-based clinical practice. This book is also a valuable resource for students at the master's and doctoral levels who want a concise review of the basic steps of the research and critiquing process. Furthermore, it is an important resource for practicing nurses who strive to use research findings as the basis for clinical decision making and development of evidence-based policies, protocols, and standards rather than tradition, authority, or trial and error. It is also an important resource for nurses who collaborate with nurse-scientists in the conduct of clinical research.

Building on the success of the fourth edition, the fifth edition of *Nursing Research: Methods, Critical Appraisal, and Utilization* prepares nursing students and practicing nurses to become knowledgeable nursing research consumers by:

- Addressing the role of the nurse as a research consumer, thereby embedding research competence in the clinical practice of every baccalaureate graduate.
- Demystifying research, which is sometimes viewed as a complex process.
- Teaching the fundamentals of the research process and critical appraisal process in a user friendly, but logical and systematic, progression.
- Promoting a lively spirit of inquiry that develops critical thinking and critical reading

skills, facilitating mastery of the critiquing process.

- Developing information literacy and research consumer competencies that prepare students and nurses to effectively locate and manage research information.
- Elevating the critiquing process and research consumership to a position of importance comparable to that of producing research. Before students become research producers, they must become knowledgeable research consumers.
- Emphasizing the role of evidence-based practice as the basis for clinical decision making and nursing interventions that support nursing practice, demonstrating quality and cost-effective outcomes of nursing care delivery.
- Presenting numerous examples of recently published research studies that illustrate and highlight each research concept in a manner that brings abstract ideas to life for students new to the research and critiquing process. These examples are a critical link for reinforcement of the research and critiquing process.
- Showcasing **Research Vignettes** by renowned nurse researchers whose careers exemplify the link between research, education, and practice.
- Providing numerous pedagogical chapter features, including **Learning Outcomes, Key Terms, Key Points, Critical Thinking Challenges, Helpful Hints, Critical Thinking Decision Paths, Critiquing Criteria,** and numerous tables, boxes, and figures.
- Introducing interactive web-based **Course Resources** to replace the print "Instructor's Manual", as well as a web-based interactive **Student Study Guide.**

In the fifth edition of *Nursing Research: Methods, Critical Appraisal, and Utilization,* the text is organized into three new parts that are preceded by an introductory section and open with an exciting "Research Vignette" by a renowned nurse researcher.

- PART ONE, RESEARCH OVERVIEW, contains five chapters: Chapter 1, "The Role of Research in Nursing," provides an exciting overview of contemporary roles, approaches, and issues in nursing research. It introduces the importance of the nurse's role as a research consumer and provides a futuristic perspective about research and evidence-based practice principles that shape clinical practice in this new millennium. Chapter 2, "Critical Reading Strategies: Overview of the Research Process," speaks directly to students by highlighting critical thinking and critical reading concepts and strategies that facilitate student understanding of the research process and its relationship to the critiquing process. The style and content of this chapter is designed to make subsequent chapters more user-friendly for students. The next three chapters address foundational components of the research process. Chapter 3, "Research Problems and Hypotheses," focuses on how research questions and hypotheses are derived, operationalized in research studies, and critically appraised. Numerous clinical examples that illustrate different types of research questions and hypotheses are used to maximize student understanding. Chapter 4, "Literature Review," showcases cutting edge information related research consumer competencies that prepare students and nurses to effectively locate, manage, and evaluate research studies and their findings. Chapter 5, the new "Theoretical Framework" chapter, addresses the importance of theoretical foundations to the design and evaluation of research studies.
- PART TWO, PROCESSES RELATED TO QUALITATIVE RESEARCH, contains three interrelated qualitative research chapters. Chapter 6, a new chapter, "Introduction to Qualitative Research," provides a framework for understanding qualitative research designs and literature. Chapter 7, "Qualitative Approaches to Research," presents and illustrates major qualitative designs and

methods using examples from the literature as exemplars. Chapter 8, "Evaluating Qualitative Research," synthesizes essential components of and criteria for critiquing qualitative research reports.

- PART THREE, PROCESSES RELATED TO QUANTITATIVE RESEARCH, contains Chapters 9 to 19. These chapters delineate essential steps of the quantitative research process, with published clinical research studies used to illustrate each step. Links between the steps and their relationship to the total research process are examined and then synthesized in Chapter 19.

- PART FOUR, APPLICATION OF RESEARCH: EVIDENCE-BASED PRACTICE, contains Chapter 20, the state-of-the-art "Use of Research in Practice" chapter, which provides an exciting conclusion to this text through its vibrant presentation of the application of nursing research in clinical practice using an evidence-based practice framework.

Critical thinking is stimulated through the presentation of the potential strengths and weaknesses in each step of the research process. Critical thinking is also enhanced by innovative chapter features such as Critical Thinking Decision Paths, Helpful Hints, and Critical Thinking Challenges, promoting development of research consumer decision-making skills. Consistent with previous editions, each chapter includes a section describing the critiquing process related to the focus of the chapter, as well as lists of Critiquing Criteria that are designed to stimulate a systematic and evaluative approach to reading and understanding qualitative and quantitative research literature.

New web-based ancillaries complement the fifth edition of the textbook and provide chapter-by-chapter interactive learning activities and strategies that promote the development of critical thinking, critical reading, and information literacy skills designed to develop the competencies necessary to produce informed consumers of nursing research. These include a passcode-protected **faculty website,** developed by Rona Levin and Harriet Feldman, that will give faculty access to all instructor materials on-line including content outlines, lecture guides, coordinating classroom activities, transparencies, and a Word or Rich Text document test bank that will allow faculty to import select questions into their on-line software. Students will have a wonderful passcode-protected **on-line study guide** designed to enhance student learning outcomes. Once registered, students are permitted re-entry to the study guide to complete exciting learning activities that enhance mastery of research consumer competencies. The **study guide** will be an interactive workbook. Students will be sent to the web to examine databases, as well as conduct library searches on CINAHL, MEDLINE, and other databases to locate select research articles for review and evaluation. In addition, crossword puzzles, interactive activities, word searches, and critical thinking exercises will challenge students.

The development and refinement of a scientific foundation for clinical nursing practice remains an essential priority for the future of professional nursing practice. The fifth edition of *Nursing Research: Methods, Critical Appraisal, and Utilization* will help students develop a basic level of competence in understanding the steps of the research process that will enable them to critically analyze research studies, judge their merit, and judiciously apply research findings in clinical practice. To the extent that this goal is accomplished, the nursing profession will have a cadre of clinicians who derive their practice from theory and research evidence specific to nursing.

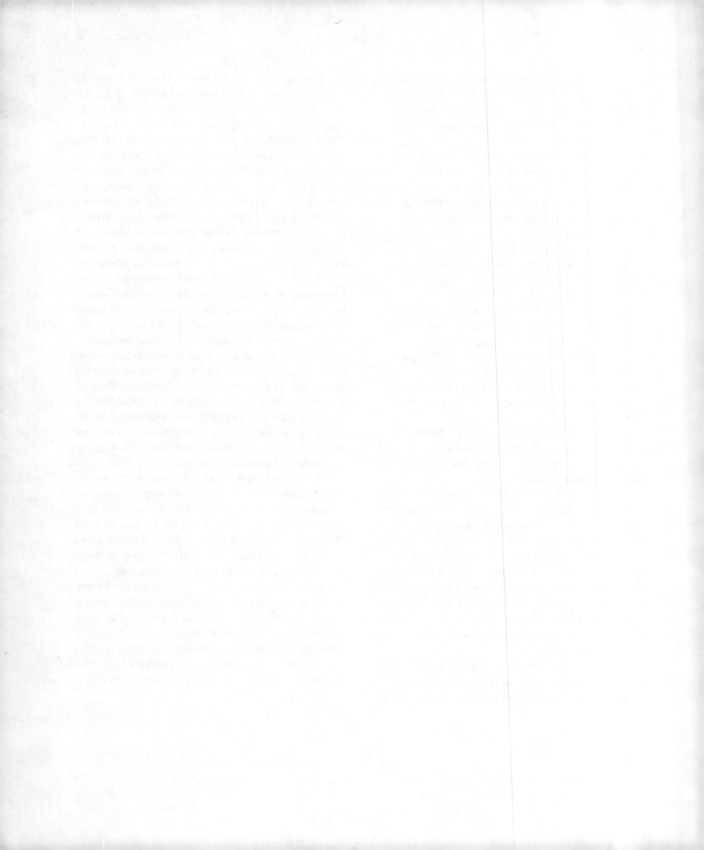

Acknowledgments

No major undertaking is accomplished alone; there are those who contribute directly and those who contribute indirectly to the success of a project. We acknowledge with deep appreciation and our warmest thanks the help and support of the following people:

- Our students, particularly the nursing students at the University of Texas—Houston Health Science Center School of Nursing and the Division of Nursing at New York University, whose interest, lively curiosity, and challenging questions sparked ideas for revisions in the fifth edition.
- Our chapter contributors, whose passion for research, expertise, cooperation, commitment and punctuality, made them a joy to have as colleagues.
- Our vignette contributors, whose willingness to share evidence of their research wisdom made a unique and inspirational contribution to this edition.
- Our foreword contributor, Carol Noll Hoskins, our former research professor and a chapter contributor to the first edition of this text, whose insightful introduction to the fifth edition lends special meaning to this text.
- Our colleagues, who have taken time out of their busy professional lives to offer feedback and constructive criticism that helped us prepare this fifth edition.
- Our editors, June Thompson, Linda Caldwell, and Eric Ham, for their willingness to listen to yet another creative idea about teaching research in a meaningful way and for their timely help with manuscript preparation and production.
- Our families: Brian Wood, who over the years as he has grown older, has sat in on classes, provided commentary, and patiently watched and waited as his mother rewrote each edition, as well as provided love, understanding, and support. Lenny and Andrew Haber and Laurie, Bob, and Michael Goldberg for their unending love, faith, understanding, and support throughout what is inevitably a consuming—but exciting—experience.

Geri LoBiondo-Wood
Judith Haber

Student Preface

We invite you to join us on an exciting nursing research adventure that begins as you turn the first page of the fifth edition of *Nursing Research: Methods, Critical Appraisal, and Utilization.* The adventure is one of discovery! You will discover that the nursing research literature sparkles with pride, dedication, and excitement about the research dimension of professional nursing practice. Whether you are a student or a practicing nurse whose goal is to use research as the foundation of your practice, you will discover that nursing research and a commitment to evidence-based practice positions our profession at the forefront of change. You will discover that nursing research is integral to meeting the challenge of providing quality biopsychosocial health care in partnership with patients and their families/significant others, as well as with the communities in which they live. Finally, you will discover the richness in the "Who," "What," "Where," "When," "Why," and "How" of nursing research and evidence-based practice, developing a foundation of knowledge and skills that will equip you for clinical practice today, as well as throughout this decade of the twenty-first century!

We think you will enjoy reading this text. Your nursing research course will be short but filled with new and challenging learning experiences that will develop your research consumer skills. The fifth edition of *Nursing Research: Methods, Utilization, and Critical Appraisal* reflects "cutting edge" trends for developing competent consumers of nursing research. The four-part organization and special features in this text are designed to help you develop your critical thinking, critical reading, information literacy, and clinical decision-making skills, while providing a "user friendly" approach to learning that expands your competence to deal with these new and challenging experiences. The innovative on-line student study guide with interactive activities will provide a companion self-paced learning tool to reinforce the chapter-by-chapter content of the text.

Remember that research consumer skills are used in every clinical setting and can be applied to every patient population or clinical practice issue. Whether your clinical practice involves primary care or specialty care and provides inpatient or outpatient treatment in a hospital, clinic, or home, you will be challenged to apply your research consumer skills and use nursing research as the foundation for your evidence-based practice. The fifth edition of *Nursing Research: Methods, Critical Appraisal, and Utilization* will guide you through this exciting adventure where you will discover your ability to play a vital role in contributing to the building of an evidence-based professional nursing practice.

Geri LoBiondo-Wood
Geri.L.Wood@uth.tmc.edu

Judith Haber
jh33@nyu.edu

Author Biographies

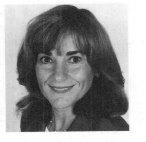

Geri LoBiondo-Wood PhD, RN, FAAN is an Associate Professor at the University of Texas Health Science Center at Houston, School of Nursing (UTHSC-Houston). She received her Diploma in nursing at St. Mary's Hospital School of Nursing in Rochester, New York and her Bachelor's and Master's degrees from the University of Rochester and a PhD in Nursing Theory and Research from New York University. Dr. LoBiondo-Wood currently teaches research and theory to undergraduate, graduate, and doctoral students at UTHSC-Houston, School of Nursing. She also holds a joint appointment for the development of nursing research at the Methodist Health Care System in Houston. She has extensive experience guiding nurses and other health care professionals in the development and utilization of research in clinical practice. Dr. LoBiondo-Wood is currently a member of the Editorial Board of *Progress in Transplantation* and a reviewer for *Nursing Research, the Journal of Advanced Nursing,* and the *Nephrology Nursing Journal.* Her research and publications focus on the impact of solid organ transplant on the child or adult recipient and their families throughout the transplant process.

Dr. LoBiondo-Wood has been active locally and nationally in many professional organizations including the Southern Nursing Research Society, the Midwest Nursing Research Society, and the North American Transplant Coordinators Organization. She has received local and national awards for teaching and contributions to nursing. In 1997, she received the Distinguished Alumnus Award from New York University, Division of Nursing Alumni Association.

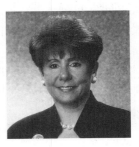

Judith Haber, PhD, APRN, CS, FAAN is Professor and Director of the Master's Program and Post-Master's Advanced Certificate Program in the Division of Nursing at New York University. She received her undergraduate nursing education at Adelphi University in New York and holds a Master's degree in Adult Psychiatric-Mental Health Nursing and a PhD in Nursing Theory and Research from New York University. Judith Haber is internationally recognized as a clinician and educator in psychiatric-mental health nursing. She has extensive clinical experience in psychiatric nursing, having been an advanced practice psychiatric nurse in private practice for over 25 years, specializing in treatment of families coping with the psychosocial sequelae of acute and chronic catastrophic illness. Dr. Haber is currently on the Editorial Board of the *Journal of the American Psychiatric Nurses Association (JAPNA)* and, as a contributing editor, writes a column on policy and politics for this journal. She is also on the Editorial Board of *Applied Nursing Research.* Her areas of research involvement include tool development, particularly in the area of family functioning. She is internationally known for developing the Haber Level of Differentiation of Self Scale. Another program of research addresses physical and psychosocial adjustment to illness, focusing specifically on women with breast cancer and their partners. Based on this research, she and Dr. Carol Hoskins have written and produced an award-winning series of psychoeducational videotapes, *Journey to Recovery: For Women with Breast Cancer and their Partners,* that they are currently testing in a randomized clinical trial.

Dr. Haber has been active locally and nationally in many professional organizations, including the American Nurses Association and the American Psychiatric Nurses Association. She has received numerous local, state, and national awards for public policy, clinical practice, and research. In 1993, she was inducted as a Fellow of the American Academy of Nursing.

Contents

PART ONE

RESEARCH OVERVIEW

Nursing Research: Impacting the Lives of the Frail Elderly

In a July 1999 issue of the *Washington Post,* the spotlight was on Clifford Lynd, Sr., a then 79-year-old retired meat cutter who was living with his wife in Philadelphia. Mr. Lynd is one of more than a thousand patients who have participated in our research team's efforts to influence, through rigorous science, the redesign of health care systems to more effectively address the complex needs of vulnerable older adults and their families.

For more than a decade, it has been my great fortune to lead a multidisciplinary team of scholars in the testing and refinement of a model of transitional care delivered by advanced practice nurses (APNs) in collaboration with patients, caregivers, physicians, and other health care providers. In contrast to most health care delivery systems, the use of the transitional care model is characterized by a number of unique features. The model incorporates state of the science interventions, relies on the professional judgment of clinical experts, and promotes a strong patient-provider relationship and continuity of care from the hospital to the patient's home.

Our team has targeted elders hospitalized with common medical and surgical conditions who are at high risk for poor post-discharge outcomes and their caregivers as the target population for testing of the model. High-risk elders include those whose treatment goals are difficult to achieve because of the nature and severity of their primary health problem, the complexity of their therapeutic regimen, and the coexistence of multiple physical and psychosocial health needs. The use of a transitional care model is based on the assumption that an acute health care problem is generally not resolved at the time

of hospital discharge in this vulnerable population and, for a definable period after discharge, these elders are at especially high risk for preventable poor outcomes, often resulting in rehospitalizations or emergency department visits.

To date, the testing of the transitional care model has been the focus of three randomized clinical trials (RCTs) funded by the National Institute of Nursing Research (NINR) and one NINR-funded secondary analysis. The science generated from these RCTs has contributed substantially to our understanding of the effective management of high-risk, cognitively intact elders throughout an acute episode of illness (Naylor et al, 1994; Naylor et al, 1999). An ongoing secondary analysis is examining the processes of care and outcomes of alternative nurse-physician models in the care of older adults over an episode of acute illness. With the support of the Alzheimer's Association, our team has expanded the testing of this model to elders whose care is further complicated by cognitive impairment.

The importance of this body of science in advancing the care of high-risk older adults making the difficult transition from hospital to home is reflected in Mr. Lynd's description of his experience in an ongoing RCT focusing on the challenging needs of elders living with heart failure. Similar to many patients at risk for poor post-discharge outcomes, Mr. Lynd experienced numerous hospitalizations for acute exacerbations of heart failure complicated by active, coexisting conditions.

Within 24 hours of a recent hospitalization, Mr. Lynd was enrolled in our study and assigned to Brian Bixby, one of a small group of clinically sophisticated, system-savvy, master's prepared nurses who are implementing our intervention protocol. Brian coordinated Mr. Lynd's preparation for discharge and assumed direct care of him when he returned home. Through home visits and telephone contacts, Brian carefully monitored Mr. Lynd's progress and—in collaboration with Mr. Lynd, his wife, and his physician—implemented a highly creative, individualized plan of care designed to improve his diet, activity, medication, and symptom management, as well as to enhance his general health status.

"He'd [Brian] sit on the sofa and we'd talk like we were buddies for years and years. . . Brian was always somebody I could always count on. If I needed anything I would call him. . . He explained everything to me and my wife. . . If it hadn't been for Brian, . . . I would have been back in the hospital" (*Washington Post,* July 20, 1999). As a result of this intervention, Mr. Lynd was very successful in managing his complex health problems and avoiding hospitalization during the study's 1-year follow-up period. He credits our project and especially Brian with "changing his life and giving him a cushion of support when he was sick" (*Washington Post,* July 20, 1999).

A central challenge to the health care system throughout the twenty-first century will be its ability to effectively respond to the needs of a growing population of older people such as Mr. Lynd who are coping with multiple, disabling, chronic illnesses. Research findings from studies are helping to inform and influence health care delivery and financing changes essential to ensure high-quality, cost-effective outcomes. Study findings are also highlighting the unique contributions of expert nurses in meeting the needs of these elders and their caregivers. Our goal is to continue advancing the science related to the care of this special group until every hospitalized elder at high risk for poor post-discharge outcomes has access to an APN to guide, coordinate, and broker their care.

Naylor M et al: Comprehensive discharge planning for the hospitalized elderly: a randomized clinical trial, *Ann Intern Med* 120(12):999-1006, 1994.

Naylor M et al: Comprehensive discharge planning and home follow-up of hospitalized elders: a randomized clinical trial, *JAMA* 281(7): 613-620, 1999. *Washington Post,* July 20, 1999, pp. 15-16; Health Section.

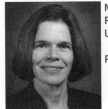

Mary Naylor, PhD, RN, FAAN
Ralston Endowed Term Professor,
University of Pennsylvania School
 of Nursing,
Philadelphia, Pennsylvania

GERI LOBIONDO-WOOD
JUDITH HABER

1

The Role of Research in Nursing

Key Terms

consumer
critique

evidence-based practice
research

research utilization
theory

Learning Outcomes

After reading this chapter, the student should be able to do the following:

- State the significance of research to the practice of nursing.
- Identify the role of the consumer of nursing research.
- Discuss the differences in trends within nursing research before and after 1950.
- Describe how research, education, and practice relate to each other.
- Evaluate the nurse's role in the research process as it relates to the nurse's level of educational preparation.
- Identify the future trends in nursing research.
- Formulate the priorities for nursing research in the twenty-first century.

We invite you to join us on an exciting nursing research adventure that begins as you read the first page of this chapter. The adventure is one of discovery! You will discover that the nursing research literature sparkles with pride, dedication, and excitement about this dimension of professional nursing practice. Whether you are a student or a practicing nurse whose goal is to use **research** as the foundation of your practice, you will discover that nursing research positions our profession at the cutting edge of change. You will also discover that nursing research is integral with meeting the challenge of achieving the goal of providing quality biopsychosocial outcomes in partnership with clients, their families/significant others, and the communities in which they live. Finally, you will discover the cutting edge "Who," "What," "Where," "When," "Why," and "How" of nursing research and developing a foundation of knowledge, evidence-based practice, and competencies that will equip you for twenty-first century clinical practice as a registered nurse.

Your nursing research adventure will be filled with new and challenging learning experiences that will develop your research consumer skills. Your critical reading, critical thinking, and clinical decision-making skills will all be expanded as you appraise the research literature and raise questions about your practice. For example, you will be encouraged to ask adventurous questions such as the following: What makes this intervention effective with one group of patients with congestive heart failure but not another? What is the effect of computer learning modules on children's self-management of asthma? What research has been conducted in the area of identifying barriers to prostate cancer screening in African-American men? What is the quality of the studies done on therapeutic touch? Are the findings from the studies done on pain management ready for use in practice? This chapter will help you begin your nursing research adventure by developing an appreciation of the significance of research in nursing and the research roles of nurses through a historical and futuristic approach.

SIGNIFICANCE OF RESEARCH IN NURSING

The health care environment is changing at an unprecedented pace. Hinshaw (2000) states that "an unprecedented explosion of nursing knowledge guided practice and advanced the health and well-being of individual clients, families, and communities." Nurses are challenged to expand their "comfort zone" by offering creative approaches to old and new health problems, as well as designing new and innovative programs that truly make a difference in the health status of our citizens. This challenge can best be met by integrating rapidly expanding evidence-based knowledge about biologic, behavioral, and environmental influences on health into nursing practice. Nursing research provides a specialized scientific knowledge base that empowers the nursing profession to anticipate and meet these constantly shifting challenges and maintain our societal relevance.

You can think of **evidence-based practice** as the conscious and judicious use of the current "best" evidence in the care of patients and delivery of health care services (Titler et al, 1999a). Through **research utilization** efforts, knowledge obtained from research is transformed into clinical practice, culminating in nursing practice that is evidence-based. For example, to help you understand the importance of evidence-based practice, think about the study by Bull, Hansen, and Gross (2000) (see Chapter 20 and Appendix A), which sought to determine whether there would be any differences in patient quality and cost outcomes related to length of stay, hospital readmission, emergency room use, satisfaction with discharge planning, perception of health, vitality, perception of care continuity, preparedness for discharge, and difficulty managing care for elders hospitalized with heart failure and caregivers who participated in a professional-patient partnership model of discharge planning compared with those who received the usual discharge planning. Findings from this quasi-experimental study indicated that elders in the intervention cohort felt more prepared to manage care, reported more continuity of information about care management and services, felt they were in better health, had fewer emergency room visits, and spent fewer days in the hospital when readmitted than the control cohort.

Caregivers in the intervention cohort also reported receiving more information about care management and having a more positive reaction to caregiving than the control cohort. Translating hospital resource use to costs using a standard charge of $800 for a 1-day uncomplicated hospital stay, $238 for an emergency room visit, and subtracting the cost of the intervention, the average cost savings per person in the partnership model was approximately $4,300 less per patient. These findings provide nurses with quality and cost-effectiveness outcome data that confirm that discharge planning managed by nurses working with patient-caregiver partnerships produces outcomes that improve the quality of clinical outcomes for elders with heart failure and their caregivers, as well as decreases the cost of providing care to this patient population. Such data support scientifically based clinical decisions about making changes in nursing care delivery models rather than adhering to traditional models of discharge planning for elderly patients. Although the data from this research study have definite potential for use in practice, changes in hospital policy will not and should not occur as a result of one study. Replication of this study is necessary to build an adequate knowledge base for implementation in practice, one that has been systematically evaluated over time.

Nurses are required to be accountable for the quality of patient care they deliver. In an era of consumerism during which the quality of health care and high health care costs are being questioned, consumers and employers—the purchasers of health insurance—are asking health professionals to document the effectiveness of their services (Hinshaw, 2000; Hinshaw, Feetham, and Shaver, 1999; Rosswurm and Larrabee, 1999; Titler, 1999a). Essentially, it is asked, "How do nursing services make a difference?" The mes-

sage can hardly be clearer; how consumers and employers perceive the value of nurses' contributions will determine the profession's role in any future delivery system (Buerhaus, 1996; Rosswurm and Larrabee, 1999). Public and private sector reimbursement groups, including insurance companies, managed-care organizations, and governmental agencies using capitated and prospective payment systems (e.g., Medicare and Medicaid) are also requiring accountability for services provided. Health care report cards that document outcomes in acute care and community-based settings related to quality and cost are increasingly common (ANA, 1997; ANA, 2000). The Joint Commission on Accreditation of Healthcare Organizations (JCAHO, 1999) standards require health care agencies to implement outcomes-management programs that demonstrate the link between quality care and cost-effective patient outcomes.

The Cabinet and Council on Nursing Research of the American Nurses Association (ANA, 1997) has recognized the need for research skills at all levels of professional nursing. The Cabinet proposes that all nurses share a commitment to the advancement of nursing science by conducting research and using research findings in practice. Scientific investigation promotes accountability, which is one of the hallmarks of the nursing profession and a fundamental concept of the ANA (2001) Code for Nurses. There is a consensus that the research role of the baccalaureate graduate calls for the skills of critical appraisal. That is, the nurse must be a knowledgeable consumer of research, one who can **critique** research and use existing standards to determine the merit and readiness of research for use in clinical practice (ANA, 1997). The remainder of this book is devoted to helping you develop that consumer expertise.

RESEARCH: LINKING THEORY, EDUCATION, AND PRACTICE

Research links **theory**, education, and practice. Theoretical formulations supported by research findings may become the foundations of theory-based practice in nursing. Your educational setting, whether it be a nursing program or health care organization where you are employed, provides an environment in which you, as students, can learn about the research process. In this setting, you can also explore different theories and begin to evaluate them in light of research findings.

A classic research study by Brooten et al (1986) illustrates a theory-based investigation that has societal relevance, is clinically oriented, is interdisciplinary, and provides research experience for student research assistants. The study sought to determine the safety, efficacy, and cost savings of early hospital discharge of very–low-birthweight infants. One group of infants (n=40) was discharged according to routine nursery criteria (i.e., weight above 2200 g). Those in the early discharge group (n=39) were discharged before they reached this weight if they met a standard set of conditions. For families of infants in the early discharge group, education, counseling, home visits, and on-call availability of a hospital-based nurse specialist for 18 months were provided. The two groups did not differ in specific outcome criteria, including the number of rehospitalizations and acute care visits and measures of physical and mental growth. The average hospital cost for the early discharge group was 27% less than that for the standard discharge group, and the average physician cost was 22% less. The average cost of the home follow-up care was $576, yielding a net savings of $18,560 for each infant in the early discharge group. Brooten et al (1986) stated that if only half of the 36,000 very–low-birthweight infants born in the United States each year were discharged according to the protocol tested, the annual health care savings could be as much as $334 million, with no adverse effect on the infants or their families. These findings have had enormous implications not only for nursing practice but also for related health care disciplines, all of which compose the interdisciplinary health care team involved in the care of very–low-birthweight infants. Using the team's quality-cost model, Brooten and other researchers have extended their work to four additional patient groups:

women with unplanned cesarean births, women with antepartum and postpartum diabetes, women who have had hysterectomies, and the frail elderly (Brooten et al, 1988; Brooten et al, 1989; Cohen, Hollingsworth, and Rubin, 1989; Graff et al, 1992; Naylor et al, 1999). The outcomes, whether for premature infants or hospitalized older adults, have consistently been higher quality outcomes (e.g., fewer rehospitalizations, greater satisfaction with the experience, and lower costs). Future research is needed to identify individuals who are at high risk during transitions in the health care systems and would particularly benefit from this type of intervention program (Hinshaw, 2000).

Another study (Cohen and Ley, 2000) examined the lived experience of cancer patients' experience of having an autologous bone marrow transplantation in order to better understand the effect of this treatment on persons' lives and how nursing care can best meet their needs (see Appendix B). Themes descriptive of the lived experience of bone marrow transplantation emerged from descriptive data obtained from interviews with autologous bone marrow transplant survivors. These themes are as follows:

- Fear of death and hope for survival
- Loss of control
- Fear of discharge
- Fear of recurrence

These themes illustrate how men and women with cancer experienced the process of undergoing the potentially life-threatening bone transplantation procedure. The informants described the survivors' fears, losses, and hopes, coupled with their sense that the bone marrow transplantation was a life-altering event. The data reveal that fear, which is a predominant reality while undergoing bone marrow transplantation, is balanced with hope for survival. The overarching fear, fear of death, was often related to the unknown, including cancer recurrence. The fear of the unknown also came from being physically and emotionally unprepared for the bone marrow transplantation procedure. Losses experienced by patients were intertwined with these fears, and included loss of both control and trust in one's body. Patients discussed their fear of leaving the hospital and not having someone to constantly look at them to make sure that the cancer has not recurred. These fears and losses changed these people's view of life and led to a need for help in bringing closure to the experience. The findings of this study highlight the need for nurses who care for patients during life-altering events (e.g., bone marrow transplantation) to be aware that these are times when people are vulnerable, open to transformation, and need to be protected, and that their actions create powerful memories. Patients identified the following nursing actions involving therapeutic communication and patient education as being helpful in allaying fear: inclusion of family and significant others, provision of knowledge and information, preparation for each step in treatment and recovery, and connecting patients to important resources (e.g., support groups). By understanding the relationship between hope and fear, nurses can use these specific strategies to decrease fear and increase hope in cancer patients undergoing bone marrow transplantation.

The preceding examples answer a question that you may have been asking: How will the theory and research content of your course relate to your nursing practice? The data from each study have clearly demonstrated societal and practice implications. The classic study by Brooten et al (1986) provided data that illustrated an innovative nursing intervention protocol that was cost-effective and maintained high-quality outcomes. In an era of continuing concern about health care costs, empirically supported programs that are cost-effective without compromising quality are essential.

Given the dramatic increase in chronic illness created by advances in technology, a national concern has emerged about the long-term impact that chronic and life-threatening illness has on individuals and families. The study by Cohen and Ley (2000) provided important data for understanding the lived experience of cancer patients undergoing bone marrow transplantation (see Appendix B). The themes that emerged from the data provide an understanding of the patients' lived experience of this life-altering passage and suggest the importance of the nurse in creating powerful healing memories for patients. The findings can be used to plan treatment that addresses the specific emotional and physical needs of cancer patients undergoing bone marrow transplantation in a manner that decreases fear and increases hope.

At this point in your nursing research adventure, you may be wondering how education in nursing research links theory and practice. The answer is twofold. First, it will provide you with an appreciation and understanding of the research process such that you will become a participant in research activities. Second, it must help you become an intelligent consumer of research. A **consumer** of research uses and applies research in an active manner. To be a knowledgeable consumer, a nurse must have a knowledge base about the relevant subject matter, the ability to discriminate and evaluate information logically, and the ability to apply the knowledge gained. It is not necessary to conduct studies to be able to appreciate and use research findings in practice. Rather, to be intelligent consumers, nurses must understand the research process and develop the critical evaluation skills needed to judge the merit and relevance of evidence provided by the findings before applying them in practice. This understanding and development will prepare each of you for evidence-based practice, in which there are many research-related activities that rely on your having excellent research consumer skills.

ROLES OF THE NURSE IN THE RESEARCH PROCESS

There is a research role for every nurse practicing in the twenty-first century. One of the marks of success in nursing research is the delineation of research competencies geared for nurses prepared in different types of educational programs (Hinshaw, 2000; Pullen, Tuck, and Wallace, 1999;

Strohschein, Schaffer, and Lia-Hoagberg, 1999). In its classic document, *Commission on Nursing Research: Education for Preparation in Nursing Research,* the American Nurses Association (ANA) (1989) identified research competencies related to the specific type of educational program a nurse has completed. Obviously, these competencies will expand over time for nurses committed to lifelong learning.

Graduates of associate degree nursing programs will demonstrate an awareness of the value or relevance of research in nursing. They may help identify problem areas in nursing practice within an established structured format, assist in data-collection activities, and—in conjunction with the professional nurse—appropriately use research findings in clinical practice (ANA, 1989). This means that as registered nurses (RNs), they will participate as team members in evidence-based practice activities, including development and revision or implementation of clinical standards, protocols, and critical paths (see Chapter 20).

Nurses with a baccalaureate education must be intelligent consumers of research; that is, they must understand each step of the research process and its relationship to every other step. Such understanding must be linked with a clear idea about the standards of satisfactory research. This comprehension is necessary when critically reading and understanding research reports, thereby determining the validity and merit of reported studies. Through critical appraisal skills that use specific criteria to judge all aspects of the research, a professional nurse interprets, evaluates, and determines the credibility of research findings. The nurse discriminates between interesting ideas that require further investigation and findings that have sufficient support before considering use of one in practice (ANA, 1989; Rosswurm and Larrabee, 1999; Titler et al, 1994, 1999). Nurses who are baccalaureate graduates will use these competencies to advance the nursing or interdisciplinary evidence-based practice projects (e.g., developing clinical standards, tracking quality-improvement data, coordinating implementation of a pilot project to test the efficacy of a new

wound-care protocol) of workplace committees of which they are members or are chairpersons.

In this context, understanding the research process and acquiring critical appraisal skills open a broad realm of information that can contribute to the professional nurse's body of knowledge and be applied judiciously to practice in the interest of providing scientifically based care (Batey, 1982; Rosswurm and Larrabee, 1999b; Stetler et al, 1998, Titler 1999a). Thus the role of the baccalaureate graduate in the research process is primarily that of a knowledgeable consumer, a role that promotes the integration of research and clinical practice.

Lest anyone think that this is an unimportant role, let us assure you that it is not. Fawcett (1984) states that we are all aware of those who assert that research is the bailiwick of "ivory tower" investigators. She goes on to state, however, that it is the staff nurse who is ultimately responsible for using the findings of nursing and other health-related research in clinical practice. To use such research findings appropriately, nurses must understand and critically appraise them. Therefore as nursing moves to a genuine research-based practice, it will be in large part up to nurses—in their role as consumers of research—to accomplish this goal.

Baccalaureate graduates also have a responsibility to identify nursing problems that require investigation and to participate in the implementation of scientific studies (ANA, 1989). Clinicians often generate research ideas or questions from hunches, gut-level feelings, intuition, or observations of patients or nursing care. These ideas are often the seeds of further research investigations. For example, a nurse working in a Pediatric Intensive Care Unit (PICU) observed that parents become accustomed to the PICU environment, and this setting—once considered threatening—becomes a source of familiarity and comfort. When a child's condition no longer warrants PICU care and the child is ready to be transferred to a regular pediatric unit, parental uncertainty and anxiety resurfaces, a phenomenon the nurse called "transfer anxiety." She discussed with her colleagues whether they could design and pilot a nursing intervention to help parents adjust to and cope with this transition by decreasing "transfer anxiety" (Bouve, Rozmus, and Giordano, 1999). Based on the Lazarus Stress and Coping Model, an educational intervention that provided information was designed to prepare parents for the transfer, thereby increasing their feeling of control. Of particular interest was whether the informational intervention made a difference in parental "transfer anxiety." In the clinical setting, nurse researchers can often lead and direct staff nurses in the systematic investigation of such an idea in an on-site clinical research project. Systematic collection of data about a clinical problem such as this one contributes to the refinement and extension of nursing practice.

Baccalaureate graduates may also participate in research projects as members of interdisciplinary or intradisciplinary research teams in one or more phases of such a project. For example, a staff nurse may work on a clinical research unit where a particular type of nursing care is part of an established research protocol (e.g., for pain management, prevention of falls, or urinary incontinence). In such a situation, the nurse administers the care according to the format described in the protocol. The nurse may also be involved in collecting and recording data relevant to the administration of and the patient response to the nursing care.

Promoting ethical principles of research, especially the protection of human subjects, is another essential responsibility of nurses with baccalaureate degrees. For example, a nurse caring for a patient who is beginning an antinausea chemotherapy research protocol would make sure that the patient had signed the informed consent and had all of his or her questions answered by the research team before beginning the protocol. A nurse who saw the patient having an adverse reaction to the medication protocol would know that his or her responsibility would be not to administer another dose before notifying an appropriate member of the research team (see Chapter 13).

Baccalaureate graduates must share research findings with colleagues. This may involve developing an article or presentation for a research or clinical conference on the findings of a study in which you participated, or it may involve sharing with colleagues the findings of a research report that you have critiqued and have found to have merit and the potential for application in your practice. In a more formal way, it may involve joining your health care agency's research committee or its quality assurance (QA) or quality improvement (QI) committee, where research study articles, integrative reviews of the literature, and clinical practice guidelines are evaluated for evidence-based clinical decision making.

Nurses who have their master's and doctoral degrees must also be sophisticated consumers of research, but they have also been prepared to conduct research as a coinvestigator or a primary investigator. At the master's level, nurses are prepared to be active members of research teams. They can assume the role of clinical expert, collaborating with an experienced researcher in proposal development, data collection, data analysis, and interpretation (ANA, 1989). Nurses with their master's degree enhance the quality and relevance of nursing research by providing not only clinical expertise about problems but also evidence-based knowledge about the way the clinical services are delivered. They facilitate the investigation of clinical problems by providing a climate that is favorable to conducting research and engaging in evidence-based practice projects. In the capacity of "change champions" (see Chapter 20), this includes collaborating with others in investigations, promoting the competency of staff nurses as research consumers, and expanding staff nurse involvement in implementing evidence-based practice projects. At the master's level, nurses conduct research investigations to monitor the quality of the practice of nursing in a clinical setting and provide leadership by helping others apply scientific knowledge in nursing practice (ANA, 1989).

Doctorally prepared nurses have the most expertise in appraising, designing, and conducting research. They develop theoretical explanations of phenomena relevant to nursing. They develop methods of scientific inquiry and use qualitative and empirical methods to discover ways to modify or extend existing knowledge so that it is relevant to nursing. In addition to their role as producers of research, doctorally prepared nurses act as role models and mentors who guide, stimulate, and encourage other nurses who are developing their research skills. They also collaborate and consult with social, educational, or health care institutions or governmental agencies in their research endeavors. Doctorally prepared nurses disseminate their research findings to the scientific community, clinicians, and—as appropriate—the lay public. Scientific journals, professional conferences, and the news media are among the mechanisms for dissemination (ANA, 1989; Brink 1995; Fitzpatrick, 2000).

The most important implication delineating research activities according to educational preparation is for maintaining a collaborative research relationship within the nursing profession. Not all nurses must or should conduct research, but all nurses must play some part in the research process. Nurses at all educational levels—whether they are consumers or producers of research or both—need to view the research process as integral to the growing professionalism in nursing.

Professionals must take time to read research studies and evaluate them using the standards congruent with scientific research. The critiquing process is used to identify the strengths and weaknesses of each study. Nurses should keep in mind that no study is perfect; although limitations should be recognized, nurses may extrapolate sound and relevant evidence from a study to be considered for potential use in clinical practice.

HISTORICAL PERSPECTIVE

The history of nursing research comprises many changes and developments. The groundwork for what has blossomed was laid late in the nineteenth century and throughout the twentieth century. To capture the essence of the development of nursing research and the works of so many excellent researchers, especially in the 1980s and 1990s, is beyond the scope of this chapter. A review of the many nursing journals available provides further support of the efforts of nursing researchers. Box 1-1 highlights key events that have set the stage for the richness of the current nursing research efforts.

NINETEENTH CENTURY—AFTER 1850

In the mid-nineteenth century, nursing as a formal discipline began to take root with the ideas and practices of Florence Nightingale. Her concepts have contributed to and are congruent with the present priorities of nursing research. Promotion of health, prevention of disease, and care of the sick were central ideas of her system. Nightingale believed that the systematic collection and exploration of data were necessary for nursing. Her collection and analysis of data on the health status of British soldiers during the Crimean War led to a variety of reforms in health care. Nightingale also noted the need for measuring outcomes of nursing and medical care (Nightingale, 1863), and she had expertise in statistics and epidemiology. Nightingale stated, "Statistics are history in repose, history is statistics in motion" (Keith, 1988). Other than Nightingale's work, there was little research during the early years of nursing's development because schools of nursing had just begun to be established and were unequal in their ability to educate, and nursing leadership had just started to develop.

TWENTIETH CENTURY—BEFORE 1950

A review of Box 1-1 reflects nursing research in the first half of the twentieth century. Research focused mainly on nursing education, but some patient- and technique-oriented research was evident. The early efforts in nursing education research were made by such leaders as Lavinia Dock (1900), Anne Goodrich (1932), Adelaide Nutting (1912, 1926), Isabel Hampton Robb (1906), Lillian Wald (1915), and Nutting and

BOX 1-1 Historical Perspective

NINETEENTH CENTURY—AFTER 1850

1852

Nightingale writes *Cassandra.*

1855

Nightingale studies and calculates mortality rates of British soldiers in the Crimean War and, on the basis of these data, develops plans to decrease military overcrowding.

1859

Nightingale's *Notes on Matters Affecting the Health, Efficiency and Hospital Administration of the British Army;* and *Notes on Hospitals* are published.

1859

Nightingale's *Notes on Nursing* is published.

1860

Nightingale founds St. Thomas's Hospital School of Nursing in England.

1861

Nightingale develops cost accounting system for the Army Medical Services.

1872

First nursing schools in United States are started: New England Hospital for Women and Children (Boston) and Women's Hospital (Philadelphia).

1893

Lillian Wald and Mary Brewster establishes Henry Street Visiting Nurse Service.

1899

International Council of Nurses is organized.

TWENTIETH CENTURY—BEFORE 1950

1900

American Journal of Nursing publication is started.

1902

Wald starts school health experiment for free child health care.

1909

Nursing programs begin at Columbia University Teacher's College and University of Minnesota.

1909

"Visiting Nursing in the United States" is conducted by Waters.

1912

American Nurses Association is established.

1913

Committee on Public Health Nursing studies infant mortality, blindness, and midwifery and calls for nursing to distinguish its role in disease prevention and health promotion.

1914

Metropolitan Life Insurance Company contracts nurses to collect data on health problems and tuberculosis.

1923

Goldmark Report (sponsored by the Rockefeller Foundation) is published.
Yale and Case Western Reserve Universities' nursing programs begin.

1924

First nursing doctoral program is started at Teacher's College, Columbia University.

1926

From 1926 to 1934, Committee on Grading of Nursing Schools convenes.

1927

Edith S. Bryan becomes first nurse to receive a PhD in psychology and counseling from The Johns Hopkins University.
Broadhurst and associates study handwashing. Clayton studies standardization of nursing techniques.

1928

Johns and Pfefferkorn publish a study on the activities of nurses.

1932

Ryan and Miller study thermometer-disinfecting techniques.

1934

Nursing doctoral program is established at New York University.
Nightingale International Foundation is established.

Continued

BOX 1-1   Historical Perspective—cont'd

1936

Sigma Theta Tau, the National Honor Society for Nursing, starts nursing research fund.

1943

U.S. Cadet Nurses Corps is created after the Nurse Practice Act is passed.

1948

Nurses for the Future (i.e., The Brown Report, a 3-year study funded by Carnegie foundation) is published.

Schwartz reports on effectiveness of nursing care for inducing sleep and decreasing medication use.

United States Public Health Service Division of Nursing conducts nursing surveys and publishes manuals for the conduct of nursing research.

TWENTIETH CENTURY—AFTER 1950

1950

American Nurses Association establishes a Master Plan for Research, 1951-1956.

1952

National League for Nursing is established.

Journal of Nursing Research, dedicated to the promotion of research, begins publication.

1953

Nursing Outlook begins publication.

Institute of Research and Service in Nursing Education is established at Teacher's College, Columbia University, focusing on the study of nurses and nursing education.

1954

ANA Committee on Research and Studies is formed, focusing on improvement of patient care and funds for nursing research.

1955

American Nurses' Foundation is formed as a center for research.

Commonwealth fund is endowed with monies to support research.

1956

United States Public Health Service begins awarding grants for nursing research.

Predoctoral fellowships for nursing research are first awarded.

1957

Department of Nursing Research is established at Walter Reed Army Hospital.

Western Council on Higher Education in Nursing (WCHEN) sponsors Western Interstate Commission for Higher Education (WICHE) to augment graduate nursing education, especially in nursing research.

1958

Abdellah and Levine publish study of nursing personnel.

1959

ANA publishes *Twenty Thousand Nurses Tell Their Story,* the results of a 5-year study of nursing functions and activities.

National League for Nursing (NLN) Research and Studies Service is established.

First faculty research grants are awarded to University of Washington and University of California at Los Angeles.

1962

American Nurses Association's Blueprint for Nursing Research is issued.

Nurse Scientist Graduate Training Grants Program is initiated. The first awards are to the Boston University and University of California Schools of Nursing.

Nursing Forum begins publication.

1963

International Journal of Nursing Studies begins publication.

Surgeon General's Consultant Group on Nursing report is issued.

Lydia Hall publishes study of chronically ill at Loeb Center.

Batey and Julian publish study on staff perceptions of state psychiatric hospital goals.

1965

American Nurses Association begins sponsoring conferences for nursing research.

1966

First Nursing Research Conference of the ANA is held; a group of nurses and nursing faculty gather to report on research and critique the findings presented.

1967

Quint publishes study on women undergoing mastectomies.

Little and Carnevali publish study about the effect of a nurse specialist on tuberculosis outcomes.

BOX 1-1 Historical Perspective—cont'd

1969

Wayne State University College of Nursing establishes the first nursing research center.

1970

Abstract for Action—Lysaught Report is published.

1971

American Nurses Association Council of Nurse Researchers is organized.

1974

Western Council on Higher Education in Nursing sets 5-year goal to triple nursing research.

ANA Commission on Nursing Research proposes involvement of students from various levels in research and a clinical trust for research.

1975

ANA representatives testify at President Gerald Ford's Panel on Biomedical Research.

1976

ANA publishes its report of nursing research trends, *Research in Nursing: Toward a Science of Health Care.*

National League for Nursing sets criteria for undergraduate nursing research course in BSN programs.

1978

Research in Nursing and Health begins publication.

Advances in Nursing Science begins publication.

1979

Western Journal of Nursing Research begins publication.

Haller, Reynolds, and Horsley publish research utilization criteria.

1980

ANA's Commission on Nursing Research sets research priorities for 1980s.

1983

Institute of Medicine completes its report, *Nursing and Nursing Education: Public and Private Action.*

1986

National Center for Nursing Research is established at the National Institutes of Health.

1987

Scholarly Inquiry for Nursing Practice and *Applied Nursing Research* begin publication.

1988

Nursing Science Quarterly and *Nursing Scan in Research* begin publication.

Conference on Research Priorities in Nursing Science (CORP No. 1) sets research priorities known as the National Nursing Research Agenda.

1989

National Center for Health Services Research becomes the Agency for Health Care Policy and Research (AHCPR).

1991

National Pressure Ulcer Advisory Panel gives its first award to Nancy Bergstrom.

Qualitative Health Research begins publication.

1992

Kathleen McCormick calls for outcome research efforts.

Conference on Research Priorities in Nursing Science (CORP No. 2) meets to set updated research priorities.

AHCPR publishes *Clinical Practice Guidelines: Urinary Incontinence in Adults, Acute Pain Management, and Pressure Ulcers in Adults.*

U.S. Public Health Service publishes *Healthy People 2000.*

1993

National Center for Nursing Research releases a report of a proposed multiyear funding mechanism to increase the integration of biologic and nursing sciences.

National Center for Nursing Research becomes the National Institute of Nursing Research (NINR).

Sigma Theta Tau International publishes *Online Journal of Knowledge Synthesis* and establishes an online computer library.

1996

ANA establishes the Nursing Information and Data Set Evaluation Center (NIDSEC).

Dock (1907). These pioneering works consist of documentation gathered for the purpose of reforming nursing education and establishing nursing as a viable profession.

The Nursing and Nursing Education in the United States Landmark Study, known as the Goldmark Report (1923), met the continued need for reform in nursing education. The report identified multiple deficiencies and disparate educational backgrounds at all levels of nursing. This study and others in the first half of the century recommended reorganizing nursing education and, most importantly, moving it into the university setting.

Clinically oriented research in the early half of the century mainly centered on the morbidity and mortality rates associated with problems such as pneumonia and contaminated milk (Carnegie, 1976). A few of these projects were instrumental in the development of patient-care protocols and the employment of nurses in community settings. An experimental project by Wald and Dock conducted in 1902 led to the employment of school nurses in the New York City school system and subsequently in other cities. Although Linda Richards, the first trained American nurse at Bellevue Hospital, did not perform formal research, she was the first nurse to keep written documentation of patient care. This documentation was used in medical investigations (Carnegie, 1976).

The 1920s saw the development and teaching of the earliest nursing research course because of the influence of Isabel M. Stewart (Henderson, 1977). The course, "Comparative Nursing Practice," first taught by Smith and later by Henderson, introduced students to the scientific method of investigation. Students were encouraged to question all aspects of nursing care and do experiments on such topics as measuring the oxygen content in an oxygen tent during a patient's bed bath to assess whether it dropped below a therapeutic level. Also during this period, case studies appeared in the *American Journal of Nursing (AJN)*. These were used as a teaching tool for students and a record of patient progress (Gort-

ner, 2000). Box 1-1 contains other practice-related research examples.

Social change and World War II affected all aspects of nursing, including research. There was an urgent need for more nurses; increased hospital admissions and military needs created a shortage of personnel. The U.S. Cadet Nurses Corps provided assistance for nurses and offered information that assisted in planning for nursing education after the war. During the war, investigations focused on hospital environments, nursing status, nursing education, and nursing shortages.

After the war, nursing, like the rest of the world, began to reassess itself and its goals. Brown's report in 1948 reemphasized the inconsistencies in educational preparation and the need to move into the university setting, and included an updated description of nursing practices. An outgrowth of Brown's report were a number of studies on nursing roles, needs, and resources.

TWENTIETH CENTURY—AFTER 1950

Nursing research blossomed in the 1950s. The developments of the 1950s laid the groundwork for nursing's current level of research skill. Nursing schools at the undergraduate and graduate levels were growing in number, and graduate programs were including courses related to research. The worth and benefit of research were appreciated by nursing leadership and beginning to filter to various levels of nursing. During the 1950s, the *Journal of Nursing Research,* which was the first journal dedicated to the promotion of research in nursing, began publication. In the mid-50s, the efforts of the ANA and the American Nurses Foundation (ANF) to fund nursing research became evident. The ANA's committee was charged with planning, promoting, and guiding research and studies relating to the Association's functions, as well as collecting and unifying nursing information that could be used to advise the ANA board about periodic inventories of nurses (See, 1977). Throughout the 1950s, organizations and other entities (e.g., the U.S. Public Health Service) put forth funds and personnel to study the characteristics of nursing members and students; the supply, organization, and distribution of nursing services; and job satisfaction.

In 1957, the first nursing-research unit at the Walter Reed Army Institute of Research was developed. Although research during this period focused on nurses and their characteristics, the fields of psychiatric nursing and maternal-child health care received monies from federal grants to develop nursing content and educational programs at the master's and doctoral levels. Grants were also conferred on individuals who studied the social context of psychiatric facilities and its influence on relations between staff and patients (Greenblatt et al, 1955; Stanton and Schwartz, 1954), as well as the role of the nurse with single mothers (Donnell and Glick, 1954).

In the late 1950s, nursing studies began to address clinical problems. In a guest editorial featured in *Nursing Research* (1956), Virginia Henderson commented that studies about nurses outnumber clinical studies 10 to 1. She stated that "the responsibility for designing its methods is often cited as an essential characteristic of a profession."

Thus in the 1960s, research priorities began to be reordered and practice-oriented research was targeted. These priorities were supported by nursing's major organizations. During the 1960s, nurses were attaining educational preparation in research design and methodology in order to teach research and conduct their own research courses. Therefore during this time, nurses primarily worked with others from related disciplines (e.g., psychology, education, and sociology) that had the expertise to teach these courses. Today this is not the case.

Consistent with this need for guidance, many of the studies during the 1950s and 1960s were coinvestigated by individuals from the social sciences and medicine. Another reason for the paucity of research was the small number of nurses with baccalaureate and higher degrees. In 1960, less than 2% of the employed registered nurses held master's degrees and less than 7% held baccalaureate degrees (ANA, 1960).

During the 1960s, studies on nurses and nursing continued while pioneers in the development of nursing theories and models (e.g., Orlando [1961], Peplau [1952], and Wiedenbach [1964]) called for the development of nursing practice based on theory. The early development of those theories spurred nurses into a more critical level of thinking about nursing practice.

Collaborative efforts in the 1960s on practice-oriented research led to follow-up research by Diers and Leonard (1966) and Dumas and Leonard (1963). These studies, done at Yale University, explored the effects of nurse-patient teaching and communication on events such as hospitalization, surgery, and labor. Another classic study, the culmination of 8 years of work by Glaser and Strauss (1965) explored various aspects of thanatology among dying patients and their caretakers.

A review of the nursing research published during the 1960s reveals that clinical studies were beginning to predominate. These studies investigated an array of nursing care issues, such as infection control, alcoholism, and sensory deprivation. Lydia Hall (1963) published the results of a 5-year study that looked at alternatives to hospitalization for a select group of elderly clients. This study gave rise to a care facility run totally by nurses, the Loeb Center in New York City, which is still in operation and run by nurses. The rich history of nursing was also recognized during the 1960s when the nursing archives at Boston University's Mugar Library were established through a federally funded grant with the goal of promoting nursing research.

In 1970, the National Committee for the Study of Nursing and Nursing Education Report, or the Lysaught Report, was published. This report, conducted with the support of the ANA, NLN, and other private foundations, surveyed nursing practice and education. It offered the conclusions that more practice- and education-oriented research was necessary and that these data must be applied to the improvement of educational organizations and curricula. The call for clinically oriented study was becoming a reality.

The 1970s also saw new growth in the number of master's and doctoral programs for nursing. These programs, along with the ANA, NLN, Sigma Theta Tau, and Western Interstate Council for Higher Education in Nursing, clearly supported nurses not only learning the research process but also producing research that could be used to enhance care quality. Box 1-1 lists the first year of publication for new journals that promoted the generation of nursing theory and research.

The 1980s were exciting and productive for research in nursing. This period saw extended growth among upper-level programs in nursing, especially at the doctoral level. By 1989, more than 5,000 of the doctorally prepared nurses held their doctorate in nursing. Consistent with the increased numbers of nurses with advanced training, federal funding and support for research increased not only in universities but also in practice settings. Many centers for nursing research developed in educational settings and hospitals. A number of these centers have programs joining education and practice that provide support and guidance for research efforts. Mechanisms for communicating research also increased. Journals and reviews now provide additional forums for communicating research. Most nursing organizations also have research sections that serve to foster the conduct and use of research.

Public Law 99-158, enacted in 1985, allowed for the development of the National Center for Nursing Research (NCNR). Established in 1986, the NCNR provided funding programs focused on studies related to health care outcomes. The efforts of the 1980s were aimed at refining and developing research and the utilization of research findings in clinical practice. The strides in research made in the 1980s suggested that nursing was ready to rise to the societal and professional demands that now confront the discipline.

During the 1990s, nursing research stood on its own through the work of many forward-thinking educators, scholars, and researchers. At the federal level, nursing leaders moved to influence policy and monies for nursing research. In 1993,

the National Institutes of Health (NIH) reauthorization bill gave the NCNR institute status. The NCNR is now the National Institute of Nursing Research (NINR). At the university level, nursing leaders developed mechanisms for faculty to develop and implement research. Centers of excellence developed in several academic settings, and leaders mentored newer nurse scientists. During the nineties, nurses and nursing students at all levels learned about research and debates about how and what type of research was appropriate ensued. Donaldson presented an important paper in 1998 entitled "Breakthroughs in Nursing Research" (1998). In this paper, Donaldson identified "pathfinders" in nursing research, who developed research programs in which they, their colleagues, and students worked.

Throughout the nineties, pathfinders and many other nurse researchers conducted research on a wide range of clinical topics, describing phenomenon and testing interventions. A review of the many nursing journals shows the growth in the number, quality, and depth of the research that is available for potential use in practice. Tracing nursing's research roots and the conduct of science to improve the health and well-being of individuals, families, and communities shows that nursing has made significant contributions to the health care in general. Nurses are far from finished with our quest to generate and test knowledge, but the nursing leaders of the twentieth century have—by example—paved the beginning of the way for the new millennium.

FUTURE DIRECTIONS—FOR THE MILENNIUM

What an exciting time to contemplate the future of nursing research. Hinshaw (2000) proposes that the unprecedented explosion of nursing knowledge during the final two decades of the twentieth century shaped nursing practice and advanced the health and well-being of individual clients, families, and communities. Now in the millennium, this explosion still provides numerous opportunities for nurses to study important research questions and issues in promoting health and ameliorating the side effects of illness and the consequences of treatment, while optimizing the health outcomes of people and their families. The growing number of nursing doctoral programs both in the United States (now totaling 79) and outside of the United States (now totaling 112), as well as the additional programs that are under development, contribute to preparing a record number of nurse researchers worldwide who are challenged to bring research-based knowledge to life by applying diverse research methods that address the compelling needs of people around the world (Hegyvary, 1999; Berlin, 2000; http://www.lib.umich.edu/hw/nursing/indoc.html).

Major shifts in the delivery of health care include the following:

- Emphasis on community-based care.
- Focus on health promotion and risk reduction.
- Increased severity of illness in inpatient settings.
- Increased incidence of chronic illness.
- Expanding number of elderly people.
- Growth of integrated health care systems using managed-care approaches.
- Emphasis on provider accountability through focus on quality and cost outcomes.

Consistent with these trends, nurse researchers are focusing on the development of clinically based outcome studies, which provide the foundation for evidence-based practice that demonstrates how nursing makes a difference. Qualitative research studies that increase our understanding of clinical phenomena and provide direction for defining research programs will continue to expand. Strategies that enhance nurses' focus on outcomes management through quality-improvement activities and use of research findings for effective clinical decision-making also are being refined and identified as priorities (see Chapter 20). Research-based practice guidelines, standards, protocols, and critical pathways will become benchmarks for cost-effective quality clinical practice (Larkin, 2000; O'Neill and Dluhy, 2000).

Nurse researchers and nurse leaders are and will be increasingly visible at the national level as they give priority to playing major roles that influence policy making, represent nursing on expert panels, provide testimony at Congressional hearings, and lobby for needed funding dollars. The extent of our research growth is evidenced by the 28.5% budget increase received by the National Institute for Nursing Research (NINR) as we enter the twenty-first century, which will allow us to capitalize on research opportunities identified by the scientific community of nurse researchers. Box 1-2 highlights NINR research priorities for 2000-2001 (Grady). Nursing has truly risen to the challenges of the development of nursing science with the ultimate goal of improving health care.

PROMOTING DEPTH IN NURSING RESEARCH

In our complex, health-oriented society, which is increasingly responsive to consumer concerns related to the cost, quality, availability, and accessibilty of health care, it is paramount to define the future direction of nursing research and establish research priorities (Chang, 2000; Hinshaw, 2000; Lynn, Layman, and Englehardt, 1998; Pullen, Tuck, and Wallace, 1999).

Nursing leaders unanimously agree that the essential priority for nursing research in the future will be promotion of excellence in nursing science (Grady, 2000; Hegyvary, 1999; Hinshaw, 2000). This priority is linked to the training and mentoring of the discipline's scholars and the studies they conduct in order to develop a knowledge base that can accurately guide nursing practice (Grady, 2000). The key to shaping our profession's destiny and directing future practice is to provide a scientific basis to guide the clinical care that nurses will deliver in the twenty-first century.

Research-based practice reflects the characteristics of the research from which it is derived. The quality of research that nursing scientists generate and the information that is provided to guide practice will be the major keys to producing predictable patient outcomes and improving patient care for

BOX 1-2   Extramural Priority Areas for Nursing Research

Integrating biological and behavioral research is a major program priority. Three dimensions—promoting health and preventing disease, managing symptoms and disability of illness, and improving environments in which care is delivered—cut across six broad science areas that include research in the following:

1. Chronic illness and long-term care, including care of individuals with arthritis, diabetes, and urinary incontinence, as well as in long-term care and family caregiving.
2. Health promotion and risk behaviors, including studies of women's health, developmental transitions (e.g., adolescence and menopause), and health and behavior research (e.g., studies of smoking cessation).
3. Cardiopulmonary health and critical care, including care of individuals with cardiac or respiratory conditions. This area also includes research in critical care, trauma, wound healing, and organ transplants.
4. Neurofunction and sensory conditions, including pain management, sleep disorders, symptom management in persons with cognitive impairment or chronic neurological conditions, this area also includes research on patient care in acute settings.
5. Immune responses and oncology, including symptoms primarily associated with cancer and AIDS (e.g., fatigue, nausea and vomiting, and cachexia); prevention research on specific risk factors, with a special focus on research at the end of life.
6. Reproductive and infant health, including prevention of premature labor; reduction of health risk factors during pregnancy; normal physiological processes of pregnancy; labor and delivery and the postpartum period; delivery of prenatal care; and care of neonates.

From the NINR: *National Institute of Nursing Research Mission Statement and Strategic Plan,* Washington, DC, 2000, The Institute.

---

our discipline (Rosswurm and Larrabee, 1999; Titler et al, 1999b). Strengthening the communication of research and practice knowledge in the nursing literature is essential to promoting linkages between the threefold mission of education, practice, and research of our educational and health care orga-nizations (O'Neill and Duffey, 2000).

The continuing development of a national and international research environment is essential to the achievement of this mission (Chang, 2000; Henry, 1998). Within this environment, an increasing number of nurses who have significant expertise in appraising, designing, and conducting research will continue to emerge within the profession. They will provide a "critical mass" of investigators who will be at the forefront of the ongoing development and refinement of our scientific knowledge base for nursing practice. The opportunities for cross-cultural and cross-national studies of problems of common interest to clinical and health care systems are consistent with this priority (Hinshaw, 2000). The nursing research priorities for many countries show many similar interests and opportunities for collaboration. Challenges associated with developing a global research community include establishing international networks, websites, and data bases; understanding different cultural perspectives and adapting the research accordingly; and obtaining funding for international projects (Henry and Chang, 1998; Hinshaw, 2000; Kitson et al, 1997).

To maximize utilization of available resources and prevent wasteful duplication, researchers must develop intradisciplinary and interdisciplinary networks in similar areas of basic and applied study across disciplines (Engebretson and Wardell, 1997; Jones, Tulman, and Clancy, 1999; O'Neill and Duffey, 2000). Clinical consortia will help delineate the common and unique aspects of patient care for various health professions. Cluster studies, multiple-site investigations, and programs of research will facilitate the accumulation of evidence supporting or negating an existing theory, thereby contributing to defining the base of nursing practice. The increasing importance of health service research will promote scientific inquiry to develop and produce knowledge of health care delivery that is applied to and addresses issues that cross disciplinary boundaries related to crucial issues such as resource utilization and policy making (Jones, Tulman, and Clancy, 1999).

Depth in nursing science will be evident when replicated, consistent findings exist in a substantive area of inquiry. Programs of research that include a series of studies in a similar area of study, each of which builds on prior investigation, both replicating and adding to the research question being studied, will promote depth in nursing science (Grady, 1999). An example of a program of research is provided by the work of Mary Naylor, the principal investigator funded by a 3-year grant from the NINR for the multisite study of the Comprehensive Discharge Planning and Home Follow-Up of Hospitalized Elders. Approximately 363 patients were enrolled in the study. The study further validated earlier studies by Naylor and colleagues that examined the effectiveness of an advanced practice nurse-centered discharge planning and home follow-up intervention for elders at risk for hospital readmissions (Brooten, Naylor, and York, 1995; Naylor et al, 1994; Naylor et al, 1999). This study led to improved patient care and ultimately to cost savings in terms of reduced readmissions, more time between discharge and readmission, and decreased cost of providing health care. In this study, the Medicare reimbursements for health services were about $1.2 million in the control group vs. $0.6 million in the intervention group, with no significant differences between groups on clinical outcome indicators such as functional status, depression, or patient satisfaction. Consistent and replicated findings across studies and sites yield a body of practice-relevant, in-depth knowledge about the effects of advanced practice, nurse-focused transitional care programs on clinical patient outcomes and cost.

The preceding example illustrates the value of replication studies that are built into programs of research that are the hallmark of research careers (Wysocki, 1998). Rosswurm and Larrabee (1999) propose that the adoption of research findings in practice, with their potential risks and benefits—including the cost of implementation, should be based on a series of replicated studies, thereby increasing how the findings can be generalized. A greater focus on "generalizability" is important if the evolving science is to be considered reliable and usable in nursing practice and influencing health policy (Hinshaw, 1999). As such, in the future, replication studies will be more credible and play a crucial role in developing depth in nursing science; the findings of such studies can then be applied in clinical practice through evidence-based practice projects.

Nursing research is increasingly addressing the biologic and behavioral aspects of nursing science, reflecting the discipline's holistic approach to health and illness for individuals and families. Investigations that reflect state-of-the-art science examine the interface of the biologic sciences with the evolving knowledge base of nursing. For example, NINR's intramural program has funded the first of three planned clinical and basic laboratories, the Laboratory of Wound Healing, which is actively investigating the cellular and molecular mechanisms responsible for defective wound healing (Grady, 1999). Two other clinical laboratories include the Laboratory of Symptom Management and the Laboratory of Health Promotion. These programs will provide direction on improving aspects of care (e.g., symptom assessment, management, and interventions) to prevent and reduce physical distress such as pain (Grady, 1999; Hinshaw, 1999).

Nurse researchers will continue to have increased methodologic expertise. They are becoming increasingly sophisticated in developing and applying computer technology to the research process (Ailinger and Neal, 1999). Measurement issues (e.g., development of tools that accurately measure clinical phenomena) will still be emphasized.

The increasing focus on the need to use multiple measures to assess clinical phenomena accurately is also apparent. The development of noninvasive methods to measure physiological parameters of interest in high-technology settings is related to this focus. These methods may be another aspect of using multiple measures to assess particular clinical phenomena. The development of qualitative measures and new qualitative computer analysis packages is also expanding as the qualitative mode of inquiry is now commonly used in research.

Nurse researchers will employ new, more diverse, and advanced methods to design research studies and analyze findings. For example, qualitative research methods are now a respected mode of scientific inquiry, contributing to theory development and providing essential descriptive data to direct clinical practice and future research studies. Consider how the findings of qualitative studies by Pollack (1990; 1993; 1995; 1996a; 1996b) on the development of a self-management model related to informational and activity needs for people with bipolar disorder have contributed to revealing the fundamental structure of patient education and therapeutic group activities for this patient population. The data from these qualitative studies provided the basis for the quantitative quasi-experimental, nonequivalent comparison group design to compare the effectiveness of the self-management group model with an interactional group model in improving the ability of people with bipolar disorder to care for themselves (Pollack and Cramer, 1999; Pollack, Cramer, and Harvin, 2000). The findings highlight the benefits of providing diagnostically homogeneous groups for this patient population when hospitalized (Pollack, 1995; Pollack and Cramer, 1999). Future research in the area is needed to test the applicability of the model in partial hospitalization and outpatient settings to ensure that the most effective treatment models are available to facilitate effective nursing management of a potentially devastating neurobiologic disorder.

INTERVENTION STUDIES

Another trend is the proliferation of intervention studies that are focused on both the patient and the delivery system (Goode and Piedalue, 1999; Omery and Williams, 1999). Stimulated by the need for cost-effective care that makes a difference without compromising quality, intervention studies will provide an unprecedented opportunity for nurses to pursue research that will contribute to the scientific basis of nursing practice.

Experimental and causal modeling designs will be increasingly used to test specific relationships between nursing interventions and patient outcomes, promoting progress toward prescribing interventions with a relatively reliable sense of predicting the outcomes (Hinshaw, 1999). Through this approach, nurses who conduct such research studies and nurses who apply the findings to practice will be adding to the body of nursing interventions that are scientifically sound and document the impact of nursing care. The intervention studies of Brooten and associates (1986), Naylor and associates (1999), and Bull, Hansen, and Gross (2000) described earlier in this chapter (each of which tested an innovative client care delivery model) are classic examples of intervention studies that document the impact of nursing care.

Through examination of outcomes related to staffing, the most cost-effective models for the delivery of high-quality collaborative care are being identified. Research by nurses has found empirical support for an inverse relationship between nurse staffing levels and adverse patient outcomes (Aiken et al, 1994; Blegen, Goode, and Reed, 1998; Harrington and Carrillo, 1998; Kovner and Gergen, 1998). It is clear that nurses must capitalize on the opportunity to lead other health care providers in ensuring that outcomes are measured fully.

PROGRAMS OF RESEARCH

Research training will increasingly become an essential component of a research career plan. In order to develop a larger cadre of nurse researchers who begin their research career at a young age, strategies must be developed to fast-track individuals through educational programs. The goal is to increase the longevity of research careers, enhance the discipline's science development, promote mentoring opportunities and prepare the next generation of researchers, and provide leadership in health care for interdisciplinary health care debates (Hinshaw, 1999).

Nurse researchers will be committed to developing research programs that are supported by public and private sources. They will also sub-scribe to a lifestyle of periodic education and re-training funded by awards, grants, and fellow-ships. For example, the NINR awards fund predoctoral, postdoctoral, midcareer, and senior scientist programs of study. These programs fa-cilitate growth in the depth and breadth of re-search expertise and recognize that some re-searchers need to be retrained as they develop or shift the emphasis of their research, seek to broaden their scientific background, acquire new research capabilities, and enlarge their command of an allied research field.

Nurses prepared to direct the conduct of re-search will head an expanding number of nursing research departments in clinical settings. Cur-rently, there are more than 100 clinical research centers in as many as 32 states. The nurse re-searchers who head these centers will involve the nursing staff in identifying nursing-sensitive out-come indicators to use in generating and con-ducting research projects and critically evaluating existing research data before using it as evidence to guide decisions about changes in clinical prac-tice. A commitment to investigating common clinical outcome indicators that link nursing practice strategies with nursing-sensitive out-comes common to acute care or community-based clinical settings nationwide should be pro-moted. Such a commitment will facilitate the merging of large data sets, the objective of which is to demonstrate how nursing interven-tion makes a difference (ANA, 1996; ANA, 1997; Titler et al, 1999b). In addition, an expanded number of centers for nursing research will be established in university settings as faculty members become qualified to direct them. Many academic centers for nursing research will partner with their clinical research depart-ment counterparts to develop and implement exciting research-related initiatives that support evidence-based practice.

AN INTERNATIONAL PERSPECTIVE

With the discipline's emphasis on cultural as-pects of nursing care and the influence of such factors on practice, increasing international re-search is a natural futuristic trend. Access to mul-tiple populations as a function of globalization allows the generation and testing of nursing sci-ence from many different perspectives. Interac-tion with colleagues from other countries pro-vides a rich context for the generation and dissemination of research issues (Henry, 1998; Hinshaw, 1999, 2000).

Alliances with international organizations committed to the goal of health for all will create natural research partnerships. For example, the World Health Organization (WHO), through the Pan-American Health Organization, has desig-nated that four WHO Collaborating Centers for Research and Clinical Training in Nursing be lo-cated in American schools and colleges of nurs-ing. These centers will provide research and clin-ical training in nursing to colleagues worldwide. The International Council of Nurses (ICN) and research conferences sponsored by ANA and other specialty organizations are examples of in-ternational nursing-research forums designed to inform nurses of the global breadth of health problems. Such forums for research dissemination will continue to increase, challenging nurse re-searchers in various regions of the world to form collaborative research relationships in which they share research expertise, educational opportuni-ties, and the ability to conduct research projects of mutual interest, as well as, perhaps, ultimately create an international research agenda (Henry, 1998; Hinshaw, 2000).

FUTURE RESEARCH PRIORITIES

In 2000, the U.S. Department of Health and Hu-man Services published the revised summary re-port, *Healthy People 2010.* The original document, *Healthy People 2000,* published in 1992, was a product of 22 expert working groups and nearly 300 national organizations—including nurs-ing—and contained 22 priority areas geared to improving the health of the nation. The current document reaffirms these priority areas. The Na-tional Research Agenda identifies priorities that are consistent with the goals of this national health agenda. By the year 2010, a cost-effective, community-based health care delivery system that emphasizes primary care and promotes prevention through risk reduction in partnership with members of a culturally diverse society will actualize a high-quality health care vision. One of the objectives, for example, is "increase the proportion of persons with long-term care needs who have access to the continuum of long-term-care services" (U.S. Department of Health and Human Services, 2000). Several nurse researchers, such as Bull, Hansen, and Gross (2000); Naylor and associates (1999); Phillips and Ayres (1999); and Roberts (1999), have been conducting research, developing theoretical perspectives, and conducting synthesis conferences in the area of maintaining the independence of elders, managing cognitive impairment and depression in the elderly, and providing supportive care environments for the elderly. Widespread use of models (e.g., the transitional care model for the elderly developed by Naylor and associates [1999]) could save significant health care dollars and influence policy to improve the quality of care for the elderly. (See Research Vignette on pages 2 and 3.)

Concern about communities and vulnerable populations will be integral to shaping the focus of a nursing-research agenda. Increasingly, the settings where care is provided will be homes, schools, workplaces, and primary care centers. Most of clinical nursing research has focused on the individual or the family, as in caregiver studies. This perspective should be expanded to include health-promotion and risk-reduction research that is population-focused and community-based (e.g., health promotion for women in the workplace, lowering cardiovascular disease in children, as well as linking interventions and outcomes in smoking-cessation and violence-reduction programs) (Hinshaw, 2000).

By the year 2010, the population will include a higher proportion of children and elderly who are chronically ill or disabled (RWJ Annual Report, 1999). The health problems of mothers and infants will continue to spur concern for dealing effectively with the maternal-infant mortality rate. Individuals of all ages who have sustained life-threatening illnesses will live by means of new life-sustaining technology that will create new demands for self-care, as well as family support that facilitates effective patient management of their conditions. Cancer, heart disease, arthritis, asthma, chronic pulmonary disease, diabetes, and Alzheimer's disease are prevalent during middle and later life and will command large proportions of the available health care resources. The impact of HIV/AIDS as a chronic illness for men, women, and children will continue to have a significant impact on the health care delivery system. As a wave of national initiatives are launched to improve end-of-life care, nurses—as clinicians and investigators—will make major contributions to end-of-life research (Matzo and Sherman, 2001).

Mental health problems will result from rapid technologic and social change; understanding of mental disorders will continue to expand as a result of the psychobiologic knowledge explosion and research initiatives. Alcohol and drug abuse will continue to be responsible for significant health care expense. Investigations that address quality of care outcomes related to nursing interventions are a top psychiatric nursing priority for the twenty-first century (Pullen, Tuck, and Wallace, 1999).

One of the most exciting research opportunities for nurses focuses on the area of genetics and the human genome, where study prospects range from basic biologic to clinical decision making and behavioral interventions. Sigmon and associates (1997) propose that nurse researchers can make significant contributions to the following:
- Understanding the gene-environment-behavior interface.
- Developing and using biological, psychosocial, and neuroimmunological markers.
- Biological psychosocial intervention.
- Counseling related to genetic health.
- Developing and testing cognitive models for decision making regarding genetic factors and genetic therapies.

- Investigating new delivery models for healthcare given the evolving genetic knowledge base.
- Addressing related ethical issues and dilemmas.

Hinshaw (2000) suggests that nurses will need to play a major role in this rapidly growing area of science so that the evolving knowledge base is structured within a "holistic" understanding of the person.

Over the next 10 years, many hard questions of cost containment and access to care will be addressed through an interdisciplinary approach and will need to address the related ethical dilemmas. An important emphasis of research studies will be related to clinical and systems issues and problems and their links to the improvement of patient outcomes (Larkin, 2000). The preeminent goal of scientific inquiry by nurses will be the ongoing development of knowledge for use in the practice of nursing. This refers to an action agenda that establishes how the quality of patient care is connected to nursing practice and how the interventions of nurses are related to patient satisfaction and important clinical outcomes. For example, the development of evidence-based approaches to reduce medication errors provides a leadership opportunity for nurses to influence solutions for a nationwide interdisciplinary systems problem identified by the Institute of Medicine (Kohn, Corrigan, and Donaldson, 1999). It also refers to patient care initiatives related to the organization and delivery of nursing care. This type of research, sometimes referred to as health-services research, would include studies that predict the future supply and demand for nursing care (Buerhaus, 1998; Kovner and Jonas, 1999; Kovner and Gergen, 1998). Consequently, priority will be given to nursing research that generates knowledge to guide practice in the areas listed in Box 1-2.

In light of the priority given to clinical research issues, the funding of investigations will increasingly emphasize clinical research projects in relation to populations of interest. For example, the historical exclusion of women from clinical research is now well-documented. Men have been the subjects in the major contemporary research studies related to adult health. The findings of such studies have been generalized from men to all adults, despite the lack of female representation (Larson, 1994). The Baltimore Longitudinal Study on Aging began in 1958 but did not include women as subjects until 1978. Although women now make up about 60% of those in the United States who are 65 or older, the study's well-respected 1984 report, "Normal Human Aging," contained no data specific to women. Minority women have been even more likely to be excluded from research studies; as a result, research data on minority women are extremely scarce. Funding for research related to women's health issues and problems (e.g., infertility, menopause, breast and ovarian cancer, and osteoporosis) has been less than equitable. Given the indisputable nature of this research bias, the Office of Research on Women's Health has been established at the NIH to redress historical inequities in research design and allocation of federal resources. Research on women's health will be a major funding focus in the future.

Based on a review of the literature focused on the research priorities identified by nine nursing specialties, Hinshaw (2000) identifies the top five American nursing research priorities as the following:

1. Quality of care outcomes and their measurement.
2. Impact/effectiveness of nursing interventions.
3. Symptom assessment and management.
4. Health care delivery systems.
5. Health promotion/risk reduction.

Areas of special research interest delineated by the NINR for 2000 to 2004 (NINR, 2000) include the following:

- **Chronic illness experiences**—managing symptoms, avoiding complications of disease and disability, supporting family caregivers, promoting adherence and self-management activities, and promoting healthy behaviors within the context of the chronic condition.

- **Cultural and ethnic considerations**—culturally sensitive interventions to decrease health disparities among groups by focusing on health-promotion activities and strategies of managing chronic illness.
- **End-of-life/palliative care research**—clinical management of physical and psychological symptom management, communication, ethics and clinical decision-making, caregiver support, and care-delivery issues.
- **Health promotion and disease prevention research**—initiatives focusing on lifestyle changes and healthy behavior maintenance across the lifespan.
- **Implications of genetic advances**—reducing factors that increase risk of disease, issues related to genetic screening, and subsequent gene-therapy techniques.
- **Quality of life and quality of care**—initiatives focusing on cost savings for the patient, health care system, and society.
- **Symptom management**—of illness and treatment (e.g., pain, cognitive impairment, fatigue, nausea and vomiting, and sleep problems).
- **Telehealth interventions and monitoring**—focus on emerging technologies to promote patient education and treatment.

Other types of research investigations (e.g., those using historical, feminist, or case study methods) embody the rich diversity of nursing-research methods. Brink (1990) states that the enormous, exponential growth in nursing research since the early 1950s seems attributable to the diversity of methodological approaches that have been used to answer the profession's research questions. The nursing profession must continue to value and promote creativity and diversity in research endeavors at all educational levels as a way of empowering nursing practice for the future. As opportunities are recognized and gaps in science are observed, nurses will engage in the conduct, critique, and utilization of nursing research in ways that give voice to how nursing care makes a difference.

Nurse researchers will have an increasingly strong voice in shaping public policy. Hinshaw (1999) states that disciplines such as nursing—because it focuses on treatment of chronic illness, health promotion, independence in health, and care of the acutely ill, all of which are heavily emphasized values for the future—are going to be central to shaping health care policy. Research data providing evidence that supports or refutes the merit of health care needs and programs focusing on these issues will be timely and relevant. Thus nursing and its science base will be strategically placed to shape health policy decisions.

Because we will continue to live in the "information age," dissemination of nursing research will become increasingly important. Research findings will continue to be disseminated in professional arenas (e.g., international, national, regional, and local electronic and print publications and conferences), as well as in consultations and staff-development programs that are implemented on-site, through web-based programs or via satellite. Dissemination of research findings in the public sector, however, is an exciting future trend that has already begun. Nurse researchers are increasingly asked to present testimony at governmental hearings and serve on commissions and task forces related to health care. Nurses are increasingly quoted in the media when health care topics are addressed, but their visibility must expand significantly (Sigma Theta Tau, 1998). Today nurses and nurse researchers are participating in teleconferences, developing their own home pages for the internet, starring in videos, and appearing in interviews on television and radio and in printed and electronic media (e.g., the internet, newspapers, and magazines). Nurses have their own radio shows and are beginning to have their own television shows. Dissemination of research through the public media provides excellent exposure to thousands of potential viewers, listeners, and readers. Practicing nurses are using technological innovations (e.g., computerized documentation systems and electronic access to databases and literature searches, interactive telecommunication educational offerings, on-line journals, and research-based practice guidelines) to make the information revolution come of age in research-related clinical practice activities (Ailinger and Neal, 1999; Carty, 2001; Deibert, 1998).

Nursing has a research heritage to be proud of and a challenging and exciting future direction.

Both consumers and producers of research will engage in a united effort to give voice to research findings that make a difference in the care that is provided and the lives that are touched by our commitment to evidence-based nursing practice.

Barbara Krainovich-Miller

Critical Thinking Challenges

➢ How will expanding your computer technology "comfort zone" to generate nursing-research data affect health care in the future?
➢ What is the assumption underlying ANA's (1989) recommendation that the role of the baccalaureate graduate in the research process is primarily that of a knowledgeable consumer?
➢ What effects will patient outcomes studies have on the practice of nursing?
➢ Discuss how research will contribute to the development of intradisciplinary and interdisciplinary networks.
➢ Discuss at least three differences between an evidence-based nursing practice and a research-based nursing practice.

Key Points

• Nursing research provides the basis for expanding the unique body of scientific knowledge that forms the foundation of nursing practice. Research links education, theory, and practice.
• Nurses become knowledgeable consumers of research through educational processes and practical experience. As consumers of research, nurses must have a basic understanding of the research process and critical appraisal skills that provide a standard for evaluating the strengths and weaknesses of research studies before applying them in clinical practice.
• In the first half of the twentieth century, nursing research focused mainly on studies related to nursing education, although some clinical studies related to nursing care were evident.
• Nursing research blossomed in the second half of the twentieth century: graduate programs in nursing expanded; research journals began to emerge; the ANA formed a research committee; and funding for graduate education and nursing research increased dramatically.
• Nurses at all levels of educational preparation have a responsibility to participate in the research process.
• The role of the baccalaureate graduate is to be a knowledgeable consumer of research. Nurses

with master's and doctorate degrees must be sophisticated consumers, as well as producers, of research studies.
• A collaborative research relationship within the nursing profession will extend and refine the scientific body of knowledge that provides the grounding for theory-based practice.
• The future of nursing research will continue to be the extension of the scientific knowledge base for nursing expertise in appraising, designing, and conducting research and will provide leadership in both academic and clinical settings. Collaborative research relationships between education and service will multiply. Cluster research studies and replication of studies will have increased value.
• Research studies will emphasize clinical issues, problems, and outcomes. Priority will be given to research studies that focus on promoting health, diminishing the negative impact of health problems, ensuring care for the health needs of vulnerable groups, and developing cost-effective health care systems.
• Both consumers and producers of research will engage in a collaborative effort to further the growth of nursing research and accomplish the research objectives of the profession.

REFERENCES

Aiken L et al: Lower medicare mortality among a set of hospitals known for good nursing care, Med Care 32(8):771-787, 1994.

Ailinger RL and Neal LJ: Developing a regional nursing research website, Image 31(3):249-250, 1999.

American Nurses Association: Facts about nursing, New York, 1960, The Association.

American Nurses Association: Code for nurses with interpretive statements, Washington, DC, 2000, The Association.

American Nurses Association: Commission on nursing research: education for preparation in nursing research, Kansas City, MO, 1989, The Association.

American Nurses Association: Nursing quality indicators: guide for implementation, Washington, DC, 1996, The Association.

American Nurses Association: Implementing nursing's report card, Washington, DC, 1997, The Association.

Batey MV: Research: a component of undergraduate education. In published proceedings: Evaluating research preparation in baccalaureate nursing education: national conference for nurse educators, published proceedings, Ames, IA, 1982, University of Iowa College of Nursing.

Berlin L: Personal communication, August 12, 2000.

Blegen M, Goode C, and Reed L: Nurse staffing and patient outcomes, Nurs Res 47(1):43-50, 1998.

Bouve LR, Rozmus CL, and Giordano, P: Preparing parents for their child's transfer from the PICU to the pediatric floor, Applied Nurs Res 12(3):114-120, 1999.

Brink P: Learning how to do research requires a mentor, West J Nurs Res 17(4):351-352, 1995.

Brink P: The discipline is the method, West J Nurs Res 22(3):432, 1990.

Brooten D et al: A randomized clinical trial of early hospital discharge and home follow-up of very–low-birth-weight infants, N Engl J Med 315(8):934-939, 1986.

Brooten D et al: Quality-cost model of early hospital discharge and nurse specialist transitional follow-up care, Image 20(2):64-68, 1988.

Brooten D et al: Development of a program grant using the quality-cost model of early discharge and nurse specialist transitional follow-up care, Nurs Health Care 10(6):315-318, 1989.

Brooten D, Naylor MD, and York R: Effects of nurse specialists transitional care on patient outcomes and cost: results of five randomized clinical trials, Am J Managed Care 1:35-41, 1995.

Buerhaus PI: The value of consumer and nurse partnerships, Nurs Policy Forum 2(2):13-20, 1996.

Bull MJ, Hansen HE, and Gross CR: A professional-patient partnership model of discharge planning with elders hospitalized with heart failure, Applied Nurs Res 13(1):19-28, 2000.

Carnegie E: Historical perspectives of nursing research, Boston, 1976, Boston University.

Carty B, editor: Nursing informatics: education for practice, New York, 2001, Springer.

Chang WY: Priority setting for nursing research, Western J Nurs Res 22(2):119-121, 2000.

Cohen MZ and Ley CD: Bone marrow transplantation: the battle for hope in face of fear, Oncology Nursing Forum 27(3):473-480, 2000.

Cohen S, Hollingsworth A, and Rubin M: Another look at psychologic complications of hysterectomy, Image 21(1):51-54, 1989.

Committee on Nursing and Nursing Education in the United States, Josephine Goldmark, Secretary, New York, 1923, Macmillan.

Deibert RJ: Virtual resources: international relations research resources on the web, International Organization 52(1): 211-221, 2000.

Diers D and Leonard RC: Interaction analysis in nursing research, Nurs Res 15:225-228, 1966.

Dock LL: What we may expect from the law, Am J Nurs 1:8-12, 1900.

Donaldson SK: Breakthroughs in nursing research, presentation, Proceedings of the 25th Anniversary of the American Academy of Nursing, Acapulco, Mexico, 1998.

Donnell H and Glick SJ: The nurse and the unwed mother, Nurs Outlook 2:249-251, 1954.

Dumas RG and Leonard RC: The effect of nursing on the incidence of postoperative vomiting, Nurs Res 12:12-15, 1963.

Engebretson J and Wardell DW: The essence of partnership in research, J Professional Nurs 13(1):38-47, 1997.

Fawcett J: Hallmarks of success in nursing research, Adv Nurs Sci 1:1-11, 1984.

Fitzpatrick JJ: A decade of applied nursing research: a new millennium and beyond, Applied Nurs Res 13(1):1, 2000.

Glaser BG and Strauss AL: Observations series: awareness of dying, Chicago, 1965, Aldine.

Goode CJ and Piedalue F: Evidence-based clinical practice, J. Nurs Admin 29(6):15-21, 1999.

Goodrich A: The social and ethical significance of nursing: a series of addresses, New York, 1932, Macmillan.

Gortner SR: Knowledge development in nursing: our historical roots and future opportunities, Nurs Outlook 48:60-67, 2000.

Grady PA: News from NINR, *Nurs Outlook* 47(2):73, 1999a.

Grady PA: News from NINR, *Nurs Outlook* 47(4):154, 1999b.

Grady PA: News from NINR, *Nurs Outlook* 47(3):73, 1999c.

Grady PA: News from NINR, *Nurs Outlook* 47(5):199, 1999d.

Graff B et al: Development of a postoperative self-assessment form, *Clin Nurs Spec* 6(1):47-50, 1992.

Greenblatt M et al: *From custodial to therapeutic patient care in mental hospitals,* New York, 1955, Russell Sage Foundation.

Hall LE: A center for nursing, *Nurs Outlook* 11:805-806, 1963.

Harrington H and Carrillo C: Nursing facilities, staffing, residents, facility, deficients, 1991 through 1996, January 1998.

Hegyvary ST: An open letter from the new editor, *Image* 31(3):203, 1999.

Henderson V: Research in nursing practice: when?, *Nurs Res* 4:99, 1956 (editorial).

Henderson V: We've "come a long way," but what of the direction?, *Nurs Res* 26:163-164, 1977 (guest editorial).

Henry B: Globalization, nursing philosophy, and nursing science, *Image* 30(4): 302, 1998.

Henry BM and Chang WY: Nursing research and priorities in Africa, Asia and Europe, *Image* 30:115-116, 1998.

Hinshaw AS: Nursing knowledge for the 21st century: opportunities and challenges, *J Nurs Scholarship* 32(2):117-123, 2000.

Hinshaw AS: Evolving nursing research traditions. In Hinshaw AS, Feetham SL, and Shaver JLF, editors: *Handbook of clinical nursing research,* Thousand Oaks, CA, 1999, Sage.

Hinshaw AS, Feetham SL, and Shaver JLF, editors: *Handbook of clinical nursing research,* Thousand Oaks, CA, 1999, Sage.

Joint Commission on Accreditation of Healthcare Organizations: Accreditation manual for hospitals, Oakbrook Terrace, IL, 1999, The Commission.

Jones CB, Tulman L, and Clancy CM: Research funding opportunities at the agency for health care policy and research, *Nurs Outlook* 47(4):156-161, 1999.

Keith JM: Florence Nightingale: statistician and consultant epidemiologist, *Int Nurs Rev* 35(5):147-149, 1988.

Kitson A et al: On developing an agenda to influence policy in health related research for effective nursing: a description of a national R & D priority setting exercise, *Nurs Times Res* 2:323-324, 1997.

Kohn L, Corrigan J, Donaldson M, editors: To err is human: building a safer health system, Washington, D.C., National Academy Press, 1999.

Kovner CT and Gergen PJ: Nurse staffing levels and adverse events following surgery in U.S. hospitals, *Image* 30(4):315-321, 1998.

Kovner AR and Jonas S, editors: *Jonas and Kovner's health care delivery in the United States,* ed 6, New York, 1999, Springer.

Larkin H: Better health outcomes possible using evidence-based medicine, *Advances* 2:1-2, 2000.

Larson E: Exclusion of certain groups from clinical research, *Image* 26(3):185-190, 1994.

National Institute of Nursing Research: About NINR, available at www.nih.gov/ninr/a mission.html, August 17, 2000.

Lynn MR, Layman EL, and Englehardt SP: Nursing administration priorities—a national Delphi study, *J Nurs Admin* 28(5):7-11, 1998.

Matzo M and Sherman DW, editors: Palliative care nursing: quality care to the end of life, New York, 2001, Springer.

Naylor M et al: Comprehensive discharge planning for the hospitalized elderly: a randomized clinical trial, *Ann Internal Med* 120:999-1006, 1994.

Naylor MD et al: Comprehensive discharge planning and home follow-up of hospitalized elders: a randomized clinical trial, *JAMA* 281(7): 613-620, 1999.

Nightingale F: *Notes on hospitals,* London, 1863, Longman Group.

Nutting MA: *Educational status of nursing (Bull No 7),* Washington, DC, 1912, US Bureau of Education.

Nutting MA: *A second economic basis for schools of nursing and other addresses,* New York, 1926, GP Putnam's Sons.

Nutting MA and Dock LL: *A history of nursing,* volumes I-IV, New York, 1907-1912, GP Putnam's Sons.

Omery A and Williams RP: An appraisal of research utilization across the United States, *J Nurs Admin* 29(12):50-56, 1999.

O'Neill AL and Duffey MA: Communication of research and practice knowledge in nursing literature, *Nurs Res* 49(4):224-230, 2000.

O'Neill ES and Dluly NM: Utility of structured care approaches in education and clinical practice, *Nurs Outlook* 48(3):132-135, 2000.

Orlando IJ: *The dynamic nurse-patient relationship,* New York, 1961, GP Putnam's Sons.

Peplau HE: *Interpersonal relations in nursing: a conceptual frame of reference for psychodynamic nursing,* New York, 1952, GP Putnam's Sons.

Phillips LR and Ayres M: Supportive and nonsupportive care environments for the elderly. In Hinshaw AS,

Feetham SL, and Shaver JLF, editors: *Handbook of clinical nursing research,* Thousand Oaks, CA, 1999, Sage.

Pollack LE: Improving relationships: groups for inpatients with bipolar disorder, *J Psychosocial Nurs Mental Health Serv* 28:17-22, 1990.

Pollack LE: Do patients with bipolar disorder evaluate diagnostically homogeneous groups?, *J Psychosocial Nurs Mental Health Serv* 31(10):26-32, 1993.

Pollack LE: Striving for stability with bipolar disorder despite barriers, *Arch Psychiatr Nurs* 9(3):122-129, 1995.

Pollack LE: Information seeking among people with manic-depressive illness, *Image* 28(3):259-265, 1996a.

Pollack LE: Inpatient self-management of bipolar disorder, *Applied Nurs Res* 9:71-79, 1996b.

Pollack LE and Cramer RD: Patient satisfaction with two models for group therapy for people hospitalized with bipolar disorder, *Applied Nurs Res* 12(3): 143-152, 1999.

Pullen L, Tuck I, and Wallace DC: Research priorities in mental health nursing, *Issues Mental Health Nurs* 20(3):217-227, 1999.

Robb IH: *Nursing: its principles and practice for hospitals and private use,* ed 3, Cleveland, 1906, EC Koeckert.

Robert Wood Johnson Foundation: Annual report 1999, Princeton, NJ, 1999, The Foundation.

Roberts BI: Activities of daily living: factors related to independence. In Hinshaw AS, Feetham SL, and Shaver JLF, editors: *Handbook of clinical nursing research,* Thousand Oaks, CA, 1999, Sage.

Rosswurm MA and Larrabee JH: A model for change to evidence-based practice, *Image* 31(4):317-322, 1999.

See EM: The ANA and research in nursing, *Nurs Res* 26:165-176, 1977.

Sigma Theta Tau: *The Woodhull study on nursing and the media,* Indianapolis, 1998, The Author.

Sigmon HD, Grady PA, and Amende LM: The National Institute of Nursing Research explores opportunities in genetics research, *Nurs Outlook* 45(5):215-219, 1997.

Stanton AH and Schwartz M: *The mental hospital,* London, 1954, Tavistock.

Stetler CB et al: Utilization-focused integrative reviews in a nursing service, *Applied Nurs Res* 11(4):195-206, 1998.

Strohschein S, Schaffer MA, and Lia-Hoagberg B: Evidence-based guidelines for public health nursing practice, *Nurs Outlook* 47(2): 84-89, 1999.

Titler MG et al: From book to bedside: putting evidence to use in the care of the elderly, *J Qual Impovement* 25(10):545-556, 1999a.

Titler MG et al: On the scene: University of Iowa hospitals and clinics: outcomes management, *Nurs Admin Q* 24:31-65, 1999b.

Titler MG et al: Infusing research into practice to promote quality care, *Nurs Res* 43(5):307-313, 1994.

US Department of Health and Human Services: *Healthy people 2000: summary report,* Pub No PH591-50213, Boston, 1992, Jones and Bartlett.

US Department of Health and Human Services: *Healthy people 2010,* Washington, DC, 2000, The Department.

Wald LD: *House on Henry Street,* New York, 1915, Henry Holt and Co.

Wiedenbach E: *Clinical nursing: a helping art,* New York, 1964, Springer.

Wysocki AB: Launching your research career through postdoctoral training opportunities, *Nurs Res* 47(3): 127-128.

WEB SITES

http://www.lib.umich.edu/hw/nursing/indoc.html Africa (number of doctoral programs outside the United States)

http://henry.ugl.lib.umich.edu/hw/nursing/usdoc. html (number of doctoral programs in the United States)

http://www.nih.gov/ninr/a_mission.html (NINR Website information)

ADDITIONAL READINGS

Abdellah FG: Overview of nursing research 1955-1968, Part I, *Nurs Res* 19:6-17, 1970a.

Abdellah FG: Overview of nursing research 1955-1968, Part II, *Nurs Res* 19:151-162, 1970b.

Abdellah FG: Overview of nursing research 1955-1968, Part III, *Nurs Res* 19:239-252, 1970c.

Acute Pain Management Guideline Panel: *Acute pain mangement: operative or medical procedures and trauma, clinical practice guideline (AHCPR Pub No 92-0032),* Rockville, Md, 1992, US Public Health Service, Agency for Health Care Policy and Research.

American Nurses Association: *Community-based quality indicators,* Washington, DC, 2001, The Association.

Batey MV and Julian J: Staff perceptions of state psychiatric hospital goals, *Nurs Res* 12:89-92, 1963.

Bavier AR: Where research and practice meet, *Nurs Policy Forum* 1(4):20-27, 1995.

Beyea S, Farley JK, and Williams-Burgess C: Teaching baccalaureate students to use research, *West J Nurs Res* 18(2):213-218, 1996.

Bidwell-Cerone S et al: Nursing research and patient outcomes: tools for managing the transformation of the health care delivery system, *J N Y State Nurs Assoc* 26(3):12-17, 1995.

Bower FL: Nursing research shapes global health, *Reflections* 4, Fall 1995.

Broadhurst J et al: Hand brush suggestions for visiting nurses, *Pub Health Nurs* 19:487-489, 1927.

Brown EL: *Nursing for the future*, New York, 1948, Russell Sage Foundation.

Buerhaus PI: Nursing's first senior scholar at the U.S. Agency for Health Care Policy and Research, *Image* 30(4):311-316, 1998.

Clayton SL: Standardizing nursing techniques: its advantages and disadvantages, *Am J Nurs* 27:939-943, 1927.

Cowan MJ et al: Integration of biological and nursing sciences: a 10-year plan to enhance research and training, *Res Nurs Health* 16(1):3-9, 1993.

Dickoff J and James P: A theory of theories: a position paper, *Nurs Res* 17:197-203, 1968.

Dickoff J, James P, and Wiedenbach E: Theory in a practice discipline, Part I, Practice-oriented theory, *Nurs Res* 17:415-435, 1968a.

Dickoff J, James P, and Wiedenbach E: Theory in a practice discipline, Part II, Practice oriented research, *Nurs Res* 17:545-554, 1968b.

Donaldson SK and Crowley DM: The discipline of nursing, *Nurs Outlook* 26:113-120, 1978.

Downs F: Informing the media, *Nurs Res* 40(4):195, 1991.

Ethridge P and Lamb G: Professional nursing case management improves quality, access and cost, *Nurs Manage* 20(1):30-37, 1989.

Gortner SR: Nursing values and science:toward a science philosophy, *Image* 22:101-105, 1990.

Gortner SR: Historical development of doctoral programs: shaping our expectations, *J Professional Nurs* 7:45-53, 1991.

Gortner SR and Nahm H: An overview of nursing research in the United States, *Nurs Res* 26:10-33, 1977.

Grady PA: News from NINR, *Nurs Outlook* 48(1):33, 2000a.

Grady PA: News from NINR, *Nurs Outlook* 48(3):127, 2000b.

Haber J et al: Shaping nursing practice through research-based protocols, *J NY State Nurs Assoc* 25(3): 4-12, 1994.

Jennings BW and Loan LA: Misconceptions among nurses about evidence-based practice, *J Nurs Schol* 33(2):122-127, 2001.

Lamb GS: Conceptual and methodological issues in nurse case management research, *Adv Nurs Sci* 15(2):16-24, 1992.

Little DE and Carnavali D: Nurse specialist effect on tuberculosis: report on a field experiment, *Nurs Res* 16:21-26, 1967.

National Commission for the Study of Nursing and Nursing Education: *An abstract for action,* New York, 1970, McGraw-Hill.

National Nursing Research Agenda: CNR invites your input, *Comm Nurs Res* 18(3):3, 1991.

Palmer I: Florence Nightingale: reformer, reactionary, researcher, *Nurs Res* 26:84-89, 1977.

Panel for the Prediction and Prevention of Pressure Ulcers in Adults: *Pressure ulcers in adults: prediction and prevention*, Clinical practice guideline (AHCPR Pub No 92-0047), Rockville, Md, 1992, Public Health Service, Agency for Health Care Policy and Research.

Parker B et al: Physical and emotional abuse in pregnancy: a comparison of adult and teenage women, *Nurs Res* 42(3):173-178, 1993.

Pollack LE, Cramer RD, and Harvin S: Inpatient group therapies for people with bipolar disorder: comparison of a self-management and an interactional model, 1999, unpublished manuscript.

Quint J: *The nurse and the dying patient*, New York, 1967, Macmillan.

Rogers M: Nursing science and the space age, *Nurs Sci Q* 5(1):27-34, 1992.

Ryan V and Miller VB: Disinfection of clinical thermometers: bacteriological study and estimated costs, *Am J Nurs* 32:197-206, 1932.

Sedham LN et al: Disseminating nursing research to the consumer, *J New York State Nurs Assoc* 31(2):21-24, 2000.

Stone PW: Dollars and sense: a primer for the novice in economic analysis (part II), *Appl Nurs Res* 14(2):100-112, 2001.

Shugars DA, O'Neil EH, Bader JD, editors: *Healthy America: practitioners for 2005: an agenda for action for US health professional schools*, Durham, NC, 1991, The Pew Health Professions Commission.

Titler MG et al: From book to bedside: putting evidence to use in the care of the elderly, *The Joint Commission Journal on Quality Improvement* 25(10):545-556, 1999.

Titler MG and Mentes JC: Research utilization in gerontological nursing practice, *J Gerontol Nurs* 25(6):6-9, 1999.

Urinary Incontinence Guideline Panel: *Urinary incontinence in adults,* Clinical practice guideline (AHCPR Pub No 92-0038), Rockville, Md, 1992, Public Health Service, Agency for Health Care Policy and Research.

Zanotti R: Overcoming national and cultural differences within collaborative international nursing research, *West J Nurs Res* 18(1):6-11, 1996.

GERI LOBIONDO-WOOD
JUDITH HABER
BARBARA KRAINOVICH-MILLER

2

Critical Reading Strategies: Overview of the Research Process

Key Terms

abstract

critical reading

critical thinking

critique

critiquing criteria

Learning Outcomes

After reading this chapter, the student should be able to do the following:

- Identify the importance of critical thinking and critical reading for the reading of research articles.
- Identify the steps of critical reading.
- Use the steps of critical reading for reviewing research articles.
- Use identified strategies for critically reading research articles.
- Use identified critical thinking and reading strategies to synthesize critiqued articles.
- Identify the format and style of research articles.

As you venture through this text, you will see the steps of the research process unfold. The steps are systematic and orderly and relate to both nursing theory and practice. Understanding the step-by-step process that researchers use will help you develop the critiquing skills necessary to judge the soundness of research studies. Throughout the chapters, research terminology pertinent to each step is identified and illustrated with many examples from the research literature. Four published research studies are found in the appendixes and used as examples to illustrate significant points in each chapter. The steps of the quantitative process generally proceed in the order outlined in Table 2-1. Highlights of the general steps of qualitative studies are outlined in Table 2-2. Remember that a researcher may vary the steps slightly, depending on the nature of the

TABLE **2-1** Steps of the Research Process and Journal Format—Quantitative Research

RESEARCH PROCESS STEPS AND/OR FORMAT ISSUE	USUAL LOCATION IN A JOURNAL HEADING OR SUBHEADING	TEXT CHAPTER
Research problem	Abstract and/or in the introduction (not labeled) or in a separate labeled heading: "Problem"	3
Purpose	Abstract and/or in the introduction or at the end of the literature review or theoretical framework section, or labeled as separate heading: "Purpose"	3
Literature review	At the end of the heading "Introduction" but not labeled as such, or labeled as a separate heading: "Literature Review," "Review of the Literature," or "Related Literature"; or not labeled but the variables reviewed appear as headings or subheadings	4
Theoretical framework (TF) and/or conceptual framework (CF)	Combined with "Literature Review" or found in a separate heading as TF or CF; or each concept or definition used in the TF or CF may appear as a separate heading or subheading	5
Hypothesis/research questions	Stated or implied near the end of the introductory section, which may be labeled or found in a separate heading or subheading: "Hypothesis" or "Research Questions"; or reported for the first time in the "Results" section	3
Research design	Stated or implied in the abstract or in the introduction or under the heading: "Methods"	9, 10, 11
Sample: type and size	"Size" may be stated in the abstract, in the methods section, or as a separate subheading under methods section as "Sample," "Sample/Subjects," or "Participants" "Type" may be implied or stated in any of previous headings described under size	12
Legal-ethical issues	Stated or implied in labeled headings: "Methods," "Procedures," "Sample," or "Subjects"	13
Instruments (measurement tools)	Found in headings labeled "Methods," "Instruments," or "Measures"	14
Validity and reliability	Specifically stated or implied in headings labeled "Methods," "Instruments," "Measures," or "Procedures"	15
Data collection procedure	Stated in methods section under subheading "Procedure" or "Data Collection," or as a separate heading: "Procedure"	14
Data analysis	Stated in methods section under subheading "Procedure" or "Data Analysis"	16, 17
Results	Stated in separate heading: "Results"	17, 18
Discussion of findings and new findings	Combined with results or as separate heading: "Discussion"	18
Implications, limitations, and recommendations	Combined in discussion or presented as separate or combined major headings	18
References	At the end of the article	2, 4
Communicating research results	Research articles, poster and paper presentations	1, 2, 18, 19, 20

research problem, but all of the steps should be addressed systematically. This chapter provides an overview of critical thinking, critical reading, and critiquing skills. It introduces the overall format of a research article and provides an overview of the subsequent chapters in the book. These topics are designed to help you read research articles more effectively and with greater understanding, making this book more "user-friendly" as you learn about the research process so that you can practice from a base of evidence and contribute to quality and cost-effective patient outcomes.

CRITICAL THINKING AND CRITICAL READING SKILLS

As you read a research article, you may be struck by the difference in style or format of a research article and a theoretical or clinical article. The terms may be new, and the focus of the content is different. You may also be thinking that the research article is too hard for you to read or that it is too technical and bores you. You may simultaneously wonder, "How will I possibly learn to evaluate (critique) all the steps of a research study, as well as all the terminology? I'm only on Chapter 2. This is not so easy; research is as hard, as everyone says."

Try to reframe these thoughts with "the glass is half-full approach." That is, tell yourself, "Yes I can learn how to read and critique research, and this chapter will provide the strategies for me to learn this skill." Remember that learning occurs with time and help. Reading research articles is difficult and frustrating at first, but the best way to become a knowledgeable consumer of research is to use critical thinking and reading skills when reading research articles. As a student, you are not expected to understand a research article or critique it perfectly the first time. Nor are you expected to develop these skills on your own. An essential objective of this book is to help you acquire critical thinking and reading skills so that you can reach this goal. Remember that becoming a competent critical thinker and reader of research, similar to learning the steps of the research process, takes time and patience.

Critical thinking is the rational examination of ideas, inferences, assumptions, principles, arguments, conclusions, issues, statements, beliefs, and actions (Paul and Elder, 2001). This means that you are engaged in the following:

- Disciplined, self-directed thinking that exemplifies the perfection of thinking appropriate to a specific domain of thinking [research];

TABLE **2-2**   Steps of the Research Process and Journal Format—Qualitative Research*

RESEARCH PROCESS STEPS AND/OR FORMAT ISSUES	USUAL LOCATION IN A JOURNAL HEADING OR SUBHEADING
Identifying the phenomenon	Abstract and/or in the introduction
Research question study purpose	Abstract and/or in the beginning or end of introduction
Literature	Abstract introduction and/or discussion
Design	Abstract and/or in the introductory section or under the method section entitled design or stated under the method section
Sample	In method section labeled "Sample" or "Subjects"
Legal-ethical issues	In the data collection or procedure's section or in the sample section
Data-collection procedure	In data collection or procedures section
Data analysis	In methods section and under subhead: "Data Analysis" or "Data Analysis and Interpretation"
Results	Stated in separate heading: "Results" or "Findings"
Discussion and recommendation	Combined in a separate section: "Discussion" or "Discussion and Implications"
References	At the end of the article

*See chapters 6, 7, and 8.

- Thinking that displays a mastery of intellectual skills and abilities [use of criteria for critiquing research];
- The art of thinking about one's thinking while thinking, to make one's thinking better (i.e., more clear, more accurate, or more defensible) [clarifying what you do understand and what you don't know].

In other words, being a critical thinker means that you are consciously thinking about your own thoughts and what you say, write, read, or do, as well as what others say, write, or do. While thinking about all of this, you are questioning the appropriateness of the content, applying standards or criteria, and seeing how things measure up.

Developing the ability to evaluate research critically requires not only critical thinking skills but also critical reading skills. Paul, a noted theorist on critical thinking, defines **critical reading** as "an active, intellectually engaging process in which the reader participates in an inner dialogue with the writer. Most people read uncritically and so miss some part of what is expressed while distorting other parts..." (Paul and Elder, 2001). This means entering into a point of view other than our own, the point of view of the writer. A critical reader actively looks for assumptions, key concepts and ideas, reasons and justifications, supporting examples, parallel experiences, implications and consequences, and any other structural features of the written text, to interpret and assess it accurately and fairly (Paul and Elder, 2001).

Actively looking for assumptions means looking at supposedly true or accepted statements that are actually unsupported by research or scientific evidence. It is perhaps easier to understand how you look for assumptions by thinking about one of the early assumptions of nursing education and practice. In the late 1950s and early 1960s, the nursing process was presented as "the" framework for practice. The formulation of a nursing diagnosis was viewed as an essential step in the nursing process. Initially, there was no scientific evidence to support this assumption, but schools of nursing began to teach these concepts and nurses began to use nursing diagnoses in practice. Nursing process eventually became a part of the American Nurses Association's (ANA, 1995) social policy statement's definition of the practice of nursing.

At the same time, assumptions related to the nursing process were introduced, nurse researchers questioned the validity of nursing diagnoses and devised studies to examine nursing diagnosis concepts in relation to nursing process (Whitley, 1999). The results of these studies provided data to support or refute the assumptions. Numerous studies conducted over the years offer evidence that these concepts are more than assumptions. In fact, in your nursing program you probably were taught to use a nursing research-based taxonomy for practice. Examples of such taxonomies are the North American Nursing Diagnosis Association's (NANDA) taxonomy of nursing diagnoses (2000) or the National Intervention Classification's (NIC) nursing intervention taxonomy (2000).

Nursing programs are mandated to develop students' critical thinking skills (Adams, 1999). Students are often introduced to critical thinking skills through the nursing process to foster diagnostic reasoning skills (Krainovich-Miller, 1997). Critical thinking and critical reading skills are further developed by learning the research process. You will find that the beginning critical thinking and reading skills used in the nursing process can be transferred to understanding the research process and reading research articles. You will gradually be able to read an entire research article and reflect on it by identifying and challenging assumptions, identifying key concepts, questioning methods, and determining whether the conclusions are based on the study's findings. Once you have obtained this research-critiquing competency, you will be ready to synthesize the findings of multiple research studies to use in developing evidence-based practice. This will be a very exciting and rewarding process for you.

PROCESS OF CRITICAL READING

To read a research study critically, you must have skilled reading, writing, and reasoning abilities. A research study commonly requires several readings. A minimum of three or four readings— or even as many as six readings—is quite common. The first helping strategy is to keep your research textbook at your side as you read. Using your research text while you read a study is necessary for you to do the following:

- Identify concepts
- Clarify unfamiliar concepts or terms
- Question assumptions and rationale
- Determine supporting evidence

Critical reading can be viewed as a process that involves various levels or stages of understanding, including the following:

- Preliminary understanding
- Comprehensive understanding
- Analysis understanding
- Synthesis understanding

PRELIMINARY UNDERSTANDING: FAMILIARITY: SKIMMING

Preliminary understanding is gained by quickly scanning or reading an article to familiarize you with its content or get a general sense of the material. During the preliminary reading, the title and abstract are read closely, but the content is skimmed. The **abstract,** a brief overview of a study, keys the reader to the main components of the study. The title keys the reader to the main variables of the study. Skimming includes reading the introduction, major headings, one or two sentences under a heading, and the summary or conclusion of the study. The preliminary reading includes use of the following strategies:

- Highlighting or underlining the main steps of the research process.
- Making notes (both comments and questions) on the photocopied article.
- Writing key variables at the top of the photocopied article.

- Highlighting or underlining new and unfamiliar terms and significant sentences on the photocopy.
- Looking up the definitions of new terms and writing them in the margins of the photocopy.
- Reviewing old and new terms before the next reading.
- Keeping a research text and a dictionary by your side.

Using these strategies enables you to identify the main theme or idea of the article and bring this knowledge to the second comprehensive reading. An illustration of how to use a number of these strategies is provided by the example in Box 2-1, which contains an excerpt from the introduction and background (conceptual framework) section of a quantitative study (Bull, Hansen, and Gross, 2000) (see Appendix A). Please note that in this particular article, the beginning section is not labeled, although a brief literature review is clearly presented to support the problem under study, as well as the aims or purpose of the study. The next section of the article is labeled *Background* and also presents a literature review to support the *Conceptual Framework* for the study. Also note that parts of the text of this section from the article were deleted to offer a number of examples within the text of this chapter.

COMPREHENSIVE UNDERSTANDING: CONTENT IN RELATION TO CONTEXT

The main purpose of reading a research study for a comprehensive understanding or skilled reading is to understand the researcher's or researchers' intent. Perhaps you have been assigned to read a research article on a topic you were interested in, but you found it difficult to understand how the study was actually conducted or what the findings were. This occurred because you could not read at a comprehension level (i.e., you probably did not know the definitions of terms the researcher used and therefore could not understand the terms in relation to the study's context or even

BOX 2-1   Example of Skimming Strategies

Significance of the Problem

More than 2 million Americans have heart failure and 400,000 new cases are diagnosed each year. Heart failure is the most common medical diagnosis in hospitalized elders and the incidence increases with advancing age (Guerra-Garcia, Taffeta, & Protas, 1977). In 1992 more than $5.6 billion was spent on hospital care for Medicare patients admitted for heart failure. An estimated $230 million was spent on medications (USDHHS, 1994). *Efforts to curtail costs have resulted in shortened lengths of hospital stays. With shortened lengths of stay, health professionals have less time in which to identify elders' needs for follow-up care and less time to arrange aftercare (National Center for Health Statistics, 1997).* Identifying these needs and arranging appropriate follow-up care are critical to helping elders maintain independent living and preventing costly hospital readmissions.

Impact on Resources

Gap in Literature

Conceptual Definition

Discharge planning, a process of identifying patient needs for follow-up care and arranging for that care, might be expected to address this problem. *Despite efforts to . . . improve the discharge-planning process and subsequent outcomes, existing mechanisms fail to accurately identify elders' needs for follow-up care; and studies report rehospitalization rates ranging from 12 to 50% (Bull, Maruyama, & Luo, 1995; Happ, Naylor, & Roe-Prio, 1997; Lockery, Dunkle, Kart, & Coulton, 1993). One study . . .*

Impact on Resources/ Literature Review

Purposes of the Study

QUESTION: What are the outcome variables? Are dependent variables the same as outcome variables?

The aims of this study were as follows:

1. **examine differences in outcomes for elders and caregivers who participated in a professional-patient partnership model of discharge planning compared to those who received the usual discharge planning, and**
2. **examine differences in costs associated with hospital readmission and use of the emergency room following hospital discharge.**

It was hypothesized that at 2 weeks postdischarge:

COMMENT: This is a quantitative study — not sure if it is an experimental design.

Dependent variable—in experimental studies the presumed effect of the independent or experimental variable on the outcome

1. Scores on perceived health will be different for clients in the intervention and control cohorts.
2. Client satisfaction with discharge planning, perceptions of care continuity, preparedness and difficulties managing care will differ for the intervention and control cohorts.
3. Caregivers' response to caregiving will be different for the experimental and control cohorts.
4. Resource use will be different for the control and intervention cohorts.

The same hypotheses were posited for 2 months postdischarge. *The professional-patient partnership model is an intervention designed to facilitate identification of elders' needs for follow-up care and to provide a mechanism for identifying those who require more in-depth assessments. It provides nursing staff with a means of getting to know the patient quickly, provides a structure for elder patient and caregivers participation in planning, and promotes interaction between health professionals and patients.*

Conceptual Definition

BACKGROUND

Conceptual Framework

The conceptual framework for this study (see Figure 1) is based on an evaluation approach that incorporates structure, process, and outcome (Donabedian, 1966). As indicated in Figure 1, the intervention occurs within the hospital's organizational context and is likely to be influenced by both patient and caregiver characteristics. *Previous research suggests that three structural factors influence the extent to which elder patients participate in discharge planning: their health status, health locus of control, and the hospital environment. . . .*

Literature Review

BOX 2-1   Example of Skimming Strategies—cont'd

Perceived lack of control over discharge decisions was associated with posthospital psychological distress for elders who scored high on the locus of control scale (Coulton, Dunkle, Haug, Chow, & Vielhaber, 1989); these patients also were more likely to take control of their health, seek health information, be knowledgeable about their diseases, and maintain their physical well-being (Wallston, Wallston, Devellis, & Peabody, 1978). Previous studies have not examined factors that influence caregiver participation in planning for discharge; however, caregivers' health status, locus of control, and demographics might influence their participation.

Gap in Literature

The discharge-planning process for elder patients is fragile and vulnerable to breakdown . . . caregivers encounter postdischarge (Bull & Kane, 1996; Jewell, 1993). In fact 80% of elders reported unmet information needs 1 week following hospital discharge (Mistriaen, Duijnhouwer, Wijkel, deBont, & Veeger, 1997). Interventions aimed at improving communication might lead to better outcomes.

More Literature Review

In previous studies, the outcomes most often examined in relation to the discharge-planning process were readmission, costs of care, and length of hospital stay. Early referral . . . (Evans, Hendricks, Lawrence-Umlauf, & Bishop, 1989; Schrager, Halmon, Myers, Nichols & Rosenblum, 1978). Hospital discharge-planning . . . programs increased lengths of stay for patients with congestive heart failure and . . Use of geriatric consultation . . . services also have resulted in fewer readmissions within 1 month of discharge (Campion, Jette, & Berkman, 1983). Use of advanced practice nurses . . . outcomes (Brooten et al., 1996). . . . Although there is lack of agreement . . . , all patients do need to have their needs for follow-up care assessed.

Although some previous studies emphasize outcomes . . . , the ability to function in their environment, having access to services to assist them with managing their care, and satisfaction with the plan of care (Bull, 1994a, Proctor, Morrow-Howell, Albaz, & Weir, 1992). Similar outcomes seem appropriate for caregivers who assist elders in managing their care following discharge. Addressing the need of caregivers is a vital component in meeting elders' needs and maintaining their independent living arrangements (Bull, Maruyama, & Luo, 1995.)

Gap in Literature

KEY

Bold italics	= Examples of student-generated comments or questions about content
Italics	= Literature Review
<u>Single underline</u>	= Significance of the Problem
<u>Double underline</u>	= Hypotheses
Wavy line	= Gap in Literature
Dotted line	= Conceptual Definition
Bold	= Purposes of the Study
Dot Dash line	= Conceptual Framework

Text from Bull, Hansen, and Gross: A professional-patient partnership model of discharge planning with elders hospitalized with heart failure, *Appl Nurs Res 13*(1): 19-28, 2000. See Appendix A.

if the terms were used appropriately). For example, when reading Cohen and Ley's (2000) qualitative study (see Appendix B) for comprehension, it is essential to understand that the purpose of a hermeneutic phenomenological study is to answer questions of meaning or the process of discovering and constructing the meaning of human experience through intensive dialogue with persons who are living the experience (see Chapters 6 and 7). To simply recall that the major variable of their study was the concept of hope is inadequate. At the comprehension level of reading, you would be able to discuss the core variables that emerged: fear of death and hope of survival, fear of the unknown, loss of control, and fear of discharge/recurrence, as well as understand that these variables or concepts represented the lived experiences of bone marrow transplantation survivors.

When reading for comprehension, keep your research text and dictionary nearby. Although some terms may seem clear during the preliminary reading, they may be unclear upon a second reading. Do not hesitate to write cues or key words on the article. If the article still does not make sense after the second reading, ask for assistance before reading it again. Indicate the unclear areas and write out specific questions on the copy. What is or is not highlighted or the comments on the copy often help the faculty person to understand your difficulty. The problem may be that further reading on the topic is necessary for you to comprehend the article. For example, if a student is unfamiliar with Martha Rogers' *Science of Unitary Human Beings* (Rogers, 1990), reading a study testing a proposition of the model may be difficult.

HELPFUL HINT   If you still have difficulty understanding a research study after using the strategies related to skimming and comprehensive reading, make another copy of your "marked up" research article, include your specific questions or area of difficulty, and ask your professor to read it.

Comprehensive understanding is facilitated by the following strategies:

- Reviewing all unfamiliar terms before reading the article for the second time.
- Clarifying any additional unclear terms.
- Reading additional sources as necessary.
- Writing cues, relationships of concepts, and questions on the photocopy.
- Making another copy of your annotated article and requesting that your faculty member read it.
- Stating the main idea or theme of the article, in your own words, in one or two sentences on an index card or on the photocopy.

Comprehensive understanding is necessary to analyze and synthesize the material. Understanding the author's perspective for the study reflects critical thinking (Paul and Elder, 2001) and facilitates the analysis of the study according to established criteria. The next reading or two allows for analysis and synthesis of the study.

ANALYSIS UNDERSTANDING: BREAKING INTO PARTS

The purpose of reading for analysis is to break the content into parts and understand each aspect of the study. Some of the questions that you can ask yourself as you begin to analyze the research article are as follows:

- Am I confident that I know the specific type of design so that I apply the appropriate criteria when critiquing the study?
- Did I capture the main idea or theme of this article in one or two sentences?
- How are the major parts of this article organized in relation to the research process?
- What is the purpose of this article?
- How was this study carried out? Can I explain it step by step?
- What are the author's or authors' main conclusions?
- Can I say that I understand the parts of this article and summarize each section in my own words?

In a sense, you are determining how the steps of the research process are presented or organized in the article and what the content related to each step is about. This is also when you begin to critique or evaluate the study by asking and answering the questions related to the research process that was used by the researcher/author. At this point of critical reading, you are ready to begin the critiquing process that will help determine the study's merit.

HELPFUL HINT Remember that not all research articles include headings related to each step or component of the research process, but that each step is presented at some point in the article.

The **critique** is the process of objectively and critically evaluating a research report's content for scientific merit and application to practice, theory, and education. It requires some knowledge of the subject matter and knowledge of how to critically read and use critiquing criteria. You will find summarized examples of critiquing questions for qualitative studies and an example of a qualitative critique in Chapter 8 and summarized critiquing questions and examples of a quantitative critique in Chapter 19. An in-depth exploration of the criteria for analysis required in quantitative research critiques is given in Chapters 9 through 19. The criteria for qualitative research critiques are presented in Chapters 6, 7, and 8. Chapters 3, 4, and 5 provide general principles for quantitative and qualitative research.

Critiquing criteria are the measures, standards, evaluation guides, or questions used to judge (critique) a product or behavior. In analyzing the research report, the reader must evaluate each step of the research process and ask questions about whether each explanation of a step of the process meets the criteria. For instance, the critiquing criteria in Chapter 4 ask if "the literature review identifies gaps and inconsistencies in the literature about a subject, concept, or problem" and if "all of the concepts and variables are included in the review." These two questions relate to critiquing the problem statement and reviewing the literature components of the research process. Box 2-1 shows at least two places that the researchers identified gaps in the literature, as well as how their study intended to fill these gaps by conducting a study for the stated aims (see Appendix A for the complete study). Therefore your answer to these posed questions might be as follows:

Bull, Hansen, and Gross (2000) clearly stated the major gaps in the literature related to the discharge problems of elders hospitalized with heart failure. The identified problems became the studied variables, and their clearly stated aims addressed the gaps in the literature.

This critiquing statement implies that reading for analysis took place. When you first begin to critique a researcher's work, you may feel inadequate, and this is expected. As a beginner, you are not expected to write a critique at the same level as a seasoned researcher who critiques a colleague's work (e.g., as published in the *Western Journal of Nursing Research*). Remember that when you are doing a critique, you are pointing out strengths, as well as weaknesses. Developing critical reading skills at the comprehension level will enable you to successfully complete a critique. The following critiquing strategies facilitate the understanding gained by reading for analysis:

- Being familiar with critiquing criteria.
- Reaching the comprehensive reading stage before applying critiquing criteria; and then rereading if necessary.
- Applying the critiquing criteria to each step of the research process in the article.
- Asking whether the content meets the criteria for each step of the research process.
- Asking fellow students to analyze the same study with the same criteria and compare results.
- Writing notes on the copy about how each step of the research process measures up against the established criteria.
- Avoiding terms in your critique that do not convey specific information (e.g., "good," "nice," "bad").

SYNTHESIS UNDERSTANDING: PUTTING TOGETHER

Synthesis is "combination or putting together; combining of parts into a whole" (*New Webster's Dictionary and Thesaurus,* 1991). The purpose of reading for synthesis is to pull all the information together to form a new whole, make sense of it, and explain relationships. Although the process of synthesizing the material may be taking place as the reader is analyzing the article, a fourth reading is recommended. It is during this synthesis reading that the understanding and critique of the whole study are put together. In this final step, you decide how well the study meets the critiquing criteria and how useful it is to practice (see Chapter 20). This is also when you decide how well each step of the research process relates to the previous step. Synthesis can be thought of as looking at a completed jigsaw puzzle. Does it form a comprehensive picture, or is there a piece out of place? In the case of reading several studies for synthesis, the interrelationship of the studies is assessed. Reading for synthesis is essential in critiquing research studies. For example, answering the previously posed critiquing questions after reading for synthesis in relation to Bull, Hansen, and Gross's (2000) study (see Appendix A), you would add the following to your critique:

Bull, Hansen, and Gross (2000) clearly stated the major gaps in the literature related to the discharge problems of elders hospitalized with heart failure. The identified problems became the studied variables, and their clearly stated aims addressed the gaps in the literature. An overall strength of this study was the researchers' literature review which clearly (1) explained Donabedian's evaluation approach, as well as (2) its use as their conceptual framework and (3) its application to the development of a professional-patient partnership model (PPPM) for discharge planning for elder patients with heart failure. They randomly selected one of the two hospitals used for the study for implementing the PPPM for discharge planning. The researchers compared the identified outcomes for elder patients with heart failure (e.g., costs associated with hospital readmission and use of the emergency room, perceived health, client satisfaction) and caregivers' outcomes (i.e., caregiver response) after 2 weeks and 2 months for those who received and delivered the usual discharge planning at Hospital #1 (control) vs. a similar dyad at Hospital #2 (intervention) who received and delivered the PPPM discharge planning.

Reading for synthesis is facilitated by the following strategies:

1. Reviewing your notes on the article on how each step of the research process compared with the established criteria.
2. Briefly summarizing the study in your own words, including the:
   a. study's components.
   b. overall strengths and weaknesses.
3. Following the suggested format of:
   a. drafting (redoing) the summary until it is limited to one page.
   b. including the citation at the top of the page in the specified reference style.

This type of summary is viewed as the first draft of a final written critique. It teaches brevity, facilitates easy retrieval of data to support the critiquing evaluation, and increases your ability to write a scholarly report. In addition, the ability to synthesize one study prepares you for the task of critiquing several studies on a similar topic and comparing and contrasting the findings (see Chapter 4).

HELPFUL HINT If you have to write a paper on a specific concept or topic that requires you to critique and synthesize the findings from several studies, you might find it useful to create a table of the data. Include the following information: author, date, type of study, design, sample, data analysis, findings, and implications.

PERCEIVED DIFFICULTIES AND STRATEGIES FOR CRITIQUING RESEARCH

Critiquing research articles is difficult for beginning consumers of research and is somewhat frustrating at first. The best way to become an intelligent consumer of research, however, is to use critical thinking and reading skills when reading. Box 2-2 presents some highlighted strategies for reading and evaluating a research report. As mentioned previously, when reading research articles for the first few times it is helpful to keep

BOX 2-2 Highlights of Critical Thinking and Reading Strategies

Read primary source data-based articles from referred journals (see Table 4-7).

Read secondary source data-based critique/response/commentary articles from referred journals (see Table 4-7).

Photocopy primary and secondary source articles; make notations directly on the copy.

While reading data-based articles:

- Keep a research text and a dictionary by your side.
- Review the chapters in a research text on various steps of the research process, critiquing criteria, unfamiliar terms, etc.
- List key variables at the top of the photocopy.
- Highlight or underline on photocopy new terms, unfamiliar vocabulary, and significant sentences.
- Look up the definitions of new terms and write them on the photocopy.
- Review old and new terms before subsequent readings.
- Highlight or underline identified steps of the research process.

- Identify the main idea or theme of the article; state it in your own words in one or two sentences.
- Continue to clarify terms that may be unclear on subsequent readings.
- Make sure you understand the main points of each reported step of the research process you identified before critiquing the article.

  Determine how well the study meets the critiquing criteria.
- Ask fellow students to analyze the same study using the same criteria and compare results.
- Consult faculty members about your evaluation of the study.

  Type a one-page summary and critique of each reviewed study.
- Cite references at the top according to APA or another reference style.
- Briefly summarize each reported research step in your own words.
- Briefly describe strengths and weaknesses in your own words.

your text nearby so that unfamiliar terms can be clarified and steps of the research process can be reviewed, if necessary. No matter how difficult it may seem, read the entire article and reflect on it. Read critically for the levels of understanding described in this chapter. Most importantly, draw on previous knowledge, common sense, and the critical thinking skills you already possess.

Another important strategy is to ask questions; remember that questioning is essential to developing critical thinking. Asking faculty members questions and sharing your thoughts about what you are reading is an effective way of developing your reading skills. Do not hesitate to write or to call a researcher if you have a question about his or her work. You will be pleasantly surprised by how willing researchers are to discuss your questions.

Throughout the text, you will find special features that will help you refine the critical thinking and critical reading skills essential to developing your competence as a research consumer. A Critical Thinking Decision Path related to each step of the research process will sharpen your

decision-making skills as you critique research articles. Look for technology icons in each chapter that will highlight computer resources that will enhance research consumer activities. Critical Thinking Challenges, which appear at the end of each chapter, are designed to reinforce your critical thinking and critical reading skills in relation to each step of the research process. Helpful Hints, designed to reinforce your understanding and critical thinking, appear at various points throughout the chapters.

When you complete your first critique, congratulate yourself; mastering these skills is not easy at the beginning, but we are confident that you can do it. Once you complete a research critique or two, you will be ready to discuss your critique with your fellow students and professor. Best of all, you can look forward to discussing the points of your critique because your critique will be based on objective data, not just personal opinion. As you continue to use and perfect critical analysis skills by critiquing studies, remember that these very skills are an expected clinical competency for delivering evidence-based nursing care.

RESEARCH ARTICLES: FORMAT AND STYLE

Before one considers the reading of research articles, it is important to have a sense of their organization and format. Many journals publish research, either as the sole type of article in the journal or in addition to clinical or theoretical articles. Although many journals have some common features, they also have unique characteristics. All journals have guidelines for manuscript preparation and submission, which generally are published in each journal. A review of these guides will give you an idea of the format of articles that appear in specific journals. It is important to remember that even though each step of the research process is discussed at length in this text, you may find only a short paragraph or a sentence in the research article that gives the details of the step in a specific study. Because of the journal's space limitations or other publishing guidelines, the published study that one reads in a journal is a shortened version of the complete work done by the researcher(s). You will also find that some researchers devote more space in an article to the results, whereas others present a longer discussion of the methods and procedures. In recent years, most authors give more emphasis to the method, results, and discussion of implications than to details of assumptions, hypotheses, or definitions of terms. Decisions about the amount to present on each step of the research process within an article are bound by the following:

- A journal's space limitations
- A journal's author guidelines
- The type or nature of the study
- An individual researcher's evaluation of what is the most important component of the study

The following discussion provides a brief overview of each step of the research process and how it might appear in an article. Table 2-1 indicates where the step can usually be located in a quantitative research article and where it is discussed in this text. Table 2-2 outlines the format of a qualitative research article. It is important to remember that a quantitative research article will differ from a qualitative research article. The components of qualitative research are discussed in Chapters 6 and 7 and summarized in Chapter 8. The primary difference is that a qualitative study seeks to interpret meaning and phenomenon and quantitative research seeks to test a hypothesis or answer research questions based on a theoretical framework.

ABSTRACT

An **abstract** is a short comprehensive synopsis or summary of a study at the beginning of an article. An abstract quickly focuses the reader on the main points of a study. A well-presented abstract is accurate, self-contained, concise, specific, nonevaluative, coherent, and readable (American Psychological Association, 1994). Abstracts vary in length from 50 to 250 words. The length of an abstract is dictated by the journal's style. Both quantitative and qualitative research studies have abstracts that provide a succinct overview of the study. An example of an abstract can be found at the beginning of the study by LoBiondo-Wood and associates (2000) (see Appendix D). It partially reads as follows:

"The purpose of the study was to explore the relationship between family stress, family coping, social support, perception of stress and family adaptation from the mother's perspective during the pretransplant period in the context of the Double ABC-X Model of Family Adaptation."

Within the first sentence of this example, the authors provide a view of the study variables. The remainder of the abstract provides a synopsis of the significance of the problem, the sample size, and the results. The studies in Appendixes A, B, C, and D all have abstracts.

HELPFUL HINT A journal abstract is usually a single paragraph that provides a general reference to the research purpose, research questions, and/or hypotheses and highlights the methodology and results, as well as the implications for practice or future research.

IDENTIFICATION OF A RESEARCH PURPOSE/PROBLEM

Early in a research article, in a section that may or may not be labeled "Introduction," the researcher presents a picture of the area researched. This is the presentation of the research purpose or problem (see Chapter 3). Reading the study by Bull, Hansen, and Gross (2000) (Appendix A), the reader can find the research problem early in the report:

"While ample evidence confirms that current discharge planning practices do not address the needs of elder heart failure patients there exists a gap in the literature that addresses these specific needs."

Another example can be found in the Cohen and Ley (2000) study (Appendix B), as follows:

"Further research is needed to explore the lived experience of patients who have undergone autologous BMT and to address the question of how nurses can provide the most effective care to these patients."

DEFINITION OF THE PURPOSE

The purpose of the study is defined either at the end of the researcher's initial introduction or at the end of the "Literature Review" or "Conceptual Framework" section. The study's purpose may or may not be labeled as such (see Chapters 3, 4, and 5). Following along in the study by Bull, Hansen, and Gross (2000) (Appendix A), at the end of the second introductory paragraph—before the Background section, the purpose is clearly stated in the aims of the study (see Box 2-1).

In the previous discussion on the components of an abstract, the purpose of LoBiondo-Wood and associates' (2000) study (see Appendix D) was found in the first sentence of the abstract and was also stated in the last sentence of the second introductory paragraph in the body of the article.

LITERATURE REVIEW AND THEORETICAL FRAMEWORK

Authors of studies and journal articles present the literature review and theoretical framework in different ways. Many research articles merge the "Literature Review" and the "Theoretical Frame-work." The section includes the main concepts investigated and may be called "Review of the Literature", "Literature Review", "Theoretical Framework", "Related Literature", "Background", or "Conceptual Framework"; or may not be labeled at all (see Chapters 4 and 5). By reviewing Appendixes A, B, C and D, the reader will find no heading indicating specific paragraphs that are in fact the literature review or introductory paragraphs. Bull, Hansen, and Gross's study (see Appendix A) has two unlabeled introductory paragraphs that are clearly a review of the literature as well as a "Background" section that discusses the conceptual framework of the study based on the reviewed literature. One style is not better than another; all of the studies in the appendixes contain all the critical elements but present the elements differently.

HYPOTHESIS/RESEARCH PROBLEM/RESEARCH QUESTION

A study's research problem, question, and hypotheses can also be presented in different ways (see Chapter 3). Research reports in journals often do not separate headings for reporting the "Hypotheses" or "Research Problem." They are often embedded in the "Introduction" or "Background" section or not labeled at all (e.g., as in the studies in the appendixes). If a study uses hypotheses, the researcher may report whether the hypotheses were or were not supported toward the end of the article in the "Results" or "Findings" section. Quantitative research studies have research problems, hypotheses, or research questions. Qualitative research studies do not have hypotheses but have research questions and purposes. Mahon, Yarcheski, and Yarcheski (2000) (Appendix C) and Bull, Hansen, and Gross (2000) (Appendix A) have hypotheses. Cohen and Ley (2000) (Appendix B) and LoBiondo-Wood and associates (2000) (Appendix D) have research questions.

RESEARCH DESIGN

The type of research design can be found in the abstract, within the purpose statement, or in the introduction to the "Procedures" or "Methods" section, or not stated at all (see Chapters 7, 10, and 11). For example, of the four studies in the appendixes, only two specifically identify the type of study design used. Cohen and Ley (2000) (see Appendix B) identified their study in the design section of the abstract and text as a hermeneutic phenomenological, descriptive, and interpretive study; and Bull, Hansen, and Gross (2000) (see Appendix A) identified their study in the text's design section as one using before and after nonequivalent control group design.

One of the first objectives is to determine whether the study is qualitative or quantitative so that the appropriate criteria are used (see Chapters 6 and 9). Although the rigor of the critiquing criteria addressed do not substantially change, some of the terminology of the questions differs for qualitative and quantitative studies. For instance, in regard to Mahon, Yarcheski, and Yarcheski's (2000) quantitative study (see Appendix C), you might be asking if the hypotheses were generated from the theoretical framework or literature review and if the design chosen was appropriate and consistent with the study's problem and purpose (see Chapters 9, 10, and 11). With a qualitative study such as Cohen and Ley's (see Appendix B), however, you might be asking if the researchers conducted the study consistent with the principles of phenomenology and therefore focused on the human experience of bone marrow transplant (see Chapters 6 and 7).

Do not get discouraged if you cannot easily determine the design. More often than not, however, the specific design is not stated or, if an advanced design is used, the details are not spelled out. One of the best strategies is to review the chapters in this text that address designs (Chapters 7, 10, and 11) and to ask your professors for assistance after you have read the chapters. Determining designs is not an easy process. The following tips will help you determine whether the study you are reading uses a quantitative design:

- Hypotheses are stated or implied (see Chapter 3).
- The terms *control* and *treatment group* appear (see Chapter 10).

- The term *survey, correlational,* or *ex post facto* is used (see Chapter 11).
- The term *random* or *convenience* is mentioned in relation to the sample (see Chapter 12).
- Variables are measured by instruments or scales (see Chapters 14).
- Reliability and validity of instruments are discussed (see Chapter 15).
- Statistical analyses are used (see Chapters 16 and 17).

In contrast, generally qualitative studies do not usually focus on "numbers." Some qualitative studies may use standard quantitative terms (e.g., subjects) rather than qualitative terms (e.g., informants). Deciding on the type of qualitative design can be confusing; one of the best strategies is to review this text's chapters on qualitative design (see Chapters 6 and 7), as well as to critique qualitative studies (see Chapter 8). Do not hesitate to ask faculty members for assistance after you have read these chapters. Although many studies may not specify the particular design used, all studies inform the reader of the specific methodology used, which can help the reader decide the type of design used to guide the study.

SAMPLING

The population from which the sample was drawn is discussed in the methods section entitled "Methods" or "Methodology" under the subheadings of "Subjects" or "Sample" (see Chapter 12). For example, LoBiondo-Wood and associates (2000) (Appendix D) and Bull, Hansen, and Gross (2000) (Appendix A) discuss the respective samples of their quantitative studies in the "Methods" section under the subheading of "Sampling." Researchers should tell you both the population from which the sample was chosen and the number of subjects that participated in the study, as well as if they had subjects who dropped out of the study. The authors of all of the studies in the appendixes discuss their samples in enough detail so that the reader is quite clear about who the subjects are and how they were selected.

RELIABILITY AND VALIDITY

The discussion related to instruments used to measure the variables of a study is usually included in a "Methods" section under the subheading of "Instruments" or "Measures" (see Chapter 14). The researcher usually describes the particular measure (i.e., instrument or scale) used by discussing its reliability and validity (see Chapter 15). LoBiondo-Wood and associates (2000) (Appendix D) discuss each of the measures used in their "Methods" section under the subheading "Instruments." They also provide the variable measured by each scale and describe the scales. The reliability and validity of each measure was presented, as was the reliability of the instruments in the study.

In some cases, researchers do not report on commonly used valid and reliable instruments (e.g., the state-trait anxiety inventory [STAI]) in an article (Spielberger et al, 1983). Seek assistance from your instructor if you are in doubt about the validity or reliability of a study's instruments.

PROCEDURES AND DATA-COLLECTION METHODS

The procedures used to collect data or the step-by-step way that the researcher(s) used the measures (instruments or scales) is generally given under the "Procedures" head (see Chapter 14). In each of the studies in Appendixes A, B, C, and D, the researchers indicate how they conducted the study in detail under the subheading "Procedure." Notice that the researchers also provided information that the studies were approved by an Institutional Review Board (see Chapter 13), thereby ensuring that each meets ethical standards.

DATA ANALYSIS/RESULTS

The data-analysis procedures (i.e., the statistical tests used in quantitative studies and the results of descriptive and/or inferential tests applied) are presented in the section labeled "Results" or "Findings" (see Chapters 16 and 17). Although qualitative studies do not use statistical tests, the procedures for analyzing the themes, concepts, and/or observational or print data are usually described in the "Method" or "Data Collection" section and reported in the "Results" or "Findings" section (see Appendix B and Chapters 7 and 8). Cohen and Ley (2000) (see Appendix B) report the data analysis method used in the "Data Analysis and Interpretation" section of their qualitative study and their results under "Findings."

Bull, Hansen, and Gross (2000) (Appendix A) have two separate sections: one that discusses the "Data Analysis" used and another that discusses the "Results." When researchers do not indicate in a separate section what statistical tests they used, the tests are presented in the "Results" section. For example, in the studies by Mahon, Yarcheski, and Yarcheski (2000) (Appendix C) and LoBiondo-Wood and associates (2000) (Appendix D), the inferential statistical tests used are reported with the results under the heading "Results."

DISCUSSION

The last section of a research study is the "Discussion" section. As you will find when you read Chapters 18 and 19, in this section, the researcher(s) tie(s) together all the pieces of the study and give(s) a picture of the study as a whole. Researchers may report the results and discussion in one section but usually report the results and the discussion in a separate section (see Appendixes A, B, C, and D). One way is no better than the other. Journal and space limitations determine how these sections will be handled. Any new findings or unexpected findings are usually described in the "Discussion" section.

RECOMMENDATIONS AND IMPLICATIONS

In some cases, a researcher reports the implications, based on the findings, for practice and education and recommends future studies in a separate section labeled "Conclusion and Recommendations" (see Appendix D); in other cases, future studies appear at the end of the "Discussion" section (see Appendixes A and C). In contrast, the qualitative study found in Appendix B presented a section on findings and then implications for practice, education, and research in a section labeled "Implications." Again, one way is not better than the other—only different.

REFERENCES

All of the references cited in a research or scholarly article are included at the end of the article. The main purpose of the reference list is to support the material presented by identifying the sources in a manner that allows for easy retrieval by the reader (APA, 1994). Journals use various referencing styles to organize references.

COMMUNICATING RESULTS

Communicating the results of a study can take the form of a research article, poster, or paper presentation (see Chapter 20). All are valid ways of providing nursing with the data and the ability to provide high-quality patient care based on research findings. Evidence-based nursing care plans and practice protocols, guidelines, or standards are outcome measures that effectively indicate communicated research.

As you develop critical thinking and reading skills by using the strategies presented in this chapter, you will become more familiar with the research and critiquing processes. Your ability to read and critique research articles will gradually improve. You will be well on your way to becoming a knowledgeable user of research from nursing and other scientific disciplines for application in nursing practice.

Critical Thinking Challenges

Barbara Krainovich-Miller

➤ It is claimed that the critical reading of research articles may require a minimum of three or four readings. Is this always the case? What assumptions underlie this claim?

➤ Why is it necessary to reach an analysis stage of critical reading before critiquing a study?

➤ To synthesize a research article, what questions must you first be able to answer?

➤ How would you answer a nursing colleague who stated the following: "Why can't I say in my critique that based on the findings of this study the researchers proved their hypotheses?"

➤ Margaret is a part-time baccalaureate nursing student who works full-time as an RN in an acute care ICU setting and is a full-time mother of two children under the age of 4 years. Discuss both the disadvantages and the advantages of Margaret using the critical thinking and reading strategies found in Box 2-1.

➤ If nurses with a baccalaureate degree are not expected to conduct research, how can nursing students be expected to critique each step of the research process or an entire study or several studies? Support either a pro or con position.

➤ Why do you think so many nursing students dread taking research and statistics courses?

➤ Discuss several reasons why practicing nurses don't read or critique research articles on a routine basis.

➤ Discuss several strategies that might motivate practicing nurses to critique research articles.

➤ What specific type of non-probability sampling did Cohen and Ley (2000) (see Appendix B) use in their study?

KEY POINTS

- The best way to develop skill in critiquing research studies is to use critical thinking and reading skills to read research articles.
- Critical thinking in learning the research process, as well as critiquing, requires disciplined, self-directed thinking.
- Critical thinking and critical reading skills will enable you to question the appropriateness of the content of a research article, apply standards or critiquing criteria to assess the study's scientific merit for use in practice, or consider alternative ways of handling the same topic.
- Critical reading involves active interpretation and objective assessment of an article, looking for key concepts, ideas, and justifications.
- Critical reading requires four stages of understanding: preliminary (skimming), comprehensive,

analysis, and synthesis. Each stage includes strategies to increase your critical reading skills.

- Critically reading for preliminary understanding is gained by skimming or quickly and lightly reading an article to familiarize you with its content or provide you with a general sense of the material.
- Critically reading for a comprehensive understanding is designed to increase your understanding of the concepts and research terms in relation to the context or the parts of the study in relation to the whole study as presented in the article.
- Critically reading for an analysis understanding is designed to break the content into parts so that each part of the study is understood; the critiquing process begins at this stage.
- Critical reading to reach the goal of synthesis understanding is to combine the parts of a research study into a whole. During this final stage the reader determines how each step relates to all of the steps of the research process, as well as how well the study meets the critiquing criteria, and the usefulness of the study for practice.
- Critiquing is the process of objectively and critically evaluating the strengths and weaknesses of a research article for scientific merit and application to practice, theory, education or the need for more research on the topic/clinical problem.
- Critiquing criteria are the measures, standards, evaluation guides, or questions used to judge the worth of a research study.
- Research articles have different formats and styles depending on journal manuscript requirements and whether they are quantitative or qualitative studies.
- Basic steps of the research process are presented in journal articles in various ways. Detailed examples of such variations can be found in chapters throughout this text.

REFERENCES

Adams B: Nursing education for critical thinking: an integrative review, *J Nurs Educat* 38(3):111-119, 1999.

American Nurses Association: *A social policy statement*, ed 2, Washington, DC, 1995, American Nurses Publishing.

American Psychological Association: *Publication manual of the American Psychological Association*, ed 4, Washington, DC, 1994, The Association.

Bull MJ, Hansen HE, and Gross CR: A professional-patient partnership model of discharge planning with elders hospitalized with heart failure, *Appl Nurs Res* 13:19-28,2000.

Cohen MZ and Ley C: Bone marrow transplantation: the battle for hope in the face of fear, *Oncol Nurs Forum* 27(3):473-480, 2000.

Krainovich-Miller B: The nursing process. In Haber J et al, editors: *Comprehensive psychiatric nursing*, ed 5, St Louis, 1997, Mosby.

New Webster's dictionary and thesaurus, New York, 1991, Book Essentials.

Paul R and Elder L: *Critical thinking: tools for taking charge of your learning and your life*, Englewood, NJ, 2001, Prentice-Hall.

Rogers ME: Nursing: science of unitary, irreducible, human beings: update 1990. In Barrett EAN, editor: *Visions of Rogers' science-based nursing*, New York, 1990, National League for Nursing.

Spielberger CD et al: *Manual for the state-trait anxiety inventory*, Palo Alto, CA, 1983, Consulting Psychologists Press.

Whitley G: Process and methodologies for research validation of nursing diagnoses, *Nursing Diagnosis* 10(1):5-14, 1999.

ADDITIONAL READINGS

Boweer FL and Timmons ME: A survey of the ways master's level nursing students learn the research process, *J Nurs Educat* 38(3):128-132, 1999.

Correa CG and de Almeida Lopes Monteiro da Cruz D: Pain: clinical validation with postoperative heart surgery patients, *Nurs Diagnosis* 11(1):5-14, 2000.

Cross KP: *Adults as learners*, San Francisco, 1987, Jossey-Bass.

Delaney C and Maas M: Reliability of nursing diagnoses documented in a computerized nursing information system, *Nurs Diagnosis* 11(3):121-134, 2000.

Morrison-Beedy D and Cote-Arsenault D: The cookie experiment revisited: broadened dimensions for teaching nursing research, *Nurse Educator* 25(6):294-296, 2000.

Rosswurm MA and Larrabee JH: A model for change to evidence-based practice, *Image: J Nurs Scholarship* 31(4):317-322, 1999.

Tanner CA: Evidence-based practice: research and critical thinking, *J Nurs Ed* 38(3):99, 1999.

JUDITH HABER

Research Problems and Hypotheses

3

Key Terms

conceptual definitions
dependent variable
directional hypothesis
hypothesis
independent variable
nondirectional hypothesis

operational definitions
population
problem statement
research hypothesis
research problem
research question

statistical hypothesis
testability
theory
variables

Learning Outcomes

After reading this chapter, the student should be able to do the following:

- Describe how the problem statement and hypothesis relate to the other components of the research process.
- Describe the process of identifying and refining a research problem.
- Identify the criteria for determining the significance of a research problem.
- Identify the characteristics of research problems and hypotheses.
- Describe the advantages and disadvantages of directional and nondirectional hypotheses.
- Compare and contrast the use of statistical vs. research hypotheses.
- Discuss the appropriate use of research questions vs. hypotheses in a research study.
- Identify the criteria used for critiquing a research problem and hypothesis.
- Apply the critiquing criteria to the evaluation of a research problem and hypothesis in a research report.

When nurses ask questions such as, "Why are things done this way?", "I wonder what would happen if. . . ?", "What characteristics are associated with. . . ?", or "What is the effect of . . . on patient outcomes?", they are often well on their way to developing a research problem, question, or hypothesis.

Formulating the research problem and developing the **research question** or hypotheses are key preliminary steps in the research process. The **research problem,** often called a **problem statement,** presents the question that is to be asked in the study and is the foundation of the research study. The **hypothesis** attempts to answer the question posed by the research problem.

Hypotheses can be considered intelligent hunches, guesses, or predictions that help researchers seek the solution or answer to the research question. Hypotheses are a vehicle for testing the validity of the theoretical framework assumptions and provide a bridge between **theory** and the real world. In the scientific world, researchers derive hypotheses from theories and subject them to empirical testing. A theory's validity is not directly examined. Instead, it is through the hypotheses that the merit of a theory can be evaluated.

Research consumers rarely see a formal statement of the research problem in a research article because this is part of the "groundwork" involved in developing the research study. More commonly, readers find research questions or hypotheses in a research article, but because of space constraints or stylistic considerations in such publications, they may be embedded in the purpose, aims, goals, or even in the results section of the research report. Nevertheless, it is equally important for both the consumer and producer of research to understand the importance of the research problem, research questions, and hypotheses as the foundational elements of the research study. This chapter provides a working knowledge of quantitative research problems, research questions, and hypotheses, as well as the standards for writing them and a set of criteria for evaluating them.

DEVELOPING AND REFINING A RESEARCH PROBLEM

A researcher spends a great deal of time refining a research idea into a testable research problem. Unfortunately, the evaluator of a research study is not privy to this creative process because it occurs during the study's conceptualization. The final problem statement usually does not appear in the research article unless the study is qualitative rather than quantitative (see Chapters 6, 7, and 8). Although this section will not teach you how to formulate a research problem, it is important to provide a glimpse of what the process of developing a research problem may be like for a researcher.

As illustrated in Table 3-1, research problems or topics are not pulled from thin air. Research problems should indicate that practical experience, critical appraisal of the scientific literature, or interest in an untested theory has provided the basis for the generation of a research idea. The problem statement should reflect a refinement of the researcher's initial thinking. The evaluator of a research study should be able to discern that the researcher has done the following:

1. Defined a specific problem area.
2. Reviewed the relevant scientific literature.
3. Examined the problem's potential significance to nursing.
4. Pragmatically examined the feasibility of studying the research problem.

DEFINING THE PROBLEM AREA

Brainstorming with teachers, advisors, or colleagues may provide valuable feedback that helps the researcher focus on a specific problem area. For example, suppose a researcher told a colleague that the area of interest was adaptation of children faced with stressful experiences. The colleague may have said, "What is it about the topic that specifically interests you?" Such a conversation may have initiated a chain of thought that resulted in a decision to explore the adaptation processes of families faced with stressful

TABLE **3-1** How Practical Experience, Scientific Literature, and Untested Theory Influence the Development of a Research Idea

AREA	INFLUENCE	EXAMPLE
Practical experience	Clinical practice provides a wealth of experience from which research problems can be derived. The nurse may observe the occurrence of a particular event or pattern and become curious about why it occurs, as well as its relationship to other factors in the patient's environment.	Although breast self-examination (BSE) has long been recommended by nurses and other health care providers as a complement to mammography and clinical breast examination, only a small percentage of U.S. women report doing a monthly BSE, and nurses observe that an even smaller percentage of women perform this health-promotion self-care procedure proficiently. Nurses working in a women's health center speculate about the effect of a structured training protocol on improving thoroughness of search using two dimensions of BSE technique (i.e., depth of palpation and duration of the BSE examination in each of two search patterns [vertical strip and concentric circle]) using biomedical instrumentation (Leight et al, 2000).
Critical appraisal of the scientific literature	The critical appraisal of research studies that appears in journals may indirectly suggest a problem area by stimulating the reader's thinking. The nurse may observe the outcome data from a single study or a group of related studies that provide the basis for developing a pilot study or quality improvement project to determine the effectiveness of this intervention in their own practice setting.	At a staff meeting where cost-effectiveness was being discussed, a nurse reported that she had read an article indicating that comprehensive discharge planning and home follow-up for hospitalized elders at risk for readmission by advanced practice nurses have demonstrated short-term reductions in readmissions of elderly patients. At 24 weeks after discharge, Medicare reimbursements for health services were about $1.2 million in the control group vs. about $0.6 million for the intervention group. There were no significant differences in post-discharge acute care visits, functional status, depression, or patient satisfaction. Another nurse said that other articles on file indicated that this model had been studied using other patient populations (i.e., very–low-birthweight babies, women having hysterectomies and unplanned cesarean births) with similar quality and cost-effectiveness outcomes (Naylor et al, 1999). The group agreed that there was a sufficient body of related research findings to use in defining their own problem focus.

Continued

TABLE **3-1** How Practical Experience, Scientific Literature, and Untested Theory
Influence the Development of a Research Idea—cont'd

AREA	INFLUENCE	EXAMPLE
Gaps in the literature	A research idea may also be suggested by a critical appraisal of the literature that identifies gaps in the literature and suggests areas for future study. Research ideas also can be generated by research reports that suggest the value of replicating a particular study to extend or refine the existing scientific knowledge base.	A nurse who had just begun working in an obstetrics clinic observed that the impact of miscarriage on the well-being of women was not a focus of attention after the miscarriage was over. She wondered whether the partners' emotional concerns (especially those related to loss, depression, and anxiety) and feelings of well-being had even been examined. Where the literature is reviewed relative to this topic, no controlled research studies are identified that demonstrated the significant effects of counseling with women who miscarry to provide a scientific basis for determining the value of caring-based counseling (early or delayed) on the integration of loss and women's emotional well-being (i.e., self-esteem and moods) in the first year subsequent to miscarrying (Swanson, 1999).
Interest in untested theory	Verification of an untested nursing theory provides a relatively uncharted territory from which research problems can be derived. Inasmuch as theories themselves are not tested, a researcher may think about investigating a particular concept or set of concepts related to a particular nursing theory. The deductive process would be used to generate the research problem. The researcher would pose questions such as, "If this theory is correct, what kind of behavior will I expect to observe in particular patients and under which conditions?" or "If this theory is valid, what kind of supporting evidence will I find?"	Development of theoretical models that are derived from nursing and related literature are conducted to provide empirical support for the accuracy of a specific theoretical model that examines the fit between the hypothesized model and the data. Using social cognitive theory, a nurse researcher sought to understand how social cognitive constructs operate together to explain condom use behavior among college students. This understanding would be useful in developing HIV and sexually transmitted disease (STD) prevention programs for college students. An estimated structural model of condom use behavior developed from the literature was tested. Overall, the findings lend support to a condom use model based on social cognitive theory, which suggests that interventions focusing on self-efficacy and reducing anxiety related to condom use increases positive perceptions about condoms and the likelihood of adopting condom use behaviors (DiIorio et al, 2000).

health care experiences (e.g., their child's need for organ transplantation). Figure 3-1 illustrates how a broad area of interest (adaptation of families faced with stressful health care experiences) was narrowed to a specific research topic (adaptation of families faced with stressful health care experiences such as their child's need for organ transplantation).

BEGINNING THE LITERATURE REVIEW

The literature review should reveal that the literature relevant to the problem area has been critically examined. Concluding sections on the recommendations and implications for practice often identify remaining gaps in the literature, the need for replication, or the need for extension of the knowledge base about a particular research focus (see Chapter 4). In the previous example about family adaptation to a child's having an organ transplant, the researcher may have conducted a preliminary review of books and journals for theories and research studies on factors apparently critical to how families adapt to the process of their child having an organ transplant. These factors, called **variables** in research language, should be potentially relevant, of interest, and measurable.

Possible relevant factors mentioned in the literature begin with an exploration of the relationship between family variables of stress, perception of stress, coping, social support, and adaptation. Other variables, such as demographical characteristics of children and their parents, the transplant process, and the phase of the transplant process, are also suggested as essential to consider. This information can then be used by the researcher to further define the research problem, address a gap in the literature, as well as extend the knowledge base related to the impact of a child's organ transplant on family adjustment. At this point, the researcher could write the following tentative research problem: What is the impact of a child's organ transplant on family adaptation? Although the research problem is not yet in its final form, readers can envision the interrelatedness of the initial definition of the problem area, the literature review, and the

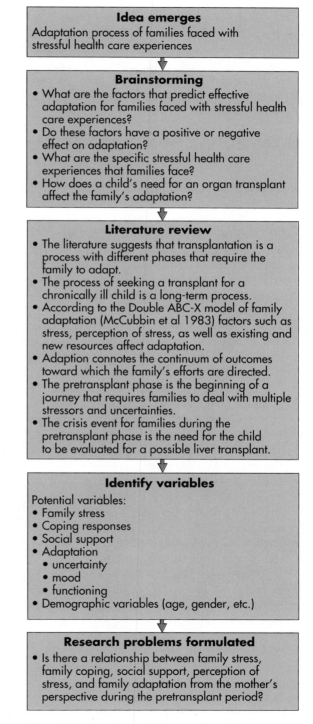

Figure 3-1   Development of a research problem.

refined research problem. Readers of research reports examine the end product of this process in the form of a research question and/or hypothesis, so it is important to have an appreciation of how the researcher gets to that point in constructing a study (LoBiondo-Wood et al, 2000; see Appendix D).

HELPFUL HINT Reading the literature review or theoretical framework section of a research article helps you trace the development of the implied research problem, research question, and/or hypothesis.

SIGNIFICANCE

Before proceeding to a final development of the research problem, it is crucial that the researcher has examined the problem's potential significance to nursing. The research problem should have the potential to contribute to and extend the scientific body of nursing knowledge. The problem does not have to be of prize-winning caliber to be significant. Guidelines for selecting research problems should meet the following criteria:

- Patients, nurses, the medical community in general, and society will potentially benefit from the knowledge derived from the study.
- The results will be applicable for nursing practice, education, or administration.
- The results will be theoretically relevant.
- The findings will lend support to untested theoretical assumptions, extend or challenge an existing theory, or clarify a conflict in the literature.
- The findings will potentially formulate or alter nursing practices or policies.

If the research problem has not met any of these criteria, it is wise to extensively revise the problem or discard it. For example, in the previously cited research problem, the significance of the problem includes the following facts:

- Organ transplantation is stressful for children and/or their families, taxing their coping skills and resources.
- Transplantation affects all aspects of individual and family life and requires families to deal with multiple stressors and uncertainties.
- Health care providers do not assess the needs of families coping with the organ transplantation process effectively.
- The perception of stress, coping, and social support may be of prime importance in family adaptational outcomes.
- This study sought to fill a gap in the related literature by beginning the exploration of the relationship between family variables of stress, perception of stress, coping, social support, and family adaptation from the mother's perspective during the pretransplantation period.
- This study sought to extend the knowledge base about this phenomenon, thereby providing a foundation for the development and testing of interventions.

FEASIBILITY

The feasibility of a research problem must be pragmatically examined. Regardless of how significant or researchable a problem may be, pragmatic considerations such as time; availability of subjects, facilities, equipment, and money; experience of the researcher; and any ethical considerations may cause the researcher to decide that the problem is inappropriate because it lacks feasibility (see Chapters 6, 9, and 13).

THE FULLY DEVELOPED RESEARCH PROBLEM

A research problem may be written in declarative or interrogative form (Table 3-2). Both are acceptable formats. The style chosen is largely a function of the researcher's preference. A good research problem exhibits the following three characteristics:

- It clearly identifies the variables under consideration.
- It specifies the population being studied.
- It implies the possibility of empirical testing.

Because each of these elements is crucial to the formulation of a satisfactory research problem, the criteria will be discussed in greater detail.

TABLE **3-2**   Components of the Research Problem and Related Criteria

VARIABLES	POPULATION	TESTABILITY
Independent variable: • Family stress • Coping responses • Social support Dependent variable: Adaptation	Mothers faced with their child's liver transplant during the pretransplant period	Differential effect of stress, coping, and social support on adaptation

VARIABLES

Researchers call the properties that they study **variables.** Such properties take on different values. Thus a variable is, as the name suggests, something that varies. Properties that differ from each other, such as age, weight, height, religion, and ethnicity, are examples of variables. Researchers attempt to understand how and why differences in one variable relate to differences in another variable. For example, a researcher may be concerned about the variable of pain in postoperative patients. It is a variable because not all postoperative patients have the same amount of pain—or any pain at all. A researcher may also be interested in what other factors can be linked to postoperative pain. It has been discovered that anxiety is associated with pain. Thus anxiety is also a variable, because not all postoperative patients have the same amount of anxiety—or any anxiety at all.

When speaking of variables, the researcher is essentially asking, "Is X related to Y? What is the effect of X on Y? How are X_1 and X_2 related to Y?" The researcher is asking a question about the relationship between one or more independent variables and a dependent variable.*

An **independent variable,** usually symbolized by X, is the variable that has the presumed effect on the dependent variable. In experimental research studies, the researcher manipulates the independent variable. For example, a nurse may study how different methods of administering pain medication effect the patient's perception of pain. The re-

searcher may manipulate the independent variable (i.e, the method of administering pain medication) by using nurse- vs. patient-controlled administration of analgesia (see Chapter 10). In nonexperimental research, the independent variable is not manipulated and is assumed to have occurred naturally before or during the study. For example, the researcher may be studying the relationship between the level of anxiety and the perception of pain. The independent variable—the level of anxiety—is not manipulated; it is just presumed to occur and is observed and measured as it naturally happens (see Chapter 11).

The **dependent variable,** represented by Y, is often referred to as the consequence or the presumed effect that varies with a change in the independent variable. The dependent variable is not manipulated. It is observed and assumed to vary with changes in the independent variable. Predictions are made from the independent variable to the dependent variable. It is the dependent variable that the researcher is interested in understanding, explaining, or predicting. For example, it might be assumed that the perception of pain (i.e., the dependent variable) will vary with changes in the level of anxiety (i.e., the independent variable). In this case, we are trying to explain the perception of pain in relation to the level of anxiety.

Although variability in the dependent variable is assumed to depend on changes in the independent variable, this does not imply that there is a causal relationship between X and Y or that changes in variable X cause variable Y to change. Let us look at an example in which nurses' attitudes toward patients with tuberculosis were

*In cases in which multiple independent or dependent variables are present, subscripts are used to indicate the number of variables under consideration.

TABLE **3-3** Research Problem Format

TYPE	FORMAT	EXAMPLE
QUANTITATIVE EXPERIMENTAL		
Correlational	Is there a relationship between **X** (independent variable) and **Y** (dependent variable) in the specified population?	Is there a correlation between trait anger and adolescent general well-being?
Comparative nonexperimental	Is there a difference in **Y** (dependent variable) between people who have **X** characteristic (independent variable) and those who do not have **X** characteristic?	Is there a difference in family adaptation between families facing their child's organ transplant who have fewer coping skills compared with those who have more coping skills?
Quantitative experimental	Is there a difference in **Y** (dependent variable) between Group A who received **X** (independent variable) and Group B who did not receive **X**?	Is there a difference in perception of pain for patients using patient-controlled analgesia (PCA) and those receiving nurse-administered analgesia?
QUALITATIVE		
Phenomenological	What is/was it like to have **X**?	What was it like to have a bone marrow transplant?

studied. The researcher discovered that older nurses had a more negative attitude about patients with tuberculosis than younger nurses. The researcher did not conclude that the nurses' negative attitudes toward patients with tuberculosis were because of their age, but at the same time it is apparent that there is a directional relationship between age and negative attitudes about patients with tuberculosis. That is, as the nurses' ages increase, their attitudes about patients with tuberculosis become more negative. This example highlights the fact that causal relationships are not necessarily implied by the independent and dependent variables; rather, only a relational statement with possible directionality is proposed. Table 3-3 presents a number of examples to help you learn how to write research problems. Practice substituting other variables for the examples in Table 3-3. You will be surprised at the skill you develop in writing and critiquing research problems with greater ease.

Although one independent and one dependent variable are used in the examples just given, there is no restriction on the number of variables that can be included in a research problem. Remember, however, that problems should not be unnecessarily complex or unwieldly, particularly in beginning research efforts. Research problems that include more than one independent or dependent variable may be broken down into subproblems that are more concise.

Finally, it should be noted that variables are not inherently independent or dependent. A variable that is classified as independent in one study may be considered dependent in another study. For example, a nurse may review an article about sexual behaviors that are predictive of risk for HIV/AIDS. In this case, HIV/AIDS is the dependent variable. When another article about the relationship between HIV/AIDS and maternal parenting practices is considered, HIV/AIDS status is the independent variable. Whether a variable is independent or dependent is a function of the role it plays in a particular study.

POPULATION

The **population** being studied must be specified in the research problem. If the scope of the problem has been narrowed to a specific focus and the variables have been clearly identified, the nature of the population will be evident to the reader of a research report. For example, a research problem that poses the question, "Is there a relationship between the type of discharge planning for elders hospitalized with heart failure and the caregivers?" suggests that the population under consideration includes elders hospitalized for heart failure and their caregivers. It is also implied that some of the elders and their caregivers were involved in a professional-patient partnership model of discharge planning in contrast to other elders who received the usual discharge planning. The researcher or reader will have an initial idea of the composition of the study population from the outset (see Chapter 12).

TESTABILITY

The statement of the research problem must imply that the problem is **testable;** that is, measurable by either qualitative or quantitative methods. For example, the research problem "Should postoperative patients control how much pain medication they receive?" is stated incorrectly for a variety of reasons. One reason is that it is not testable; it represents a value statement rather than a relational problem statement. A scientific or relational problem must propose a relationship between an independent and a dependent variable and do this in such a way that it indicates that the variables of the relationship can somehow be measured. Many interesting and important questions are not valid research problems because they are not amenable to testing.

The question "Should postoperative patients control how much pain medication they receive?" could be revised from a philosophic question to a research question that implies testability. Two examples of the revised research problem might be the following:

- Is there a relationship between patient-controlled analgesia (PCA) vs. nurse-administered analgesia and perception of postoperative pain?
- What is the effect of PCA on pain ratings by postoperative patients?

These examples illustrate the relationship between the variables, identify the independent and dependent variables, and imply the testability of the research problem.

Now that the elements of the formal research problem have been presented in greater detail, this information can be integrated by formulating a formal research problem about the adaptation of families faced with stressful health care experiences (e.g., their child's need for organ transplantation). Earlier in this chapter, the following unrefined research problem was formulated: What is the effect of a child's organ transplant on family adaptation? This problem statement was originally derived from a general area of interest—the adaptation of families faced with stressful health care experiences. The topic was more specifically defined by delineating a particular problem area—the adaptation of families facing stressful health care experiences (e.g., their child's need for organ transplantation). The problem crystallized further after a preliminary literature review and emerged in the unrefined form just given. With the four criteria inherent in a satisfactory research problem, it is now possible to propose a refined research problem; that is, one that specifically states the problem in question form and specifies the relationship of the key variables in the study, the population being studied, and the empirical testability of the problem. Congruent with these three criteria, the following research problem can then be formulated: Is there a relationship between family stress, family coping, social support, perception of stress, and family adaptation from the mother's perspective during the pretransplant period (LoBiondo-Wood et al, 2000)? Table 3-2 identifies the components of this research problem as they relate to and are congruent with the three research problem criteria.

STATEMENT OF THE PROBLEM IN PUBLISHED RESEARCH

A formal research problem is not included in most current research articles. Formal research problems are used in developing grant proposals, theses, and dissertations when greater detail is required. A statement of purpose, which is usually stated in the introductory paragraph or at the beginning or end of the literature review section, is used more commonly in articles. As such, it is important for research consumers to be clear about the difference between these two components of the research process.

> **HELPFUL HINT** Remember that research problems are often not explicitly stated. The reader has to infer the research problem from the title of the report, the abstract, the introduction, or the purpose.

PURPOSE STATEMENT

The purpose of the study encompasses the aims or goals the investigator hopes to achieve with the research, not the problem to be solved. For example, a nurse working with rehabilitation patients with bladder dysfunction may be disturbed by the high incidence of urinary tract infections. The nurse may propose the following research question: "What is the optimum frequency of changing urinary drainage bags in patients with bladder dysfunction to reduce the incidence of urinary tract infection?" If this nurse were to design a study, its purpose might be to determine the differential effect of a 1-week and 4-week urinary drainage bag change schedule on the incidence of urinary tract infections in patients with bladder dysfunction. The purpose communicates more than just the nature of the problem. Through the researcher's selection of verbs, the purpose statement suggests the manner in which the researcher sought to study the problem. Verbs like *discover, explore,* or *describe* suggest an investigation of a little researched topic that might appropriately be guided by research questions rather than hypotheses. In contrast, verb statements indicating that the purpose is to test the effectiveness of an intervention or compare two alternative nursing strategies suggest a study with a better-established knowledge base that is hypothesis testing in nature. Box 3-1 provides other examples of purpose statements.

> **HELPFUL HINT** The purpose statement often provides the most information about the intent of the research problem and hypotheses.

> **BOX 3-1** Examples of Purpose Statements
>
> - The purpose of this study was to examine outcomes of the existing brief psychiatric treatment program (Tucker, Moore, and Luedtke, 2000).
> - The aim of this study was to determine whether a nursing intervention could reduce the transfer anxiety experienced by parents when they are faced with the imminent transfer of their child from the PICU to the general pediatric floor (Bouve, Rozmus, and Giordano, 1999).
> - The purpose of this study was to examine women's concerns about recovery from CABG and about living with CAD (King, Rowe, and Zerwic, 2000).
> - The objective of the present study was to examine the effectiveness of an advanced practice nurse-centered discharge planning and home follow-up intervention for elders at risk for hospital readmission (Naylor et al, 1999).
> - The purpose of this study was to test an intervention to help postpartum women avoid or manage smoking lapses, thereby enhancing their likelihood of maintaining continuous smoking abstinence and reducing their risk of daily smoking after the birth of their babies (Johnson et al, 2000).

DEVELOPING THE RESEARCH HYPOTHESES

Like the research problem, hypotheses are often not stated explicitly in a research article. The evaluator will often find that the hypotheses are embedded in the data analysis, results, or discussion section of the research report. It is then up to the reader to discern the nature of the hypotheses being tested. For example, in the study by LoBiondo-Wood and associates (2000), the hypotheses are embedded in the *Results* section of the article; the reader must interpret that the statement, "Coping as measured by the CHIP was negatively and significantly related to family adaptation," represents the hypothesis that tests the relationship between coping and adaptation in families facing their child's organ transplantation. In light of that stylistic reality, it is important to be acquainted with the components of hypotheses, how they are developed, and the standards for writing and evaluating them.

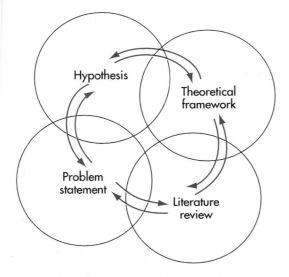

Figure 3-2   Interrelationships of problem statement, literature review, theoretical framework, and hypothesis.

Hypotheses flow from the research problem, literature review, and theoretical framework. Figure 3-2 illustrates this flow. A **hypothesis** is a statement about the relationship between two or more variables that suggests an answer to the research question. A hypothesis converts the question posed by the research problem into a declarative statement that predicts an expected outcome. It explains or predicts the relationship or differences between two or more variables in terms of expected results or outcomes of a study.

Each hypothesis represents a unit or subset of the research problem. For example, a research problem might pose the question "What is the effect of psychological distress on the initial onset/exacerbation of gastrointestinal symptoms in individuals with irritable bowel syndrome?" (Jarrett et al, 1998). This problem can be broken down into the following two subproblems:

1. What is the effect of psychological distress on the onset of gastrointestinal symptoms in individuals with irritable bowel syndrome?
2. What is the effect of psychological distress on the exacerbation of gastrointestinal

symptoms in individuals with irritable bowel syndrome?

A hypothesis can then be generated for each unit of the research problem (i.e., the subproblems). The hypotheses of the research problem already mentioned might be stated in the following way:

Hypothesis 1: There will be a positive relationship between measures of recalled psychological distress and gastrointestinal symptom distress.

Hypothesis 2: There will be a positive relationship between daily psychological distress and gastrointestinal symptom distress.

The critiquer of a research report will want to evaluate whether the hypotheses of the study represent subsets of the main research problem as illustrated by the examples just given.

Hypotheses are formulated before the study is actually conducted because they provide direction for the collection, analysis, and interpretation of data. Hypotheses have the following three purposes:

1. To provide a bridge between theory and reality, in this sense, unifying the two domains.
2. To be powerful tools for the advancement of knowledge because they enable the researcher to objectively enter new areas of discovery.
3. To provide direction for any research endeavor by tentatively identifying the anticipated outcome.

HELPFUL HINT   When hypotheses are not explicitly stated by the author at the end of the *Introduction* section or just before the *Methods* section, they will be embedded or implied in the *Results* or *Discussion* sections of a research article.

CHARACTERISTICS

Nurses who are conducting research or critiquing published research studies must have a working knowledge about what constitutes a "good" hypothesis. Such knowledge will enable them to have a standard for evaluating their own work or the work of others. The following discussion about the characteristics of hypotheses presents criteria to be used when formulating or evaluating a hypothesis.

RELATIONSHIP STATEMENT

The first characteristic of a hypothesis is that it is a declarative statement that identifies the predicted relationship between two or more variables. This implies that there is a systematic relationship between an independent variable and a dependent variable. The direction of the predicted relationship is also specified in this statement. Phrases such as *greater than; less than; positively, negatively,* or *curvilinearly related* (i.e., shaped like ∩ or ∪); and *difference in* connote the directionality that is proposed in the hypothesis. In the following example of a directional hypothesis, "The rate of continuous smoking abstinence (dependent variable) at 6 months postpartum, based on self-report and biochemical validation, will be significantly higher in the treatment group (postpartum counseling intervention) than in the control group (independent variable)." The two variables are explicitly identified, and the relational aspect of the prediction is contained in the phrase *significantly higher than.*

The nature of the relationship, either causal or associative, is also implied by the hypothesis. A causal relationship is one in which the researcher can predict that the independent variable **(X)** causes a change in the dependent variable **(Y).** In research, it is rare that one is in a firm enough position to take a definitive stand about a cause-and-effect relationship. For example, a researcher might hypothesize that relaxation training would have a significant effect on the physical and psychological health status of patients who have suffered myocardial infarction. It would be difficult for a researcher to predict a strong cause-and-effect relationship, however, because of the multiple intervening variables (e.g., age, medication, and lifestyle changes) that might also influence the subject's health status.

Variables are more commonly related in noncausal ways; that is, the variables are systematically related but in an associative way. This means that there is a systematic movement in the associated values of the two phenomena. For example, there is strong evidence that asbestos exposure is related to lung cancer. It is tempting to state that there is a causal relationship between asbestos exposure and lung cancer. Do not overlook the fact, however, that not all of those exposed to asbestos will have lung cancer and not all of those who have lung cancer have had asbestos exposure. Consequently, it would be scientifically unsound to take a position advocating the presence of a causal relationship between these two variables. Rather, one can say only that there is an associative relationship between the variables of asbestos exposure and lung cancer, a relationship in which there is a strong systematic association between the two phenomena.

TESTABILITY

The second characteristic of a hypothesis is its **testability.** This means that the variables of the study must lend themselves to observation, measurement, and analysis. The hypothesis is either supported or not supported after the data have been collected and analyzed. The predicted outcome proposed by the hypothesis will or will not be congruent with the actual outcome when the hypothesis is tested. Hypotheses advance scientific knowledge by confirming or refuting theories.

Hypotheses may fail to meet the criteria of testability because the researcher has not made a prediction about the anticipated outcome, the variables are not observable or measurable, or the hypothesis is couched in terms that are value-laden. Table 3-4 illustrates each of these points and provides a remedy for each problem.

HELPFUL HINT When a hypothesis is complex (i.e., it contains more than one independent or dependent variable), it is difficult for the findings to indicate unequivocally that the hypothesis is supported or not supported. In such cases, the reader must infer which relationships are significant in the predicted direction from the *Findings* or *Discussion* section.

TABLE **3-4**   Hypotheses that Fail to Meet Criteria of Testability

PROBLEMATIC HYPOTHESIS	PROBLEMATIC ISSUE	REVISED HYPOTHESIS
Social support related to adaptation.	No predictive statement about the relationship is made; so the relationship is not verifiable.	Social support is positively related to adaptation.
Patients who receive preoperative instruction have less postoperative stress than have patients who do not.	The "postoperative stress" variable must be specifically defined so that it is observable or measurable, or the relationship is not testable.	Patients who attend preoperative education classes have less postoperative emotional stress than patients who do not attend.
Small-group teaching will be better than individualized teaching for dietary compliance in patients with coronary artery disease (CAD).	"Better than" is a value-laden phrase that is not objective. Moral and ethical questions containing words such as *should, ought, better than,* and *bad for* are not scientifically testable.	Dietary compliance will be greater in patients with CAD receiving diet instruction in small groups than in CAD patients receiving individualized diet instruction.
Nurses' attitudes toward patients with AIDS cause changes in the patients' mood state.	Causal relationships are proposed without sufficient evidence.	Nurses' attitudes toward AIDS patients will be positively related to the emotional status of the AIDS patient.

THEORY BASE

A sound hypothesis is consistent with an existing body of theory and research findings. Whether a hypothesis is arrived at inductively or deductively (see Chapter 5), it must be based on a sound scientific rationale. Readers should be able to identify the flow of ideas from the research problem to the literature review, to the theoretical framework, and through the research question(s) or hypotheses (see Chapters 4 and 5). Table 3-5 illustrates this process in relation to the research problem, "What is the effect of a child's need for organ transplantation on family adapatation?" (LoBiondo-Wood et al, 2000; see Appendix D). In this example, it is clear that there is an explicitly developed, relevant body of scientific data that provides the theoretical grounding for the study. The hypotheses, as stated in Table 3-5, are logically derived from the theoretical framework. The research consumer, however, should be cautioned about assuming that the theory-hypothesis link will always be present.

WORDING THE HYPOTHESIS

As you read the scientific literature and become more familiar with it, you will observe that there are a variety of ways to word a hypothesis. Regardless of the specific format used to state the hypothesis, the statement should be worded in clear, simple, and concise terms. If this criterion is met, the reader will understand the following:

- The variables of the hypothesis.
- The population being studied.
- The predicted outcome of the hypothesis.

Information about hypotheses may be further clarified in the *Instruments, Sample,* or *Methods* sections of a research report (see Chapters 12, 14, and 15).

DIRECTIONAL VS. NONDIRECTIONAL HYPOTHESES

Hypotheses can be formulated directionally or nondirectionally. A **directional hypothesis** is one that specifies the expected direction of the relationship between the independent and dependent

TABLE **3-5**   Flow of Data among Problem Statement, Literature Review, Theoretical Framework, and Hypotheses

PROBLEM	LITERATURE REVIEW	THEORETICAL FRAMEWORK	HYPOTHESES
What is the effect on family adaptation of a child's need for organ transplantation?	1. Studies related to the impact of the child's liver transplant on the mother during the post operative period as a significant variable influencing adaptation. 2. A study related to the description of the feelings of parents whose children had or were awaiting a heart or liver transplant that contribute to understanding the family coping process related to this phenomenon. 3. The Double ABC-X Model of Family Adaptation proposes that factors such as stress, perception of stress, resources, and coping responses would be variables that contribute to family adaptation. 4. The pretransplant phase has not been studied in relation to these variables.	1. Gap in the literature related to the impact of a child's organ transplant during the preoperative stage. 2. The process of seeking a transplant for a chronically ill child is a long-term process that has identifiable phases. 3. The definition of stress and stressors is a perceptual experience derived from the meaning that family members give. Stress is evidenced by uncertainty, mood, and functioning. 4. Existing and new resources include social support as manifested by the family's ability to meet its demands and needs, as well as include existing and expanded family support and resources. 5. How family members cope is related to their adaptation. 6. Family adaptation is the component of the ABC-X framework that denotes the continuum of outcomes toward which the family's efforts are directed.	1. Coping was predicted to be positively related to adaptation. 2. Overall family stress was predicted to be negatively related to adaptation. 3. Resources were predicted to be positively related to adaptation. 4. Perception of stress, as evidenced by mood state, was predicted to be negatively related to adaptation. 5. Perception of stress, as evidenced by uncertainty, was predicted to be negatively related to adaptation.

variables. The reader of a directional hypothesis may observe not only that a relationship is proposed but also the nature or direction of that relationship. The following is an example of a directional hypothesis: "Trait anger and state anger each are positively related to change in early adolescents"(Mahon, Yarcheski, and Yarcheski, 2000). Examples of directional hypotheses can also be found in examples 2 to 5, 6, and 7 in Table 3-6.

Whereas a **nondirectional hypothesis** indicates the existence of a relationship between the variables, it does not specify the anticipated direction of the relationship. The following is an example of a nondirectional hypothesis: "Client satisfaction with discharge planning, perceptions of care conti-

nuity, and preparedness, as well as difficulties managing care will differ for the intervention and control cohorts" (Bull, Hansen, and Gross, 2000). Other examples of nondirectional hypotheses are illustrated in examples 1 and 8 in Table 3-6.

Nurses who are learning to critique research studies should be aware that both the directional and nondirectional forms of hypotheses statements are acceptable. They should also be aware that there are definite pros and cons pertaining to each one.

Proponents of the nondirectional hypothesis state that this format is more objective and impartial than the directional hypothesis. It is argued that the directional hypothesis is potentially biased, because the researcher, in stating an

TABLE **3-6**   Examples of How Hypotheses Are Worded

HYPOTHESIS	VARIABLES*	TYPE OF HYPOTHESIS	TYPE OF DESIGN SUGGESTED
1. There will be a difference in fatigue between two groups of caregivers of preterm infants (i.e., on vs. not on apnea monitors) during three time periods (i.e., prior to discharge, 1 week post-discharge, and 1 month post-discharge).	IV: Apnea monitor DV: Fatigue	Nondirectional, research	Nonexperimental
2. There will be a positive relationship between phase-specific telephone counseling and emotional adjustment in women with breast cancer and their partners.	IV: Telephone counseling DV: Emotional adjustment	Directional, research	Experimental
3. There will be a greater decrease in state anxiety scores for patients receiving structured informational videos prior to abdominal or chest tube removal than for patients receiving standard information.	IV: Preprocedure structured videotape information IV: Standard information DV: State anxiety	Directional, research	Experimental
4. The incidence and degree of severity of subject discomfort will be less after administration of medications by the Z-track intramuscular injection technique than after administration of medications by the standard intramuscular injection technique.	IV: Z-track intramuscular injection technique IV: Standard intramuscular injection technique DV: Subject discomfort	Directional, research	Experimental
5. Specialized oncology home care services provided to terminally ill patients will have a positive effect on bereavement psychological distress among survivors compared with other models of care.	IV: Specialized oncology home care services IV: Other models of care DV: Bereavement psychological distress	Directional, research	Experimental
6. Hospitals with higher registered nurse-to-patient ratios will have fewer adverse patient events.	IV: Registered nurse-to-patient ratio DV: Adverse patient events	Directional, research	Nonexperimental
7. There will be a positive effect from a social support, boosting intervention on levels of stress, coping and social support among caregivers of children with HIV/AIDs.	IV: Social support boosting intervention DV: Stress DV: Coping DV: Social support	Directional, research	Experimental
8. There will be a difference in posttest state anxiety scores in subjects treated with noncontact therapeutic touch than in subjects treated with contact therapeutic touch.	IV: Noncontact therapeutic touch IV: Contact therapeutic touch DV: State anxiety	Nondirectional, research	Experimental

*IV, Independent variable; DV, dependent variable

anticipated outcome, has demonstrated a commitment to a particular position.

On the other side of the coin, proponents of the directional hypothesis argue that researchers naturally have hunches, guesses, or expectations about the outcome of their research. It is the hunch, the curiosity, or the guess that initially leads them to speculate about the problem. The literature review and the conceptual framework provide the theoretical foundation for deriving the hypothesis. Consequently, it might be said that a deductive hypothesis derived from a theory is most always directional (see Chapter 5). The theory will provide a critical rationale for proposing that relationships between variables will have particular outcomes. When there is no theory or related research to draw on for rationale or when findings in previous research studies are ambivalent, a nondirectional hypothesis may be appropriate.

In summary, the evaluator of a hypothesis should know that there are several advantages to directional hypotheses, making them appropriate for use in most studies. The advantages are as follows:

- Directional hypotheses indicate to the reader that a theory base has been used to derive the hypotheses and that the phenomena under investigation have been critically thought about and interrelated. The reader should realize that nondirectional hypotheses may also be deduced from a theory base. Because of the exploratory nature of many studies utilizing nondirectional hypotheses, however, the theory base may not be as developed.
- They provide the reader with a specific theoretical frame of reference, within which the study is being conducted.
- They suggest to the reader that the researcher is not sitting on a theoretical fence, and as a result, the analyses of data can be accomplished in a statistically more sensitive way.

The important point for the critiquer to keep in mind about the directionality of the hypotheses is whether there is a sound rationale for the choice the researcher has proposed regarding directionality.

STATISTICAL VS. RESEARCH HYPOTHESES

Readers of research reports may observe that a hypothesis is further categorized as either a research or a statistical hypothesis. A **research hypothesis,** also known as a scientific hypothesis, consists of a statement about the expected relationship of the variables. A research hypothesis indicates what the outcome of the study is expected to be. A research hypothesis is also either directional or nondirectional. If the researcher obtains statistically significant findings for a research hypothesis, the hypothesis is supported. For example, in a study exploring the relative effectiveness of one intervention, Coping Skills Training (CST), Grey and associates (1999) hypothesized that diabetic adolescents who participated in CST would have better metabolic control and psychosocial outcomes than adolescents who received routine intensive management. The authors reported that after 6 months, subjects who had received CST combined with intensive management had significantly better metabolic control (HbA1c) and general self-efficacy than subjects who received intensive therapy alone. Subjects reported significantly less negative impact from diabetes on their quality of life and had fewer worries about diabetes. As such, the hypothesis is supported; that is, the study findings supported the predicted outcome. The examples in Table 3-6 represent research hypotheses.

A **statistical hypothesis,** also known as a null hypothesis, states that there is no relationship between the independent and dependent variables. The examples in Table 3-7 illustrate statistical hypotheses. If, in the data analysis, a statistically significant relationship emerges between the variables at a specified level of significance, the null hypothesis is rejected. Rejection of the statistical hypothesis is equivalent to acceptance of the research hypothesis. For example, in the study by Swanson (1999), the effects of caring-based counseling, measurement, and time on the integration of loss (i.e., miscarriage loss) and women's emotional well-being (i.e., moods and self-esteem) were tested using a statistical or null hypothesis. One example of a null hypothesis is "There will be

TABLE **3-7** Examples of Statistical Hypostheses

HYPOTHESIS	VARIABLES*	TYPE OF HYPOTHESIS	TYPE OF DESIGN SUGGESTED
Oxygen inhalation by nasal cannula of up to 6 L/min does not affect oral temperature measurement taken with an electronic thermometer.	IV: Oxygen inhalation by nasal cannula DV: Oral temperature	Statistical	Experimental
There will be no difference in the performance accuracy of adult nurse practitioners (ANP) and family nurse practitioners (FNP) in formulating accurate diagnoses and acceptable interventions for suspected cases of domestic violence.	IV: Nurse Practitioner (ANP or FNP) category DV: Diagnosis and intervention performace accuracy	Statistical	Non-experimental

*_IV,_ Independent variable; _DV,_ dependent variable.

no difference in miscarriage impact, disturbed moods, or self-esteem at 4 months and 1 year after the loss." Swanson (1999) reported that there were significant differences in patient outcomes in relation to these variables. Because the difference in outcomes was greater than expected by chance, the null hypothesis was rejected (see Chapter 17).

Some researchers refer to the null hypothesis as a statistical contrivance that obscures a straightforward prediction of the outcome. Others state that it is more exact and conservative statistically, and that failure to reject the null hypothesis implies that there is insufficient evidence to support the idea of a real difference. Readers of research reports will note that when hypotheses are stated, research hypotheses are generally used more often than statistical hypotheses because they are more desirable to state the researcher's expectation. Readers then have a more precise idea of the proposed outcome. In any study that involves statistical analysis, the underlying null hypothesis is usually assumed without being explicitly stated.

RELATIONSHIP BETWEEN THE HYPOTHESIS AND THE RESEARCH DESIGN

Regardless of whether the researcher uses a statistical or a research hypothesis, there is a suggested relationship between the hypothesis and the research design of the study. The type of design, experimental or nonexperimental (see Chapters 10 and 11), will influence the wording of the hypothesis. For example, when an experimental design is used, the research consumer would expect to see hypotheses that reflect relationship statements, such as the following:

- X_1 is more effective than X_2 on Y.
- The effect of X_1 on Y is greater than that of X_2 on Y.
- The incidence of Y will not differ in subjects receiving X_1 and X_2 treatments.
- The incidence of Y will be greater in subjects after X_1 than after X_2.

Such hypotheses indicate that an experimental treatment (i.e., independent variable X), will be used and that two groups of subjects, experimental and control groups, are being used to test whether the difference in the outcome (i.e., dependent variable Y) predicted by the hypothesis actually exists. Hypotheses reflecting experimental designs also test the effect of the experimental treatment (i.e., independent variable X) on the outcome (i.e., dependent variable Y).

In contrast, hypotheses related to nonexperimental designs reflect associative relationship statements, such as the following:

- X will be negatively related to Y.
- There will be a positive relationship between X and Y.

Table 3-7 provides additional examples of this concept. The Critical Thinking Decision Path will help you determine the type of hypothesis

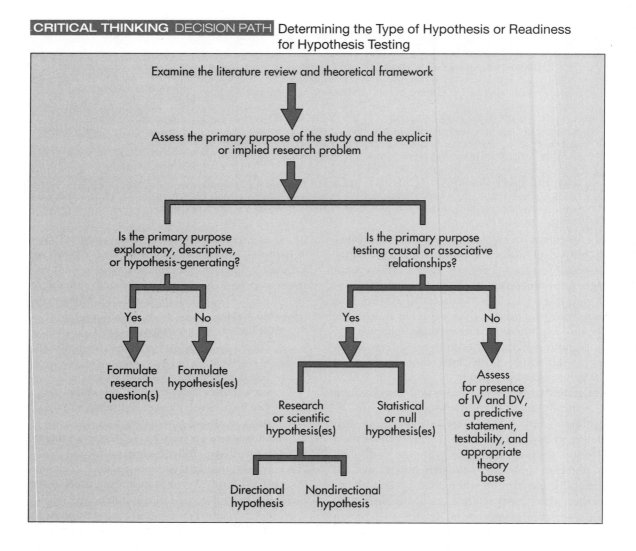

CRITICAL THINKING DECISION PATH Determining the Type of Hypothesis or Readiness for Hypothesis Testing

Examine the literature review and theoretical framework

Assess the primary purpose of the study and the explicit or implied research problem

Is the primary purpose exploratory, descriptive, or hypothesis-generating?

Is the primary purpose testing causal or associative relationships?

Yes — Formulate research question(s)

No — Formulate hypothesis(es)

Yes — Research or scientific hypothesis(es) / Statistical or null hypothesis(es)

No — Assess for presence of IV and DV, a predictive statement, testability, and appropriate theory base

Research or scientific hypothesis(es): Directional hypothesis / Nondirectional hypothesis

presented in a study, as well as the study's readiness for a hypothesis-testing design.

RESEARCH QUESTIONS

Research studies do not always contain hypotheses. As you become more familiar with the scientific literature, you will notice that exploratory studies usually do not have hypotheses. This is particularly common when there is a dearth of literature or related research studies in a particular area that is of interest to the researcher. The re-

searcher, interested in finding out more about a particular phenomenon, may engage in a fact- or relationship-finding mission, guided only by research questions. The outcome of the exploratory study may be that data about the phenomenon are amassed, so the researcher can then formulate hypotheses for a future study. This is sometimes called a hypothesis-generating study.

A study by McDonald and associates (2000) examined how patients communicate their pain and pain-management needs after surgery. The research question, which includes the following vari-

BOX 3-2 Examples of Research Questions

- Do nurses with greater empathy have patients experiencing less pain and receiving adequate analgesia (Watt-Watson et al, 2000)?
- To what extent do women engage in risk factor modification activities after CABG surgery (King, Rowe, and Zerwic, 2000)?
- What are nurses' perceptions of people who are homeless (Minick et al, 1998)?
- What are the self-care strategies used by patients with heart failure to manage their symptoms (Bennett et al, 2000)?
- Do gender, race, or both affect the relationship between patterns of anger expression as measured

by the Jacobs Pediatric Anger Expression Scale and blood pressure readings (BPR) (Hauber et al, 1998)?
- Does continuous light or very light handrail support reduce oxygen uptake and/or heart rate compared with no handrail support in women during submaximal step treadmill exercise (Christman et al, 2000)?
- Is the incidence of depression greater among adolescents who are legally blind than among adolescents who are sighted (Koenes and Karshmer, 2000)?

ables, pain (independent variable X) and postoperative caregiver pain communication (dependent variable Y), illustrates how an investigation designed to generate relationships and fill a gap in the literature was guided by research questions.

- How do postoperative patients communicate their pain and pain-management needs to their health care providers?
- How are demographical variables (e.g., race and gender) related to pain and the communication of pain-management needs to health care providers?

Because there has been little research on the effectiveness of postoperative communication of pain, research questions—rather than hypotheses—are appropriate for this baseline phase of a study. The findings of the study highlighted the importance of effective patient communication of pain as a variable related to effective pain management by health care providers. Reasons for decreased pain communication include the following:

- Not wanting to complain.
- Not wanting to take the provider away from other patients.
- Avoiding unpleasant analgesic side effects.
- Not wanting to take "drugs."

The problems in the communication of pain management identified in this study could be used to design nursing-intervention studies to improve pain communication and the consequent pain relief in postoperative patients.

Qualitative research studies also are guided by research questions rather than hypotheses. The

descriptive findings of qualitative studies also can provide the basis for future hypothesis-testing studies. "What is it like to go through depression as a Black West-Indian Canadian woman" is an example of a research question from a qualitative study by Schreiber and associates (2000) that sought to enrich understanding about how women from a nondominant cultural background (i.e., West Indian) experience and manage depression (see Chapters 6, 7, and 8).

As you can see, research questions tend to be more specific than the research problems discussed in the research problem section of this chapter. The more specific research questions are, however, the more they provide direction for the study.

In other studies, research questions are formulated in addition to hypotheses to answer questions related to ancillary data. Such questions do not directly pertain to the proposed outcomes of the hypotheses. Rather, they may provide additional and sometimes serendipitous findings that enrich the study and provide direction for further study. Sometimes they are the kernels of new or future hypotheses. The evaluator of a research study must determine whether it was appropriate to formulate a research question rather than a hypothesis given the nature and context of the study. Box 3-2 provides examples of research questions.

HELPFUL HINT Remember that research questions are most often used in exploratory, descriptive, qualitative, or hypothesis-generating studies.

CRITIQUING the Research Problem and Hypotheses

The care that a researcher takes when developing the research problem, the research question, or the hypotheses is often representative of the overall conceptualization and design of the study. A methodically formulated research problem or question provides the basis for hypothesis development. In a quantitative research study, the remainder of a study revolves around testing the hypotheses or, in some cases, the research questions. In a qualitative research study, the objective is to answer the research question. This may be a time-consuming, sometimes frustrating endeavor for the researcher, but in the final analysis, the product, as evaluated by the consumer is most often worth the struggle. Because this text focuses on the nurse as a critical consumer of research, the following sections will primarily pertain to the evaluation of research problems, research questions, and hypotheses in published research reports.

CRITIQUING THE RESEARCH PROBLEM

The Critiquing Criteria box provides several criteria for evaluating this initial phase of the research process—the research problem. Because the research problem represents the basis for the study, it is usually introduced at the beginning of the research report to indicate the focus and direction of the study to the readers. Readers will then be in a position to evaluate whether the rest of the study logically flows from its base. The author will often begin by identifying the general problem area that originally represented some vague discontent or question about an unsolved problem. The experimental and scientific background that led to the specific problem is briefly summarized; and the purpose, aim, or goal of the study is identified. Finally, the research problem and any related subproblems are proposed in the same places as they are used in an article.

CRITIQUING CRITERIA

The Research Problem

1. Was the research problem introduced promptly?
2. Is the problem stated clearly and unambiguously in declarative or question form?
3. Does the research problem express a relationship between two or more variables or at least between an independent and a dependent variable, implying empirical testability?
4. Does the research problem specify the nature of the population being studied?
5. Has the research problem been substantiated with adequate experiential and scientific background material?
6. Has the research problem been placed within the context of an appropriate theoretical framework?
7. Has the significance of the research problem been identified?
8. Have pragmatic issues, such as feasibility, been addressed?
9. Have the purpose, aims, or goals of the study been identified?

The Hypotheses

1. Does the hypothesis directly relate to the research problem?
2. Is the hypothesis concisely stated in a declarative form?
3. Are the independent and dependent variables identified in the statement of the hypothesis?
4. Are the variables measurable or potentially measurable?
5. Is each of the hypotheses specific to one relationship so that each hypothesis can be either supported or not supported?
6. Is the hypothesis stated in such a way that it is testable?
7. Is the hypothesis stated objectively, without value-laden words?
8. Is the direction of the relationship in each hypothesis clearly stated?
9. Is each hypothesis consistent with the literature review?
10. Is the theoretical rationale for the hypothesis explicit?
11. Are research questions appropriately used (i.e., exploratory, descriptive or qualitative study or in relation to ancillary data analyses)?

The purpose of the introductory summary of the theoretical and scientific background is to provide the reader with a contextual glimpse of how the author critically thought about the research problem's development. The introduction to the research problem places the study within an appropriate theoretical framework and sets the stage for the unfolding of the study. This introductory section should also include the significance of the study (i.e., why the investigator is doing the study). For example, the significance may be to solve a problem encountered in the clinical area and thereby improve patient care, to resolve a conflict in the literature regarding a clinical issue, or to provide data supporting an innovative form of nursing intervention that is of equal or better quality and is also cost-effective.

In reality, readers often find that the research problem is not clearly stated at the conclusion of this section. In some cases, it is only hinted at, and the reader is challenged to identify the research problem under consideration. In other cases, the research problem is embedded in the introductory text or purpose statement. To some extent, this depends on the style of the journal. Nevertheless, the evaluator must remember that the main research problem should be implied if it is not clearly identified in the introductory section—even if the subproblems are not stated or implied.

The reader looks for the presence of three key elements that are described and illustrated in an earlier section of this chapter. They are the following:

- Does the research problem express a relationship between two or more variables, or at least between an independent and a dependent variable?
- Does the research problem specify the nature of the population being studied?
- Does the research problem imply the possibility of empiric testing?

The reader uses these three elements as criteria for judging the soundness of a stated research problem. It is likely that if the problem is unclear in terms of the variables, the population, and the implications for testability, then the remainder of the study is going to falter. For example, a research study contained introductory material on anxiety in general, anxiety as it relates to the perioperative period, and the potentially beneficial influence of nursing care in relation to anxiety reduction. The author concluded that the purpose of the study was to determine whether selected measures of patient anxiety could be shown to differ when different approaches to nursing care were used during the perioperative period. The author did not go on to state the research problems. A restatement of the problem in question form might be as follows:

$$(Y_1) \qquad (X_1, X_2, X_3)$$

What is the difference in patient anxiety level in relation to different approaches to nursing care during the perioperative period?

If this process is clarified at the outset of a research study, all that follows in terms of the design can be logically developed. Readers will have a clear idea of what the report should convey and can knowledgeably evaluate the material that follows.

CRITIQUING THE HYPOTHESIS

As illustrated in the Critiquing Criteria box, several criteria for critiquing the hypotheses should be used as a standard for evaluating the strengths and weaknesses of the hypotheses in a research report.

1. When reading a research study, research consumers may find the hypotheses clearly delineated in a separate hypothesis section of the research article (i.e., after the literature review or theoretical framework section[s]). In many cases, the hypotheses are not explicitly stated and are only implied in the *Results* or *Discussion* section of the article. As such, readers must infer the hypotheses from the purpose statement and the type of analysis used. Readers must also be cognizant of this variation and not think that because hypotheses do not appear at the beginning of the article, they do not exist in the particular study. Even when hypotheses are stated at the beginning of an article, they are reexamined in the *Results* or *Discussion* section as the findings are presented and discussed. Readers should expect hypotheses to be appropriately reflected depending on the purpose of the study and format of the article.

2. If a research problem was posed at the beginning of the report, the hypothesis should directly answer it. Its placement in the research report logically follows the literature review, and the theoretical framework, because the hypothesis should reflect the culmination and expression of this conceptual process. It should be consistent with both the literature

review and the theoretical framework. The flow of this process, as depicted in Table 3-7, should be explicit and apparent to the reader. If this criterion is met, the reader feels reasonably assured that the basis for the hypothesis is theoretically sound.

3. As readers examine the actual hypothesis, several aspects of the statement should be critically appraised. First, the hypothesis should consist of a declarative statement that objectively and succinctly expresses the relationship between an independent and a dependent variable. In wording a complex vs. a simple hypothesis, there may be more than one independent and dependent variable.

Second, readers can expect that there may be more than one hypothesis, particularly if there is more than one independent and dependent variable. This is a function of the type of study being conducted.

Third, the variables of the hypothesis should be understandable to the reader. In the interest of formulating a succinct hypothesis statement, the complete meaning of the variables is often not apparent. Readers must realize that sometimes a researcher is caught between the "devil and the deep blue sea" on that issue. It may be a choice between having a complete but verbose hypothesis paragraph or a less complete but concise hypothesis. The solution to this dilemma is for the researcher to have a definition section in the research report. The inclusion of **conceptual definitions** and **operational definitions** (see Chapter 5) provides the complete explication of the variables. Readers can then examine the hypothesis alongside the definitions and determine the exact nature of the variables under consideration. An excellent example of this process appears in a research article by Mahon, Yarcheski, and Yarcheski (2000), who hypothesized the following:

Trait anger and state anger each are positively related to change in early adolescents.

and

Trait anger has a direct effect on state anger.

and

Both trait anger and state anger have a direct effect on vigor and inclination to change

These are appropriately worded hypotheses. It is not completely clear, however, what the variables "Trait anger," "State anger," "Vigor," or "Inclination to change" imply. It is only upon examination of the definitions of these variables, which are included in the literature review section, that the exact nature of the variables becomes clear to readers. (See Appendix C.)

- Trait Anger: "The disposition of individuals to perceive a wide range of situations as annoying, tending to respond to such situations with elevations in state anger."
- State Anger: "An emotional state marked by subjective feelings that vary in intensity from mild annoyance or irritation to intense fury and rage."
- Vigor: "A mood of vigorousness, ebullience, and high energy."
- Inclination to Change: "Seeking new and different, readily changing opinions or values in different circumstances, and adapting readily to change in the environment."

The context of the variables is now revealed to the evaluator.

Fourth, although a hypothesis can legitimately be nondirectional, it is preferable to indicate the direction of the relationship between the variables in the hypothesis. Readers will find that when there is a dearth of data available for the literature review (i.e., the researcher has chosen to study a relatively undefined area of interest), the nondirectional hypothesis may be appropriate. There simply may not be enough information available to make a sound judgment about the direction of the proposed relationship. All that could be proposed is that there will be a relationship between two variables. Essentially, readers want to determine the appropriateness of the researcher's choice regarding directionality of the hypothesis.

4. The notion of testability is central to the soundness of a hypothesis. One criterion related to testability is that the hypothesis should be stated in such a way that it can be clearly supported or not supported. Although the previous statement is very important to keep in mind, readers should also understand that ultimately theories or hypotheses are never proven beyond the shadow of a doubt through hypothesis testing. Researchers who claim that their data have "proven" the validity of their hypothesis should be regarded with grave

reservation. Readers should realize that, at best, findings that support a hypothesis are considered tentative. If repeated replication of a study yields the same results, more confidence can be placed in the conclusions advanced by the researchers. An important thing to remember about testability is that although hypotheses are more likely to be accepted with increasing evidence, they are ultimately never proven.

Another point about testability for research consumers to consider is that the hypothesis should be objectively stated and devoid of any value-laden words. Value-laden hypotheses are not empirically testable. Quantifiable words such as greater than; less than; decrease; increase; and positively, negatively, and curvilinearly related convey the idea of objectivity and testability. Readers should immediately be suspicious of hypotheses that are not stated objectively.

5. The evaluator of a research study should be cognizant of the fact that how the proposed relationship of the hypothesis is phrased suggests the type of research design that will be appropriate for the study. For example, if a hypothesis proposes that treatment X_1 will have a greater effect on Y than treatment X_2, an experimental or quasiexperimental design is suggested (see Chapter 10). If a hypothesis proposes that there will be a positive relationship between variables X and Y, a nonexperimental design is suggested (see Chapter 11). A review of Table 3-6 provides you with additional examples of hypotheses and the type of research design that is suggested by each hypothesis. The reader of a research report should evaluate whether the selected research design is congruent with the hypothesis. This factor has important implications for the remainder of the study in terms of the appropriateness of sample selection, data collection, data analysis, interpretation of findings, and—ultimately— the conclusions advanced by the researcher.

6. If the research report contains research questions rather than hypotheses, the reader will want to evaluate whether this is appropriate to the study. The criterion for making this decision, as presented earlier in this chapter, is whether the study is of an exploratory, descriptive, or qualitative nature. If it is, then it is appropriate to have research questions rather than hypotheses. Ancillary research questions should be evaluated as to whether they answer additional questions secondary to the hypotheses. Sometimes, the substance of an additional research question is more appropriately posed as another hypothesis in that it relates in a major way to the original research problem.

Critical Thinking Challenges

Barbara Krainovich-Miller

➤ Do you agree or disagree with the following statement: A research study published in a journal does not clearly state the research problem, then it fails to meet the critiquing criteria for problem statements as presented in this chapter. Justify your answer.

➤ Is it possible for "level of anxiety" to be the independent variable in one study and the dependent variable in another study? Support your position.

➤ Is it possible for a research hypothesis not to be theory derived? Support your answer with examples.

➤ What is the difference between your friend predicting that students who don't study will not do well on a test and a research study's hypothesis on the topic? Justify your answer.

Key Points

• Formulation of the research problem, research question, and stating the hypothesis are key preliminary steps in the research process.

• The research problem is refined through a process that proceeds from the identification of a general idea of interest to the definition of a more specific and circumscribed topic.

- A preliminary literature review reveals related factors that appear critical to the research topic of interest and helps to further define the research problem.
- The significance of the research problem must be identified in terms of its potential contribution to patients, nurses, the medical community in general, and society. Applicability of the problem for nursing practice, as well as its theoretical relevance, must be established. The findings should also have the potential for formulating or altering nursing practices or policies.
- The feasibility of a research problem must be examined in light of pragmatic considerations (e.g., time); availability of subjects, money, facilities, and equipment; experience of the researcher; and ethical issues.
- The final research problem consists of a statement about the relationship of two or more variables. It clearly identifies the relationship between the independent and dependent variables; specifies the nature of the population being studied; and implies the possibility of empirical testing.
- A hypothesis attempts to answer the question posed by the research problem. When testing the validity of the theoretical framework's assumptions, the hypothesis bridges the theoretical and real worlds.
- A hypothesis is a declarative statement about the relationship between two or more variables that predicts an expected outcome. Characteristics of a hypothesis include a relationship statement, implications regarding testability, and consistency with a defined theory base.
- Hypotheses can be formulated in a directional or a nondirectional manner. Hypotheses can be further categorized as either research or statistical hypotheses.
- Research questions may be used instead of hypotheses in exploratory, descriptive, or qualitative research studies. Research questions may also be formulated in addition to hypotheses to answer questions related to ancillary data.
- The critiquing criteria provide a set of guidelines for evaluating the strengths and weaknesses of the problem statement and hypotheses as they appear in a research report.
- The critiquer assesses the clarity of the research problem, as well as the related subproblems, the specificity of the population, and the implications for testability.
- The interrelatedness of the research problem, the literature review, the theoretical framework, and the hypotheses should be apparent.
- The appropriateness of the research design suggested by the research problem is also evaluated.
- The purpose of the study (i.e., why the researcher is doing the study) should be differentiated from the research problem or the research question.
- The reader evaluates the wording of the hypothesis in terms of the clarity of the relational statement, its implications for testability, and its congruence with a theory base. The appropriateness of the hypothesis in relation to the type of research design suggested by the design is also examined. In addition, the appropriate use of research questions is evaluated in relation to the type of study conducted.

REFERENCES

Bennett SJ et al: Self-care strategies for symptom management in patients with chronic heart failure, *Nurs Res* 49(3):139-145, 2000.

Bouve LR, Rozmus CL, and Giordano P: Preparing parents for their child's transfer from the PICU to the pediatric floor, *Appl Nurs Res* 12(3):114-120, 1999.

Bull MJ, Hansen HE, and Gross CR: Professional-patient partnership model of discharge planning with elders hospitalized with heart failure, *Appl Nurs Res* 13(1):19-28, 2000.

Christman SK et al: Continuous handrail support, oxygen uptake, and heart rate in women during submaximal step treadmill exercise, *Res Nurs Health* 23:35-42, 2000.

Dilorio C et al: A social cognitive-based model for condom use among college students, *Nurs Res* 49(4):208-214, 2000.

Grey M et al: Coping skills training for youths with diabetes on intensive therapy, *Appl Nurs Res* 12(1):3-12, 1999.

Hauber RP et al: Anger and blood pressure readings in children, *Appl Nurs Res* 11(1):2-11, 1998.

Jarrett M et al: The relationship between psychological distress and gastrointestinal symptoms in women with irritable bowel syndrome, *Nurs Res* 47(3):154-161, 1998.

Johnson JL et al: Preventing smoking relapse in postpartum women, *Nurs Res* 49(1): 44-52, 2000.

King K, Rowe M, and Zerwic J: Concerns and risk factor modification in women during the year after coronary artery surgery, *Nurs Res* 49(3): 167-172, 2000.

Koenes SG and Karshmer JF: Depression: a comparison study between blind and sighted adolescents, *Iss Mental Health Nurs* 21(2):269-279, 2000.

Leight SB et al: The effect of structured training on breast self-examination search behaviors as measured using biomedical instrumentation, *Nurs Res* 49(5):283-289, 2000.

LoBiondo-Wood G et al: Family adaptation to a child's transplant: pretransplant phase, *Progress in Transplantation* 10(2):1-8, 2000.

Mahon NF, Yarcheski A, and Yarcheski TJ: Positive and negative outcomes of anger in early adolescents, *Res Nurs Health* 23(1):17-24, 2000.

McDonald DD et al: Communicating pain and pain management needs after surgery, *Appl Nurs Res* 13(2):70-75, 2000.

Minick P et al: Nurses' perceptions of people who are homeless, *Western J Nurs Res* 20(3):356-369, 1998.

Naylor MD et al: Comprehensive discharge planning and home follow-up of hospitalized elders: a randomized clinical trial, *JAMA* 281(7):999-1000, 1999.

Schreiber R, Noerager-Stern P and Wilson C: *Being strong: how Black West-Indian Canadian women manage depression and its stigma, J Nurs Scholarship* 32(1): 39-45, 2000.

Swanson KM: Effects of caring measurement, and time on miscarriage impact and women's well-being, *Nurs Res* 48(6):288-298, 1999.

Tucker S, Moore W, and Luedtke C: Outcomes of a brief inpatient treatment program for mood and anxiety disorders, *Outcomes Management for Nursing Practice* 4(3):117-123, 2000.

Watt-Watson J et al: The impact of nurses' empathic responses on patients' pain management in acute care, *Nurs Res* 49(4):191-200, 2000.

ADDITIONAL READINGS

Campbell DT and Stanley JC: *Experimental and quasi-experimental designs for research,* Chicago, 1963, Rand-McNally.

Kerlinger FN: *Foundations of behavioral research,* New York, 1986, Holt, Rinehart, and Winston.

Pedhazur EJ and Schmelkin LP: *Measurement, design, and analysis: an integrated approach,* Hillsdale, NJ, 1991, Lawrence Erlbaum Associates.

Van Dalen DB: *Understanding educational research,* New York, 1979, McGraw-Hill.

BARBARA KRAINOVICH-MILLER

Literature Review

4

Key Terms

computer databases
conceptual literature
Cumulative Index to Nursing
  and Allied Health Literature
  (CINAHL)
data-based literature
electronic database
empirical literature
integrative review

Internet
literature
MEDLINE
primary source
print databases
print indexes
quantitative research
refereed, or peer-reviewed,
  journals

research literature
review of the literature
scholarly literature
scientific literature
secondary source
theoretical literature
web browser
world wide web (www)

Learning Outcomes

After reading this chapter, the student should be able to do the following:

- Discuss the relationship of the literature review to nursing theory, research, education, and practice.
- Discuss the purposes of the literature review from the perspective of the research investigator and the research consumer.
- Discuss the use of the literature review for quantitative designs and qualitative approaches.
- Discuss the purpose of reviewing the literature in development of evidence-based practice protocols.
- Differentiate between conceptual (theoretical) and data-based (research) literature.
- Differentiate between primary and secondary sources.
- Compare the advantages and disadvantages of the most commonly used on-line databases and traditional print database sources for conducting a relevant literature review.
- Identify the characteristics of a relevant literature review.
- Critically read, critique, and synthesize conceptual and data-based resources for the development of a literature review.
- Apply critiquing criteria to the evaluation of literature reviews in selected research studies.

You may wonder why an entire chapter of a research text is devoted to the **review of the literature.** The main reason is because the literature review is not only a key step in the research process, but it is also used in all steps of the process. A more personal question you might ask is, "Will knowing more about the literature review really help me in my student role or later in my research consumer role as a practicing professional nurse?" The answer is that it most certainly will. The ability to review the literature is a skill essential to your role as a student and your future role as a research consumer (ANA, 1993, 1995, 2000).

The **review of the literature** is considered a systematic and critical review of the most important scholarly literature on a particular topic. The term scholarly literature can refer to published and unpublished **data-based (research) literature,** as well as **conceptual (theoretical)** literature. **Data-based literature** comprises reports of research studies. **Conceptual** or **theoretical literature** are reports of theories, some of which underlie reported research. An article that discusses a particular theory or reviews the research and nonresearch literature related to a concept such as anxiety is considered conceptual rather than data-based.

As Figure 4-1 shows, this chapter introduces the review of the literature as a component of the research process that is essential to theory research, education, and practice. The review of the literature section of a published study often contains both data-based or **research literature,** as well as conceptual or theoretical literature, but the entire research article is categorized as data-based literature. A critical review of the literature does the following:

- Uncovers conceptual and data-based knowledge related to a particular subject, concept, or clinical problem and is used in all aspects of the research process.
- Uncovers new knowledge that can lead to the development, validation, or refinement of theories.
- Reveals research questions for the discipline.
- Provides the latest knowledge for education.
- Uncovers research findings that support evidenced-based practice.

The purpose of this chapter is to introduce you to the review of the literature as it is used in research and other scholarly activities. The primary focus of the discussion is on using your critical thinking and reading competencies (see Chapter 2) for developing the necessary skills for critically appraising the literature.

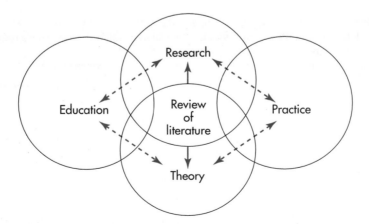

Figure 4-1　Relationship of the review of the literature to theory, research, education, and practice.

REVIEW OF THE LITERATURE

OVERALL PURPOSE: KNOWLEDGE

The overall purpose of a review of the literature is to develop a strong knowledge base for the conduct of research and evidenced-based practice. Before you can critique the literature review in a research study, it is important to understand what purpose the review of the literature serves in a research study. Box 4-1 outlines the overall purposes of a literature review for a research study. The knowledge uncovered from a critical review of the literature contributes to the development, implementation, and results of a research study.

RESEARCH STUDY: PURPOSE OF THE LITERATURE REVIEW

All 10 objectives listed in Box 4-1 reflect the purposes of a literature review for the conduct of quantitative research. Critically reading the literature is essential to meeting these objectives. The main goal of a literature review is to develop the foundation of a sound study. Table 4-1 summarizes the main focus of the literature review for use in the steps of the research process for quantitative and qualitative designs. Box 4-2 lists the characteristics of a literature review that meet cri-

tiquing criteria; these characteristics are discussed throughout the chapter.

RESEARCH CONSUMER: REVIEW OF LITERATURE PURPOSES

The major reason to review the literature on a given topic is to uncover knowledge for use in education and practice. Box 4-1 and Table 4-2 illustrate a few examples of research consumer activities. For example, a student assignment might involve retrieving and critically reviewing a number of data-based (research) articles and conceptual (theoretical) articles listed for a practice protocol, standard, or policy to determine the degree of support found in the data-based and conceptual literature. A critical review of the literature essentially uncovers data that contribute evidence to support current practice, clinical decision making, and changes in practice.

RESEARCH CONDUCT AND CONSUMER OF RESEARCH PURPOSES: DIFFERENCES AND SIMILARITIES

How does the literature review differ when it is used for research purposes vs. consumer of research purposes? The literature review in a research study is used to develop a sound research proposal. In a research study, the literature review

---

BOX 4-1 Overall Purposes of a Review of Literature

Major Goal

To develop a strong knowledge base to carry out research and other scholarly educational and clinical practice activities.

Objectives

A review of the literature does the following:
1. Determines what is known and unknown about a subject, concept, or problem.
2. Determines gaps, consistencies, and inconsistencies in the literature about a subject, concept, or problem.
3. Discovers unanswered questions about a subject, concept, or problem.
4. Discovers conceptual traditions used to examine problems.

5. Uncovers a new practice intervention(s), or gains support for current intervention(s), protocols, and policies.
6. Promotes revising and development of new practice protocols, policies, and projects/activities related to nursing practice.
7. Generates useful research questions and hypotheses for nursing.
8. Determines an appropriate research design, methodology, and analysis for answering the research question(s) or hypothesis(es) based on an assessment of the strengths and weaknesses of earlier works.
9. Determines the need for replication of a study or refinement of a study.
10. Synthesizes the strengths and weaknesses and findings of available studies on a topic/problem.

TABLE **4-1**   Examples of the Uses of Literature Review for Research Process:
Quantitative and Qualitative

QUANTITATIVE PROCESS	QUALITATIVE PROCESS

The review of the literature is used for all **quantitative research** designs.
The review of the literature is defined as a step of the research process. When a research study is written as a proposal or published, the literature review is often written as a separate aspect of the study—*even if it isn't labeled as such.* The actual review of the literature (i.e., the results of the review), however, is used in developing all steps of the research process.
The review of the literature is essential to the following steps of the research process:
    Problem
    Need/significance
    Question/hypothesis(es)
    Theoretical/conceptual framework
    Design/methodology
    Specific instruments (validity and reliability)
    Data-collection method
    Type of analysis
    Findings (interpretation)
    Implications of the findings
    Recommendations based on the findings
	The use of the literature review depends on the selected qualitative approach/method, designs/types, and phases. An extensive database is usually not available and conceptual data are somewhat limited, so a qualitative design is used.
	The following examples highlight the predominant use of the literature review for the particular qualitative approach:
	    Phenomenologic—compare findings with information from the review of the literature (Cohen and Ley, 2000, Appendix B)
	    Grounded theory—constantly compare literature with the data being generated (Northington, 2000)
	    Ethnographic—more conceptual than data-based; provides framework for study (Haglund, 2000)
	    Case study—conceptual and data-based literature embedded in the report (Offredy, 2000)
	    Historical—review of literature is source of data (Aita, 2000)

BOX **4-2**   Characteristics of a Written "Relevant" Review of Literature

Each reviewed source of information reflects critical thinking and scholarly writing and is relevant to the study/topic/project, and the content satisfies the following criteria:
- Purposes of a literature review were met.
- Summary is succinct and adequately represents the reviewed source.
- Critiquing (objective critical evaluation) reflects analysis and synthesis of material(s).
- Application of accepted critiquing criteria to analyze for strengths, weaknesses, or limitations and conflicts or gaps in information as it relates directly and indirectly to the area of interest.

- Evidence of synthesis of the critiques of each source of information. Putting the parts (i.e., each critique) together to form a new whole or connecting link for what is to be studied, replicated, developed, or implemented.
- Review consists of mainly primary sources.
- Sufficient number of sources are used, especially data-based sources.
- Material is synthesized rather than presented as a series of quoted contents.
- Summaries/critiques of studies are presented in a logical flow ending with a conclusion or synthesis of the reviewed material that reflects why the study or project should be implemented.

includes a critical evaluation of both data-based and conceptual literature related to the proposed study. The literature review in a study concludes with a statement relating the proposed study's purpose to the reviewed research. This statement is not a rehash or simple paraphrasing of the reviewed studies.

From a broader perspective, the major focus of reviewing the literature as a consumer is to uncover multiple sources on a given topic. From a

TABLE **4-2**   Examples of the Uses of the Literature for Research Consumer Purposes:
Educational and Practice Settings

EDUCATIONAL SETTING	CLINICAL/PROFESSIONAL SETTING
UNDERGRADUATE STUDENTS Develop academic scholarly papers (i.e., researching a topic, problem, or issue) Prepare oral presentations or debates of a topic, problem, or issue; prepare clinical projects **GRADUATE STUDENTS (MASTER'S AND DOCTORAL)** Develop research proposals Develop research- or evidence-based practice protocols and other scholarly projects **FACULTY** Develop and revise curricula Develop theoretical papers for presentations and/or publication Develop research proposals	**NURSES IN THE CLINICAL SETTING** Implement research-based nursing interventions and evidence-based practice protocols Develop hospital-specific nursing protocols or policies related to patient care Develop, implement, and evaluate hospital-specific quality assurance projects or protocols related to patient outcome data **PROFESSIONAL NURSING ORGANIZATIONS/GOVERNMENTAL AGENCIES** Develop ANA's major documents (e.g., *Social Policy Statement*, 1995; *Nursing Care Report Card for Acute Care*, 1995; *Women's Primary Health Care: Protocols for Practice*, 1995; *Standards of Clinical Practice*, 1995; *Scope and Standards of Home Health Nursing Practice*, 2000; *Scope and Standards of Practice for Nursing Professional Development*, 2000; *Scope and Standards of Public Health Nursing Practice*, 2000) Develop AHCPR's practice guidelines (e.g., *Evaluation and Management of Early HIV Infection*, 1994)

student perspective, a critical review of the literature is essential to acquiring knowledge for the development of scholarly papers, presentations, debates, and evidence-based practice. Students use data-based and conceptual literature resources to support rationale for nursing interventions written for a nursing diagnosis. The first six objectives in Box 4-1 address consumer purposes.

Both types of review are similar in that both reviews should be critical, framed in the context of previous data-based and conceptual literature, and pertinent to the objectives presented in Box 4-1. The amount of literature required to be reviewed, however, may differ between a research proposal and an academic paper or clinical project. Table 4-2 lists a number of research consumer projects conducted in educational and clinical settings.

A critical literature review is central to developing and implementing activities for research consumers. A practice protocol or nursing interventions implemented in a health care setting should be based on a critical review of data-based (research) literature. For example, the interdisciplinary Agency for Healthcare Research and Quality (AHRQ), formerly the Agency for

Health Care Policy and Research (AHCPR), has published a number of guidelines for frequently occurring health problems. One such guideline is the *Evaluation and Management of Early HIV Infection* (1994). For the development of these practice guidelines, a large team of researches and clinicians conducted an extensive review/critique of all of the available data-based and conceptual literature on each topic.

LITERATURE REVIEW: UNDERSTANDING THE PERSPECTIVE OF THE RESEARCH INVESTIGATOR

The literature review is essential to all steps of the quantitative research process. From this perspective, the review is broad and systematic, as well as in-depth, but not usually exhaustive; it is a critical collection and evaluation of the important published literature in journals, monographs, books, and/or book chapters, as well as unpublished data-based print and computer accessed materials (e.g., doctoral dissertations and master's theses), audiovisual materials (e.g., audiotapes and videotapes), and sometimes personal communications (e.g., conference presentations and one-on-one interviews).

From the perspective of a producer of research, objectives 1 to 5 and 7 to 10 of Box 4-1 represent different ways of thinking about the literature. These objectives direct the questions the researcher asks while reading the literature to determine a useful research question(s) and implementation of a particular study.

As a consumer of research, the following brief overview of the use of the literature review in relation to the steps of the quantitative research process will help you to understand the researcher's focus. (Chapters 6, 7, and 8 provide an in-depth presentation related to qualitative research.) A critical review of relevant literature impacts the steps of quantitative research process as follows:

- *Theoretical or conceptual framework:* A critical literature review reveals conceptual traditions, concepts, and/or theories or conceptual models from nursing and other related fields that can be used to examine problems. This framework presents the context for studying the problem and can be viewed as a map for understanding the relationships between or among the variables in quantitative studies. The literature review provides rationale for the variables and explicates linkages or relations of the individual variables for the theoretical framework of the study. The literature review should demonstrate use of primary and secondary sources, but will mainly demonstrate the use of primary sources. A **primary source** is written by a person or persons who developed a theory or conducted the research. A **secondary source** is written by a person or persons other than the individual(s) who developed the theory or conducted the research.
- *Problem statement and hypothesis:* The literature review helps to determine what is known and not known; to uncover gaps, consistencies, or inconsistencies; and/or to reveal unanswered questions in the literature about a subject,

concept, theory, or problem. The review allows for refinement of research problems and questions and/or hypotheses.

- *Design and method:* The literature review reveals the strengths and weaknesses of designs and methods of previous research studies. The review is crucial to choosing an appropriate design, data-collection method, sample size, valid and reliable instruments, and effective data analysis method(s), as well as in helping to develop an appropriate consent form that addresses ethical concerns. A review of the critical literature reveals the appropriateness of a study's design and can help the researcher determine whether a previous study should be replicated and/or refined. It also can uncover instruments that lack validity and reliability, thus identifying the need for instrument refinement or development through research testing.
- *Outcome of the analysis (i.e., findings, discussion, implications, and recommendations):* The literature review is used to accurately interpret and discuss the results/findings of a study. The researcher returns to the literature and uses conceptual and data-based literature to accomplish this goal (see Chapter 18). The researcher then indicates in this section of the journal article that a particular finding was supported by one or several prior research studies (i.e., data-based articles), as well as by several theories on anxiety (i.e., conceptual articles or books) documented in the literature review. The literature review also helps to develop the implications of the findings for practice, education, and further research. Figure 4-2 relates the literature review to all aspects of the quantitative research process.

REVIEW OF THE LITERATURE: RESEARCH CONSUMER PERSPECTIVE

As a consumer of research, you are not expected to write a complete review of the literature on your own but are expected to know how to con-

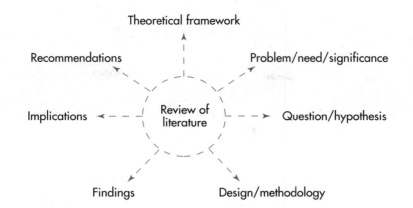

Figure 4-2   Relationship of the review of the literature to the steps of the quantitative research process.

duct a literature review and critically evaluate it (ANA, 1993). Understanding the purpose(s) of a literature review for research and research-consumer purposes will enable you to meet this outcome. Embedded in the purposes is the ability to do the following:

- Efficiently retrieve an adequate amount of scholarly literature using **electronic databases.** Such electronic databases can be retrieved via CD-ROM or on-line (i.e., via the internet) programs such as **Cumulative Index to Nursing and Allied Health Literature (CINAHL)** database, as well as traditional print resources for material not entered into the common databases.
- Critically evaluate data-based and conceptual material based on accepted critiquing criteria for reviewing the respective literature.
- Synthesize the critically evaluated literature (e.g., the entire compilation of conceptual and data-based literature about patient-controlled analgesia [PCA]).

The objectives in Box 4-1 reflect both academic and professional expectations for a beginning consumer of research (see Chapter 1). Table 4-3 presents an overview of the steps for conducting a literature search. In the right-hand column, you will find some useful tips/strategies or rationales for successfully completing these steps. This process is the same whether the purpose is critiquing or

writing a literature review; it reflects the cognitive processes and manual techniques of retrieving and critically reviewing literature sources. The remainder of this chapter presents the essential material for accomplishing these goals.

SCHOLARLY LITERATURE

CONCEPTUAL AND DATA-BASED LITERATURE: SYNONYMS AND SOURCES

Synonyms for conceptual and data-based scholarly literature are presented in Table 4-4. The term *theoretical literature* is most often interchanged with *conceptual literature;* while the terms *empirical literature, scientific literature,* or *research literature* are interchanged with *data-based literature.* Table 4-5 presents definitions and examples of conceptual and data-based literature.

The usual sources of conceptual literature are books, chapters of books, and journal articles. The most common sources of data-based literature are journal articles, critique reviews, abstracts published in conference proceedings, professional and governmental reports, and unpublished doctoral dissertations. More data-based and conceptual articles are available on-line in full-text format. Note, however, that although a number of journals initially made their respective articles available for free on the **world wide web,** currently very few—if any—are free, except as noted

TABLE **4-3** Steps and Strategies for Searching for Literature

STEPS OF LITERATURE REVIEW	STRATEGY
Step I: Determine concept/issue/topic/problem	Keep focused on the types of patients/clients you deal with in your work setting. You know what works and does not work in the delivery of nursing care. In your student role, keep focused on the assignment's objective; use the literature to support opinions or develop a concept under discussion.
Step II: Identify variables/terms	Ask your reference librarian for help, and read the data-based guide books usually found near the computers used for student searches; include "research" as one of your variables.
Step III: Conduct computer search using fee-based recognized databases (electronic [inline or CD-ROM] and/or print)	Do it yourself or with the help of your librarian; it is essential to use at least two health-related databases, such as CINAHL, MedLine, or PubMed.
Step IV: Weed out irrelevant sources before printing	Scan through your search, read the abstracts provided, and mark only those that fit your topic; select "references", as well as "search history" and "full-text articles" if available, prior to printing your search or downloading it to a disk or e-mailing it to yourself.
Step V: Organize sources from printout for retrieval	Organize by journal type and year and reread abstracts to determine if the articles chosen are relevant and worth retrieving.
Step VI: Retrieve relevant sources	If an article is available on-line or in journals or microfiche, scan its abstract before printing or copying it to determine if it is worth your time and money to retrieve it.
Step VII: Copy articles	Save yourself time and money; buy a library copying card ahead of time or bring plenty of change, so that you avoid wasting time midway to secure change. Copy the entire article (including the references), making sure that you can clearly read the name of the journal, year, volume number, and pages; this can save you an immense amount of time when you are word processing your paper.
Step VIII: Conduct preliminary reading and weed out irrelevant sources	Review critical reading strategies (see Chapter 2) (e.g., read the abstract at the beginning of the article; see the example in this chapter).
Step IX: Critically read each source (summarize and critique each source)	Use the critical reading strategies from Chapter 2 (e.g., use a standardized critiquing tool); take the time to word process each summary, no more than 1 page long, include the reference in APA style at the top or bottom of each abstract, and staple copied article to back of summary.
Step X: Synthesize critical summaries of each article	Decide how you will present your synthesis of the reviewed articles (e.g., chronologically, according to type—data-based or conceptual), and word process the synthesized material and a reference list.

TABLE **4-4** Literature Review Synonyms

CONCEPTUAL LITERATURE	DATA-BASED LITERATURE
Theoretical literature	Empirical literature
Scholarly nonresearch literature	Scientific literature
Scholarly literature	Research literature
Soft- vs. hard-science	Scholarly research literature
Literature review article	Research study
Analysis article	Concept analysis (as methodology)
Integrative review	Study

TABLE **4-5** Types of Information Sources for a Review of Literature*

CONCEPTUAL LITERATURE	DATA-BASED LITERATURE
Published articles; documents; chapters in books; or books discussing theories, conceptual frameworks, and/or conceptual models, concept(s), constructs, theorems.	Published quantitative and qualitative studies, including concept analysis and/or methodology studies on a concept. Such material is found in journals, monographs, or books that are directly or indirectly related to the problem of interest.
Literature reviews of a concept that include both conceptual and data-based critiques.	Unpublished studies: master's theses and doctoral dissertations.
Proceedings and audiotapes and videotapes from scholarly conferences containing abstracts of a conceptual paper or the entire conceptual presentation.	Unpublished research abstracts or entire studies from print, audio, on-line: proceedings of conferences, compendiums, professional organizations' home pages, or listservs (see library/computer activities section in text).

*Many of the examples given are or will be available on-line.

in Table 4-8. Less-common and less-used sources of scholarly material are audiotapes, videotapes, personal communications (e.g., letters or telephone or in-person interviews), unpublished doctoral dissertations, and master's theses. Most computer searches have the feature of including the abstract (see Chapter 2) for the reference, as well as all of the references used in the article.

HELPFUL HINT The critical reading strategy (see Chapter 2) of scanning an article's abstract is very useful in helping to determine if the article is data-based or conceptual.

EXAMPLES OF THEORETICAL MATERIAL

Some conceptual or theoretical articles do not use the term *conceptual* in the title, yet on close review these articles are actually extensive literature reviews of both conceptual and data-based articles on a specific concept or variables. In other conceptual articles that literature reviews, you may see the following terms used interchangeably: *literature review, review of the literature,* and ***integrative review.*** The article by Neabel, Fothergill-Bourbonnais, and Dunning (2000), "Family assessment tools: A review of the literature from 1978-1997," illustrates this point. The authors state that they reviewed literature that was retrieved using electronic databases. Key words used for the search were: "acute care," "critical care," "tertiary care," "family needs," "family assessment," "family interventions," and "research instruments."

Determining whether an article is conceptual or data-based is discussed later in this chapter in the presentation on electronic search strategies. An example of a conceptual article is Lanuza, Lefaiver, and Farcas' (2000) paper entitled "Research on the quality of life of lung transplant candidates and recipients: an integrative review." Early in the article, the authors indicate that they used **CINAHL, MEDLINE,** and PubMed electronic databases and also conducted a hand "search of references cited in each relevant publication (from 1980 to early 1999)." The authors also included the key words used in their search. The reasons for conducting a hand or manual search when using electronic databases are discussed later in this chapter.

Another example of a conceptual article is Redeker's (2000) "Integrative review of sleep in acute care settings." The abstract clearly states that the purpose of the paper is to present a critique of the research related to the acutely ill hospitalized adults in relation to sleep pattern and intervention variables. In addition, it discusses the problems related to studying sleep in acute care settings and suggests future research. The title of Redeker's article suggested that it was a conceptual rather than a research article. For example, if the article's title were, "A study to determine the sleep patterns of hospitalized adults in the acute care setting," this would suggest that the article was data-based.

Do not assume that because an article's abstract uses terms such as *purpose, organizing framework, findings* and *conclusions* that it is a research study. For example, theses were used as subtitles or headings in Redeker's conceptual article.

HELPFUL HINT The differences between data-based and conceptual articles will become clear to you as you learn about the various types of quantitative and qualitative designs and become more familiar with the fact that some research journals include theoretical articles, as well as research articles.

As a rule of thumb, even if a research study does not obtain significant findings, it is still considered a data-based article. Also, conceptual articles do not use terminology such as *design, sample, experimental and control group, or methodology* as headings. When in doubt, ask your reference librarian or a faculty member to help you. Asking for clarification is a true sign of a critical thinker (Paul and Elder, 2001).

DATA-BASED MATERIAL

Nursing has an ever-growing body of data-based or research literature that focuses on testing various concepts, theories, or models, as well as a variety of variables related to the practice of nursing. Data-based articles are *primary sources.* For example, there are studies that tested components of Peplau's theory of "Interpersonal relations in nursing" (1952, 1991), such as the work of Forchuk (1993, 1994), Forchuk and Voorberg (1991), Forchuk and associates (2000), and Peden (1993, 1996, 1998)

Other examples of data-based articles and their foci are as follows:

- Mahon, Yarcheski, and Yarcheski (2000) investigated negative and positive outcomes of anger in early adolescents (see Appendix C). *Focus*—population problem.
- Cohen, Dunn, and Ley's (2000) phenomenological study generated specific nursing actions that bone marrow patients identified as helpful in decreasing their fear and helping them maintain hope (see Appendix B). *Focus*—Generation of theory.
- Bull, Hansen, and Gross (2000) compared the differences in outcomes for elderly hospital-

ized heart failure patients and their caregivers, as well as the costs related to hospital readmission and use of ER services after discharge between subjects who received the professional-patient partnership model of discharge planning and those who did not (see Appendix A). *Focus*—Nursing care delivery system.
- LoBiondo-Wood and associates' (2000) study explored the relationship between family stress, family coping, and family adaptation (see Appendix D). *Focus*—Exploration of population-specific problem.

Data-based articles may specifically indicate in their title that a study was conducted, but more often they do not. There are several ways to determine if an article is data-based. First, read the title and look for key words that suggest testing (e.g., effect, relationship, evaluation, exploration, cross-sectional, or longitudinal). Next, see which journal published the article. There are a number of journals that predominately publish research articles (e.g., *Nursing Research, Applied Nursing Research,* and *Research In Nursing and Health*). These hints are a beginning; the only way to determine if an article is actually a research study is to read the abstract and the article itself. A review of the abstracts of the studies that appear in Appendixes A, B, C, and D indicates that all of the articles are reports of completed studies.

REFEREED JOURNALS

A major portion of most literature reviews consists of journal articles. Journals are a ready source of the latest information on almost any conceivable subject. Unfortunately, books and texts—despite the inclusion of multiple data-based sources—take much longer to publish than journals. Therefore journals are the preferred mode of communicating the latest theory or results of a research study. As a beginning consumer of research, you should use **refereed** or **peer-reviewed journals** as your first source of primary scholarly literature. A refereed journal has a panel of external and internal reviewers (i.e., peer-reviewed) or editors who review sub-

TABLE **4-6**   Primary and Secondary Sources

PRIMARY: ESSENTIAL	SECONDARY: USEFUL
The person who conducted the study, developed the theory (model), or prepared the scholarly discussion on a concept, topic, or issue of interest (i.e., the original author).	Someone other than the original author (i.e., the person who conducted the original work—whether it's data-based or conceptual) writes or presents the author's original work. These are usually in the form of a summary and critiques (i.e., analysis and synthesis) of someone else's scholarly work.
Primary sources can be published or unpublished.	Secondary sources can be published or unpublished.
Data-based examples: An investigator's report of his or her research study (i.e., purpose or aims, questions/hypothesis[es], design/method, sample/setting, findings, results [e.g., articles in Appendixes A, B, C, and D]) is a primary source of data-based reports; McCloskey and Bulechek's (2000) book is a primary source for the data-based nursing intervention classification (NIC) system; Johnson and Maas's (2000) article is a primary source for this nursing outcomes classification (NOC) system. NANDA's taxonomy of nursing diagnoses (2001) is a primary source of these diagnoses and defining characteristics, many of which have been refined through research studies.	Response/commentary/critique articles of a research study, a theory/model, or a professional view of an issue; review of literature article published in a refereed scholarly journal; abstracts of a published work written by someone other than the original author; a doctoral dissertation's review of the literature.
Conceptual or theoretical example: A theorist's work reported in the literature by the author in an article, chapter of a book, or a book (Peplau, 1952, 1991).	Clark (1999) discusses standardized medical and nursing language with emphasis on the six ANA-approved taxonomies (i.e., NANDA, OMHAH, HHCC, NIC, NOC, Ozbolt Patient Care Dataset) included in the Unified Medical Language System (UMLS). Powelson and McGahan (2000) discuss how to introduce nursing language (taxonomies) in educational settings. Both articles are secondary sources of nursing taxonomies.
HINT: Critical evaluation of mainly primary sources is essential to a thorough and relevant review of the literature.	HINT: Use secondary sources sparingly; however, secondary sources—especially of studies that include a research critique—are a valuable learning tool for a beginning consumer of research.

mitted manuscripts for possible publication. The external reviewers are drawn from a pool of nurse scholars who are experts in various fields. In most cases, these reviews are "blind"; that is, the manuscript (i.e., research study or conceptual article) to be reviewed does not include the name of the author(s). The review panels use a set of scholarly criteria to judge whether a manuscript is worthy of publication that are similar to those used to judge the strengths and weaknesses of a study (see Chapter 19). The credibility of the reported research or conceptual article is enhanced through this peer-review process.

PRIMARY AND SECONDARY SOURCES

A credible literature review reflects the use of mainly *primary sources*. Table 4-6 gives the general definition and examples of these sources. Most primary sources are found in published literature. A *secondary source* often represents a response to or a summary and critique of a theorist's or researcher's work or an in-depth analysis of a topic/issue/problem/concept.

Box 4-3 lists journals that contain both primary and secondary articles. Table 4-6 highlights

BOX 4-3   Examples of Nursing Journals for Literature Reviews*

Advances in Nursing Science	Journal of Nursing Scholarship (formerly Image: Journal
American Journal of Critical Care	of Nursing Scholarship)
AORN Journal (Association of Operating Room Nurses)	Journal of Obstetric, Gynecologic and Neonatal Nursing
Applied Nursing Research	Journal of Professional Nursing
Archives of Psychiatric Nursing	Journal of Qualitative Research
Cancer Nursing	Journal of the American Psychiatric Nurses Association
Clinical Nurse Specialist	Journal of Transcultural Nursing
Clinical Nursing Research	Nurse Educator
Evidence Based Nursing	Nursing Diagnosis: The International Journal of Nurs-
Geriatric Nursing	ing Language and Classification (formerly Nursing
Heart & Lung	Diagnosis)
International Journal of Nursing Studies	Nursing Management
Issues in Comprehensive Pediatric Nursing	Nursing Outlook
Issues in Mental Health Nursing	Nursing Research
Journal of the American Psychiatric Nurses Association	Nursing Science Quarterly
Journal of Advanced Nursing	Oncology Nursing Forum
Journal of Clinical Nursing	Pediatric Nursing
Journal of Neonatal Nursing	Public Health Nursing
Journal of Nursing Administration (JONA)	Research in Nursing & Health
Journal of Nursing Care Quality	Scholarly Inquiry for Nursing Practice
Journal of Nursing Education	Western Journal of Nursing Research
Journal of Nursing Measurement	

*Main focus: Peer-reviewed journals, primary sources of research studies and conceptual articles; sources of some secondary sources (e.g., extensive reviews of literature on a particular concept) and issues, as well as responses or critiques of data-based and conceptual articles; most are refereed journals; all can be searched through CINAHL, PubMed, and MEDLINE, as well as other health-related computer and print databases.
Note: Many articles found in these journals are available on-line.

the differences between primary and secondary sources. Table 4-7 gives examples of primary and secondary print sources. There are two general reasons for using secondary sources. The first reason is that a primary source is literally unavailable. This is rarely the case in this age of computer searches and interlibrary loan. In addition, most libraries have the ability to copy an article and send or fax it to the person requesting the information. Also, many articles are available today as full-text articles on an electronic database. Another reason to use a secondary source is because it can provide different ways of looking at an issue or problem. Secondary sources can help you develop the ability to see things from another person's point of view, which is an essential aspect of critical reading (Paul and Elder, 2001). Secondary sources should not be over-

used, however—especially for literature reviews, although they can be very valuable to the beginning consumer of research.

Secondary sources published in refereed journals usually provide a critical evaluation of or a response to a theory or research study. These sources usually include implications for practice and/or the work's contributions to the development of nursing science. Some issues of the *Western Journal of Nursing Research* contain a critique, entitled "Commentary," that follows a published study. The *Annual Review of Nursing Research* (Fitzpatrick and Goeppinger, 2000) is another source of critiqued research.

Another secondary source that contains research evidence information presented in a distilled format is *Evidence-Based Nursing*, a publication of study abstracts. Each abstract includes a

TABLE **4-7**   Conceptual and Data-Based Examples of Primary and Secondary Journal Articles, Books, Chapters in Books, or Documents

PRIMARY	SECONDARY
JOURNAL ARTICLE Mahon NE, Yarcheski A, and Yarcheski TJ: Positive and negative outcomes of anger in early adolescents, *Research in Nursing & Health* 23:17-24, 2000 (see Appendix C). (Data-based)	**JOURNAL COMMENTARY** Cheater FM: Nursing home residents used 6 strategies to manage urinary incontinence...Commentary on Robinson, JP: Managing urinary incontinence in the nursing home: residents' perspectives, *Journal of Advanced Nursing* 31:68-77, 2000, *Evidence-Based Nursing* 3(4):136, 2000.
BOOK Peplau HE: *Interpersonal relations in nursing: a conceptual frame of reference for psychodynamic nursing,* New York, 1991, Springer. (Conceptual)	**BOOK** Fawcett J: *Contemporary nursing knowledge: nursing models and theories,* Philadelphia, 2000, FA Davis.
CHAPTER IN A BOOK Krainovich-Miller B and Rosedale M: Behavioral health home care. In Shea C et al, editors: *Advanced practice nursing in psychiatric and mental health care,* St Louis, 1999, Mosby.	**CHAPTER IN A BOOK** Belcher JR and Fish LJB: Hildegard E Peplau. In George JB, editor: *Nursing theories: the base for profession nursing practice,* ed 5, Norwalk, CT, in revision, 2001, Appleton & Lange.
DOCTORAL DISSERTATION Allison MJ: *The effect of a social cognitive theory-based intervention on self-efficacy and physical activity in older adults post coronary event,* The University of Texas Health Science Center at San Antonio, Dissertation Abstracts, 9967580, 2000.	**DOCUMENTS** Agency for Health Care Research and quality: *Garlic: effects on cardiovascular risks and disease, protective effects against cancer, and clinical adverse effects,* Evidence Report/Technology Assessment No. 20.2000 (AHRQ 01-E023), Rockville, MD, 2000, The Agency. Early HIV Infection Guideline Panel: *Evaluation and management of early HIV infection,* AHCPR Pub No 94-0572, Rockville, Md, 1994, Agency for Health Care Policy and Research, Public Health Service, US Department of Health and Human Services.
DOCUMENT American Nurses Association: *Scope and Standards of Practice for Nursing Professional Development,* Washington, DC, 2000, The Association.	

commentary relating the study's findings to practice. Secondary sources, especially those mentioned, are an important credible and time-saving measure that can help nurses keep up with the latest evidence for practice. As stressed earlier, to develop research critiquing competencies, research consumers must read primary sources and use standardized critiquing criteria (see Chapters 8 and 19). Consulting faculty, advisors, or librarians about secondary sources is an effective way to secure an appropriate resource.

HELPFUL HINT

- Remember that a secondary source of a theory or data-based study usually does not include all of the theory's concepts or aspects of a study, and/or definitions may not be fully presented.

- If concepts or variables are included, the definitions may be collapsed or paraphrased to such a degree that it no longer represents the theorist's actual work.
- Perhaps the critique (whether positive or negative) is based on the condensed summary or abstract; as such, it is less useful to the consumer.
- Read a primary data-based study, as well as a secondary source critique on the same study; compare your critique with the critique of the secondary source.

CONDUCTING A SEARCH AS A CONSUMER OF RESEARCH

Most students who are preparing an academic paper read the required course materials, as well as additional literature retrieved from the library.

Students often state, "I know how to do research." Perhaps you have thought the same thing because you researched a topic for a paper in the library. In this situation, however, it would be more accurate for you to say that you have been "searching" the literature to uncover knowledge to prepare an academic term paper on a certain topic.

Although reviewing the literature for research purposes and research consumer activities requires the same critical thinking and reading skills, a literature review for a research proposal is usually much more extensive. From an academic standpoint, requirements for a literature review for a particular assignment differ depending on the level and type of course, as well as the specific objective of the assignment. These factors determine whether a student's literature search requires a minor, selected, or cursory review (i.e., a limited review or a major or extensive review). Regardless, discovering knowledge is the goal of any "search;" therefore a consumer of research must know how to search the literature. Box 4-2 summarizes the important steps of a relevant review of the literature. Reference librarians are excellent people to ask about various sources of scholarly literature. If you are unfamiliar with the process of conducting a scholarly computer search, your reference librarian can certainly help.

TYPES OF RESOURCES

PRINT DATABASES

Before the 1980s, a search was usually done by hand using **print indexes** or **print databases.** This was a tedious and time-consuming process. Print indexes are actually a small portion of what is available electronically because the electronic format has virtually unlimited space. Print indexes (e.g., CINAHL's "red books" and *Index Medicus*) contain brief citations (e.g., those in a card catalog) and do not usually contain abstracts. Everything in the print index is in the **electronic database,** but the electronic database contains many more fields and much more information (Pravikoff and Donaldson, 2001). The

print indexes, however, are useful for finding sources that have not been entered into electronic databases. Print indexes and/or electronic databases are used to find journal sources (periodicals) of data-based and conceptual articles on a variety of topics (e.g., doctoral dissertations), as well as the publications of professional organizations and various governmental agencies.

Card catalogues are used to secure books, monographs, conference proceedings, master's theses, and doctoral dissertations. Box 4-4 lists examples of the more commonly used print indexes that are still published; noted next to each print database is its electronic counterpart. Today, databases are accessed by computer either using the web for on-line direct or via a vendor service or using a CD-ROM version. These electronic databases include sources from whatever date the particular database added an electronic version, as well as from a few years before the database became electronic (e.g., the CINAHL database via the computer access [on-line or CD-ROM] contains sources from 1982 to the present, whereas the print index covers 1956 to the present). The most relevant and frequently used print source for nursing literature remains the **Cumulative Index to Nursing and Allied Health Literature** print index, which is also known as the "Red Books." It covers all nursing and related literature from 1956 to the present. Print resources are still necessary if a search requires materials not entered into an electronic database before a certain year or if a library does not have electronic databases.

INTERNET: ON-LINE DATABASES

The **internet** is a global resource, which is a rather broad term that describes an international network that links a cadre of participating networks (e.g., commercial, educational, and governmental agencies). These resources share computer power, software, and information. Many uses for the internet are beyond the objectives of this chapter, although the internet's main objective of communication is in concert with the ob-

BOX 4-4   Common Print Databases

INDEXES

Cumulative Index to Nursing and Allied Health Literature (CINAHL)
- Initially called Cumulative Index to Nursing Literature
- First published in 1956
- Print version known as the "Red Books"
- Electronic version available as part of the OVID on-line service

Index Medicus (IM)
- Published by the National Library of Medicine in the United States
- Oldest health-related index, first published in 1879
- Includes literature from medicine, allied health, biophysical sciences, humanities, veterinary medicine, and nursing from 1960 to the present
- The electronic version, MEDLINE, covers 1966 to the present and is available on the web via OVID or PubMed

Psychological Abstracts
- Cover 1927 to the present
- Electronic version, PsychINFO, is available via the web

International Nursing Index (INI)
- Quarterly publication of American Journal of Nursing Company in cooperation with National Library of Medicine
- Started in 1966
- Includes over 200 journals of all languages, includes nursing publications in nonnursing journals

Nursing Studies Index
- Developed by Virginia Henderson
- Publishes nursing literature, as well as from other disciplines (see INI above), from 1900 to 1959

Hospital and Health Administration Index (HHAI)
- Formerly known as *Hospital Literature Index (HLI)*
- Published in 1945 by the American Hospital Association in cooperation with the National Library of Medicine (NLM)
- Included over 700 journals and related journals from the IM
- Main focus is hospital administration and delivery of care

Current Index to Journals in Education (CIJE)
- First published in 1969 in cooperation with the Educational Resources Information Center (ERIC)
- An electronic version, ERIC, is available on the web

CARD CATALOGUES

List books, monographs, theses, dissertations, audiovisuals, and conference proceedings

ABSTRACT REVIEWS

Dissertation Abstracts International, Master's Abstracts, Nursing Abstracts, Psychological Abstracts, and *Sociological Abstracts*

---

jectives of this chapter. Table 4-8 presents several internet sites and their usefulness for conducting a literature review.

E-mail and searching the world wide web (www), which is commonly referred to as the "web," are important to learn but have varying levels of usefulness for research consumers. When you access a **web browser** (e.g., Netscape Communicator or Internet Explorer), you can search the various web sites listed in Table 4-8. Basically, communication software allows computers to talk to each other. The web, in addition to text capabilities, also has video, audio, and nontext capabili-

ties because of its hypertext interface. There is little quality control over what is put on various web sites, so beginning consumers of research should not consider this a primary way of searching the literature (McKibbon and Marks, 1998). It is the internet, however, that enables you to access potentially useful health-related databases (e.g., CINAHL and MEDLINE), as well as other consumer health-education web sites.

Table 4-8 presents a number of web sites and indicates both the strengths and weaknesses of each in terms of meeting the objectives of a scholarly literature search. Many of these on-line

TABLE **4-8**   Selected Examples of Web Sites and Outcomes
              for Literature Searches

SITE	SOURCES	OUTCOMES FOR LITERATURE REVIEW
Online Journal of Issues in Nursing: Site can be linked from *www.ana.org* and visa-versa; online journal owned by Kent University College of Nursing and published in partnership with the American Nurses Association's (ANA) *Nursing World*	Service offered without charge, simply join by entering your e-mail address; site will keep you posted of new articles; peer-reviewed electronic journal providing a fee forum of discussion of issues in nursing	Limited for scholarly review of data-based literature when used as only source; only able to access literature that is published on the *Online Journal of Issues in Nursing;* source of complete articles from this site's journal, can be printed; interesting site for students in beginning courses in nursing (especially in courses in issues and trends) or practicing nurses; able to link to nursing's professional nursing association (ANA); journal can be accessed via CINAHL
AORN Online (Association of Operating Room Nurses, Inc., *www.aorn.org:* able to many other sites	General information about AORN, events, research activities and funding, has numerous nursing and health-related links; library has limited direct access to sources; some theses, dissertations, research papers available but in PDF format, which requires Adobe's Acrobat Reader to launch and display	Very limited for scholarly review of data-based literature if used as only source; links to Medline database, but anything published related to nursing is in CINAHL database, so both are needed; interesting way to keep up with a specialty; able to discuss research projects AORN is currently involved in; offers additional services to members
Sigma Theta Tau International (STTI): *www.nursingsociety. org,* Honor Society of Nursing	Visit and update on news and activities of the society; three online research sources available through links to Virginia Henderson International Library: *Registry of Nursing Research (RNR), Journal of Knowledge Synthesis for Nursing (OJKSN),* and *Nursing Knowledge Indexes*	For a fee, an online literature search via Medline can be requested (see Box 4-6 for advantages of CINAHL with MEDLINE); limited for scholarly review of data-based literature if used as the only search tool; OJKSN literature limited to studies published in STTI on-line journal; RNR contains over 11,000 English language international nursing studies, which are not peer-reviewed
National Institute of Nursing Research: *www.nih.gov/ninr*	Promotes science for nursing practice, funding for nursing and interdisciplinary research, and nurse scientist training programs; provides links to many nursing organizations and search sites; excellent site for graduate students	Although able to link to CRISP (Computer Retrieval of Information on Scientific Projects) and PubMed (National Library of Medicine's search service), which accesses literature via Medline and PreMEDLINE and other related material from on-line journals, this is a LIMITED site for the beginning consumer of research for conducting scholarly review of nursing data-based literature because MEDLINE alone does not include all nursing literature; searching CINAHL and MedLine on your own would be your first choice; useful site for graduate students in addition to CINAHL and MEDLINE and a third database related to topic
Graduate Research in Nursing: *www. graduateresearch.com*	On-line journal and search site; provides other opportunities to join listserv groups, employment opportunities and practice products; subscribe using e-mail address; graduate students might find it worth exploring	Limited site for the beginning consumer of research for scholarly electronic data-based searches; valuable site for graduate students for networking; potential source of additional data-based material not found in CINAHL and MedLine

SITE	SOURCES	OUTCOMES FOR LITERATURE REVIEW
Midwest Nursing Research Society (MNRS) www.mnrs.org	Web page: site/members share information on nursing research, funding, and its organization; links to other nursing sites as well as related health care sites.	Limited site for the beginning consumer of research for scholarly electronic data-based searches; graduate students may seek research grant information (see Box 4-6)
www.Allnurses.com	Offers discussions, ability to browse nursing web sites, and join discussions; connects to search tools and nursing literature, as well as student organizations and nursing specialties; can subscribe to a free nursing newsletter	Limited site for the beginning consumer of research for scholarly electronic data-based searches; students and practicing nurses may find the discussion/chat room interesting; reported that nurses use this site for surfing (see Box 4-6)
Clinical Evidence: www.clinical evidence.org	Fee-based subscription from British Medical Journal Publishing Group. On-line full-text compendium of summaries of current knowledge on clinical conditions based on literature sources and reviews; updated and expanded every 6 months; each issue is peer-reviewed by renowned group of international experts	Costly for individuals to subscribe; determine if your institution's (work or school) library is a subscriber; limited site for the beginning consumer of research because this is a "secondary" source of information; instead choose CINAHL, MEDLINE, and another electronic database (see Box 4-6)
Agency for Health Research and Quality (formerly Agency for Health Care Policy and Research) www.ahrq.gov	AHRQ supports the development of evidence reports through its 12 evidence-based Practice Centers and the dissemination of evidence-based guidelines through the Agency's National Guideline Clearinghouse for the improvement of health outcomes	Free source of primary sources of clinical guidelines; can be printed; latest research activities, newest evidence-based guidelines, and previous clinical practice guidelines developed when it was known as AHCPR; important source of latest governmental documents for both consumers and conductors of research; these governmental guidelines are not available through CINAHL and other electronic databases
Cochrane Library www.cochrane.org includes Cochrane Database of Systematic Reviews (COCH), Database of Abstracts of Reviews of Effectiveness, the Cochrane Controlled Trials Register, the Cochrane Methodology Register, Health Technology Assessment database (HTA), and the NHS Economic Evaluation Database (NHS EED); considered a database rather than a website	An electronic publication designed to supply high-quality evidence to inform people providing and receiving care, and those responsible for research, teaching, funding and administration at all levels	Abstracts of Cochrane Reviews are available without charge and can be browsed or searched; uses many databases in its reviews including CINAHL and MEDLINE; some are primary sources (e.g., systematic reviews/meta-analyses), others (if commentaries of single studies) are a secondary source; important source for clinical evidence but limited as a provider of primary documents for literature reviews

Continued

TABLE **4-8**   Selected Examples of Web Sites and Outcomes
for Literature Searches—cont'd

SITE	SOURCES	OUTCOMES FOR LITERATURE REVIEW
Intelihealth: *www.intelihealth.com*	Group of individuals interested in promoting good health who review trusted sources of information, including Harvard Medical School's consumer health information; funded by Aetna U.S. Healthcare	Limited as a source of primary data-based studies; free site that summarizes clinical information for the consumer drug search; medical dictionary; provides government sources of information on a variety of topics
Net Med: *www.netmed.com*	Provides a link of medical topics and disciplines; able to link to primary and secondary sources of information	Limited as a primary source of data-based studies of a literature review; free site; provides links to other sources of information

services require some type of additional cost to individuals in order to subscribe, as well as additional software program(s) so that information can be read when downloaded.

HELPFUL **HINT**

- Find someone who is experienced in using the internet in order to learn how to more easily access your academic institution's or health care agency's library's electronic databases. Watch what they do. Make sure you find time to learn it and do it.
- Make sure you have enough hard drive space to accommodate new software browser programs.
- As a student, find out what electronic library resources you can access on-site, as well as from home.

The number of nursing sites, web home pages, and chat rooms available via the web is growing daily. Many schools of nursing and individual nurses and nursing organizations have web sites, but they are too numerous to list in this chapter. Although you may find that some of these sites provide interesting information, surfing the web can be time-consuming and is not an effective use of your time because health-information and/or nursing sites and chat rooms generally do not provide scholarly literature search-and-retrieval capabilities anywhere similar to that of the CINAHL database or the other fee-based databases, several examples of which are listed in Table 4-9.

Most electronic databases require a subscription fee for access, as well as additional computer software programs. The most important strategy that you can use in conducting a scholarly literature search is to familiarize yourself with the electronic databases that are listed in Box 4-5.

PERFORMING A COMPUTER SEARCH

WHY A COMPUTER SEARCH?

Perhaps you are still not convinced that computer searches are the best way to acquire information for a review of the literature. Maybe you have gone to the library, taken out a few of the latest journals and tried to find a few related articles. This is an understandable temptation, especially if your assignment only requires you to use five articles. Try to think about it once again from another perspective and ask yourself the following question: "Is this the most appropriate and efficient way to find out what is the latest research on a topic that impacts patient care?" If you take the time to learn how to do a sound electronic search, you will have the essential competency needed for your career in nursing.

If you are still intimidated by the computer, it would be better for you to use CINAHL Information Systems' print indexes (the "Red Book"),

TABLE **4-9** On-Line Databases: Examples of Fee-Based Databases

ELECTRONIC DATABASE	SOURCES: DATA-BASED AND CONCEPTUAL LITERATURE
CINAHL (Cumulative Index to Nursing and Allied Health Literature) • 1982 to present • Available as part of OVID on-line service	Citations articles in journals in the nursing and allied health fields (e.g., medical technology, health care administration) and publications of the ANA and NLN
MEDLINE (medical literature analysis and retrieval system on-line) • 1966 to present • Available as part of OVID online service • On the web via PubMed search service	Produced by the National Library of Medicine; citations and some abstracts to articles on health-related topics for over 3,600 biomedical and nursing journals; search service provides access to over 11 million citations in MEDLINE and PreMEDLINE and other related databases, with links to participating on-line journals
PsychINFO	Covers professional and academic literature in psychology and related disciplines; worldwide coverage of over 1300 journals in 20 languages; books and chapters in books in English

BOX 4-5 Advantages of Using Multiple On-Line Fee-Based Databases: CINAHL and MEDLINE for Nurse Consumers of Research*

QUICK

On-line information can be instantly accessed, especially if you have a LAN/cable connection (as opposed to a modem/telephone connection). Internet access depends on a number of factors (e.g., the server may be "down" or the number of users can affect your ability to access the information [i.e., the number of users slows down access]). CD-ROM versions can be faster and more dependable than on-line access.

MULTIPLE DATABASES INCREASES ACCESS TO MULTIPLE SOURCES

Using multiple databases allows you to cover a broad scope of sources. CINAHL accesses more than 600,000 records from 1982 to the present (e.g., journals, books, chapters in books, abstracts, software, audiovisual). MEDLINE provides access to over 3,600 biomedical and nursing and related journals (i.e., over 11 million citations).

ALLOWS KEYWORD SEARCHING

Synonyms and related terms are considered; you can use the thesaurus for each database. For data-based literature include the terms *systematic reviews* and *meta analysis.* Keep refining your search by combining terms with Boolean connectors (e.g., *and, or,* and *not*). CINAHL

uses ANA-approved taxonomy terms (*NANDA, NIC, NOC, OMAHA,* and *HHC*) (McCormick et al, 1994).

SOURCE OF ABSTRACTS AND SOME FULL-TEXT ARTICLES AVAILABLE

IMPORTANT SOURCES OF DATA-BASED LITERATURE

Access to clinical trials, meta-analysis, systematic reviews, methodologies, conceptual frameworks, and variables. All research instruments are identified.

FREQUENT UPDATES

These databases are updated monthly or weekly.

DOCUMENT RETRIEVAL

Documents can be retrieved via e-mail, downloaded to disk, and/or delivered via fax or mail for CINAHL direct and PubMed.

SAVES TIME AND INCREASES CREDIBILITY OF SEARCH

*Access time and all features are not available with print index. (From CINAHL Information Systems: *Recent statistics for the CINAHL database,* Glendale, CA, 2000, CINAHL Information Systems. Retrieved 1/10/01 from www.cinahl.com/prodsvcs. cinahldb.htm and the National Library of Medicine. PubMed information from www.ncbi.nlm.nih.gov/PubMed/

even though you will have to write out each relevant reference you find unless you have access to a copier, in which case, you could copy each page an entry is on. This can be a very time-consuming and costly proposition, how-

ever, but at least you would have all of the necessary information for retrieving the articles. If you are doing your search by hand and cannot photocopy the CINAHL entry, determine your library's protocol for retrieving journals and

CRITICAL THINKING DECISION PATH | Consumer of Research Literature Review

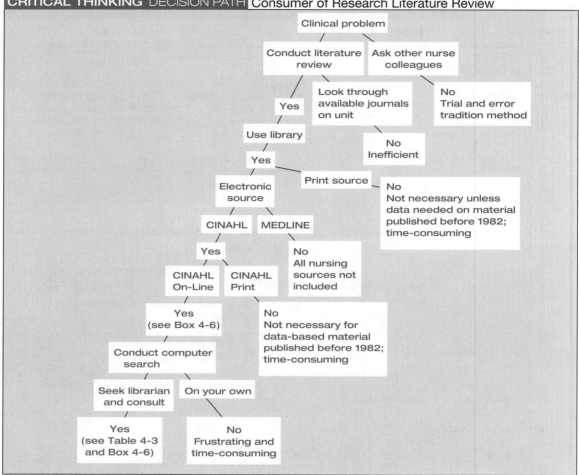

books (i.e., what type of call slip is used) and write the information from the print index directly on to the appropriate "call slip." It is strongly suggested that you *try at least once* to do a CINAHL computer search; you will see how easy it is to do and feel confident that you did a thorough search. You will also avoid the pitfall of missing important studies that may not appear in just the past few journals taken off the library shelf or borrowed from a friend. The critical-thinking decision path illustrates how to conduct a research consumer-focused computer literature search.

HELPFUL HINT First think of a CINAHL computer search. It can facilitate all steps of critically reviewing the literature, especially Steps III, IV, and V (see Table 4-3).

HOW FAR BACK MUST THE SEARCH GO?

Students often ask questions such as "How many articles do I need?," "How much is enough?," and "How far back in the literature do I need to go?" When conducting a search, you must specify the range of years for the search (e.g., 1991 to 2001), as well as the variables (i.e., key words) and other factors (e.g., "research," "abstract," or "full text"), or you may end up with hundreds or thousands of citations. Ending up with so many citations is usually a sign that there was something wrong with your search technique. Each electronic database offers an explanation of each feature; it is worth your time to click on each icon and explore the explanations offered because this will increase your confidence.

A general timeline for most academic or evidenced-based practice papers/projects is to go back in the literature at least 3 but preferably 5 years; although a research project may warrant going back 10 or more years. Extensive literature reviews on particular topics or a concept clarification methodology study helps you to limit the length of your search.

As you scroll through and mark the citations you wish to include in your downloaded or printed search, make sure you review all the fields of the citation manager. In addition to indicating which citations you want and choosing which fields to search (e.g., citation plus abstract or ASCII full text [if available]), there is an opportunity to indicate if you want the "search history" included. It is always a good idea to include this information. It is especially helpful if your instructor suggests that some citations were missed because you can then produce your search and together figure out what variable(s) you missed so that you do not make the same error next time. This is also your opportunity to indicate if you want to e-mail the search to yourself.

WHAT DO I NEED TO KNOW?

Each database usually has a specific search guide that provides information on the organization of the entries and the terminology used. The following suggestions and strategies incorporate general search strategies, as well as those related to CINAHL and MEDLINE. Finding the right variables/concepts/terms to "plug in" as key words for a computer search is an important aspect of conducting a search. Both databases are very user friendly in regard to this aspect of your search; they have "explode" features (i.e., you can search multiple headings with a single command). Another feature of this program is its mapping capability. If the term you use is not exactly the same as is in the database, the program maps or connects you to a term nearest to what you typed in (CINAHL, 2001). Both databases have assigned index terms known in CINAHL as medical headings and in MEDLINE as MeSH. It is important to combine index terms and to expect to do a number of search histories. This may sound like it will take a great deal of time, but it does not. Once you type in your keywords and choose "perform search," the results come up almost instantly. If you are still having difficulty, do not hesitate to ask your reference librarian.

Box 4-6 offers a quick overview of how user friendly using these two databases can be; it provides a number of helpful hints that literally walk you through the steps of a search. This particular protocol is based on using CINAHL and MEDLINE. Of course the specifics may differ in your institution but there are more similarities than differences. The example given in Table 4-10 indicates the number of citations retrieved using two databases at once, CINAHL and MEDLINE. After choosing the tab on the menu "Choose more than one database," the keywords *depression* and *treatment* were entered and the search performed. As indicated in Table 4-10, the first search revealed 6,679 citations, which is a very good indication that you did not narrow your keywords sufficiently. This is far too many citations to scroll through. In addition to the number of citations retrieved, the first few citations usually appear. In this example, the first few were found in the CINAHL database. In the next search, the keywords were combined (e.g. "depression and treatment" and "nursing intervention and adults"). The publication years were limited to six (1995 to 2001), and "research" and "full-text available" were checked off. Table 4-10 indicates that the next search history (indicated as numbers 2 to 5 in Table 4-10) revealed a more useful number of retrievals. Search history number 2 indicates 109 research citations; number 3 indicates 11 research citations are available as full text; and per search histories number 4 and 5, eight citations resulted. A review of the actual citations in

BOX 4-6   Helpful Hints: Using CINAHL and MEDLINE On-Line via OVID

- Connect to your library's electronic databases via your internet server. Choose "Health Sciences Related Database" or determine which general category houses CINAHL on the menu. Then hit "Enter."
- An alphabetical list of databases usually appears. Scroll down to "CINAHL." In the next column, the source of the database is indicated (e.g., on the web); place your cursor on this term and hit "Enter."
- The "Choose a Database" menu will appear. You can either choose one database or choose the tab that indicates that you can choose more than one database. It is recommended that you use at least two databases. Choose "Select more than one database to search."
- Once the next menu pops up, mark each of the databases you wish to search (e.g., CINAHL [1982 to December 2000] and MEDLINE [1997 to December Week 4 2000]).
- Your next screen will indicate at the top that you are using CINAHL and MEDLINE databases. It asks you to type in the keyword or phrase for your search history. Don't hesitate to explore the various icons that appear at the top of the menu. You can search by author, title, or particular journal. Another useful icon is the "?" or "Help" icon.
- Type in your keyword or phrase (e.g., "nursing intervention and depression"). Do not use complete sentences. (Ask your librarian for the manual guide for each database.)

- Each word is searched separately, and "hits" (i.e., a set of corresponding items) are created for each word.
- Before choosing "Perform search," make sure you mark "Save search history," limit the years of publication according to the objectives of your assignment, and indicate if you are limiting it to "Research" and/or "Abstracts" or "Full text available."
- See the results in Table 4-10 that used the terms *treatment* and *depression:* 6,679 citations were retrieved. This first history did not "limit," as was suggested here. Before performing the search, the program may ask you to limit your search by providing various keywords or phrases for you to mark either "focus" or "explode" (i.e., narrowing or broadening your search).
- Add additional variables to narrow your search (e.g., "nursing intervention"). Mark any additional limitations by typing in the "Keyword" box "#1" and "nursing intervention" and marking the appropriate "limit to" categories.
- Using the Boolean connector "and" between each of the above words you wish to use plus additional variables narrows your search. Using the Boolean "or" broadens your search.
- Boolean connectors save time because you don't have to retype each search word.
- Once the search results appear and you determine that they're manageable, you can decide whether to review them on screen, print them, save them to disk, or e-mail them to yourself (i.e., in the NYU, Bobst Library, CINAHL, MEDLINE OVID Search).

searches number 4 and 5 were exactly the same. At this point, the choice is whether to scroll through the 109 research entries and mark off those that best meet your assigned objective, or to download this search to a disk or e-mail it to your home e-mail address or print it at this time. The advantage is that you have not only the choice but also the ability to retrieve 11 of these citations as full-text articles.

This is a typical computer search using two databases (CINAHL and MEDLINE). The main focus of this search was on retrieving nursing research related to nursing interventions for adults diagnosed with depression. Using the Boolean connector "and" with nursing interventions re-

sulted in 109 entries (see the explanation of the Boolean connector "and" in Box 4-6). This was a manageable number to review on screen by quickly reading over the abstracts and marking some for print retrieval. Do not forget to mark off the appropriate circles in the "citation," "fields," "citation format," and "action" columns, as well as to check off the box "include search history" before printing your search. The "complete reference" option should be checked in the "fields" column; although this makes for a long print job, you will often come across some classic document or one that was not entered in the computer database because it was published before 1982. If you intend to download your search to a 3.5″ mi-

TABLE **4-10** Example of CINAHL, MEDLINE, OVID Search

STEP 1: INITIAL TRY

#	Search History	Results	Display
1	(depression and treatment). mp. [mp = ti, sh, ab, it, rrw]	6,679	Display

0 Saved Searches   0 Save Search History   0 Delete Searches   0 Remove Duplicates

Enter Keyword or Phrase

	Perform Search

Limit to:
    Abstracts   Consumer Health Journals   English Language
    Full Text Available   Review Articles Human   Latest Update   Research
Publication Year

	⇩		⇧	

Ask A Librarian

STEP 2: SECOND TRY

#	Search History	Results	Display
2	(nursing interventions and adults).mp	109	Display
3	Limit 4 to full text available	11	Display
4	Limit 5 to research [Limit not valid in: MEDLINE; records were retained]	8	Display
5	Limit 6 to yr = 1995-2001	8	Display

Modified from CINAHL, MEDLINE, OVID search

crodisk, make sure you include this option. When you upload it on your PC, you will be able to retrieve all of your references, as well as the references of each entry, into your word processing program. Think how much time you will save! Your reference list will be typed, and you will only have to do some editing to put it into the style required by your instructor.

If, as suggested, you did your preliminary reading of available abstracts as you marked an entry before printing your search, you should be ready to retrieve and photocopy each article you select except for the 11 that were available as full text. Having a copy of each article will allow you to organize them for priority critical reading.

HOW DO I COMPLETE THE SEARCH?

Now the truly important aspect of the search begins: your critical reading of the retrieved materials. Critically reading scholarly material, especially data-based articles, requires several readings and the use of critiquing criteria (see Chapters 2, 8, and 19). Do not be discouraged if all of the retrieved articles are not as useful as you first thought; this happens to the most experienced researcher. If most of the articles are not useful, be prepared to do another search, but discuss the variables you will use next time with your instructor and/or the reference librarian and you may very well want to add a third database. In the previous example of interventions with adults diagnosed with depression, the third database of choice may be PsychINFO (see Table 4-9). Remind yourself how quickly you will be able to do it, now that you are experienced. It is also a good idea to review the references of your articles; if any seem relevant, you can retrieve them.

LITERATURE REVIEW FORMAT: WHAT TO EXPECT

Becoming familiar with the format of the literature review helps research consumers use critiquing criteria to evaluate the review. To decide which style you will use so that your review is presented in a logical and organized manner, you must consider the following:

- The research question/topic.
- The number of retrieved sources reviewed.
- The number and type of data-based vs. conceptual materials.

Some reviews are written according to the variables being studied and presented chronologically under each variable. Others present the material chronologically with subcategories or variables discussed within each period. Still others present the variables and include subcategories related to the study's type or designs or related variables.

An example of a literature review that is logically presented according to the variables under study was completed by Bull, Hansen, and Gross (2000, Appendix A). The researchers stated that they were examining the differences in several outcomes noted in elderly patients with heart failure and caregivers and the type of discharge planning that was used. The authors did not label the first four introductory paragraphs as a review of the literature, but literature was presented related to the problem under study. The next section of the paper was labeled "background." In these four paragraphs, a review of the research, as well as conceptual literature on the variables under study, were presented.

In contrast to the styles of previous quantitative studies, the literature reviews of qualitative studies are usually handled in a different manner (see Chapters 6, 7, and 8). There is often little known about the topic under study, or the very nature of the qualitative design dictates that a review of the literature be conducted after the study is completed; then the researchers compare the literature review with their findings. In some cases, the reviewed literature is used during the analysis process. For example, Cohen and Ley's (2000, Appendix B) phenomenological study presented the experiences of patients undergoing bone marrow transplantation and their views of specific nursing actions that would assist them during this process. These researchers used the reviewed literature related to the study in their "discussion," "implications," and "conclusion" sections.

CRITIQUING Criteria for a Review of the Literature

As you analyze (critique) a scholarly report, you must use appropriate criteria. If you are reading a research study, it must be evaluated in terms of each step of the research process. The characteristics of a relevant review of the literature (see Box 4-2) and the purposes of the review of the literature (see Box 4-1) provided the framework for developing the evaluation criteria for a literature review. Difficulties that research consumers might have regarding this task and related strategies are presented after a discussion of the critiquing criteria. For a more in-depth discussion of critiquing criteria see Chapters 8 and 19.

Critiquing the literature review of data-based or conceptual reports is a challenging task for the research consumers. Critiquing criteria have been developed for all aspects of the quantitative research process, for various quantitative designs and qualitative approaches, and for research consumer projects for educational and clinical settings. Critiquing criteria for the review of the literature are usually presented from the quantitative research

---

CRITIQUING CRITERIA

1. What gaps or inconsistencies in knowledge does the literature review uncover?
2. How does the review reflect critical thinking?
3. Are all of the relevant concepts and variables included in the review?
4. Does the summary of each reviewed study reflect the essential components of the study design (e.g., in a quantitative design: type and size of sample, instruments; validity and reliability; in a qualitative design: does it indicate the type [e.g., phenomenologic])?
5. Does the critique of each reviewed study include strengths, weaknesses, or limitations of the design; conflicts; and gaps or inconsistencies in information related to the area of interest?
6. Are both conceptual and data-based literature included?
7. Are primary sources mainly used?
8. Is there a written summary synthesis of the reviewed scholarly literature?
9. Does the synthesis summary follow a logical sequence that leads the reader to reason(s) why the particular research or nonresearch project is needed?
10. Does the organization of the reviewed studies (e.g., chronologically, according to concepts/variables, or by type/design/level of study) flow logically, enhancing the reader's ability to evaluate the need for the particular research or nonresearch project?
11. Does the literature review follow the purpose(s) of the study or nonresearch project?

---

process perspective. Because the focus of this book is on the baccalaureate nurse in the research consumer role, the critiquing criteria for the literature review incorporate this frame of reference. The processes used in qualitative studies are specifically presented in Chapter 8, and Chapter 19 presents an overview of evaluating quantitative research studies. The important issue is for the reader to determine the overall value of the data-based or conceptual report. Does the review of the literature permeate the report? Does the review of the literature contribute to the significance of the report in relation to nursing theory, research, education, or practice (see Figure 4-1)? The overall question to be answered is, "Does the review of the literature uncover knowledge?" This question is based on the overall purpose of a review of the literature, which is to uncover knowledge (see Box 4-1). The major goal turns into the question, "Did the review of the literature provide a strong knowledge base to carry out the reported research or scholarly educational or clinical practice setting project?" The Critiquing Criteria box provides questions for the consumer of research to ask about literature review.

Questions related to the logical presentation of the reviewed articles are somewhat more challenging for beginning consumers of research. The more

you read scholarly articles, the easier this question is to answer. At times, the type of question being asked in relation to the particular concept lends itself to presenting the reviewed studies chronologically (i.e., perhaps beginning with early or landmark data-based or conceptual literature).

Questions must be asked about whether each explanation of a step of the research process met or did not meet these guidelines (criteria). For instance, Box 4-1 illustrates the overall purposes of a literature review. The second objective listed states that the review of the literature is to determine gaps, consistencies, and inconsistencies in the literature about a subject, concept, or problem. The guide questions in Table 19-1 (see Chapter 19) is, "What gaps or conflicts in knowledge about the problem are identified? How does this study intend to fill those gaps or resolve those conflicts?" In this example, the purpose or objective of the literature review became the evaluation question or criterion for critiquing the review of the literature.

Two other important questions to ask are, "Were both conceptual and data-based literature included?" and "Does the review consist of mainly primary sources?" Other sets of critiquing criteria may phrase these questions differently or more broadly. For instance, the question may be, "Does the literature search seem adequate?" or "Does the report demonstrate scholarly writing?" These may seem to be difficult questions for you to answer; one place to begin, however, is by determining whether the source is a refereed journal. It is fairly reasonable to assume that a scholarly refereed journal publishes manuscripts that are adequately searched, use mainly primary sources, and are written in a scholarly manner. This does not mean, however, that every study reported in a refereed journal will meet all of the criteria in an equal manner. Because of style differences and space constraints, each citation summarized is often very brief or related citations may be summarized as a group and lack a critique. You still must answer the critiquing questions. Consultation with a faculty advisor may be necessary to develop skill in answering this question.

A literature review in a research article should reflect a synthesis or putting together of the main points or value of all the sources reviewed in relation to the study's research question (see Box 4-1). The relationship between and among these studies must be explained. The synthesis of a written review of the literature usually appears at the end of the review section before the research question or hypothesis reporting section. If not labeled as such, it is usually evident in the last paragraph. Therefore demonstrating synthesis becomes an essential critiquing criterion for the review of the literature.

Although Bull, Hansen, and Gross (2000) (see Appendix A) do not label their reviewed data-based literature as a review of the literature, the last paragraph of the section labeled as "background" is a summary and synthesis of the reviewed studies relating to their study. They stated the following:

"Although some previous studies emphasize outcomes in terms of resource consumption, others emphasized outcomes important to the elder patients such continuity of information, the ability to function in their environment, having access to services to assist them with managing their care and satisfaction with the plan of care (Bull, 1994a; Proctor et al, 1992). Similar outcomes seem appropriate for caregivers who assist elders in managing their care following discharge. Addressing the needs of caregivers is a vital component in meeting elders' needs and maintaining their independent living arrangements (Bull, Maruyama, and Luo, 1995)."

The preceding summary synthesis meets the objective of uncovering knowledge, determining what is known and not known, and finding gaps and inconsistencies in the literature. The synthesis was brief, yet it provided enough data to conclude that their literature review reflected critical thinking and scholarly writing, as well as provided the bridge or reason for carrying out the study. This example specifically addresses a number of the questions found in the Critiquing Criteria box.

Critiquing a review of the literature is an acquired skill. Continue reading and rereading, as well as seeking advice from faculty. Think about using the literature review as your essential key to implementing a research-based practice.

Critical Thinking Challenges

Barbara Krainovich-Miller

- ➤ How is it possible that the review of the literature can be both an individual step of the research process and a research component used in each of the steps of the process? Support your answer with specific examples.
- ➤ How does a researcher justify using both conceptual and data-based literature in a literature review; and would you—for research consumer purposes (e.g., developing an academic scholarly paper)—use the same types of literature?
- ➤ A classmate in your research class tells you that she has access to the internet and can do all of her searches from home. What essential questions do you need to ask her to determine if database sources can be accessed?
- ➤ An acute care agency's nursing research committee is developing a research-based practice protocol for patient-controlled analgesia (PCA). One suggestion is to use AHCPR's *Pain Guideline* (1992), and another is to conduct a review of the literature from the past 6 years on pain control. How would you settle the question—which one of these suggestions will most effectively contribute to the goal of a research-based protocol?

Key Points

- The review of the literature is defined as a broad, comprehensive, in-depth, systematic critique of scholarly publications, unpublished scholarly print and on-line materials, audiovisual materials, and personal communications.
- The review of the literature is used for development of research studies, as well as other consumer of research activities such as development of evidence-based practice protocols and scholarly conceptual papers for publications.
- The main objectives for the consumer of research in relation to conducting and writing a literature review are to acquire the ability to do the following: (1) conduct an appropriate electronic data-based and/or print data-based search on a topic; (2) efficiently retrieve a sufficient amount of scholarly materials for a literature review in relation to the topic and scope of project; (3) critically evaluate (i.e., critique) data-based and conceptual material based on accepted critiquing criteria; (4) critically evaluate published reviews of the literature based on accepted standardized critiquing criteria; and (5) synthesize the findings of the critique materials for relevance to the purpose of the selected scholarly project.
- Primary data-based and conceptual resources are essential for literature reviews.
- Secondary sources, from peer-reviewed journals, are part of a learning strategy for developing critical evaluation skills.
- It is more efficient to use electronic rather than print databases for retrieving scholarly materials.
- Strategies for efficiently retrieving scholarly literature for nursing include consulting the reference librarian and using at least two **computer databases** (e.g., CINAHL and MEDLINE).
- Literature reviews are usually organized according to variables, as well as chronologically.
- Critiquing criteria for scholarly literature reflect the purposes and characteristics of a relevant literature review and are presented in the form of questions.

REFERENCES

Agency for Health Care Policy and Research, Public Health Service, US Department of Health and Human Services: *Guideline for the evaluation and management of early HIV infection*, AHCPR Pub No 94-0572, Rockville, MD, 1994, The Department.

Agency for Healthcare Research and Quality: Garlic: effects on cardiovascular risks and disease, protective effects against cancer, and clinical adverse effects evidence report/technology assessment, No. 20. 2000 (AHRQ 01-E023), Rockville, MD, 1994, The Agency.

Aita VA: Science and compassion: vacillation in nursing ideas 1940s-1960, *Scholarly Inquiry for Nursing Practice* 14(2):115-141, 2000.

Allison MJ: The effect of a social cognitive theory-based intervention on self-efficacy and physical activity in older adults post coronary event, The University of Texas Health Science Center at San Antonio, Dissertation Abstracts, 9967580, 2000, The University of Texas.

American Nurses Association (ANA): *Education for participation in nursing research*, Washington, DC, 1993, American Nurses Publishing.

American Nurses Association (ANA): *Nursing care report card for acute care*, Washington, DC, 1995, American Nurses Publishing.

American Nurses Association (ANA): *Nursing's social policy statement*, Washington, DC, 1995, American Nurses Publishing.

American Nurses Association (ANA): *Standards of clinical nursing practice*, Washington, DC, 1995, American Nurses Publishing.

American Nurses Association (ANA): *Scope and standards of home health nursing practice*, Washington, DC, 2000, American Nurses Publishing.

American Nurses Association (ANA): *Scope and standards of practice for nursing professional development*, Washington, DC, 2000, American Nurses Publishing.

American Nurses Association (ANA): *Scope and standards of public health nursing practice*, Washington, DC, 2000, American Nurses Publishing.

American Nurses Association (ANA): *Women's primary health care: protocols for practice*, Washington, DC, 1995, American Nurses Publishing.

Belcher JR et al: In George JB, editor: *Nursing theories: the base for profession nursing practice*, ed 5, Norwalk, CT, 2001, Appleton and Lange.

Bull MJ, Hansen HE, and Gross CR: A professional-patient partnership model of discharge planning with elders hospitalized with heart failure, *Appl Nurs Res* 13(1):19-28, 2000.

Cheater FM: Nursing home residents used 6 strategies to manage urinary incontinence, *Evidence-Based Nursing* 3(4):136, 2000.

CINAHL: *Reload News*, 2000, CINAHL Information Systems, *www.cinahl.com*.

Clark DJ: A language for nursing, *Nursing Standard* 13(31):21-27, 1999.

Cohen MZ and Ley CD: Bone marrow transplantation: the battle for hope in the face of fear, *Oncology Nursing Forum* 27(3):473-480, 2000.

Fawcett J: Contemporary nursing knowledge: nursing models and theories, Philadelphia, 2000, FA Davis.

Fitzpatrick J and Goeppinger J: *Annual review of nursing research,* Vol 18, New York, 2000, Springer.

Forchuk C and Voorberg N: Evaluating a community mental health program, *Canadian J Nurs Admin* 4(6):16-20, 1991.

Forchuk C: *Hildegard E. Peplau: interpersonal nursing theory,* Newbury Park, CA, 1993, Sage.

Forchuk C: The orientation phase of the nurse-client relationship: testing Peplau's theory, *J Advance Nurs Pract* 20:532-537, 1994.

Forchuk C et al: The developing nurse-client relationship: nurses' perspectives, *J Am Psychiatr Nurs Assoc* 6(1):3-10, 2000.

Johnson M and Maas M: *Nursing outcomes classification (NOC): Iowa outcomes project,* St Louis, 2000, Mosby.

Krainovich-Miller B and Rosedale M: Behavioral health home care. In Shea C et al, editors: *Advanced practice nursing in psychiatric and mental health care,* St Louis, 1999, Mosby.

LoBiondo-Wood G et al: Family adaptation to a child's transplant: pretransplant phase, *Progress in Transplantation* 10(2):81-87, 2000.

Mahon NE, Yarcheski A, and Yarcheski TJ: Positive and negative outcomes of anger in early adolescents, *Res Nurs Health* 23:17-24, 2000.

McCloskey JC and Bulechek GM, editors: *Iowa intervention project: nursing interventions classification (NIC),* ed 3, St Louis, 2000, Mosby.

McKibbon KA and Marks S: Searching for the best evidence, Part 1: where to look, *Evidence-Based Nursing* 1(3):68-70, 1998a.

Neabel B, Fothergill-Bourbonnais F, and Dunning J: Family assessment tools: a review of the literature from 1978-1997, *Heart and Lung* 29(3):196-209, 2000.

North American Nursing Diagnosis Association (NANDA): *Nursing diagnoses: definitions and classification 2000-2001,* Philadelphia, 2001, The Association.

Northington L: Chronic sorrow in caregivers of school age children with sickle cell disease: a grounded theory approach, *Iss Comprehensive Pediatr Nurs* 23(3): 141-54, 2000.

Offredy M: Advanced nursing practice: the case of nurse practitioners in three Australian states, *J Adv Nurs* 31(2):274-281, 2000.

Paul R and Elder L: *Critical thinking: tools for taking charge of your learning and your life,* NJ, 2001, Prentice-Hall.

Peden AR: Recovering in depressed women: research with Peplau's theory, *Nurs Sci Q* 6(3):140-6, 1993.

Peden AR: Recovering from depression: a one-year follow-up, *J Psychiatr Mental Health Nurs* 3: 289-295, 1996.

Peden AR: Evolution of an intervention—the use of Peplau's process of practice-based theory development, *J Psychiatr Mental Health Nurs* 5(3):173-178, 1998.

Peplau HE: Interpersonal relations in nursing: a conceptual frame of reference for psychodyamic nursing, New York, 1952, Putnum and Sons.

Peplau HE: Interpersonal relations in nursing: a conceptual frame of reference for psychodyamic nursing, New York, 1991, Springer.

Powelson SA and McGahan SA: Viewpoint: where to start? Introducing standardized nursing languages in educational settings, *Nurs Diagnosis* 11(3):135-138, 2000.

Pravikoff D and Donaldson N: The online journal of clinical innovations, *Online J ISS Nurs* 5(1): www.nursingworld.org/ojin/topic11/tpc11_6c.htm.

Redeker NS: Sleep in acute care settings: an integrative review, *J Nurs Scholarship* 32(1):31-38, 2000.

ADDITIONAL READINGS

American Nurses Association: The scope of practice for nursing informatics, Washington, DC, 1994, The Association.

American Psychological Association: *Publication manual of the American Psychological Association,* ed 4, Washington, DC, 1994, The Association.

Andrews MM: How to search for information on transcultural nursing and health subjects: internet and CD-ROM resources, *J Transcultural Nurs* 10(1):69-74, 1999.

Brazier H and Begley CM: Selecting a database for literature searches in nursing: MEDLINE or CINAHL?, *J Adv Nurs* 24(4):868-875, 1996.

Forchuk C: The orientation phase: how long does it take?, *Perspectives Psychiatr Care* 28(4):7-10, 1992.

Gentz CA: Perceived learning needs of the patient undergoing coronary angioplasty: an integrative review of the literature, *Heart and Lung* 29(3):161-172, 2000.

Haglund K: Patenting a second tome around: an ethnography of African American grandmothers parenting grandchildren due to parental cocaine abuse, *J Fam Nurs* 6(2): 120-35, 2000.

Hendry C and Farley A: Reviewing the literature: a guide for students, *Nurs Standard* 12(44):46-48, 1998.

Hek G, Langton H, and Blunden G: Systematically searching and reviewing literature, *Nurse Researcher* 7(3):40-57, 2000.

Hyde CJ, Fry-Smith A, and Young J: Finding literature on pre-hospital emergency care, *Pre-Hospital Immediate Care* 3(1):22-32, 1999.

Kibirige HM and DePalo L: The internet as a source of academic research information: findings of two pilot studies, *Information Technology and Libraries* 19(1): 11-16, 2000.

Lamond D and Thompson C: Intuition and analysis in decision making and choice, *J Nurs Scholarship* 32(4):411-414, 2000.

Leasure AR, Davis L, and Thievon SL: Comparison of student outcomes and preferences in a traditional vs. world wide web-based baccalaureate nursing research course, *J Nursing Ed* 39(4):149-154, 2000.

McCormick KA et al: Toward standard classification schemes for nursing language: recommendations of the American Nurses Association Steering Committee on databases to support clinical nursing practice, *JAMA* 1(6):421-427, 1994.

McKibbon KA and Marks S: Searching for the best evidence, Part 2: searching CINAHL and MEDLINE, *Evidence-Based Nursing* 1(4):105-107, 1998b.

New York University, Bobst Library Information Literacy Competencies, Unpublished document, 2000.

Oermann MH and Wilson FL: Quality of care information for consumers on the internet, *J Nurs Care Quality* 14(4):45-54, 2000.

Rankin M and Esteves MD: How to assess a research study, *Am J Nurs* 96(12):32-36, 1996.

Seers K: Sound out the clinical evidence, *Practice Nurse* 14(3):177-8, 180, 1997.

Segedy A: Making the web work for you: on-line research resources, *Rehab Management: The Interdisciplinary Journal of Rehabilitation* 13(1):46, 2000.

Sigma Theta Tau International (STTI): The on-line journal of knowledge synthesis for nursing, www.nursingsociety.org, 2001.

Woods A: Web monitor: sites to sharpen nursing research, *Dimensions Crit Care Nurs* 18(5):49, 1999.

Wright S: Review: both Gram stain and urine dipstick analysis were accurate in diagnosing urinary tract infection in children, *Evidence-Based Nurs* 33:86, 2000.

Zhou J: The internet, the world wide web, library web browsers, and library web servers, *Information Technology and Libraries* 19(1):50-2, 2000.

PATRICIA LIEHR
MARY JANE SMITH

5

Theoretical Framework

Key Terms

concept
conceptual definition
conceptual framework
deductive reasoning
empirical

grand theory
hypothesis
inductive reasoning
microrange theory
midrange theory

model
operational definition
theoretical framework
theory

Learning Outcomes

After reading this chapter, the student should be able to do the following:

- Compare inductive and deductive reasoning.
- Differentiate between conceptual and theoretical framework.
- Identify the purpose and nature of conceptual and theoretical frameworks.
- Describe how a framework guides research.
- Differentiate between conceptual and operational definitions.
- Describe the relationship between theory and research and practice.
- Discuss levels of abstraction related to frameworks guiding research.
- Differentiate among grand, midrange, and microrange theories in nursing.
- Describe the points of critical appraisal used to evaluate the appropriateness, cohesiveness, and consistency of a framework guiding research.

As an introduction to frameworks for research, put yourself in the shoes of Kate and thoughtfully listen to her story by attending to the message it brings for the practicing nurse who wishes to critique, understand, and do research.

Kate works in a coronary care unit (CCU). She has worked in this unit for nearly 3 years since she graduated with a baccalaureate degree in nursing. She has grown more comfortable over time and now believes that she can readily manage whatever comes her way with the complexities of patient care in the CCU. Recently, she has been observing the pattern of blood pressure (BP) change when health care providers enter a patient's room. This observation began when Kate noticed that one of her patients, a 62-year-old black woman who had continuous arterial monitoring, had dramatic increases in BP, as much as 100%, each time the health care team made rounds in the CCU. Furthermore, this elevated BP persisted after the team left her room and slowly decreased to reach preround levels within the following hour. Conversely, when the nurse manager visited this same patient on her usual daily rounds, the patient engaged calmly in conversation and was often left with lower BP when the nurse manager moved on to the next patient. Kate thought about what was happening and adjusted her work so that she could closely observe the details of this phenomenon over several days.

Team rounds were led by the attending cardiologist and included nurses, pharmacists, social workers, medical students, and nursing students. The nurse manager's visit occurred one-on-one. During team rounds, the patient was discussed and occasionally she was asked to respond to a question about her history of heart disease or her current experience of chest discomfort. Participants took turns listening to her heart and students responded to questions related to her case. During the nurse manager's visit, the patient had the nurse's attention. Kate noticed that the nurse manager was especially attentive to the patient's experience. In fact, the nurse usually sat and spent time talking to the patient about how her day was going, what she was thinking about while lying in bed, and what feelings were surfacing as she began to consider how life would be when she returned home.

Kate decided to talk to the nurse manager about her observation. The nurse manager, Alison, was pleased that Kate had noticed these BP changes associated with interaction. She told Kate that she, too, noticed these change during her 8-year experience of working in the CCU. Her observation led her to the theory of *attentively embracing story* (Liehr and Smith, 2000; Smith and Liehr, 1999), which seemed applicable to the observation. Alison had learned the theory as a first-year master's student, and she was applying it in practice and beginning plans to use the theory to guide her thesis research. *Attentively embrac-*

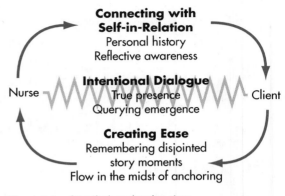

Figure 5-1   Attentively embracing story.

ing story proposes that intentional nurse-client dialogue, which engages the human story, enables connecting with self-in-relation to create ease (Figure 5-1). As depicted by the theory model, the central concept of the theory is intentional dialogue, which is what Kate had first observed when she noticed Alison interacting with the patient. Alison was fully attentive to the patient, following her lead and pursuing what mattered most to the patient. Alison seemed to get a lot of information in a short time, and the patient seemed willing to share things she wasn't sharing with other people.

According to the theory, each of the three concepts—intentional dialogue, connecting with self-in-relation, and creating ease—is intricately connected. So, when Kate observed intentional dialogue, she also observed connecting with self-in-relation as the patient reflected on her experience in the moment, and creating ease, when she saw lowered BP as the nurse manager left the room. Alison and Kate shared an understanding that there was a relationship between patient-health care provider interaction and BP. They discussed several possible issues that might be affecting this relationship. They identified research questions related to each issue (Table 5-1). You may be able to think of other issues that could generate a research question contributing to understanding of the relationship between patient–health care provider interaction and BP. The list developed by Kate and Alison only serves as a reflection of the complexity of the relationship. The list highlights the fact that the relationship cannot be understood with one study, but a series of studies may enhance understanding and offer suggestions for change. For instance, a thorough understanding may lead to testing different approaches for conducting team rounds.

TABLE **5-1** Issues Affecting BP Change and Related Research Questions

ISSUES	RESEARCH QUESTIONS
Number of people in patient's room	Is there a difference in BP for patients in CCU when interacting with one person as compared with interacting with two people or a group of three or more people?
Involvement of patient	For the patient in CCU, what is the relationship between BP and the amount of time spent listening to the health care team's discussion of personal qualities during routine rounds?
	What is the effect of nurse-patient intentional dialogue on BP within the hour after the dialogue?
Continuing effect of experience on BP over the next hour	What is the BP pattern of patients in CCU from the beginning of routine health care rounds until 1 hour after the completion of rounds?
Content of dialogue	What is the relationship between issues discussed during intentional dialogue and BP?
Meaning of experience for the patient	What is the patient experience of being the object of routine health care rounds?
	What is the patient experience of sharing personal matters with a nurse while in the CCU?

BP, blood pressure; *CCU;* coronary care unit.

PRACTICE-THEORY-RESEARCH LINKS

Several important aspects of frameworks for research are embedded in the story of Kate and Alison. First, it is important for the reader to notice the links among practice, theory, and research. Each is intricately connected with the other to create the knowledge base for the discipline of nursing. (Figure 5-2). **Theory** is a set of interrelated concepts that provides a systematic view of a phenomenon. Theory guides practice and research; practice enables testing of theory and generates questions for research; research contributes to theory-building and establishing practice guidelines. So, what is learned through practice, theory, and research interweaves to create the knowledge fabric of the discipline of nursing. From this perspective, each reader is in the process of contributing to the knowledge base of the discipline. For instance, if you are practicing, you can use focused observation (Liehr, 1992) just as Kate did to consider the nuances of situations that matter to patient health. Kate noticed the change in BP occurring with interaction and systematically began to pay close attention to the effect of varying interactions. This inductive

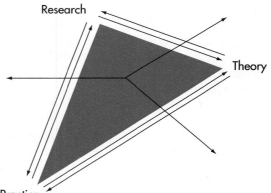

Figure 5-2 Discipline knowledge: theory-practice-research connection.

process often generates the questions that are most cogent for enhancing patient well-being.

APPROACHES TO SCIENCE

Another major theme of the story of Kate and Alison can be found in each nurse's way of approaching the phenomenon of the relationship between health care provider–patient interaction and BP. Each nurse was using a different approach for looking at the situation, but both were systematically evaluating what was observed. This is the essence of science—systematic collection, analysis, and interpretation of data. Kate was using **inductive reasoning,** a process of starting with details of experience and moving to a general picture. Inductive reasoning involves the observation of a particular set of instances that belong to and can be identified as part of a larger set. Alison told Kate that she, too, had begun with inductive reasoning and now was using **deductive reasoning,** a process of starting with the general picture, in this case the theory of *attentively embracing story,* and moving to a specific direction for practice and research. Deductive reasoning uses two or more related concepts, that when combined, enable suggestion of relationships between the concepts. Inductive and deductive reasoning are basic to frameworks for research. Inductive reasoning is the pattern of "figuring out what's there" from the details of the nursing practice experience. Inductive reasoning is the foundation for most qualitative inquiry (see Chapters 6, 7, and 8). Research questions related to the issue of the meaning of experience for the patient (see Table 5-1) can be addressed with the inductive reasoning of qualitative inquiry. Deductive reasoning begins with a structure that guides one's searching for "what's there." All but the last two research questions listed in Table 5-1 would be addressed with the deductive reasoning of quantitative inquiry.

Given Alison's use of deductive reasoning guided by the theory of attentively embracing story, it can be assumed that she has read and critiqued the literature on theoretical frameworks and has chosen *attentively embracing story* to guide her master's thesis research. In order for Kate to move on in her thinking about research to study the way changes in blood pressure are related to health care provider–patient interaction, she needs to become well versed on the importance of theoretical frameworks. As she reads the literature and reviews research studies, she will critique the theoretical frameworks guiding those studies. In critiquing existing frameworks, she will develop the knowledge and understanding needed to

choose an appropriate framework for research. As a beginning, Kate is reading this chapter, recognizing that she is critiquing nursing research.

HELPFUL HINT Investigators may not always provide a detailed explicit statement of the observation(s) that led them to their conclusion(s) when using inductive reasoning; likewise, you will not always find a clear picture of the structure guiding the study when deductive reasoning has been used.

FRAMEWORKS AS STRUCTURE FOR RESEARCH

Whether evaluating a qualitative or a quantitative study, it is wise to look for the framework that guided the study. Generally, when the researcher is using qualitative inquiry and inductive reasoning methods, the critical reader will find the framework at the end of the manuscript in the discussion section (see Chapters 6, 7, and 8). From the findings of the study, the researcher builds a structure for moving forward. In the study on bone marrow transplantation in Appendix B (Cohen and Ley, 2000), the researchers obtained stories about what it was like to have a bone marrow transplant. These stories were analyzed and the findings were synthesized at the theoretical level. The researchers moved from *particulars* of the bone marrow transplant experience to a *general* structure of concepts that included fears, losses, hopes, and a sense of transitioning through a life-altering event. These concepts were described in the context of the subjects' stories and relevant literature, creating a conceptual structure that could be modeled.

A **model** is a symbolic representation of a set of concepts that is created to depict relationships. Figure 5-1 is the model of *attentively embracing story.* It represents the nurse-client connection through the rhythmic symbol labeled *intentional dialogue.* The model depicts process by connecting the concepts through nurse-client dialogue with linking arrows. This model could be the basis for deductive reasoning. An example of a deductive question that could be derived from the model is as follows:

"What is the difference in salivary cortisol (an indicator of ease) for cancer patients who engage with participants (connecting with self-in-relation) in a nurse-led (intentional dialogue) cancer support group?"

HELPFUL HINT   When an investigator has used a deductive approach, the theoretical framework should be described to substantiate how the research question emerged.

When the researcher uses quantitative inquiry and deductive reasoning methods, the critical reader will find the framework at the beginning of the paper before a discussion of study methods. In the study of a model for discharge planning for elders with heart failure in Appendix A, Bull, Hansen, and Gross (2000) present a model they derived from a broader evaluation perspective. Their model, which depicts inputs, process, and outputs, is a framework for structuring the research questions and accompanying hypotheses. The inputs they identify are elder and family-caregiver characteristics. The process is the partnership model, which proposes that discharge planning should be a collaborative interaction among professionals, patients, and family caregivers. The partnership model is the intervention administered to the experimental group in their research. The outputs or outcomes they measure are health status satisfaction, perception of care continuity, difficulties of managing care, and resource use for both the elderly patient and the family caregiver. The researchers have identified questionnaires or medical record sources that will bring these outcomes to a measurable level. Their model and the related literature lead Bull, Hansen, and Gross (2000) to form the following hypotheses:

1. Scores on perceived health will be different for clients in the intervention and control cohorts.
2. Client satisfaction with discharge planning, perceptions of care continuity, preparedness, and difficulties managing care will differ for the intervention and the control cohorts.
3. The caregiver's response to caregiving will be different for the experimental and control cohorts.
4. Resource use will be different for the control and intervention cohorts.

The researchers used deductive reasoning to move from their model, which they substantiated with literature, to the hypotheses (see Chapter 3), or best guesses, regarding what they will find. Their model provided a framework to guide their research from theory to hypotheses, or from the abstract to the concrete. This is in contrast to Cohen and Ley (2000) who moved from the concrete experience of bone marrow transplant to the abstract structure of the concepts.

THE LADDER OF ABSTRACTION

The ladder of abstraction is a way for the reader to gain a perspective when reading and thinking about frameworks for research. When critiquing the framework of a study, imagine a ladder (Figure 5-3). The highest level on the ladder includes beliefs and assumptions, what is sometimes called the worldview of the researcher. Although the worldview is not always explicitly stated in a manuscript, it is there. In the study on outcomes of anger (Mahon, Yarcheski, and Yarcheski, 2000) (see Appendix C), the researchers hold beliefs that there is a relationship between mind and body and that emotions do indeed influence health. The middle level on the ladder includes the frameworks, theories, and concepts the researcher uses to articulate the problem, purpose, and structure for research. Mahon, Yarcheski, and Yarcheski (2000) studied the problem of positive and negative outcomes of anger in early adolescents. As defined by the authors, the purpose of their study was to examine symptom patterns and diminished well-being as negative outcomes of trait and state anger and vigor and willingness to change as

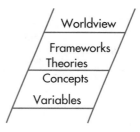

Figure 5-3   The ladder of abstraction.

positive outcomes of trait and state anger. Using the literature base, specifically Spielberger's theory of anger, they created frameworks of the positive and negative outcomes of state and trait anger. The negative outcomes framework depicts relationships among the concepts of state anger, trait anger, diminished well-being, and symptom patterns. The positive outcomes framework outlines links among state anger, trait anger, vigor, and willingness to change. The researchers used these literature-derived frameworks, presented as models, to logically structure their study.

This "middle of the ladder" position of frameworks, theories, and concepts moves to a lower rung where **empirical** factors are located. Empirical factors refer to those things that can be observed through the senses and include the variables measured and described in quantitative research studies and the story that is described in qualitative studies. Table 5-2 outlines the con-

TABLE **5-2** Concepts and Variables: Conceptual and Operational Definitions

CONCEPT	CONCEPTUAL DEFINITION	VARIABLE	OPERATIONAL DEFINITION
Trait anger	Disposition of individuals to perceive a wide range of situations as frustrating or annoying, tending to respond to such situations with elevations in state anger (p. 17)	Trait anger	Spielberger Trait Anger Scale Ten items that assess how angry one generally feels
State anger	Emotional state marked by subjective feelings that vary in intensity from mild annoyance or irritation to intense fury and rage (p. 17)	State anger	Spielberger State Anger Scale Ten items that assess how angry one is feeling right now
General well-being	Holistic, multidimensional construct incorporating mental/psychological, physical and social dimensions (p. 18)	General well-being	Short version of Adolescent General Well-Being Questionnaire Thirty-nine items that assess the social, physical, and mental dimensions of well-being
Symptom patterns	Physical, psychological and psychosomatic patterns (p. 18)	Symptom patterns	Symptom Pattern Scale Seventeen items that measure physical, psychological, and psychosomatic manifestations of psychological distress
Vigor	Mood or vigorousness, ebullience and high energy (p. 19)	Vigor-activity	Vigor-activity subscale of the Profile of Moods States Eight-item adjective checklist used to measure vigor
Inclination to change	Seeking new and different experiences, readily changing opinions or values in different circumstances, and adapting readily to changes in the environment (p. 19)	Change	Change subscale of the Personality Research Form-E Sixteen true-false items assessing inclination to change

From Mahon NE, Yarcheski A, and Yarcheski T J: Positive and negative outcomes of anger in early adolescents, *Res Nurs Health* 23: 17-24, 2000. (See Appendix B).

NOTE : Page numbers refer to the actual article.

cepts with their conceptual definitions and the accompanying variables with their operational definitions from the Mahon, Yarcheski, and Yarcheski (2000) study (Appendix C).

A **conceptual definition** is much like a dictionary definition, conveying the general meaning of the concept. However, the conceptual definition goes beyond the general language meaning found in the dictionary by defining the concept as it is rooted in the theoretical literature. The **operational definition** specifies how the concept will be measured—that is, what instruments will be used to capture the variable. In looking closely at the language used to describe conceptual and operational definitions (see Table 5-2), the reader will notice that operational definitions are lower on the ladder of abstraction than conceptual definitions. The language of the operational definition is closer to the ground.

HELPFUL HINT Some reports of research embed conceptual definitions in the literature review. It is wise for the reader to seek and find the conceptual definitions so that the logical fit between the conceptual and operational definitions can be determined.

THE MIDDLE OF THE LADDER: FRAMEWORKS, THEORIES, AND CONCEPTS

It is important to consider the middle of the ladder of abstraction where concepts, theories, and frameworks are located. Pretend to look at the middle section through a magnifying glass so that what is located there can be distinguished and clarified. Concepts, theories, and frameworks can be compared to each other from the perspective of abstraction, with concepts being the lowest on the ladder and frameworks the highest. However, some concepts are closer to the ground than others. The same is true for theories and frameworks. For instance, the concept of pain relief is closer to the ground than the concept of caring. The idea of varying levels of abstraction within the middle of the ladder is emphasized in the section addressing theories, but it has relevance for concepts and frameworks as well.

CONCEPTS

A **concept** is an image or symbolic representation of an abstract idea. Chinn and Kramer (1999) define a concept as a "complex mental formulation of experience." Concepts are the major components of theory and convey the abstract ideas within a theory. In this chapter, you have been introduced to several concepts, such as trait and state anger, well-being, and vigor. The concepts of the theory of attentively embracing story, intentional dialogue, connecting with self-in-relation, and creating ease have been defined and their relationship has been modeled. Each concept creates a mental image that is explained further through the conceptual definition. For instance, pain is a concept whose mental image means something based on experience. The experiential meaning of the concept of pain is different for the child who has just fallen off a bike, for the elderly person with rheumatoid arthritis, and for the doctorally prepared nurse who is studying pain mechanisms using an animal model. These definitions and associated images of the concept of pain incorporate different experiential and knowledge components, all with the same label—pain. Therefore, it is important to know the meaning of the concept for the person. In the case of the reader, it is important to know the meaning that the researcher gives to the concepts in a research study. As outlined in Table 5-2, Mahon, Yarcheski, and Yarchesi (2000) clearly defined the concepts of interest in their study.

THEORIES

A theory is a set of interrelated concepts that structure a systematic view of phenomena for the purpose of explaining or predicting. A theory is like a blueprint, a guide for modeling a structure. A blueprint depicts the elements of a structure and the relation of each element to the other, just as a theory depicts both the concepts that compose it and how they are related. Chinn and Kramer (1999) define a theory as an "expression of knowledge. . . . a creative and rigorous structuring of ideas that project a tentative, purposeful, and systematic view of phenomena." Theories are located on the ladder of abstraction relative to their scope. An often-used label in nursing is "grand theory," which suggests a broad scope, covering major areas of importance to the discipline. Grand theories arose at a time when nursing was addressing its nature, mission, and goals (Im and Meleis, 1999), so it is historically important. However, its significance extends beyond history to have implications for guiding the discipline today and in the future. For the purpose of introducing the reader to theory as a framework for nursing research, grand theory, midrange theory, and microrange theory are discussed. As is suggested by the names of these theory categories, grand theories are highest and microrange theories are lowest in level of abstraction.

GRAND THEORY

Theories unique to nursing help the discipline define how it is different from other disciplines. Nursing theories reflect particular views of person, health, environment, and other concepts that contribute to the development of a body of knowledge specific to nursing's concerns. **Grand theories** are all-inclusive conceptual structures that tend to include views on person, health, and environment to create a perspective of nursing. This most abstract level of theory has established a knowledge base for the discipline and is critical for further knowledge development in the discipline.

The grand theories of several well-known nursing theorists have served as a basis for practice and research. Among these theories are Rogers' (1990, 1992) science of irreducible human beings, Orem's (1995) theory of self-care deficit, Newman's theory of health as expanding consciousness (1997), Roy's adaptation theory (1991), Leininger's culture care diversity and universality theory (1996), King's goal attainment theory (1997), and Parse's theory of human becoming (1997). Each of these grand theories addresses the phenomena of concern to nursing from a different perspective. For example, Rogers views the person and the environment as energy fields coextensive with the universe. So, she recognizes the person-environment unity as a mutual process. In contrast, King (1997) distinguishes the personal system from the interpersonal and so-

cial systems, focusing on the interaction among systems and the interaction of the systems with the environment. For King, person and environment are interacting as separate entities. This is different from the person-environment mutual process described by Rogers.

If a researcher uses Roger's theory to guide plans for a study, the research question will reflect different values than if the researcher had used King. The researcher using Roger's theory might study the relationship of therapeutic touch to other phenomena that reflect a valuing for energy fields and pattern appreciation, whereas the one using King might study outcomes related to nurse-patient shared goals or other phenomena related to interacting systems. It is important for the reader to realize that one grand theory is not better than another. Rather, these varying perspectives allow the nurse researcher to select a framework for research that facilitates movement of concepts of interest down the ladder of abstraction to the empirical level, where they can be measured as study variables. What is most important about the use of theoretical frameworks for research is the logical connection of the theory to the research question and the study design.

MIDRANGE THEORY

Midrange theory is a focused conceptual structure that synthesizes practice-research into ideas central to the discipline. Merton (1968), who has been the original source for much of nursing's description of midrange theory, says that midrange theories lie between everyday working hypotheses and all-inclusive grand theories. The reader might notice that Merton's view of the "middle" allows for a great deal of space between grand theories and hypotheses. This expansive view of the "middle" has been noted and efforts have been made to more clearly articulate the middle and to distinguish the characteristics of midrange theory. In a 10-year review of nursing literature using specific criteria, Liehr and Smith (1999) identified 22 midrange theories. Following the suggestion of Lenz (1996), they considered the scope of the 22 midrange theories and grouped them into high-middle, middle-middle, and low-middle categories using the theory names (Table 5-3). The reader will recognize that the groupings move from a higher to a lower level of abstraction. Because midrange theories are lower in level of abstraction than grand theories, they offer a more direct application to research and practice. As the level of abstraction decreases, translation into practice and research simplifies. In their conclusion, Liehr and Smith (1999) recommend that nurses thoughtfully construct midrange theory weaving practice and research threads to create a whole fabric that is meaningful for the discipline. Hamric, Spross, and Hanson (2000) in their text on advanced nursing practice call midrange theories to the attention of advanced practice nurses:

"Middle-range theories address the experiences of particular patient populations or a cohort of people who are dealing with a particular health or illness issue. . . . Because middle range theories are more specific in what they explain, practitioners often find them more directly applicable. . . ."

The theory of attentively embracing story, introduced at the beginning of this chapter, is a midrange theory. The theory was generated from nursing practice and research experience (Smith and Liehr, 1999).

MICRORANGE THEORY

Microrange theory is a linking of concrete concepts into a statement that can be examined in practice and research. Higgins and Moore (2000) distinguish two levels of microrange theory, one at a higher level abstraction than the other. They suggest that microrange theories at the higher level of abstraction are closely related to midrange theories, comprised of a limited number of concepts and applicable to a narrow issue or event (Higgins and Moore, 2000) The low-middle theory in Table 5-3 may fit this category. Hypotheses are an example of low abstraction microrange theories. The reader will recall that a hypothesis is a best guess or prediction about what one expects to find. Chinn and Kramer (1999) define a **hypothesis** as a "tentative statement of relationship between two or more variables that can be empirically tested." Higgins and Moore (2000) emphasize the value of microrange theory, noting that the "particularistic approach is invaluable for scientists and practitioners as they work to describe, organize and test their ideas."

As you read this text, you could articulate a microrange theory at the level of a hypothesis. At the beginning of this chapter, Kate formulated a hypothesis about the relationship between patient-health care provider interaction

TABLE **5-3**   Middle Range Theory by Level of Abstraction

HIGH-MIDDLE	MIDDLE-MIDDLE	LOW-MIDDLE
Caring	Uncertainty in illness	Hazardous secrets and reluctantly taking charge
Facilitating growth and development	Unpleasant symptoms	Affiliated individuation as a mediator of stress
Interpersonal perceptual awareness	Chronic sorrow	Women's anger
Self-transcendence	Peaceful end of life	Nurse-midwifery care
Resilience	Negotiating partnerships	Acute pain management
Psychological adaptation	Cultural brokering	Balance between analgesia and side effects
	Nurse-expressed empathy and patient distress	Homelessness-helplessness
		Individualized music intervention for agitation
		Chronotherapeutic intervention for postsurgical pain

From Liehr P and Smith MJ: Middle range theory: spinning research and practice to create knowledge for the new millennium, *Adv Nurs Sci* 21(4):81-91, 1999.

and blood pressure. Although Kate didn't label her idea as a hypothesis, it was a best guess based on observation. If you would take a minute to think about it, some experience from nursing practice that has provoked confusion could be stated as a hypothesis. A mismatch between what is known or commonly accepted as fact and what one experiences creates a hypothesis-generating moment. Every nurse experiences such moments. Cultivating hypothesis-generating moments requires noticing them, focusing observation to untangle details, and allowing time for creative thinking and dialogue (Liehr, 1992), leading to possibilities for creating low-level microrange theory, or hypotheses.

HELPFUL HINT The reader of research will find conflicting views regarding levels and placement of theory. While one author labels a particular theory "grand," another author will label the same theory "midrange." The reader can evaluate the theory and assign its level the ladder of abstraction. If a theory is at the more concrete level on the ladder, then it falls into microtheory.

FRAMEWORKS FOR RESEARCH

The critical thinking decision path takes the reader through the thinking of a researcher who is about to begin doing research. It is reasonable for the reader to expect to find some but not all of the phases of decision-making addressed in a research manuscript. Beginning with the view of the world, the highest rung on the ladder of abstraction, the researcher is inclined to approach a research problem from a perspective of inductive or deductive reasoning. If the researcher pursues an inductive reasoning approach, he or she generally will not present a framework before beginning discussion of the methods. This is not to say that literature will not be reviewed before introducing methods. As an example, consider the Cohen and Ley (2000) manuscript in Appendix B. The authors provide a brief overview of the increasing prevalence of bone marrow transplant as a treatment for cancer, and they describe several studies that examined dimensions of life for persons undergoing transplant. The point of their literature review is to establish a case for doing the research they are reporting. They do not provide a framework for the study because they are planning an inductive approach to study the problem. Their intent is to be free of the structures that may limit what they learn and to be open to the experience of the person who is living through a bone marrow transplant.

Conversely, if the researcher's view of the world is guided by deductive reasoning, he or she must choose between a conceptual or a theoretical framework. The reader will notice when reading the theory literature that these terms are used interchangeably (Chinn and Kramer, 1999). However, in the case presented in the Critical Thinking Decision Path, each term is being distinguished from the other on the basis of whether the researcher is creating the structure or whether the structure has already been created by someone else. Generally, each of these terms refers to a structure that will provide guidance for research. A **conceptual framework** is a structure of concepts and/or theories pulled together as a map for the study. A **theoretical framework** is a structure of concepts that exists in the literature, a ready-made map for the study.

To better understand these differences, refer to the study by Mahon, Yarcheski, and Yarcheski (2000) in Appendix C. The authors create a conceptual framework for their study incorporating Spielberger's anger theory with the four concepts of well-being, symptom patterns, vigor, and willingness to change. This framework is shared as a model, and the reader is able to follow the logic of the study by referring to the conceptual framework. In contrast, the study by LoBiondo-Wood and associates (2000) (see Appendix D) uses a theoretical framework to guide its research, the Double ABC-X Model of Family Adaptation. Although not a nursing theory, the Model of Family Adaptation is a tested structure that some would label a midrange theory. The authors focus on one piece of the model, the postcrisis period, which includes the five concepts of pile-up, existing new

CRITICAL THINKING DECISION PATH Choosing a Theoretical Path

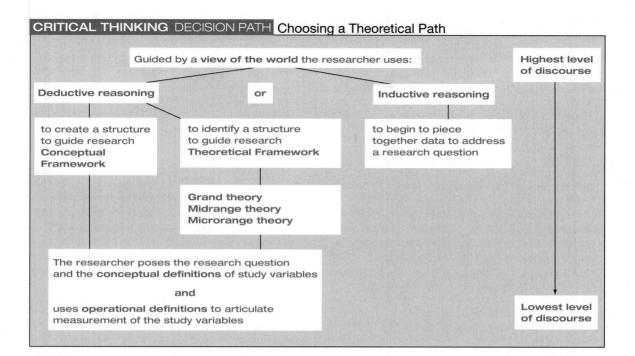

resources, coping, perception of stressor, and adaptation. Each of these concepts is presented with clear indication of how it was measured in this sample of mothers of children who undergo organ transplantation. The Double ABC-X Model of Family Adaptation logically guides the choice of variables and measures. Instead of creating a structure, these authors used a theoretical framework that already existed in the literature.

HELPFUL HINT When researchers use conceptual frameworks to guide their studies, you can expect to find a system of ideas, synthesized for the purpose of organizing thinking and providing study direction.

From the perspective of the Critical Thinking Decision Path, theoretical frameworks can incorporate grand, midrange, or microrange theories. Whether the researcher is using a conceptual or theoretical framework, conceptual and then operational definitions will emerge from the framework. The decision path moves down the ladder of abstraction from the philosophical to the empirical level, tracking thinking from the most abstract to the least abstract for the purposes of planning a research study.

CRITIQUING the Framework

The framework for research provides guidance for the researcher as study questions are fine-tuned, methods for measuring variables are selected, and analyses are planned. Once data are collected and analyzed, the framework is used as a base of comparison. Did the findings coincide with the framework? If there were discrepancies, is there a way to explain them using the framework? The reader of research needs to know how to critically appraise a framework for research (Critiquing Criteria box).

The first question posed is whether a framework is presented. Sometimes, a structure may be guiding the research, but a diagrammed model is not included in the manuscript. The reader must then look for the study structure in the narrative description of the study concepts. When the framework is identified, it is important to consider its relevance for nursing. The framework doesn't have to be one created by a nurse but the importance of its content for nursing should be clear. The question of how the framework depicts a structure congruent with nursing should be addressed. For instance, although the Double ABC-X Model was not created by a nurse, it is clearly related to nursing practice with families. Sometimes, frameworks from very different disciplines, such as physics or art, may be relevant. It is the responsibility of the author to clearly articulate the meaning of the framework for the study and to link the framework to nursing.

Once the meaning and nursing-relatedness are articulated, the reader will be able to determine whether the framework is appropriate to guide the research. For instance, if a researcher is studying students' responses to the stress of being in the clinical setting for the first time and presents a framework of stress related to recovery from chronic illness, this is a blatant mismatch, which generally won't occur. However, subtle versions of mismatch will occur. So, the reader will want to look closely at the framework to determine if it is "on target" and the "best fit" for the research question and proposed study design.

Next, focus on the concepts being studied. Does the reader know which concepts are being studied and how they are defined and translated into measurable variables? Is there literature to support the choice of concepts? Concepts should clearly reflect the area of study; for example, using the general concept of stress when anxiety is more appropriate to the research focus creates difficulties in defining variables and determining methods of measurement. These issues have to do with the logical consistency between the framework, the concepts being studied, and the methods of measurement. All along the way, from view of the world to operational definitions, the reader is evaluating fit. Consider once more the paper by LoBiondo-Wood and associates (2000) (see Appendix D). The authors provide a logically consistent link among the Double ABC-X Model of Family Adaptation, the concepts diagrammed in the postcrisis phase of the model, and the measures used to address each concept. Finally, the reader will expect to find a discussion of the findings as they relate to the model. This final point enables evaluation of the framework for use in further research. It may suggest necessary changes to enhance the relevance of the framework for continuing study, and thus serves to let others know where one will go from here.

CRITIQUING CRITERIA

1. Is the framework for research clearly identified?
2. Is the framework consistent with a nursing perspective?
3. Is the framework appropriate to guide research on the subject of interest?
4. Are the concepts and variables clearly and appropriately defined?
5. Was sufficient literature presented to support study of the selected concepts?
6. Is there a logical consistent link between the framework, the concepts being studied, and the methods of measurement?
7. Are the study findings examined in relationship to the framework?

Evaluating frameworks for research requires skill that can only be acquired through repeated critique and discussion with others who have critiqued the same manuscript. The novice reader of research must be patient as these skills are developed. With continuing education and a broader knowledge of potential frameworks, one builds a repertoire of knowledge to judge the foundation of a research study, the framework for research.

Critical Thinking Challenges

Barbara Krainovich-Miller

➤ You are taking an elective course in advanced pathophysiology. The professor compares the knowledge of various disciplines and states that nursing is an example of a nonscientific discipline. She supports this assertion by citing that nursing's knowledge has been generated with unstructured methods such as intuition, trial and error, tradition, and authority. What assumptions has this professor made? Would you defend or support her position?

➤ Nurse researchers claim that a theoretical framework is essential for systematically identifying the relationship between the chosen variables. If this is true, why do nonnursing research studies not identify theoretical frameworks?

➤ How would you as a consumer of research use computer databases to verify tools for measuring operational definitions?

➤ How would you argue against the following statement: "As a beginning consumer of research it is ridiculous to expect me to determine if a researcher's study has an appropriate theoretical framework; I only had Nursing Theory 101."

➤ Is it possible for a research study's theoretical framework and variables to be the same?

Key Points

- The scientific approaches used to generate nursing knowledge reflect both inductive and deductive reasoning.
- The interaction among theory, practice, and research is central to knowledge development in the discipline of nursing.
- Conceptual frameworks are created by the researcher, whereas theoretical frameworks are identified in the literature.
- The use of a framework for research is important as a guide to systematically identify concepts and to link appropriate study variables with each concept.
- Conceptual and operational definitions are critical to the evolution of a study whether or not they are explicitly stated in a manuscript
- In developing or selecting a framework for research, knowledge may be acquired from other disciplines or directly from nursing. In either case, that knowledge is used to answer specific nursing questions.
- Theory is distinguished by its scope. Grand theories are broadest in scope and at the highest level of abstraction, and microrange theories are most narrow in scope and at the lowest level of abstraction; midrange theories are in the middle.
- Midrange theories are at a level of abstraction that enhances their usefulness for guiding practice and research.
- In critiquing a framework for research, it is important that one examine the logical consistent link among the framework, concepts for study, and the methods of measurement.

REFERENCES

Bull MJ, Hansen HE, and Gross CR: A professional-patient partnership model of discharge planning with elders, *Appl Nurs Res* 13:19-28, 2000.

Chinn PL and Kramer MK: *Theory and nursing: a systematic approach,* ed 5, St Louis, 1999, Mosby.

Cohen MZ and Ley CD: Bone marrow transplantation: The battle for hope in the face of fear, *Oncol Nurs Forum* 27(3):473-480, 2000.

Hamric AB, Spross JA, and Hanson CM: *Advanced nursing practice,* Philadelphia, 2000, WB Saunders.

Higgins PA and Moore SM: Levels of theoretical thinking in nursing, *Nurs Outlook* 48(4):179-183, 2000.

Im E and Meleis AI: Situation-specific theories: philosophical roots, properties and approach, *Adv Nurs Sci* 22(2):11-24, 1999.

King IM: King's theory of goal attainment in practice, *Nurs Sci Q* 10(4):180-185, 1997.

Leininger MM: Culture care theory, *Nurs Sci Q* 9(2): 71-78, 1996.

Lenz E: Middle range theory—role in research and practice. In *Proceedings of the sixth Rosemary Ellis Scholar's Retreat, nursing science implications for the 21st century*, Cleveland, Ohio, 1996, Frances Payne Bolton School of Nursing, Case Western Reserve University.

Liehr P: Prelude to research, *Nurs Sci Q* 5(3):102-103, 1992.

Liehr P and Smith MJ: Middle range theory: Spinning research and practice to create knowledge for the new millennium, *Adv Nurs Sci* 21(4):81-91, 1999.

Liehr P and Smith MJ: Using story to guide nursing practice, *Int J Hum Caring* 4(2):13-18, 2000.

LoBiondo-Wood G et al: Family adaptation to a child's transplant: Pretransplant phase, *Prog Transplant* 10:81-87, 2000.

Mahon NE, Yarcheski A, and Yarcheski TJ: Positive and negative outcomes of anger in early adolescents, *Res Nurs Health* 23:17-24, 2000.

Merton RK: *Social theory and social structure*, New York, 1968, Free Press.

Newman MA: Evolution of the theory of health as expanding consciousness, *Nurs Sci Q* 10(1):22-25, 1997.

Orem DE: *Nursing: concepts of practice*, ed 5, St Louis, 1995, Mosby.

Parse RR: Transforming research and practice with the human becoming theory, *Nurs Sci Q* 10(4):171-174, 1997.

Rogers ME: Nursing: Science of unitary, irreducible human beings: Update 1990. In E. Barrerr, editor: *Visions of Rogers' science-based nursing*, New York, 1990, National League for Nursing.

Rogers ME: Nightingale's notes on nursing: prelude to the 21st century. In Rogers ME: *Notes on nursing: what it is and what it is not*, commemorative ed, Philadelphia, 1992, Lippincott.

Roy C and Andrews HA: *The Roy adaptation model: the definitive statement*, Norwalk, 1991, Appleton & Lange.

Smith MJ and Liehr P: Attentively embracing story: a middle range theory with practice and research implications, *Sch Inq Nurs Pract* 13(3):3-27, 1999.

ADDITIONAL READINGS

Marriner-Tomey A and Alligood MR:, *Nursing theorists and their works*, ed 4, St Louis, 1998, Mosby.

Nicoll LH: *Perspectives on nursing theory*, ed 3, Philadelphia, 1997, J.B. Lippincott.

Rodgers BL and Knafl KA: *Concept development in nursing: foundations, techniques, and applications*, ed 2, Philadelphia, 2000, W.B. Saunders.

TWO

PROCESSES RELATED TO QUALITATIVE RESEARCH

Research Vignette

The Challenge of Historical Research

I never intended to become a researcher specializing in military nursing history, but I enjoyed teaching nursing, and I wanted a doctoral degree. In 1980 I began my studies at New York University without a clue about a dissertation topic. After reading a book on Vietnam War veterans that contained stories from nurses, I went to the library to gather material on these nurses whose stories I had found so intriguing. I found nothing in NYU's library. The thought that their amazing experiences would soon be forgotten was so troublesome that I decided to record and analyze these nurses' experiences for my dissertation. This study changed my life.

I quickly learned that you do not decide to conduct oral history interviews in 1 week. I was fortunate to find a mentor at NYU, a professor who spent 7 months working with me on my interview schedule. A historian has to be as fully informed as possible before interviewing a subject. Nothing will make an interview fail more quickly than when a person senses an interviewer is disorganized or unprepared. This fact is especially true with war veterans who are about to share the most intense times of their lives.

Using a snowball sampling technique, I found 50 women who agreed to be interviewed. Armed with a map of Vietnam, two tape recorders (in case one broke), and questions, I began. Speaking with these women, some of whom were still in uniform, others who had become civilians, was interesting and exhilarating. The deep commitment to their patients, their courage under fire, and their compassion made me proud to be a nurse. I remember thinking that if people such as these were nurses, I was in the right profession.

Speaking with these veterans was also stressful and often very sad. I came to see that nurses truly see the consequences of war. The combat soldier is too busy fighting and trying to stay alive to recognize the true extent of the slaughter. It is the nurse standing by the bloody gurneys who knows war like no one else. Their stories of loss—youth, health, naiveté—were hard to hear over and over. Many women cried as they recalled particular patients or the less than warm welcome our country gave the Vietnam veterans when they came home. They made me look at the world and at war in a much more meaningful way than I ever had.

I transcribed and analyzed each tape; however, I collected so much detail that I used only about one quarter of my data in my dissertation. After I graduated in 1986, I decided to write a book and in 1990 published *Women at War: The Story of Fifty Military Nurses who Served in Vietnam 1965-1973* (University of Pennsylvania Press). To celebrate I had a party for these nurses. Several of them have become good friends because bonds can be formed between oral historian and subject as war experiences are shared. Many scholars are not aware of these friendships, but they are a nice reward for this type of research.

About the time my book was published, I decided to organize another wartime nursing study. This time I wanted to research the 77 military nurses who were captured in the Philippines in 1942 and became the largest group of female prisoners of war (POWs) in the history of our country. I felt that the prison experience would add another dimension to my wartime study. Using a contact I had made during the Vietnam study, I found these women and began the process again: reading, organizing my questions, and reviewing archival material. (As an aside, another secret to historical work is that archivists in private and federal libraries are the most friendly and helpful resource people you will ever meet in your work).

Several of the former WWII POWs, like their Vietnam counterparts, only agreed to speak with me because I was a nurse. They felt that I would understand the difficult decisions they often had to make in a way that someone who was not a nurse would not. These interviews took on a familiar pattern. War veterans almost always begin the interviews by asking you a few personal questions, then they tell you one or two funny stories from the war. I begin my interview with general questions about their youth, a time period that is generally easy to discuss. Slowly we work our way to the difficult questions about fear, death, triage, courage, and cowardice. The process is similar to peeling an onion, but I always end the sessions by discussing the present, not only to get important data but also to help them recover from their intense memories. Rarely do I conduct just one interview with each subject, usually I return many times. The multiple interviews combined with photos, diaries, and letters the veterans share provide a rich source of material and research data.

The WWII veterans taught me something else about nursing. For them, the ability to keep working whether on the battlefield or in prison camp was life-sustaining. Nursing gave them a reason to get up every morning, and their coworkers became family who helped them get through the despair and loneliness of prison camp. Once again, I found myself proud to be a nurse.

During the course of this study, which took 8 years, I often experienced another joy of historical research—the hunt for long-lost but important material. Historians can spend weeks going through archival boxes or calling relatives of deceased subjects looking for a particular piece of information. When you find it, there is a feeling of "eureka" and a moment to be savored. This reaction happened when I found a diary on microfilm that no one knew existed or a series of essential memorandum in a box stored in a garage.

This group's story was so compelling that I decided to write a book for the general public, and in 1999 Random House published the hard cover and in 2000 Pocket Books the paperback of *We Band of Angels: The Untold Story of American Nurses Trapped on Bataan by the Japanese*. My current project is a book about the men who served on Bataan. I became so absorbed with their story and plight that I wanted to study them before they were all gone. I am working with a coinvestigator for the first time, and together with Michael Norman I have traveled to Asia four times to interview former Filipino and Japanese soldiers and across our country to speak with American veterans for a book we call *Tears in the Darkness*. We are still organizing and analyzing this data, but already I can see the value of looking at historical experiences through the lens of three different cultures.

We all have much to learn about war and its aftermath. I hope that researchers just starting their careers will consider historical work so that more of our past does not vanish before we learn its valuable secrets and lessons.

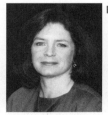

Elizabeth Norman, PhD, RN, FAAN
Professor and Director,
Doctoral Program,
Division of Nursing,
New York University,
New York, NY

MARLENE ZICHI COHEN

Introduction to Qualitative Research

6

Key Terms

case studies
context
empirical analytical
epistemology
ethnographic research

ethnographies
grounded theory
naturalistic research
ontology
paradigm

phenomenological research
philosophical beliefs
qualitative research
text
worldview

Learning Outcomes

After reading this chapter, the student should be able to do the following:

- Define key concepts in the philosophy of science.
- Identify assumptions underlying the received view and the perceived view of research.
- Identify assumptions underlying quantitative (empirical analytical) and the qualitative methods of grounded theory, case study, ethnographic, and phenomenological approaches to research.

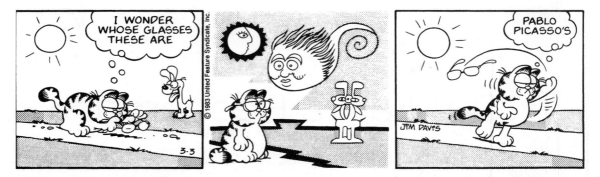

Figure 6-1   Shifting perspectives: seeing the world as others see it. (GARFIELD ©1983 Paws, Inc. Reprinted with permission of UNIVERSAL PRESS SYNDICATE. All rights reserved.)

Qualitative research is an important term to understand because it is a broad label that includes many approaches. Qualitative research can mean the analysis of open-ended questions respondents are asked to write on a survey. It also can refer to what is thought of as **naturalistic research,** a general label for qualitative research methods that involve the researcher going to a natural setting, that is, to where the phenomenon being studied is taking place. Qualitative research includes many methods: **grounded theory, case study, ethnography, phenomenology,** and many others. These methods share both similarities and differences. Because all methods involve data that are **text** rather than numbers, all include some means of doing content analysis on the text. Text means data are in a textual form, that is, narrative or words written from interviews that were recorded and then transcribed or notes written from observations of the researcher. However, the methods differ in the philosophical bases upon which they are built and in purpose and outcome. This chapter addresses the philosophies underlying the qualitative research methods most commonly used by nurses.

The first question nurse researchers must answer when they decide to begin research is what approach they will use. Beginning is never easy and requires many forms of preparation. Beginning research is like beginning a marriage. With luck, both are worth the time and trouble, and what you learn about yourself along the way is often the most important part of the process. In research, as in marriage, having a wonderful partner with whom to share the process is both useful and helpful. This partner will make the journey more fun and a better and richer experience for having been there. Nursing research, like nursing itself, concerns many different and complex phenomena. Good research is seldom simple, and therefore, conducting research alone is seldom feasible. As a nurse you will be in an ideal position to identify practice problems. When these problems require research solutions, if you find a team to help solve them, both your patients and your nursing practice will be the better for it.

So, as you begin your research "marriage," how might you choose among the many different qualitative research methods? Of course, the first lesson learned in research classes is that the research design should match the question being asked. Another important consideration is the philosophy that underlies a research method and how it matches the objectives of the study. Both are addressed in this chapter. Understanding the philosophy upon which research is based also is important in evaluating research as a consumer and user of research in your nursing practice.

Figure 6-1 illustrates one of the reasons your research "marriage" might lead you to select a qualitative method. As this cartoon shows, Garfield is putting on glasses, and the scene changes as he realizes the glasses belong to Picasso. This is the goal of qualitative methods, to be able to see the world as those who are having the experience you are studying see it.

THE NATURE OF KNOWLEDGE

Of course, qualitative research is not the only way to obtain answers to questions. When you have clinical questions, many ways of knowing are important in providing answers to consider in guiding your practice. You are taught rituals and traditions in nursing. We also learn from experts who have experience and wisdom to share. We learn from other disciplines, which is why nursing students take courses in chemistry, philosophy, psychology, and other fields. We also learn from our intuition and sometimes know what to do from trial and error, although this is not a very efficient way to solve problems. We also learn from scientific problem solving.

Science is an important way to learn, and the knowledge from research is an important guide to be used in nursing practice. Knowledge from scientific reasoning or research is less vulnerable to individual skill level. On a good day what you do by "instinct" and naturally may be effective, but on a day when you are tired or have just experienced an upsetting event your performance may be adversely affected. If what we do is based on sound and logically derived research, we will do the same thing when we are tired or distracted as when we are more alert.

We sometimes learn in research that what we believe is helpful and what we have learned from experts may not in fact be helpful to a particular group of patients. An example of this is the now outmoded practice that experts taught for many years of not providing patients with information. Early nursing research clearly showed that providing patients with information of various types did improve their health in many ways (see for example, Johnson et al, 1997).

Belenky and associates (1986) interviewed women to describe their ways of knowing. The questions that interested them included: What is truth? What is authority? To whom do I listen? What counts for me as evidence? How do I know what I know?" Although their focus was women, these questions are relevant to all people. The answers to these basic questions are important guides to our nursing practice as they shape how we see the world and our roles in it. How we provide nursing care and how we conduct research differs depending on how we answer these questions.

PHILOSOPHIES OF RESEARCH

Every specialized field uses characteristic language to communicate important features of the work that are not as pertinent to those outside that field. Learning a new language is part of what students do in nursing school and part of what researchers do when they learn research methods and skills. Each research method and all philosophies of science have special language that you will encounter as you read. A few words are important to clarify so you can read the literature with a good understanding.

The word science comes from a word meaning "knowledge," and the word philosophy comes from one meaning "wisdom" (Brown, 1993). All research is based on *philosophical beliefs* about the world, also called a **worldview** or **paradigm. Paradigm** is from a Greek word meaning "pattern." Thomas Kuhn (1962) first applied this word to science to describe the way people in society think about the world.

Although those who conduct qualitative research are more likely to explicitly describe their beliefs and assumptions, all research is based on these beliefs. Therefore it is important to know and comprehend these beliefs in order to understand and use research findings. These views are not right or wrong, but rather they represent different ways of viewing the world that may be more or less useful, depending on the goals of the research. Table 6-1 compares two paradigms that are the basis for research. The perceived view is the basis for *naturalistic* (qualitative) research, while the received view is the basis of *empirical analytic* (quantitative) research. These paradigms can be thought of as extremes. That is, research approaches fall along a continuum, with these extremes at either end. Later in this chapter, five research approaches are discussed in the order they would fall along this continuum.

TABLE **6-1** Basic Beliefs of Research Paradigms

	PERCEIVED PARADIGM	RECEIVED PARADIGM
Epistemology	"Truth" determined by the individual or cultural group Subjectivism valued	Truth sought via replicable observation Objectivism valued
Ontology	Multiple realities exist, influenced by culture and environment	One reality exists "out there" Driven by natural laws
Context	Emphasized, value placed on rich details of context in which phenomenon occurs Time and place are important	Minimized, value placed on generalizability across contexts
Inquiry aims	Description (narrative), understanding, transformation, reconstruction	Description (statistical), explanation; prediction and control
Values	Included, add to understanding of phenomenon	Excluded, detract from inquiry aim
Voice of researcher	Active participant	Neutral observer
Methodology	Dialogic, transformative	Experimental, controlled

Adapted from Guba E, and Lincoln Y: *Competing paradigms in qualitative research.* In Denzin NK and Lincoln YS, editors: *Handbook of qualitative research,* Thousand Oaks, Calif, 1994, Sage.

HELPFUL **HINT** All research is based on a paradigm, but this is seldom specifically stated in a research report.

The philosophical language in Table 6-1 needs to be clarified. **Epistemology** deals with what it is we know, that is, what is "truth." The origins, nature, and limits of knowledge are included. It deals with why and how we know some things and what constitutes our knowing. **Ontology** (from the Greek *onto,* meaning "to be") is the science or study of being or existence and its relation to nonexistence. Existentialists and phenomenologists discuss Being and non-Being or Nothingness as categories. Ontology deals with what is real (versus fiction or appearance), what is the nature of reality, or matter. Whereas in the received view, one reality exists and we seek to learn the laws of nature, in the perceived view, reality is constructed differently by different people. For example, what is real and important to patients may be unnoticed by nurses. **Context** is where something occurs. Context can include physical settings such as the hospital or homes or less concrete "environments" such as the context cultural understandings and beliefs bring to an experience. The *aims of inquiry,* or the goals of

the research, also vary with the paradigm. The *researchers' role* or *voice* and how their *values* are viewed and *methodology* used also vary with different paradigms.

The "perceived paradigm," is the basis of most qualitative research (Suppe and Jacox, 1985) (see Chapters 7 and 8). The "received paradigm" is the basis of most empirical analytical or quantitative research (see Chapters 9 through 19). An example from oncology research may make it clear that some types of research are more congruent with the "received paradigm" than the "perceived paradigm" and vice versa. Consider the example of chemotherapy for cancer. When studying the efficacy of a drug for the treatment of cancer, it seems quite logical that experimental research should be used. This approach, based on the received paradigm, is guided by the ontological view that there is one reality. That is, that all people will respond in the same way to this drug. Of course, it is also true that responses to drugs may vary by age, gender, ethnicity, and so on, but those features can be considered by doing research that includes persons of diverse ethnicity and both genders and looking at the effect of the drugs by group. Epistemology leads to seeking truth in an objective, replicable way. That is, the way the drug is prepared and provided to people will be the same for each person, and other researchers in other parts of the world would do the research in the same way. In this framework, the emphasis is on studying parts, so the focus might be on the responses of tumor cells rather than the whole person. The context is not central in this research, which is why researchers would expect to find the same response to drugs in different parts of the world.

The goal of quantitative or empirical research is to control or cure the cancer and predict the outcome for patients, which is that the cancer would be eliminated or at least its growth slowed. The goal of research guided by the received view is to statistically describe; explain; predict; and finally, to control the cancer. In the received view, the basis of most quantitative research, researchers are neutral observers. That means that researchers do not have a vested interest in showing that the drug is better than another drug. Values are thought to detract from the inquiry. If someone who owned a company producing the drug ran a study, concerns would be raised about whether a profit motive was involved in how the research was done. Of course, values are always a part of what we do—we would not study something we did not believe is important, or that we value. The goal is to keep the values as separate from the research as possible.

However, when we are interested in what it means to people to have cancer or cancer treatment, a qualitative study is more appropriate. Qualitative studies, based on the perceived paradigm, are guided by the ontological view that there are multiple realities. The meaning of cancer will likely be different for a young mother than for a grandmother. The meaning of cancer also may be different in the United States than in Japan. Epistemology includes the view that truth varies and is subjective. Context is important, and description is the goal. When seeking to understand patients' experiences of a treatment, we would expect that what is important, and "true," for one person may not be for another. Some of the differences may result from context. The experience may well vary according to where the

person is treated and various features of the persons such as age, gender, ethnicity, and so on. Having cancer may well be different for someone whose parent died a painful death from cancer than for someone who knew people whose cancer was cured. The values of all involved are acknowledged. Researchers work to be sure their values do not cloud their view and prevent them from understanding how others view experiences. What is valued and important also helps us understand experiences. Qualitative research is conducted in a dialogue or interview with the participant who is seen as an active part of the research. In fact, while research is done with "subjects" in the received view, these people would more likely be called "informants" or "participants" to recognize their active role in the perceived paradigm. The research results would be useful in describing, understanding, and leading to a way to transform or change situations.

HELPFUL HINT Values are involved in all research. It is important, however, that they not influence the results of the research.

Another way of thinking about these views and linking them to research is illustrated in the critical thinking decision path. This decision algorithm illustrates that beliefs lead to different questions, which lead to selecting different research approaches. Different research methods have different assumptions that are consistent with that method but more specific than these global worldviews. These beliefs and approaches lead to different research activities as is illustrated in the critical thinking path.

This chapter provides an overview of the five research traditions commonly used in qualitative nursing research. These traditions are the quantitative methods or empirical analytical research and the qualitative approaches of grounded theory, case study, ethnographic, and phenomenological research. Each of these is discussed as shown in Figure 6-2, and they are based on views that move along a continuum from the received view to the perceived view.

CRITICAL THINKING DECISION PATH Selecting A Research Process

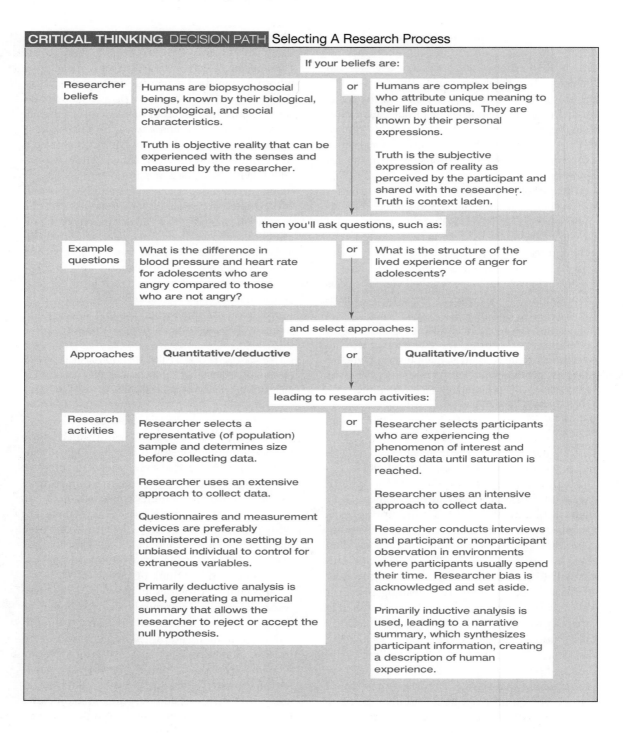

If your beliefs are:

Researcher beliefs

Humans are biopsychosocial beings, known by their biological, psychological, and social characteristics.

Truth is objective reality that can be experienced with the senses and measured by the researcher.

or

Humans are complex beings who attribute unique meaning to their life situations. They are known by their personal expressions.

Truth is the subjective expression of reality as perceived by the participant and shared with the researcher. Truth is context laden.

then you'll ask questions, such as:

Example questions

What is the difference in blood pressure and heart rate for adolescents who are angry compared to those who are not angry?

or

What is the structure of the lived experience of anger for adolescents?

and select approaches:

Approaches   **Quantitative/deductive**   *or*   **Qualitative/inductive**

leading to research activities:

Research activities

Researcher selects a representative (of population) sample and determines size before collecting data.

Researcher uses an extensive approach to collect data.

Questionnaires and measurement devices are preferably administered in one setting by an unbiased individual to control for extraneous variables.

Primarily deductive analysis is used, generating a numerical summary that allows the researcher to reject or accept the null hypothesis.

or

Researcher selects participants who are experiencing the phenomenon of interest and collects data until saturation is reached.

Researcher uses an intensive approach to collect data.

Researcher conducts interviews and participant or nonparticipant observation in environments where participants usually spend their time. Researcher bias is acknowledged and set aside.

Primarily inductive analysis is used, leading to a narrative summary, which synthesizes participant information, creating a description of human experience.

QUANTITATIVE/EMPIRICAL ANALYTICAL RESEARCH

Empirical analytical is a general label for quantitative research approaches that test hypotheses. These methods are discussed in detail in Part 3. In this chapter about philosophical foundations of qualitative research, it is important to note that although all research is based on philosophy, researchers who use quantitative approaches are less aware of, or at least often make less explicit, the philosophy underlying the research. The philosophical basis, which is the "received" view, is also called positivism. This approach to research focuses on testing hypotheses that are derived from theories or conceptual frameworks. The goal is to support the research hypothesis, and therefore reject the null hypothesis with the data from the study (see Chapter 17). In addition to the received view beliefs already discussed, Weiss (1995) argued that three assumptions underlie contemporary empiricism in nursing (Box 6-1).

The remainder of this chapter focuses on four qualitative research methods and their philosophical foundations. The methods are described in the order they appear on the continuum in Figure 6-2.

GROUNDED THEORY

Grounded theory is a research method designed to inductively develop a theory based on observations of the world of selected people. In an example of a grounded theory study, oncology patients were interviewed about their care experiences in order to develop a theory of what constitutes quality nursing care (Radwin, 2000). Grounded theory moves along the philosophical continuum from the received view toward the perceived view (see Figure 6-2). It is a method based on the sociological tradition of the Chicago School of Symbolic Interactionism. Glaser and Strauss (1967) developed the method of grounded theory, which has changed over time, but three major premises continue to underlie grounded theory research (Box 6-2) (Blumer, 1969).

The purpose of grounded theory, as the name implies, is to generate a theory from data. Qualitative data are gathered through interviews and observation. Analysis generates substantive codes that are clustered into categories. Propositions about the relationships among and between the categories create a conceptual framework, which guides further data collection. Additional data thought likely to answer generated hypotheses are collected until all categories are "saturated," meaning no new information is generated (see Chapter 7). The goal of

---

BOX 6-1 Assumptions of Contemporary Empiricism

1. The world is to some extent predictable. Reality has order to it that is driven by laws of nature.
2. The purpose of research is to develop the basis for nursing care.
3. Human responses to health and illness can be identified, measured, and understood.

Continuum of research and methods

Paradigm:
Received view ——————————————————————→ Perceived view

Research tradition:
Quantitative research / grounded theory / case study / ethnographic / phenomenological
(Empiric analytic)

Approach to research:
Falsify hypotheses— generate theory— describe— describe and interpret

Figure 6-2 Continuum of philosophical foundations and qualitative research methods.

BOX 6-2

Major Premises of Grounded Theory

1. Humans act toward objects on the basis of the meaning those objects have for them. Meaning is in, and cannot be separated from, the context or from the consequences of the meanings in a particular setting.
2. Social meanings arise from social interactions with others over time and are embedded socially, historically, culturally, and contextually. The focus of grounded theory is therefore social interactions.
3. People use interpretive processes to handle and change meanings in dealing with their situations.

generating a theory implies that laws drive at least some portion of reality. The truth is sought from relevant groups, for example, those who are dying. The context is very important, as was shown in a classic work by Glaser and Strauss (1965). They noted that at the time of this work Americans were unwilling to talk openly about the process of dying, American physicians were unwilling to disclose impending death to patients, and nurses were expected not to make these disclosures. This lack of communication led Glaser and Strauss (1965) to their study of the problem of awareness of dying. They described various types of awareness contexts, problems of awareness, and practical uses of awareness theory. Their early fieldwork led to hypotheses and the gathering of additional data, and the framework was refined with further analysis until they formed a systematic substantive theory.

CASE STUDY

Case study as a research method involves an in-depth description of essential dimensions and processes of the phenomenon being studied. Case study research has been given several definitions and can be thought of as the collection of detailed, relatively unstructured information from several sources, usually including the reports of those being studied.

Case studies can be used in a variety of ways, including as a way to present data gathered with another method, as a teaching device, or as a research method (Yin, 1994). Hammersley (1989) linked case studies to the Chicago School of Sociology, where grounded theory was developed. Case studies have been used in various disciplines, including nursing, political science, sociology, business, social work, economics, and psychology. Nurses have a long and continuing tradition of using case studies for teaching and learning about patients (e.g., Parsons, 1911). Nightingale (1969) stressed the importance of coming to know patients and of basing practice on experience. She noted that knowing how to provide care "must entirely depend upon an inquiry into all the conditions in which the patient lives." In case studies, these details are described and lessons that can be learned from the particular patient are made clear. The *American Journal of Nursing* recently introduced case studies as a regular feature. The editor noted that case studies are a way of providing in-depth, evidence-based discussion of clinical topics along with practical information and guidelines for improving practice (Mason, 2000). The journal features actual case studies, written by staff nurses, and includes a commentary on some aspect of the case. A case study on advocacy by Miller, Cohen, and Kagan, (2000) was the first example of this new feature.

Case studies allow us to understand complex phenomena about which little is known. They can be exploratory and descriptive, as in Whyte's famous example (1943/1955) describing one neighborhood. They also can be explanatory, as in Allison's (1971) case of the Soviet Union and the United States confrontation over placement of missiles in Cuba. They can involve one case or multiple cases.

When used as research, case studies have the following characteristics (Yin, 1994):
- Case studies investigate contemporary phenomenon within real life context.
- Case studies are used when the boundaries between phenomenon and context are not clear.
- Case studies are used when there are more features of interest (or variables) than "data points."

- Case studies use multiple sources of evidence and converge or triangulate data. Both quantitative and qualitative data can be used.
- Data collection and analysis are guided by theory.

An example of a case study described a 32-year-old black woman who was diagnosed with an abnormal Pap smear (Shireen, 1998). This woman did not follow through with the recommended treatment. The understanding her case provides can perhaps be used to help identify ways to motivate women to obtain needed treatment.

ETHNOGRAPHIC RESEARCH

Anthropologists developed **ethnographic research,** a tradition viewed as beginning with the British anthropologist Bronislaw Malinowski, who was influenced by Rivers, a physician-anthropologist-psychologist (Stocking, 1983). Scotch (1963) first described medical anthropology as the field of research that focuses on health and illness within a cultural system. Nurses conduct medical ethnographies (Roper and Shapira, 2000). Although early work was done on "foreign" cultures, nurses now often do focused ethnographies, which are the study of distinct problems within a specific context among a small group of people or the study of a groups' social construction and understanding of a health or illness experience (Roper and Shapira, 2000). **Ethnographies** describe cognitive models or patterns of behavior of people within a culture. They seek to understand another way of life from the "native's" perspective.

The following values underlie ethnography:
- Culture is fundamental to ethnographic studies. Culture includes behavioral/materialist and cognitive perspectives. The behavioral/materialist perspective sees culture as observed through a group's patterns of behavior and customs, their way of life, and what they produce. In the cognitive perspective, culture consists of beliefs, knowledge, and ideas people use as they live. Culture is the structures of meaning through which we shape experiences.
- Understanding culture requires a holistic perspective that captures the breadth of beliefs, knowledge, and activities of the group being studied.
- Context is important for an understanding of a culture. Understanding this context requires intensive face-to-face contact over an extended time. People are studied where they live, in their natural settings, or where an experience occurs, such as in a hospital or in a community setting.
- The aim of ethnographies is to combine the emic perspective—the insider's view of the world—with the etic perspective—the view the researcher (outsider) brings—to develop a scientific generalization about different societies. That is, generalizations are drawn from special examples or details from participant observation.

An example of ethnographic work that has been useful to nurses is the idea of explanatory models. This idea was most developed by cognitive anthropologists, especially Kleinman and associates (Kleinman, 1980). Explanatory models use an interactive approach, emphasizing variations between patients' and practitioners' models of illness. They offer explanations of sickness and treatment, guide choices among available therapies and therapists, and give social meaning to the experience of sickness. These cognitive models vary over time and in response to a particular illness episode. Allan (1998) recently used this idea to explore women's explanatory models of being overweight and the congruence of these models with professional models and the professionally recommended treatment for being overweight. This information can guide nursing interventions with those who need treatment for being overweight.

PHENOMENOLOGICAL RESEARCH

Phenomenological research is used to answer questions of meaning. This method is most useful when the task is to understand an experience as those having the experience understand it. Phenomenological research is an important method with which to begin when studying a new topic or a topic that has been studied but for which a fresh perspective is needed.

Phenomenological research is based on phenomenological philosophy, which has changed over time and with philosophers. Various and differing phenomenological methods exist, including eidetic phenomenology, which is descriptive and based on Husserl's philosophy; Heideggerian phenomenology, which is interpretive and based on Heidegger's philosophy; and hermeneutical phenomenology, which is both descriptive and interpretive and is based on the Dutch phenomenologists (Cohen, Kahn, and Steeves, 2000).

There are five important concepts or values in phenomenological research (Cohen, 1987):

1. Phenomenological research was developed to understand meanings. The goal was to develop a rigorous science in the service of humanity. This science seeks to go to the roots or foundations of a topic to be clear about what the basic concepts are and what they mean.
2. Phenomenology was based on a critique of positivism, or the received view, which was seen as inappropriate to the study of some human concerns. Carefully considering representative examples was the test of knowledge.
3. The object of study is the life-world (*Lebenswelt*), or lived experience, not contrived situations. That is, as Husserl said, we go to the things themselves. We are concerned with the appearance of things (phenomena) rather than the things themselves (noumena). For example, think about a desk in a classroom. There is a real physical object, the noumena, which we all see. If that were not the case, we would bump into the desk every time we passed it. In addition, there is your view of that desk, the phenomena, that changes as you move in the room. If you sit at the desk, you only see the top of it. However, as you move away you can see the desk's legs and so on.

Nurses are often interested in various aspects of peoples' experiences or views of health, illness, and treatment.

4. Intersubjectivity, the belief that others share a common world with us, is an important tenet in phenomenology. Although phenomena differ, they also share similarities based on the similarities in people. The most fundamental of those similarities is that we all have a body in space and time. That is, our physical bodies and historical sense lead to similarities in how we experience phenomena.
5. The phenomenological reduction, also called bracketing, is more important in some phenomenological approaches than in others. It is the statement that researchers must be aware of and examine their prejudices or values. The term bracketing comes from the mathematical metaphor of putting "brackets" around our beliefs so they can be put aside and we can "see" the experience as the person having it sees it rather than as it changes as filtered through our prejudices.

For example, in a study of persons who had had blood and marrow transplantation (BMT), patients described spiritual aspects in their experiences. Their illness and its treatment led them to a search for meaning and purpose in life that went beyond (transcended) the individual (Cohen, Headley, and Sherwood, 2000). Understanding these experiences can assist nurses to provide comprehensive care to whole persons, rather than focusing only on fragmented tasks that need to be accomplished in providing nursing care. Our goal is to come to understand the world as the person who has had the experience sees it. We shift our perspective to see the world as patients see it—something that is central to providing competent nursing care to meet patient needs.

MATCHING RESEARCH GOALS WITH RESEARCH PHILOSOPHY

Some researchers have written about "qualitative" and "quantitative" research as incompatible approaches. The value of one over the other has been argued. However, others have recognized that different research methods accomplish different goals, and they advocate using the method appropriate to the research question and combining methods when this best suits the research goals. Understanding the philosophy underlying each method can help researchers use the method that best meets the intended purpose and can guide the reader to use the research findings in appropriate ways. In the example regarding chemotherapy used at the beginning of this chapter, when studying the effectiveness of a drug for cancer, it would be foolish to ignore measuring changes in tumor size. It would be equally foolish to ignore what patients tell us is important to them when taking this drug when we want to understand what it means to them. Because meanings may well determine needs that can be met with nursing interventions, such as the need for information or the need to talk about fear of death, this information is vital to guide effective nursing practice.

CRITIQUING the Foundation of Qualitative Research

A final example illustrates the differences in the methods discussed in this chapter and provides you with the beginning skills of how to critique qualitative research. The information in this chapter coupled with the information presented in Chapter 7 will provide the underpinnings of critical analysis of qualitative research. Consider the question of nursing students learning how to conduct research. The empirical analytical approach (quantitative research) might be used in an experiment to see if one teaching method led to better learning outcomes than another. The students' knowledge might be tested, the teaching conducted, and then a posttest of knowledge given. Scores on these tests would be analyzed statistically to see if the different methods produced a difference in the results.

The grounded theorist would be interested in the process, and for this example, would consider the process of learning research. The researcher might attend the class to see what occurs, and interview students to ask them to describe how their learning changed over time. They might be asked to describe becoming researchers or becoming more knowledgeable about research. The goal would be to describe the stages or process of this learning.

A case study could be written about a particular research class to provide a detailed description of the class or perhaps a particular individual in the class. The case would then be used to explicate what is important in this setting.

Ethnographers would consider the class as a culture and could join to observe and interview students. Questions would get at the students' values, behaviors, and beliefs in learning research. The goal would be to understand and describe the group members' shared meanings.

Phenomenologists would be interested in the meaning of the students' experiences. They would get at this by asking students to describe learning research, that is, to give concrete specific examples. The goal would be to understand and describe the meaning of this experience for the students.

Many other research methods exist. Although it is important to be aware of the basis of the research methods used, it is most important that the method chosen is the one that will provide the best approach to answering the question being asked. Some research methods, such as focus groups developed from marketing research, are not explicitly based on philosophy, but they have been useful as a method of collecting data to answer nursing research questions. An example of focus group research was a study conducted with groups of black women to explore their beliefs, attitudes, and practices related to

CRITIQUING CRITERIA

- Is the philosophical basis of the research method consistent with the study's purpose?
- Are the researchers' values apparent and influencing the research or the results of the study?
- Is the phenomenon focused on human experience within a natural setting?

breast cancer screening (Phillips, Cohen, and Moses, 1999). This approach was chosen because little qualitative research related to breast cancer screening had been conducted with black women. This area is important to study because black women have lower survival rates and more breast cancers detected at a later stage than other groups. Therefore, this type of information is needed to develop interventions to increase screening in a way that will take into account cultural factors.

A helpful metaphor about the need to use a variety of research methods was used by Seymour Kety, a key figure in the development of biological research in psychiatry who was the scientific director to the U.S. National Institute of Mental Health (NIMH) for many years. He invited readers to think about a civilization whose inhabitants, although very intelligent, had never seen a book (Kety, 1960). On discovering a library, they set up a scientific institute for studying books, which included anatomists, physical chemists, molecular biologists, behavioral scientists, and psychoanalysts. Each discipline discovered important facts, such as the structure of cellulose, the frequency of collections of letters of varying length, and so on. But the meaning of a "book" continued to escape them. As he put it: "We do not always get closer to the truth as we slice and homogenize and isolate." He argued that a truer picture of a topic under study would emerge only from research by a variety of disciplines and techniques, each with its own virtues and particular limitations. Qualitative research methods could be added to understand how books are used by different groups, the meaning of books for individuals, and so on.

This idea can serve as summary of an important point of this chapter. It is not that one research method is better than others, but rather that there are a variety of methods, based on different worldviews. Considering what we need to know to do the important and complex work of nursing, we need to guide our practice with knowledge from both nonscientifical and scientifical realms, and within science, from a wide variety of methods.

Critical Thinking Challenges
Barbara Krainovich-Miller

➤ Explain the differences between research that uses a "perceived paradigm" vs. a "received paradigm" as the basis of the respective study.

➤ Discuss how a researcher's values could influence the results of a study. Include an example in your answer.

➤ If a grounded theory research study developed a theory, for example, on why certain cultural groups do not use pain medication, why is it necessary to test it with empirical methods?

➤ Can the metaphor "We do not always get closer to the truth as we slice and homogenize and isolate [it]" be applied to both qualitative and quantitative methods? Justify your answer.

Key Points

- All research is based on philosophical beliefs or a paradigm.
- Paradigms are useful or not useful in reaching research goals, but are not correct or incorrect.
- Values should be kept as separate as possible from the conduct of research.
- Grounded theory is based on Symbolic Interactionism and is focused on processes or social interactions.
- Case studies are based on the Chicago School of Sociology and are ways to study complex real life situations.
- Ethnographical research, developed by anthropologists, is used to understand cultures.
- Phenomenological research is based on phenomenological philosophy and is designed to understand the meaning of a lived experience.

REFERENCES

Allan J: Explanatory models of overweight among African American, Euro-American, and Mexican American women, *West J Nurs Res* 20(1):45-66, 1998.

Allison G: *Essence of decision: explaining the Cuban missile crisis,* Boston, 1971, Little, Brown.

Belenky M et al: *Women's ways of knowing: the development of self, voice, and mind,* New York, 1986, Basic Books.

Blumer H: *Symbolic interactionism: perspective and method,* Englewood Cliffs, NJ, 1969, Prentice Hall.

Brown L, editor: *The new shorter Oxford English dictionary,* Oxford, 1993, Clarendon Press.

Cohen MZ: A historical overview of the phenomenological movement, *Image* 19(1):31-34, 1987.

Cohen MZ, Headley J, and Sherwood G: Spirituality in bone marrow transplantation: When faith is stronger than fear, *Int J Hum Caring* 4(2):40-46, 2000.

Cohen MZ, Kahn D, and Steeves R: *Hermeneutic phenomenological research: a practical guide for nurse researchers,* Thousand Oaks, Calif, 2000, Sage.

Glaser B and Strauss A: *Awareness of dying,* Chicago, 1965, Aldine De Gruyter.

Glaser B and Strauss A: *The discovery of grounded theory: strategies for qualitative research,* New York, 1967, Aldine De Gruyter.

Guba E and LincolnY: Competing paradigms in qualitative research. In Denzin NK and Lincoln YS, editors: *Handbook of qualitative research,* Thousand Oaks, Calif, 1994, Sage.

Hammersley M: *The dilemma of qualitative research,* Routledge, London, 1989, Herbert Blumer and the Chicago Tradition.

Johnson J et al: *Self-regulation theory: applying theory to your practice,* Pittsburgh, 1997, Oncology Nursing Press.

Kety S: A biologist examines mind and behavior, *Science* 132(3443):1861-1870, 1960.

Kleinman A: *Patients and healers in the context of culture,* Berkeley, 1980, University of California Press.

Kuhn T: *The structure of scientific revolutions,* Chicago, 1962, The University of Chicago Press.

Marcus M and Liehr P: Qualitative approaches to research. In LoBiondo-Wood G and Haber J, editors: *Nursing research: methods, critical appraisal, and utilization,* ed 4, St Louis, 1998, Mosby.

Mason D: On centennials and millennia, *Am J Nurs* 100(1):7, 2000 (editorial).

Miller SH, Cohen MZ, and Kagan SH: The measure of advocacy, *Am J Nurs* 100(1):61-64, 2000.

Nightingale F: *Notes on nursing: what it is and what it is not,* New York, 1969, Dover.

Parsons S: The case method of teaching nursing, *Am J Nurs* 11(11):1009-1011, 1911.

Phillips JM, Cohen MZ, and Moses G: Breast cancer screening and African-American women: fear, fatalism, and silence, *Oncol Nurs Forum* 26(3), 561-571, 1999.

Radwin L: Oncology patients' perception of quality nursing care, *Res Nurs Health* 23(3):179-190, 2000.

Roper J and Shapira J: *Ethnography in nursing research,* Thousand Oaks, Calif, 2000, Sage.

Scotch N: Medical anthropology, *Biennial Rev Anthropol* 3:30-68, 1963.

Shireen R: Nonadherence to follow-up treatment of an abnormal Pap smear: a case study, *Cancer Nurs* 21(5):342-348, 1998.

Stocking G: *Observers observed: essays on ethnographic fieldwork,* Madison, 1983, University of Wisconsin Press.

Suppe F and Jacox A: Philosophy of science and the development of nursing theory. In Werley H and Fitzpatrick J, editors: *Annual review of nursing research,* 3:241-267, 1985.

Weiss S: Contemporary empiricism. In Omery A, Kasper C, and Page G, editors: In *Search of nursing science,* Thousand Oaks, Calif, 1995, Sage.

Whyte W: *Street corner society: the social structure of an Italian slum,* Chicago, 1955, (original publication 1943), University of Chicago Press.

Yin R: *Case study research: design and methods,* ed 2, Thousand Oaks, Calif, 1994, Sage.

PATRICIA R. LIEHR
MARIANNE TAFT MARCUS

7

Qualitative Approaches to Research

Key Terms

auditability
bracketing
case study method
constant comparative
  method
credibility
culture
data saturation
domains
emic view

ethnographic method
etic view
external criticism
fittingness
grounded theory method
historical research method
internal criticism
instrumental case study
intrinsic case study
key informants

life context
lived experience
phenomenological method
primary sources
qualitative research
secondary sources
theoretical sampling
triangulation

Learning Outcomes

After reading this chapter, the student should be able to do the following:

- Distinguish the characteristics of qualitative research from those of quantitative research.
- Recognize the uses of qualitative research for nursing.
- Identify the processes of phenomenological, grounded theory, ethnographic, and case study methods.
- Recognize appropriate use of historical methods.
- Identify research methodology emerging from nursing theory.
- Discuss significant issues that arise in conducting qualitative research in relation to such topics as ethics, criteria for judging scientific rigor, combination of research methods, and use of computers to assist data management.
- Apply the critiquing criteria to evaluate a report of qualitative research.

Nursing is a body of knowledge that provides the foundation for practice and research. It is both a science and an art. **Qualitative research** combines the scientific and artistic natures of nursing to enhance understanding of the human health experience. It is a general term encompassing a variety of philosophic underpinnings and research methods. According to Denzin and Lincoln (2000), "qualitative researchers study things in their natural settings, attempting to make sense of, or interpret, phenomena in terms of the meanings people bring to them." Naturalistic settings are ones that people live in everyday. So, the researcher doing qualitative research goes wherever the participants are—in their homes, schools, communities, and sometimes in the hospital or an outpatient setting.

This chapter focuses on four of the most commonly used qualitative research methods: grounded theory, ethnography, phenomenology, and case study. Each of these methods, although distinct from the others, shares characteristics that identify it as a method within the qualitative research approach. In the previous chapter, Cohen located these qualitative methods along a continuum ranging from the "received" to the "perceived" view paradigm. She emphasized the importance of one's paradigmatic perspective, sometimes called a worldview. Embedded in one's worldview are beliefs that guide the choice of an issue for research study and the creation of a research study question. For instance, if your view fits best with the received paradigm, it is likely that you believe in the composite nature of humans, allowing isolation of body systems for accurate measurement purposes. If you hold this perspective, you will pose a research question to be addressed by an empiric/analytic method. If, on the other hand, your view fits best with the perceived paradigm, it is likely that you believe in the unitary nature of human life—that humans are intricately connected to each other and their environment. If you hold this perspective, you will most often pose a research question that can be best addressed with a qualitative method.

It is important to understand that one research method is not better than another; one is not good while another is excellent and yet another poor. The only judgment of excellence has to do with the fit between one's worldview, the research question, and the research method. If there is congruence between worldview, question, and method, then the researcher has made an excellent choice of method. For instance, if a researcher's worldview comes from the received view paradigm and a question about the effect of slow stroke back massage on blood pressure is posed, there is a good fit between the worldview and the research question. Massage is an intervention that can be manipulated by the researcher, and blood pressure is an outcome variable that can be measured. When researchers study the effects of an intervention on an outcome variable, they generally use empiric/analytic methods, grounded in the received worldview.

In this chapter, you are invited to look through the lens of the perceived view to learn about grounded theory, ethnographic, phenomenological, and case study methods. You are encouraged to change glasses as each method is introduced—to imagine how it would be to study an issue of interest from the perspective of each of these methods. No matter which methods a researcher uses, there is a demand to embrace the wholeness of humans, focusing on human experience in natural settings. The researcher using these methods believes that unique humans attribute meaning to their experience, and experience evolves from life context. **Life context** is the matrix of human-human-environment relationships emerging over the course of day-to-day living. So, one person's experience of pain is distinct from another's and can be known by the individual's subjective description of it. The researcher interested in studying the lived experience of pain for the adolescent with rheumatoid arthritis will spend time in the adolescent's natural settings, such as the home and school. Effort will be directed to uncover the meaning of pain as it extends beyond the facts of the number of medications taken or a rating on a reliable and valid scale. These methods are grounded in the belief that factual objective data do not capture the human experience. Rather, the meaning of the ado-

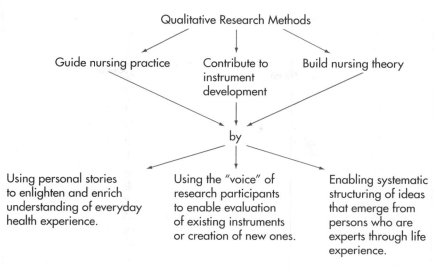

Figure 7-1   Qualitative approach and nursing science

lescent's pain emerges within the context of personal history, current relationships, and future plans as the adolescent lives daily life in dynamic interaction with environment.

The researcher using qualitative methods begins collecting bits of information and piecing them together, building a mosaic or a picture of the human experience being studied. As with a mosaic, when one steps away from the work, the whole picture emerges. This whole picture transcends the bits and pieces and cannot be known from any one bit or piece. In presenting study findings, the researcher strives to capture the human experience and present it so that others can understand it. Often, findings are shared as a summary story.

QUALITATIVE APPROACH AND NURSING SCIENCE

Qualitative research is particularly well suited to study the human experience of health, a central concern of nursing science. Because qualitative methods focus on the whole of human experience and the meaning ascribed by individuals living the experience, these methods extend understanding of health beyond traditionally measured units

to include the complexity of the human health experience as it is occurring in everyday living. This closeness to what is "real" and "everyday" promises guidance for nursing practice; it is also important for instrument and theory development (Figure 7-1). Three examples are cited to emphasize the capacity of qualitative methods to (1) guide nursing practice, (2) contribute to instrument development, and (3) develop nursing theory.

QUALITATIVE RESEARCH GUIDING PRACTICE

In a study of caring for dying patients who have air hunger, Tarzian (2000) suggests that "understanding is the first step toward a more consistent and informed response by health care providers to dying patients who suffer from air hunger, and to their family members who witness their distress." Because of the ethical and practical problems of studying patients enduring air hunger, Tarzian (2000) studied the experience of nurses caring for these patients and family members who had witnessed air hunger. Twelve nurses and two family members participated. Family members' descriptions were used to enhance what was shared by the nurses.

An interpretive phenomenologic method was used to analyze the data. Tarzian (2000) identified three major themes related to caring for dying patients who have air hunger: patient's look-panic beckons, surrendering and sharing control, and fine tuning dying. The first theme highlights the interactive patient-nurse relationship. Nurses described their own unsettled feelings when confronting a dying air hungry patient. The second theme continues to emphasize the interactive nurse-patient relationship, describing the balance of surrendering and controlling as choices are made to ease discomfort. The final theme, fine tuning dying, provides the substance of guidance for practice. Within this theme, the author synthesizes a caring direction: (1) attend to both patient and family needs for comfort; (2) plan ahead to decide what will be done when air hunger occurs; (3) prepare patients and family ahead of time so that they know what to expect; (4) be prepared to deal with barriers, such as the failure of physicians to order or the failure of nurses to provide comfort-inducing medication.

In this study the author has provided a description of the human experience of air hunger and has derived guidance for health care providers. The importance of the interactive nurse-patient/family relationship during the suffering of air hunger surfaces as implicit guidance in addition to the explicit direction emerging from the third theme. That is, the ability of the nurse to "be with" the patient and family is a critical dimension in the stories shared by nurses and family members. The consumer of nursing research reading this study can use the information to plan care for persons suffering air hunger. The information enables thoughtful consideration of the challenges to be encountered in this nursing situation.

QUALITATIVE RESEARCH CONTRIBUTING TO INSTRUMENT DEVELOPMENT

As part of a larger study evaluating the reliability and validity of the adolescent version of the Cook-Medley Hostility Scale, Liehr and associates (2000) used qualitative analysis to assess the content validity of the scale. The scale had been tested and used often with adults but there was little information about the adolescent version of the scale, and all the available information had been collected with Anglo-American children and adolescents.

Fifty-seven male and female African-, Anglo-, and Mexican-American adolescents were studied. Each adolescent was asked to recall a time when he/she felt angry and to share it with the data collector in as much detail as could be recalled. Remembered circumstances that provoked anger were ones that were likely to be accompanied by hostile attitudes. Data were analyzed using a content analysis procedure outlined by Waltz, Strickland, and Lenz (1991).

Five themes were synthesized to capture the adolescents' descriptions of circumstances that made them angry: aggression, unfulfilled personal expectations, mistrust/lying, criticism of effort, and rejection. These five themes were used to evaluate the comprehensiveness of the 23-item hostility scale. The researchers were interested in whether the hostility scale addressed all the themes presented by the adolescents. Eight hostility scale items were linked with mistrust/lying, four with rejection, three with aggression, and only one each with unfulfilled personal expectations and criticism of effort. To improve the comprehensiveness of the scale's content and therefore improve content validity, the authors suggest adding an additional four items: two to tap unfulfilled personal expectations and two to tap criticism of effort. This would result in a minimum of three hostility items for each anger/hostility theme. In this instance, qualitative research was used to strengthen an existing instrument, making it more relevant to the population for whom it was intended.

QUALITATIVE RESEARCH CONTRIBUTING TO THEORY BUILDING

As a consumer of nursing research, you will notice that the qualitative method most readily linked with theory building is the grounded theory method. Schreiber, Stern, and Wilson (2000) studied depression in twelve black West-Indian Canadian women (see Chapter 8). They asked participants the question "What is it like to go through depression as a black West-Indian Canadian? In addition to interviews, participant observation occurred, in keeping with the grounded theory method. The authors emphasize that this experience was heavily influenced by major contexts: visible minority status in a Eurocentric society, social stigma of depression imposed by their own cultural group, gender expectations within their cultural group, and Christian up-bringing.

"The goal of the women was to be able to manage their depression with grace and to live up to the cultural imperative to be strong." Being strong was the overarching social process used by these women in managing their depression. Being strong included the subprocesses of "dwelling on it," "diverting myself," and "regaining my composure." Dwelling on it referred to the women's recognition that suffering and struggle were integral with being a woman and there was little they could do about it. As a way of dwelling on it, the authors describe patterns of separating from others; gaining a sense of competence by showing compassion when confronted with insensitive behavior; and recognizing the depression for what it was, which enabled them to divert themselves. Diverting self, the second subprocess, was the beginning of efforts to manage depression. These efforts included seeking God's comfort, professional help, socializing, exercising, and thinking positively. The author's suggest that diverting self led to the third subprocess, regaining composure. Regaining composure was characterized by "recognizing God's strength within" and moving on with everyday living.

These central subprocesses of being strong were enhanced by the willingness of some women to consider other ways to manage their depression. The authors labeled this willing effort "trying new approaches." They emphasize the challenging nature of new approaches for women embedded in the black West-Indian Canadian cultural context. The authors provide a model of "being strong," depicting the relationships between subprocesses and contexts. This qualitative study enabled creation of the structure of "being strong," which contributes to nursing's knowledge base and offers guidance for further research and practice.

FOUR QUALITATIVE RESEARCH METHODS

Thus far an overview of the qualitative research approach has been presented, attending to its importance for nursing science. An effort has been made to highlight how choice of a qualitative approach is reflective of one's worldview and research question and how qualitative methods contribute to guiding practice, testing instruments, and building theory. These topics provide a foundation for examining the four qualitative methods discussed in this chapter. The Critical Thinking Decision Path introduces the consumer of nursing research to a process for recognizing differing qualitative methods by distinguishing areas of interest for each method and noting how the research question might be introduced for each distinct method. The phenomenological, grounded theory, ethnographic, and case study methods are described for the consumer of nursing research.

Parse, Coyne, and Smith (1985) suggested that research methods, whether quantitative or qualitative, include the following five basic elements:
1. Identifying the phenomenon
2. Structuring the study
3. Gathering the data
4. Analyzing the data
5. Describing the findings

Each qualitative method is defined, followed by a discussion of these five basic elements. The factors that distinguish the methods are highlighted, and research examples are presented, providing critiquing direction for the beginning research consumer.

PHENOMENOLOGICAL METHOD

The **phenomenological method** is a process of learning and constructing the meaning of human

CRITICAL THINKING DECISION PATH Selecting a Qualitative Research Method

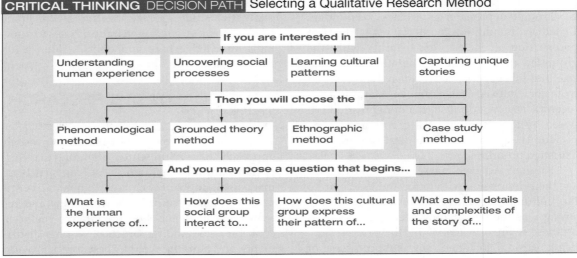

experience through intensive dialogue with persons who are living the experience. The researcher's goal is to understand the meaning of the experience as it is lived by the participant. Meaning is pursued through a dialogic process, which extends beyond a simple interview and requires thoughtful presence on the part of the researcher. In the previous chapter, Cohen introduced the nurse research consumer to the traditional philosophical bases, which provide a foundation for phenomenological research. Each philosopher-guided (Husserl's eidetic phenomenology; Heidegger's interpretive phenomenology; Dutch hermeneutical phenomenology) base directs slight differences in research methods. Further, Caelli (2000) has distinguished American forms of phenomenological research from the traditional forms. She suggests that nursing tends to use American forms, which focus on understanding the reality of experience for *the person* as they engage with the phenomenon, rather than focusing on the more objective *phenomenon itself*, as is the case in traditional forms of phenomenological research. Whatever the form of phenomenological research, the consumer of nursing research will find the researcher asking a question about lived experience.

IDENTIFYING THE PHENOMENON

Because the focus of the phenomenological method is the **lived experience,** the researcher is likely to choose this method when studying some dimension of day-to-day existence for a particular group of individuals. For instance, the nurse may be interested in the experience of anger for persons who have heart disease or the experience of success for baccalaureate nursing students. Chiu (2000) studied the lived experience of spirituality for Taiwanese women with breast cancer, and Burton (2000) studied the experience of living with stroke. Each of these authors used the phenomenological method to explore dimensions of health as it was lived day-to-day. Cohen and Ley (2000) (see Appendix B) studied the experience of having an autologous bone marrow transplant. They subtitled their work: "The battle for hope in the face of fear. The researchers used the hermeneutical phenomenological method. Their research report is used to guide understanding of the phenomenological method.

STRUCTURING THE STUDY

For the purpose of describing structuring, the following topics are addressed: the research question, the researcher's perspective, and sample selection. The issue of human subjects' protection has been suggested as a dimension of structuring (Parse, Coyne, and Smith, 1985); this issue is discussed generally with ethics in a subsequent section of the chapter.

Research Question

The question that guides phenomenological research always asks about some experience of everyday living. It guides the researcher to ask the participant about some past or present experience. The research question is not exactly the same as the question used to initiate dialogue with the participant, but often, the research question and the question used to begin dialogue are very similar. For instance, Orne and associates (2000) posed the research question: What is the lived experience of being employed but medically uninsured? The statement that introduced their research dialogue with participants was: "Please describe for me as thoroughly as you can, what it is like to be working without medical insurance." It is important that the question used to begin dialogue be understandable for the participant. Cohen and Ley's (2000) research question was, "What is the human experience of having an autologous bone marrow transplant?" Participants were volunteers who had undergone and survived an autologous bone marrow transplant. The question the researcher posed to the participants was, "What was it like to have a bone marrow transplant?"

HELPFUL HINT   Although the research question may not always be explicitly reported, it may be identified by evaluating the study purpose or the question/statement posed to the participants.

Researcher's Perspective

When using the phenomenological method, the researcher's perspective is **bracketed.** That is, the researcher identifies personal biases about the phenomenon of interest to clarify how personal experience and beliefs may color what is heard and reported. The researcher is expected to set aside personal biases—to bracket them—when engaged with the participants. By becoming aware of personal biases, the researcher is more likely to be able to pursue issues of importance as introduced by the participant, rather than leading the participant to issues the researcher deems important.

In the previous chapter, Cohen suggested that bracketing was more important for some phenomenologic methods than others. However, the researcher using phenomenologic methods always uses some strategy to identify personal biases and hold them in abeyance while querying the participant. The reader may find it difficult to identify bracketing strategies because they are seldom explicitly identified in a research manuscript. Sometimes, the researcher's view of the world provides insight into biases that have been considered and bracketed. In the Cohen and Ley (2000) paper, the authors let the reader know that they are interested in understanding the experience of autologous bone marrow transplant so that nursing care can be adjusted to best meet the needs of these patients. From the perspective of bracketing, their nursing practice perspective will be held in abeyance as they come to understand the meaning of the experience from the perspective of the person living it.

Sample Selection

The reader of a phenomenological study report will find that the selected sample either is living the experience the researcher is querying or has lived the experience in their past. Because phenomenologists believe that each individual's history is a dimension of the present, a past experience exists in the present moment. Even when a participant is describing an experience occurring in the present, remembered information is being gathered. The participants in Cohen and Ley's (2000) study were an average of 16 months posttransplant. However, because the range of time after transplant was 2 to 49.5 months, a broad range of posttransplant experience was sampled.

DATA GATHERING

Written or oral data may be collected when using the phenomenological method. The researcher may pose the query in writing and ask for a written response or may schedule a time to interview the participant and tape-record the interaction. In either case the researcher may return to ask for clarification of written or tape-recorded transcripts. To some extent, the particular data-collection procedure is guided by the choice of a specific analysis technique. Different analysis techniques require a differing number of interviews. Data saturation usually guides decisions regarding how many interviews are enough. **Data saturation** is the situation of "having heard the themes before." The researcher knows that saturation has been reached when the ideas surfacing in the dialogue are ones previously heard from other participants. Cohen and Ley (2000) collected data from 20 participants.

DATA ANALYSIS

Several techniques are available for data analysis when using the phenomenological method. For detailed information about specific techniques, the reader is referred to original sources (Colaizzi, 1978; Giorgi, Fischer, and Murray, 1975; Spiegelberg, 1976; van Kaam, 1969). Although the techniques are slightly different from each other, there is a general pattern of moving from the participant's description to the researcher's synthesis of all participants' descriptions. The steps generally include the following:

1. Thorough reading and sensitive presence with the entire transcription of the participant's description
2. Identification of shifts in participant thought resulting in division of the transcription into thought segments
3. Specification of the significant phrases in each thought segment, using the words of the participant
4. Distillation of each significant phrase to express the central meaning of the segment in the words of the researcher
5. Grouping together of segments that contain similar central meanings for each participant

6. Preliminary synthesis of grouped segments for each participant with a focus on the essence of the phenomenon being studied
7. Final synthesis of the essences that have surfaced in all participant's descriptions, resulting in an exhaustive description of the lived experience

Cohen and Ley (2000) analyzed data using the hermeneutic phenomenological method based on the Utrecht School. The audiotape of each dialogue was reviewed simultaneously while reading the typed transcript. They moved from the line-by-line generation of themes to a synthesis of themes across participants.

DESCRIBING THE FINDINGS

When using the phenomenological method, the nurse researcher provides the research consumer with a path of information leading from the research question, through samples of participant's words, researcher's interpretation, and leading to the final synthesis that elaborates the lived experience as a narrative. When reading the report of a phenomenological study, the reader will find that detailed descriptive language is used to convey the complex meaning of the lived experience. Cohen and Ley (2000) provide quotes from participants to support their findings. They synthesize three themes that describe the experience of having an autologous bone marrow transplant: fear of death and hope for survival, loss of control, fear of discharge/fear of recurrence. Direct participant quotes enable the reader to evaluate the connection between what the participant said and how the researcher labeled what was said.

GROUNDED THEORY METHOD

The **grounded theory method** is an inductive approach involving a systematic set of procedures to arrive at theory about basic social processes. The emergent theory is based on observations and perceptions of the social scene and evolves during data collection and analysis in the actual research process (Strauss and Corbin, 1994). The aim of the grounded theory approach is to discover underlying social forces that shape human behavior. This method is used to construct theory where no theory exists or in situations when existing theory fails to explain a set of circumstances. According to Denzin (1998), grounded theory is the qualitative perspective most widely used by social scientists today, largely because it sets forth clearly defined steps for the researcher.

Developed originally as a sociologist's tool to investigate interactions in social settings (Glaser and Strauss, 1967), the grounded theory method is not bound to that discipline. Investigators from different disciplines may study the same phenomenon from varying perspectives (Denzin and Lincoln, 1998; Strauss and Corbin, 1994, 1997). As an example, in an area of study such as chronic illness, a nurse might be interested in coping patterns within families, a psychologist in personal adjustment, and a sociologist in group behavior in health care settings. King and colleagues (2000) studied organizational characteristics and issues affecting the longevity of self-help groups for parents of children with special needs. Their research team included a social psychologist, a psychologist, and two occupational therapists. Pharmacologists, Volume and Farris (2000), studied the concept of hope and the discontinuation of anorexiant medications in a secondary analysis of data from an earlier study. In the earlier study, Volume (1998) described bridging the gap, a grounded theory of the experiential process of taking prescription medications for weight loss. Theory generated by each discipline will reflect the discipline and serve it in explaining the phenomenon.

IDENTIFYING THE PHENOMENON

Researchers typically use the grounded theory method when they are interested in social processes from the perspective of human interactions, or "patterns of action and interaction between and among various types of social units" (Denzin and Lincoln, 1998). The basic social process is often expressed as a *gerund*, indicating change across time as social reality is negotiated. For example, Mallory and Stern (2000) studied

awakening as a change process for woman at risk for HIV, or the developmental process that occurs when women become sex workers out of economic necessity. Marcus (1998) studied the process of recovery from substance abuse in a long-term residential therapeutic community (TC), likening that process to changing careers. Marcus' study is used to introduce the research consumer to the grounded theory method.

STRUCTURING THE STUDY
Research Question

Research questions appropriate for the grounded theory method are those that address basic social process. They tend to be action or change oriented such as, "How do obstetricians and gynecologists identify and intervene with patients who are victims of domestic violence?" (Rittmayer and Roux, 1999) or "How do individuals with type I diabetes explicate the structure and process of transformation within chronic illness (Paterson et al, 1999)? In a grounded theory study, the research question can be a statement or a broad question that permits in-depth explanation of the phenomenon. For example, the reader will recognize Marcus' question implied in the statement that her study "explores the lived experience of recovery in a TC" (Marcus, 1998).

Researcher's Perspective

In a grounded theory study, the researcher brings some knowledge of the literature to the study, but the consumer will notice that an exhaustive literature review is not done. This allows theory to emerge directly from data. For example, Marcus (1998) allows TC participants to give voice to their experience and illuminate the more subjective aspects of recovery inherent in their worldview and self-image. Factors such as the social circumstances and structured behavior modification inherent in the TC approach to recovery also are investigated to provide sufficient depth for theory generation. Thus, grounded theory is more likely to be sensitive to contextual values and not merely to the researcher's values (Strauss and Corbin, 1997).

Another important aspect of the researcher's perspective is concern that theory remains connected to or "grounded in" the data. Marcus (1998) noted that while other researchers had identified the goal of treatment in a TC to be a global change or transformation of the individual, her data indicate that the nature of change in the TC experience is one of translation rather than transformation—a redirection of skills to more constructive activities.

Sample Selection

Sample selection involves choosing participants who are experiencing the circumstance and selecting events and incidents related to the social process under investigation. Marcus recruited individuals who were, or had been, residents in one of a network of three TCs managed by one foundation. The number of years of substance abuse among the participants ranged from 6 to 27. The overall time spent in the TC ranged from 4 to 28 months; 3 participants had graduated from the program. Thus, the participants had a sufficient period of learning about TC method and activities and about the overall experience of being drug-free.

DATA GATHERING

In the grounded theory method, the consumer will find that data are collected through interviews and through skilled observations of individuals interacting in a social setting. Interviews are audiotaped and then transcribed, and observations are recorded as field notes. Open-ended questions are used initially to identify concepts for further focus. Marcus (1998) interviewed each participant for approximately 1.5 to 2 hours. The interviews took place in a private area within the residential facility. The interview guide was formulated based on Marcus' prior naturalistic observations as a primary care provider in the facility. Questions were developed to probe aspects of uncertainty in the process of recovery in the TC setting. Examples of questions include the following:

"What is it like to be in recovery in a program such as this?"

"What is it like not to have drugs?"
"How do you experience recovery in this setting?"
"How do you learn to be drug-free?"
"What strategies do you use to cope with the restrictions of the program?"
"What information and support are needed for recovery?"
"Why do residents remain in the program?"
"Why do they leave?"
"What aspects of your sense of self contribute to or detract from the recovery process?"

DATA ANALYSIS

A major feature of the grounded theory method is that data collection and analysis occur simultaneously. The process requires systematic, detailed record keeping using field notes and transcribed interview tapes. Hunches about emerging patterns in the data are noted in memos, and the researcher directs activities in the field by pursuing these hunches. This technique, called **theoretical sampling,** is used to select experiences that will help the researcher test ideas and gather complete information about developing concepts. The researcher begins by noting indicators or actual events, actions, or words in the data. Concepts, or abstractions, are developed from the indicators (Charmaz, 2000; Strauss, 1987).

The initial analytic process is called open *coding* (Strauss, 1987). Data are examined carefully line by line, broken down into discrete parts, and compared for similarities and differences (Strauss and Corbin, 1990). Data are compared with other data continuously as they are acquired during research. This is a process called the **constant comparative method.** Codes in the data are clustered to form categories. The categories are expanded and developed or collapsed into one another. Theory is constructed through this systematic process. As a result, data collection, analysis, and theory generation have a direct reciprocal relationship (Charmaz, 2000; Strauss and Corbin, 1990).

Related literature, both technical and nontechnical, is reviewed continuously throughout data collection and analysis. All literature is treated as data and is compared with the researcher's developing theory as it progresses. When critiquing a study using grounded theory, expect to find, at the end of the report, the researcher's grounded theory formally related to and incorporated with existing knowledge. For example, Marcus (1998) noted that recovery in a TC had some similarities to the social process of conversion in religious movements, another way that individuals seek to resolve personal crisis (Lofland and Richardson, 1984). She distinguished conversion from alternation, also an experience associated with religious movements. Individuals who join a religious movement and do not undergo radical changes are said to alternate rather than convert (Travisano, 1970). Marcus' study participants are seen as alternators, individuals who, "although retaining elements of their previous worldview and personality, adopt prescribed behaviors to solve the problems of an addictive lifestyle" (Marcus, 1998). Marcus also compared the stages of her theory of recovery in this setting to those of DeLeon (1996) and Denzin (1987), other researchers who have studied recovery from substance use disorders. The study thus contributes to understanding of the developmental processes of change in recovery advanced by others.

According to study participants, recovery in the TC setting was like "changing careers," translating the strenuous and demanding life of an addict to the equally demanding career of ex-addict. The process of changing careers has four progressive stages (1) entering the program, (2) learning the program, (3) working the program, and (4) gaining control. The theory further defined strategies or properties common to each stage.

> **HELPFUL HINT**   In a report of research using the grounded theory method, the consumer can expect to find a diagrammed model of a theory that synthesizes the researchers' findings in a systematic way.

DESCRIBING THE FINDINGS

Grounded theory studies are reported in sufficient detail to provide the reader with the steps in the process and the logic of the method. Marcus (1998) takes the reader through the steps of data collection, theoretic sampling, constant comparisons, and three levels of coding to a schematic model that depicts the process of changing careers or becoming clean and sober in a TC. Reports of grounded theory studies use descriptive language and diagrams of the process to ensure that the theory reported in the findings remains connected to the data.

ETHNOGRAPHIC METHOD

Derived from the Greek term *ethnos*, meaning people, race, or cultural group, the **ethnographic method** focuses on scientific description and interpretation of cultural or social groups and systems (Creswell, 1998). The reader should know that the goal of the ethnographer is to understand the natives' view of their world or the **emic view.** The emic (insiders') view is contrasted to the **etic** (outsiders') **view** obtained when the researcher uses quantitative analyses of behavior. The ethnographic approach requires that the researcher enter the world of the study participants to watch what happens, listen to what is said, ask questions, and collect whatever data are available. The term *ethnography* is used to mean both the research technique and the product of that technique, the study itself (Creswell, 1998; Tedlock, 2000). Steward (1998) indicates that ethnographies share the following characteristics: participant observation, holism, context, sensitivity, and sociocultural description. Vidick and Lyman (1998) trace the history of ethnography, with roots in the disciplines of sociology and anthropology, as a method born out of the need to understand "other" and "self." Nurses use the method to study cultural variations in health and patient groups as subcultures within larger social contexts.

IDENTIFYING THE PHENOMENON

The phenomenon under investigation in an ethnographic study varies in scope from a long-term study of a very complex culture, such as that of the Aborigines (Mead, 1949), to a shorter-term study of a phenomenon within subunits of cultures. For example, a researcher may study the health and healing philosophies of nurses and alternative healers (Engebretson, 1996); ways Jewish seniors adapt to the nursing home environment (Kahn, 1999); or cross-cultural comparison of health perceptions, concerns and coping strategies among Asian and Pacific Islander American elders (Torsch and Ma, 2000). Kleinman (1992) notes the clinical utility of ethnography in describing the "local world" of groups of patients who are experiencing a particular phenomenon, such as suffering. The local worlds of patients have cultural, political, economical, institutional, and social-relational dimensions in much the same way as larger complex societies. Kahn's (1999) study of the shared meanings held by residents of a nursing home as they adapt to the setting is used as an example to introduce the reader to ethnography.

STRUCTURING THE STUDY
Research Question

When reviewing the report of ethnographic research, notice that questions are asked about lifeways or particular patterns of behavior within the social context of a culture or subculture. **Culture** is viewed as the system of knowledge and linguistic expressions used by social groups that allows the researcher to interpret or make sense of the world (Aamodt, 1991). Ethnographic nursing studies address questions that concern how cultural knowledge, norms, values, and other contextual variables influence one's health experience. Torsch and Ma (2000) asked, "What are the health perceptions, concerns, and coping strategies of Asian and Pacific Islander American elders?" Other possible ethnographic questions include "What does comforting mean in Hispanic families?" "What are patient and nurse roles like in intensive care units?" and "What are the meanings of health and illness care to migrant workers?" Often the research question is implied in the purpose statement. As an example, Kahn (1999) constructed his study to ask, "How do residents adapt to the dual nature of the nursing home as institution and as home?"

Researcher's Perspective

When using the ethnographic method, the researcher's perspective is that of an interpreter entering an alien world and attempting to make sense of that world from the insider's point of view (Agar, 1986). Like phenomenologists and grounded theorists, ethnographers make their own beliefs explicit and *bracket*, or set aside, their personal biases as they seek to understand the worldview of others. Although Kahn (1999) identifies the object of description and interpretation in this study as the larger cultural discourse of the nursing home, knowledge of this domain was approached through "thick description" (Geertz, 1983) or interpretive examination of microscopic phenomena in the domain. In his first field note, Kahn wrote "what is strange about this place is that it reminds me of a hospital but is not quite a hospital—people live here, not just stay for a short time while they are treated" (Kahn, 1999). This observation identifies for the first time the dialectic between home and institution that becomes a major focus of the study.

Sample Selection

The ethnographer selects a cultural group that is living the phenomenon under investigation. The researcher gathers information from general informants and from key informants. **Key informants** are individuals who have special knowledge, status, or communication skills and who are willing to teach the ethnographer about the phenomenon (Creswell, 1998). Kahn spent 9 months doing fieldwork in a 145-bed nursing home for older Jewish people located in the western United States. The nursing home was recognized for its high standards of care. The informants were a convenience sample of 21 individuals who needed nursing home care because of physical problems but who had no cognitive impairment.

HELPFUL HINT Managing personal bias is an expectation of researchers using all the methods discussed in this chapter.

DATA GATHERING

Ethnographic data gathering involves participant observation or immersion in the setting, informant interviews, and interpretation by the researcher of cultural patterns (Crabtree and Miller, 1992). According to Boyle (1991), ethnographic research in nursing as in other disciplines always involves "face-to-face interviewing, with data collection and analysis taking place in the natural setting." Thus fieldwork is a major focus of the method. Other techniques may include obtaining life histories and collecting material items reflective of the culture. Photographs and films of the informants in their world can be used as data sources. Spradley (1979) identified three categories of questions for ethnographic inquiry: descriptive, or broad, open-ended questions; structural, or in-depth questions that expand and verify the unit of analysis; and contrast questions, or ones that further clarify and provide criteria for exclusion.

Data gathering for Kahn's study consisted of multiple audiotaped ethnographic interviews with the 21 key informants and participant observations of the activities of nursing home life. The interviews were conversational in nature and not directed toward specific probes. Informants were told that Kahn was interested in who they were and what their lives were like in the nursing home. No specific questions were asked about adaptation to their living circumstances. The interviews varied from 20 minutes to an hour, depending on the stamina of the informant. The number of interviews with each individual ranged from 5 to 18. The participant observation component of the study consisted of non-recorded conversations and observations captured through field notes.

DATA ANALYSIS

As with the grounded theory method, data are collected and analyzed simultaneously. Data analysis proceeds through several levels as the researcher looks for the meaning of cultural symbols in the informants' language. Analysis begins with a search for **domains** or symbolic categories that include smaller categories. Language is analyzed for semantic relationships, and structural questions are formulated to expand and verify data. The informants in Kahn's study (1999) used the phrase "making the best of it" frequently to summarize their feelings and beliefs about living in the nursing home. Analysis proceeds through increasing levels of complexity and includes taxonomical analysis, or in-depth verification of domains; componential analysis, or analysis for contrasts among categories; and theme analysis, or uncovering of cultural themes. Four dimensions of "making the best of it" emerged as themes: "recognizing the ambivalence of the situation, downplaying negative aspects, having no other options, and using volition or will to transcend the institutional environment and create a home" (Kahn, 1999). The data, grounded in the informants' reality and synthesized by the researcher, lead eventually to hypothetical propositions about the cultural phenomenon under investigation. Kahn (1999) hypothesizes in his conclusion that the nursing home residents recognized the ambiguity of the setting as a place in which "they had to live until they died, getting as much satisfaction as possible from what remained of their lives" (Kahn, 1999). Making the best of it represented a continual effort to reframe the social environment and, in a sense, symbolized the outcome of their struggle with old age. The reader is encouraged to consult Creswell (1998) for detailed description of the ethnographic analysis process.

DESCRIBING THE FINDINGS

Ethnographic studies yield large quantities of data amassed as field notes of observations, interview transcriptions, and other artifacts such as photographs. Creswell (1998) describes three aspects of the process of transforming data into findings. One aspect is description or chronicling a "day in the life," a key event, or a "story" that captures the perspectives of members of the group. A second aspect is an analysis of building taxonomies in search of patterned regularities. The third aspect of transforming ethnographic data is referred to as interpretation of the culture-sharing group, or drawing inferences from the data to structure the study incorporating the ethnographer's perspective. Charmaz' (2000) guidelines for ethnographic writing provide an excellent framework for the consumer of nursing research wishing to critique descriptions of ethnographic studies. The five techniques recommended in Charmaz' guidelines are: pulling the reader in, recreating experiential mood, adding surprise, reconstructing ethnographic experience, and creating closure for the study. When critiquing, be aware that the report of findings usually provides examples from data, thorough description of the analytical process, and statements of the hypothetical propositions and their relationship to the ethnographer's frame of reference. Complete ethnographies may be published as monographs.

CASE STUDY

Case study research, which is rooted in sociology, is currently described slightly differently by Yin, Stake, Merriam, and Creswell, major thinkers who write about this method (Aita and McIlvain, 1999). For the purposes of introducing the nurse consumer to this research method, Stake's view is emphasized. **Case study** is about studying the peculiarities and the commonalities of a specific case—familiar ground for practicing nurses. Stake (2000) notes that case study is not a methodological choice, but rather a choice of what to study. Case study can include quantitative and/or qualitative data, but it is defined by its focus on uncovering an individual case. Stake (2000) distinguishes intrinsic from instrumental case study. **Intrinsic case study** is undertaken to have a better understanding of the case—nothing more or nothing less. "The researcher at least temporarily subordinates other curiosities so that the stories of those "living the case" will be teased out" (Stake, 2000). **Instrumental case study** is defined as research that is done when the researcher is pursuing insight into an issue or wants to challenge some generalization.

In spite of the potential salience of case study research for the discipline of nursing, the consumer will seldom find published case study research in nursing journals. Its location nearest the perceived view on the continuum provided by Cohen in Chapter 6 may threaten its legitimacy in some people's eyes and contribute to this paucity of case study research in the nursing literature. In contrast, the consumer will find case reports. Case report is a familiar format for sharing information, long used by health care professionals. Case reports enable in-depth description of individual commonalities and nuances often related to a particular diagnosis or health circumstance. The format of the report is often a story that captures the complexity of the health experience beyond what is possible with empiric data.

Engebretson (2000) shares a case report story that details the experience of a nursing student who sits in silence with a mom through the death of her newborn son. She provides a picture of the experience from the perspective of the student; the mom; the intensive care environment; and for her, the nursing instructor. By documenting the lessons learned from the experience with a story, Engebretson (2000) enables continued opportunity for sharing the lesson of the experience with other students and faculty. Familiarity with case report establishes a base for understanding case study. Like case reports, case studies "draw together many elements needed to understand the complex nature of a problem" (Aita and McIlvain, 1999).

IDENTIFYING THE PHENOMENON

Although some definitions of case study demand that the focus of research be contemporary, Stake's (1995, 2000) defining criterion of attention to the single case broadens the scope of phenomenon for study. By a single case, Stake is designating a focus on an individual, a family, a community, an organization—some complex phenomenon that demands close scrutiny for understanding. For our purposes, we are interested in examining a case study that uses a qualitative approach. The example manuscript is one that also is characterized as historical research. Nichols and Hammer (1998) studied a case of institution-building exemplified by the Baby Hospital in Oakland California. They were especially interested in the roles of nurse Bertha Wright and colleagues.

STRUCTURING THE STUDY
Research Question

The research question for case study is one that provokes the curiosity of the researcher. Stake (2000) suggests that research questions be developed around issues that serve as a foundation to uncover complexity and pursue understanding. The questions posed by Nichols and Hammer (1998) were as follows:

Who was Bertha Wright?

How did her idea become the reality of the Baby Hospital?

With whom did she work to realize her dream?

What was Baby Hospital and what was its significance?

Although the researchers pose these questions to begin, the beginning questions are never all-inclusive. Rather, the researcher uses an iterative process of "growing questions" in the field. That is, as data are collected to address these questions, other questions will emerge to guide the researcher down another path in the process of untangling the complex story. So, research questions evolve over time and recreate themselves in case study research.

Researcher's Perspective

When the researcher begins with questions developed around suspected issues of importance, the perspective of the researcher is reflected in the questions; this is sometimes referred to as an etic perspective. As the researcher begins engaging the phenomenon of interest, the story unfolds and leads the way, shifting from an etic (researcher) to an emic (story) perspective (Stake, 2000). The reader may recognize a shift from etic to emic perspective when stories spin off of the original questions posed by the researcher. For example, questions in the Nichols and Hammer study provided detail about the caring relationship between Bertha Wright and Mabel Weed, cofounders of the Baby Hospital. Although this direction was not one posed in the original research

questions, it provided insight into the humanness of the cofounders and shed a different light on the institution-building endeavor.

Sample Selection

This is one of the areas where scholars in the field present differing views, ranging from only choosing the most common cases to only choosing the most unusual cases (Aita and McIlvain, 2000). Stake (2000) advocates selecting cases that may offer the best opportunities for learning. For instance, if there are several heart transplant patients the researcher may study, practical factors will influence who offers the best opportunity for learning. Persons who live in the area and can be easily visited at home or in the medical center would be a better choice than someone living in another country. The researcher may want to choose someone who has an actively participating family, since most transplant patients exist in a family setting. No choice is perfect when selecting a case. There is much to learn about any one individual, situation, or organization when doing case study research, regardless of the contextual factors influencing the unit of analysis.

It is difficult to know how Nichols and Hammer (1998) chose their institution-building case study. The first sentence of the manuscript suggests that the impetus for choice came from a photograph: "At Children's Hospital in Oakland, California, in a clinic hallway, there hangs a large photograph of a stern-looking Victorian woman holding two babies, one balanced in each arm. The description identifies her as Bertha Wright." If the photograph was the impetus, the case *presented itself* (as often happens in practice situations) rather than *being selected*. Instead of selecting a case for study, the case of the Baby Hospital presented itself to the researchers through the curiosity generated when they viewed the photograph.

DATA GATHERING

Data are gathered using interview, observation, document review, and any other methods that enable understanding of the complexity of the case. The researcher will do what is needed to get a sense of the environment and the relationships that provide the context for the case. Stake (1995) advocates development of a data-gathering plan to guide the progress of the study from definition of the case through decisions regarding reporting. The consumer of research may find little or no explicit information about data gathering in the report of research. Nichols and Hammer (1998) cite personal interviews, meeting minutes, and organization annual reports as some of the sources for their case study. Often, sources of data are most easily found in the reference list of the manuscript.

DATA ANALYSIS/DESCRIBING FINDINGS

Data analysis is closely tied to data gathering and description of findings as the case study story is generated. "Qualitative case study is characterized by researchers spending extended time, on site, personally in contact with activities and operations of the case, reflecting, revising meanings of what is going on" (Stake, 2000). Reflecting and revising meanings are the work of the case study researcher, who has recorded data, searched for patterns, linked data from multiple sources, and arrived at preliminary thoughts regarding the meaning of collected data. This reflective dynamic evolution is the iterative process of creating the case study story. The reader of a qualitative case study will have difficulty determining how data analysis was conducted because the research report generally does not list research activities. Findings are embedded in (1) a chronologic development of the case, (2) the researcher's story of coming to know the case, (3) one-by-one description of case dimensions, and (4) vignettes that highlight case qualities (Stake, 1995).

Nichols and Hammer (1998) provide the story of the Baby Hospital chronologically from its female-driven origin in 1912 through its male-dominated transition to Children's Hospital in 1930. Although the researcher's perspective of coming to know the story is not explicitly stated, the authors weave institution-building and contextual information with thoughtful interpretation to create a report that reflects their perspective. Case dimensions, such as the stories of the four women who were most critical to the creation of the Baby Hospital are documented, as are influencing environmental factors, such as the influx of refugees made homeless by the San Francisco earthquake and Great Fire. Vignettes acquired from personal communication and published writings are used by Nichols and Hammer (1998) to clarify the picture of institution-building they report.

HISTORICAL RESEARCH

The **historical research method** is a systematic approach for understanding the past through collection, organization, and critical appraisal of facts. One of the goals of the researcher using historical methodology is to shed light on the past so that it can guide the present and the future. Nursing's attention to historical methodology was initiated by Teresa E. Christy. Christy elaborated the method (1975) and the need (1981) for historical research long before most nurse scholars accepted it as a legitimate research method. More recently, Lusk (1997) summarized important information for the nurse interested in understanding historical research. She provided guidance for choosing a topic, acquiring data, addressing ethical issues, analyzing data, and reporting findings.

When critiquing a study that used the historical method, expect to find the research question embedded in the phenomenon to be studied. The question is stated implicitly rather than explicitly. Data sources provide the sample for historical research. The more clearly a researcher delineates the historical event being studied, the more specifically data sources can be identified. Data may include written or video documents, interviews with persons who witnessed the event, photographs, and any other artifacts that shed light. Sometimes pivotal information cannot be retrieved and must be eliminated from the list of possible sources. To determine which data sources were used when reviewing a published study, the reader will look at the reference list. Sources of data may be primary or secondary. **Primary sources** are eyewitness accounts pro-

> **BOX** **7-1**   Establishing Fact, Probability, and Possibility with the Historical Method
>
> | | |
> |---|---|
> | **FACT** | **PROBABILITY** |
> | Two independent primary sources that agree with each other | One primary source that receives critical evaluation and no substantive conflicting data |
> | *or* | *or* |
> | One independent primary source that receives critical evaluation and one independent secondary source that is in agreement and relieves critical evaluation and no substantive conflicting data | Two primary sources that disagree about particular points |
> | | **POSSIBILITY** |
> | | One primary source that provides information but is not adequate to receive critical evaluation |
> | | *or* |
> | | Only secondary or tertiary sources |

Modified from Christy TE: The methodology of historical research: a brief introduction, *Image J Nurs Sch* 24(3): 189-192, 1975.

vided by varying sorts of communication appropriate to the time. **Secondary sources** provide a view of the phenomenon from another's perspective rather than a first-hand account.

Validity of documents is established by external criticism; reliability is established by internal criticism. **External criticism** judges the authenticity of the data source. The researcher seeks to ensure that the data source is what it seems to be. For instance, if the researcher is reviewing a handwritten letter of Florence Nightingale, some of the validity issues are the following:

- Are the ink, paper, and wax seal on the envelope representative of Nightingale's time?
- Is the wax seal one that Nightingale used in other authentic data sources?
- Is the writing truly Nightingale's?

Only if the data source passes the test of external criticism does the researcher begin internal criticism. **Internal criticism** concerns the reliability of information within the document (Christy, 1975). To judge reliability, the researcher must familiarize self with the time in which the data emerged. A sense of the context and language of the time is essential to understanding a document. The meaning of a word in one era may not be equivalent to the meaning in another era. Knowing the language, customs, and habits of the historical period is critical for judging reliability. The researcher assumes that a primary

source provides a more reliable account than a secondary source (Christy, 1975). The further a source moves from providing an eyewitness account, the more questionable is its reliability. The researcher using historical methods attempts to establish fact, probability, or possibility (Box 7-1).

HELPFUL HINT   When critiquing the historical method, do not expect to find a report of data analysis but simply a description of findings synthesized into a continuous narrative.

QUALITATIVE APPROACH: NURSING METHODOLOGY

The qualitative methodologies elaborated throughout this chapter are derived from other disciplines such as sociology, anthropology, and philosophy. The discipline of nursing borrows these methodologies to conduct research. However, as the discipline matures, methodology based on nursing ontology (belief system) is emerging. Madeleine Leininger (1996), Rosemarie Rizzo Parse (1997), and Margaret Newman (1997) are examples of nurse theorists who have created research methods specific to their theories. Table 7-1 compares the methodology of these theorists. Each method was developed over years and tested by other researchers. Each attempts to advance nursing knowledge through inquiry that is congruent with the specific nursing theory.

TABLE **7-1** Nursing Research Methodology

	LEININGER	PARSE	NEWMAN
Theory	Culture Care	Human Becoming	Health As Expanding Consciousness
Research Methodology	Ethnonursing is centered on learning from people about their beliefs, experiences, and culture care information (Leininger, 1996).	Parse's research methodology is the study of universal health experiences through true presence both with participants sharing life stories and with transcribed data to uncover meaning (Parse, 1997).	Newman's method focuses on pattern recognition and uses multiple interviews, involving interviewer-interviewee collaboration to arrive at recognized life patterns (Newman, 1997).
Research Example	Use of culture care theory with Anglo- and African-American elders in a long-term care setting(McFarland, 1997).	The lived experience of serenity: Using Parse's research method (Kruse, 1999).	Pattern of expanding consciousness in midlife women: creative movement and narrative as modes of expression (Picard, 2000)

ISSUES IN QUALITATIVE RESEARCH

ETHICS

Inherent in all research is the demand for the protection of human subjects. This demand exists for both quantitative and qualitative research approaches. Human subjects' protection as applicable to the quantitative approach is discussed in Chapter 13. These basic tenets hold true for the qualitative approach. However, several characteristics of qualitative methodologies outlined in Table 7-2 generate unique concerns and necessitate an expanded view of protecting human subjects.

NATURALISTIC SETTING

The central concern that arises when research is conducted in naturalistic settings focuses on the need to gain consent. The need to acquire informed consent is a basic researcher responsibility, but it is not always easy in naturalistic settings. For instance, when research methods include observing groups of people interacting over time, the complexity of gaining consent is apparent. These complexities generate controversy and debate among qualitative researchers. The balance between respect for human participants and efforts to collect meaningful data must be continuously negotiated. The reader should look for information that the researcher has addressed this issue of balance by recording attention to human participant protection.

EMERGENT NATURE OF DESIGN

The emergent nature of the research design emphasizes the need for ongoing negotiation of consent with the participant. In the course of a study, situations change and what was agreeable at the beginning may become intrusive. Sometimes, as data collection proceeds and new information emerges, the study shifts direction in a way that is not acceptable to the participant. For instance, if the researcher were present in a family's home during a time that marital discord arose, the family may choose to renegotiate the consent. From another perspective, Morse (1998) discusses the increasing involvement of participants in the research process, sometimes resulting in their request to have their name published in the findings or be included as a coauthor. If the participant originally signed a consent form and then chose an active identified role, Morse (1998) suggests that the participant then sign a "release for publication" form. The underlying nature of this discussion is that the emergent qualitative research process demands ongoing negotiating of researcher-participant relationships, including the consent relationship. The opportunity to

TABLE **7-2** Characteristics of Qualitative Research Generating Ethical Concerns

CHARACTERISTICS	ETHICAL CONCERNS
Naturalistic setting	Some researchers using methods that rely on participant observation may believe that consent is not always possible or necessary.
Emergent nature of design	Planning for questioning and observation emerges over the time of the study. Thus it is difficult to inform the participant precisely of all potential threats before he or she agrees to participate.
Researcher-participant interaction	Relationships developed between the researcher and participant may blur the focus of the interaction.
Researcher as instrument	The researcher is the study instrument, collecting data and interpreting the participant's reality.

renegotiate consent establishes a relationship of trust and respect characteristic of the ethical conduct of research.

RESEARCHER-PARTICIPANT INTERACTION

The nature of the researcher-participant interaction over time introduces the possibility that the research experience becomes a therapeutic one. It is a case of research becoming practice. There are basic differences between the intent of the nurse when conducting research or engaging in practice (Smith and Liehr, 1999). In practice, the nurse has caring-healing intentions. In research, the nurse intends to "get the picture" from the perspective of the participant. "Getting the picture" may be a therapeutic experience for the participant. Sometimes, talking to a caring listener about things that matter energizes healing, even though it was not intended. From an ethical perspective, the qualitative researcher is promising only to listen and to encourage the other's story. If this experience is therapeutic for the participant, it becomes an unplanned benefit of the research.

RESEARCHER AS INSTRUMENT

The responsibility to remain true to the data requires that the researcher acknowledge any personal bias, interpreting findings in a way that accurately reflects the participant's reality. This is a serious ethical obligation. To accomplish this, the researcher may return to the subjects at critical interpretive points and ask for clarification or validation.

CREDIBILITY, AUDITABILITY, AND FITTINGNESS

Quantitative studies are concerned with reliability and validity of instruments, as well as internal and external validity criteria, as measures of scientific rigor (see the Critical Thinking Decision Path), but these are not appropriate for qualitative work. The rigor of qualitative methodology is judged by unique criteria appropriate to the research approach. Credibility, auditability, and fittingness are scientific criteria proposed for qualitative research studies by Guba and Lincoln in 1981. Although these criteria were proposed two decades ago, they still capture the rigorous spirit of qualitative inquiry and persist as reasonable criteria for evaluation. The meanings of **credibility, auditability,** and **fittingness** are briefly explained in Table 7-3.

TRIANGULATION . . . OR IS IT CRYSTALLIZATION?

Triangulation has become a "buzzword" in qualitative research over the past several years. The buzz has progressed from viewing triangulation as merely a strategy for ensuring data accuracy (more than one data source presents the same picture) to viewing it as an opportunity to more fully address the complex nature of the human

TABLE **7-3**   Criteria for Judging Scientific Rigor: Credibility, Auditability, Fittingness, and Confirmability

CRITERIA	CRITERIA CHARACTERISTICS
Credibility	Truth of findings as judged by participants and others within the discipline. For instance, you may find the researcher returning to the participants to share interpretation of findings and query accuracy from the perspective of the persons living the experience.
Auditabililty	Accountability as judged by the adequacy of information leading the reader from the research question and raw data through various steps of analysis to the interpretation of findings. For instance, you should be able to follow the reasoning of the researcher step-by-step through explicit examples of data, interpretations, and syntheses.
Fittingness	Faithfulness to everyday reality of the participants, described in enough detail so that others in the discipline can evaluate importance for their own practice, research, and theory development. For instance, you will know enough about the human experience being reported that you can decide whether it "rings true" and is useful for guiding your practice.

experience. From this perspective, **triangulation** can be defined as the expansion of research methods in a single study or multiple studies to enhance diversity, enrich understanding, and accomplish specific goals. Richardson (2000) has suggested that the triangle be replaced by the crystal, as a more appropriate metaphor for the multimethod approach. Although there is support for the use of multiple research methods, controversies still exist about the appropriateness of combining qualitative and quantitative research approaches and even about combining multiple qualitative methods in one study (Barbour, 1998). It will not take the serious reader of nursing research very long to figure out that approaches and methods are being combined to contribute to theory building, guide practice, and facilitate instrument development. Table 7-4 synthesizes three manuscripts reporting multimethod analyses. The table notes the conceptual focus of the work, the study purposes and whether the manuscript suggests implications for theory, practice, and instrument development.

From the perspective of crystallization, Swanson's work is most complete (see Table 7-4) because she has addressed implications for practice, instrument development, and theory building focused on the issue of caring for women who have had a miscarriage. Her research program has included an initial theory building phase (studies 1 and 2), an instrument development phase (studies 3, 4, and 5) and a phase of testing a practice intervention (study 6). Swanson (1999) used the phenomenological method for studies 1 and 2 and quantitative methods for each of her other studies. In no study does she use more than one method, but her use of multimethods during the course of her 15-year research program can be likened to examining different facets of one crystal—in this case the experience of miscarrying. The crystallization process has contributed to theory building, nursing practice, and instrument development. Her practice contribution is highlighted by a case exemplar (Swanson, 1999), which synthesizes her years of work with women living through the life experience of miscarrying their baby.

Both Hunter and Chandler (1999) and Liehr and colleagues (2000) are reporting pilot studies that include qualitative findings. Each study indicates plans for further investigation, based on the qualitative findings. Hunter and Chandler's study (1999) combined qualitative (phenomenological method, using focus groups, interview, and written stories) and quantitative (Wagnild and Young's resiliency scale) methods to address their twofold study purpose (see Table 7-4). Data from the quantitative methods provided a different perspective than the one emerging from the qualitative methods—like differing facets of a

TABLE 7-4 Research Using Multimethod Approaches

AUTHOR/DATE	CONCEPTUAL FOCUS	MULTIMETHOD APPROACH	STUDY PURPOSE	THEORY-BUILDING IMPLICATIONS	PRACTICE IMPLICATIONS	INSTRUMENT DEVELOPMENT IMPLICATIONS
KM Swanson, 1999	Miscarriage and caring	Six studies, each using one method	**Study 1:** Define common themes for women who had recently miscarried	Yes	Yes	
			Study 2: Describe the human experience of miscarriage and describe the meaning of caring	Yes	Yes	
			Study 3: Use descriptive data to create a survey instrument based on women's experience of miscarriage			Yes
			Study 4: Evaluate the relevance of the survey items to create miscarriage scale			Yes
			Study 5: Assess reliability and validity of the miscarriage scale			Yes
			Study 6: Test the effects of caring, measurement, and time on women's well-being in the first year after miscarriage.	Yes	Yes	Yes
AJ Hunger and GE Chandler, 1999	Adolescent resilience	1 study using multimethods	Pilot study to explore the meaning of resilience for adolescents, and evaluate a resilience instrument	Yes	Yes	Yes
P Liehr, et al., 2000	Adolescent hostility	1 study using multimethods	Pilot study to test the reliability and validity of the adolescent version of the Cook-Medley Hostility scale with multiethnic sample			Yes

crystal. The authors synthesize these differing perspectives in a model, entitled "Continuum of resilience in adolescents." They pose questions for further study related to (1) the health-promoting potential of resilience and (2) the likelihood of capturing adolescent resilience with a single paper and pencil measure.

The study reported by Liehr and associates (2000) (see Table 7-4) has a narrow focus. The purpose of the study was focused on instrument development. Within a quantitative context of reliability and validity testing, these researchers used a qualitative method (content analysis of adolescents' remembered descriptions of a time they experienced feeling angry) to evaluate the content validity of the adolescent version of the Cook-Medley Hostility Scale. The researchers note that the findings from this pilot study have led to changes in the scale for use in ongoing research.

These three manuscripts (see Table 7-4) present a range of approaches for combining methods in research studies, but the combining-methods picture is broader and growing. The consumer of nursing research is encouraged to follow the ongoing debate about combining methods as nurse researchers strive to determine which research combinations promise enhanced understanding of human complexity and substantial contribution to nursing science.

COMPUTER MANAGEMENT OF QUALITATIVE DATA

At the completion of data collection, the qualitative researcher is faced with volumes of data requiring sorting, coding, and synthesizing. The researcher may use one of many computer programs available to assist with the task of data management. Meadows and Dodendorf (1999) categorize computer programs into three types:

- Code and retrieve, which assist in organizing and grouping data;
- Theory builders, which move to a different level of data organization by connecting themes and categories; and
- Conceptual network builders, which incorporate graphics with theory building capabilities.

Unlike computer programs used with quantitative data, these programs do not actually analyze data. Data analysis and interpretation remain largely the task of the researcher. However, orderly organization and grouping of data make the job of analysis and interpretation much easier for the researcher.

CRITIQUING Qualitative Research

Although general criteria for critiquing qualitative research are proposed in the Critiquing Criteria box, each qualitative method has unique characteristics that influence what the research consumer may expect in the published research report. The criteria for critiquing are formatted to evaluate the selection of the phenomenon, the structure of the study, data gathering, data analysis, and description of the findings. Each question of the criteria focuses on factors discussed throughout the chapter. Critiquing qualitative research is a useful activity for learning the nuances of this research approach.

The reader is encouraged to identify a qualitative study of interest and apply the criteria for critiquing.

In summary, the term "qualitative research approach" is an overriding description of multiple methods with distinct origins and procedures. In spite of distinctions, each method shares a common nature that guides data collection from the perspective of the participants to create a story that synthesizes disparate data pieces into a comprehensible whole and promises direction for building nursing knowledge.

CRITIQUING CRITERIA

Identifying the Phenomenon

1. Is the phenomenon focused on human experience within a natural setting?
2. Is the phenomenon relevant to nursing and/or health?

Structuring the Study

Research Question

3. Does the question specify a distinct process to be studied?
4. Does the question identify the context (participant group/place) of the process that will be studied?
5. Does the choice of a specific qualitative method fit with the research question?

Researcher's Perspective

6. Are the biases of the researcher reported?
7. Do the researchers provide a structure of ideas that reflect their beliefs?

Sample Selection

8. Is it clear that the selected sample is living the phenomenon of interest?

Data Gathering

9. Are data sources and methods for gathering data specified?
10. Is there evidence that participant consent is an integral part of the data gathering process?

Data Analysis

11. Can the dimensions of data analysis be identified and logically followed?
12. Does the researcher paint a clear picture of the participant's reality?
13. Is there evidence that the researcher's interpretation captured the participant's meaning?
14. Have other professionals confirmed the researcher's interpretation?

Describing the Findings

15. Are examples provided to guide the reader from the raw data to the researcher's synthesis?
16. Does the researcher link the findings to existing theory or literature, or is a new theory generated?

Critical Thinking Challenges

Barbara Krainovich-Miller

➢ Discuss how the qualitative researcher knows when "data saturation" has occurred. Offer explanations from your life experience that are similar to the experience of data saturation.
➢ How would you answer your classmate in research class who insists that it is impossible for researchers to "bracket" their personal biases about the phenomenon they are going to study. Use examples from your own clinical experience in your response.
➢ You are asked to defend why qualitative studies do not include hypotheses. Include in your argument whether or not you think qualitative studies warrant the same recognition as true experimental studies.
➢ How would the researcher use information gathered via computer-based searches and the internet in various qualitative designs?
➢ Do you think that it would be legitimate qualitative research to conduct an interview using an internet chat room? Justify your position and address ethical considerations.

Key Points

- Qualitative research is the investigation of human experiences in naturalistic settings, pursuing meanings that inform theory, practice, instrument development, and further research.
- Qualitative research studies are guided by research questions.
- Data saturation occurs when the information being shared with the researcher becomes repetitive.
- Qualitative research methods include five basic elements: identifying the phenomenon, structuring the study, gathering the data, analyzing the data, and describing the findings.
- The phenomenological method is a process of learning and constructing the meaning of human experience through intensive dialogue with persons who are living the experience.
- The grounded theory method is an inductive approach that implements a systematic set of procedures to arrive at theory about basic social processes.
- The ethnographic method focuses on scientific descriptions of cultural groups.
- The case study method focuses on a selected phenomenon over a short or long time to provide an in-depth description of its essential dimensions and processes.
- The historical research method is the systematic compilation of data and the critical presentation, evaluation, and interpretation of facts regarding people, events, and occurrences of the past.
- Ethical issues in qualitative research involve issues related to the naturalistic setting, emergent nature of the design, researcher-participant interaction, and researcher as instrument.
- Credibility, auditability, and fittingness are criteria for judging the scientific rigor of a qualitative research study.
- Triangulation has shifted from a strategy for combining research methods to assess accuracy to expansion of research methods in a single study or multiple studies to enhance diversity, enrich understanding, and accomplish specific goals. A better term may be crystallization.
- Multimethod approaches to research are controversial but promising.
- Qualitative research data can be managed through the use of computers, but the researcher must interpret data.

REFERENCES

Aamodt AA: Ethnography and epistemology: generating nursing knowledge. In Morse JM, editor: *Qualitative nursing research: a contemporary dialogue,* Newbury Park, Calif, 1991, Sage.

Agar MH: *Speaking of ethnography,* Beverly Hills, Calif, 1986, Sage.

Aita VA and McIlvain HE: An armchair adventure in case study research. In Crabtree B and Miller WL, editors: *Doing qualitative research,* ed 2, Thousand Oaks, Calif, 1999, Sage.

Barbour RS: Mixing qualitative methods: quality assurance or qualitative quagmire?, *Qual Health Res* 8(3):352-361, 1998.

Boyle JS: Field research: a collaborative model for practice and research. In Morse JM, editor: *Qualitative nursing research: a contemporary dialogue,* Newbury Park, Calif, 1991, Sage.

Burton CR: Living with stroke: a phenomenological study, *J Adv Nurs* 32(2):301-309, 2000.

Caelli K: The changing face of phenomenological research: traditional and American phenomenology in nursing, *Qual Health Res* 10(3):366-377, 2000.

Charmaz K: Grounded theory: objectivist and constructivist methods. In Denzin NK and Lincoln YS, editors: *Handbook of qualitative research,* ed 2, Thousand Oaks, Calif, 2000, Sage.

Chiu L: Lived experience of spirituality in Taiwanese women with breast cancer, *West J Nurs Res* 22(1):29-53, 2000.

Christy TE: The methodology of historical research: a brief introduction, *Image J Nurs Sch* 24(3):189-192, 1975.

Christy TE: The need for historical research in nursing, *Image J Nurs Sch* 4:227-228, 1981.

Cohen MZ and Ley CD: Bone marrow transplantation: the battle for hope in the face of fear, *Oncol Nurs Forum* 27(3):473-480, 2000.

Colaizzi P: Psychological research as a phenomenologist views it. In Valle RS and King M, editors: *Existential phenomenological alternatives for psychology,* New York, 1978, Oxford University Press.

Crabtree BF and Miller WL: *Doing qualitative research,* Newbury Park, Calif, 1992, Sage.

Creswell JW: *Qualitative inquiry and research design: choosing among five traditions,* Thousand Oaks, Calif, 1998, Sage.

DeLeon G: Integrative recovery: a stage paradigm, *Substance Abuse* 17(1):51-63, 1996.

Denzin NK: The art and politics of interpretation. In Denzin NK and Lincoln YS, editors: *Collecting and interpreting qualitative materials,* Thousand Oaks, Calif, 1998, Sage.

Denzin NK: *The recovering alcoholic,* Newbury Park, Calif, 1987, Sage.

Denzin NK and Lincoln YS: *The landscape of qualitative research,* Thousand Oaks, Calif, 1998, Sage.

Denzin NK and Lincoln YS: Introduction: the discipline and practice of qualitative research. In Denzin NK and Lincoln YS, editors: *Handbook of qualitative research,* ed 2, Thousand Oaks, Calif, 2000, Sage.

Engebretson J: Comparison of nurses and alternative healers, *Image J Nurs Sch* 28(2):95-99, 1996.

Engebretson J: Caring presence: a case study, *Int J Hum Caring* 4(2):33-39, 2000.

Geertz C: *Local knowledge: further essays in interpretive anthropology,* New York, 1983, Basic Books.

Giorgi A, Fischer CL, and Murray EL, editors: *Duquesne studies in phenomenological psychology,* Pittsburgh, 1975, Duquesne University Press.

Glaser BG and Strauss AL: *The discovery of grounded theory: strategies for qualitative research,* Chicago, 1967, Aldine.

Guba E and Lincoln Y: *Effective evaluation,* San Francisco, 1981, Jossey-Bass.

Hunter AJ and Chandler GE: Adolescent resilience, *Image J Nurs Sch* 31(3):243-247, 1999.

Kahn DL: Making the best of it: adapting to the ambivalence of a nursing home environment, *Qual Health Res* 9(1):119-132, 1999.

King G, et al: Organizational characteristics and issues affecting the longevity of self-help groups for parents of children with special needs, *Qual Health Res* 10(2):225-241, 2000.

Kleinman A: Local worlds of suffering: an interpersonal focus for ethnographies of illness experience, *Qual Health Res* 2(2):127-134, 1992.

Kruse BG: The lived experience of serenity: using Parse's research method, *Nurs Sci Q* 12(2):143-150, 1999.

Leininger MM: Culture care theory, *Nurs Sci Q* 9(2):71-78, 1996.

Liehr P et al: Psychometric testing of the adolescent version of the Cook-Medley Hostility Scale, *Issues in Comprehensive Pediatric Nursing* 23(2):103-116, 2000.

Lofland J and Richardson JT: Religious movement organizations: elemental forms and dynamics, *Research in Social Movements, Conflict and Change* 7:29-51, 1984.

Lusk B: Historical methodology for nursing research, *Image J Nurs Sch* 29(4):355-359, 1997.

Mallory C and Stern PN: Awakening as a change process among women at risk for HIV who engage in survival sex, *Qual Health Res* 10(5):581-594, 2000.

Marcus MT: Changing careers: Becoming clean and sober in a therapeutic community, *Qual Health Res* 8(4):466-480, 1998.

McFarland MR: Use of culture care theory with Anglo- and African-American elders in a long term care setting, *Nurs Sci Q* 10(4):186-192, 1997.

Mead M: *Coming of age in Samoa,* New York, 1949, New American Library, Mentor Books.

Meadows LM and Dodendorf DM: Data management and interpretation using computers to assist. In Crabtree B and Miller WL, editors, *Doing qualitative research,* ed 2, Thousand Oaks Calif, 1999, Sage.

Morse JM: The contracted relationship: ensuring protection of anonymity and confidentiality, *Qual Health Res* 8(3):301-303, 1998.

Newman MA: Evolution of the theory of health as expanding consciousness, *Nurs Sci Q* 10(1):22-25, 1997.

Nichols DJ and Hammer MS: Case study of institution-building by nurse Bertha Wright and colleagues, *Image J Nurs Sch* 30(4):385-389, 1998.

Orne RM, et al: Living on the edge: a phenomenological study of medically uninsured working Americans, *Res Nurs Health* 23(3):204-212, 2000.

Parse RR: Transforming research and practice with the human becoming theory, *Nurs Sci Q* 10(4):171-174, 1997.

Parse RR, Coyne AB, and Smith MJ: *Nursing research: qualitative and quantitative methods,* Bowie MD, 1985, Brady.

Paterson B, et al: Living with diabetes as a transformational experience, *Qual Health Res* 9(6):786-802, 1999.

Picard C: Pattern of expanding consciousness in midlife women: creative movement and narrative as modes of expression, *Nurs Sci Q* 13(2):150-157, 2000.

Richardson L: Writing: a method of inquiry. In Denzin NK and Lincoln YS, editors: *Handbook of qualitative research,* ed 2, Thousand Oaks, Calif, 2000, Sage.

Rittmayer J and Roux G: Relinquishing the need to "fix it": medical intervention with domestic abuse, *Qual Health Res* 9(2):166-181, 1999.

Schreiber R, Stern PN, and Wilson C: Being strong: how black West-Indian Canadian women manage depression and its stigma, *J Nurs Sch* 32(1):39-45, 2000.

Smith MJ and Liehr P: Attentively embracing story: a middle range theory with practice and research implications, *Scholarly Inquiry for Nursing Practice: An International Journal* 13(3):187-204, 1999.

Spiegelberg H: *The phenomenological movement,* vols I and II, The Hague, 1976, Martinus Nijhoff.

Spradley JP: *The ethnographic interview,* New York, 1979, Holt, Rinehart, and Winston.

Stake RE: *The art of case study research,* Thousand Oaks, Calif, 1995, Sage.

Stake RE: Case studies. In Denzin NK and Lincoln YS, editors: *Handbook of qualitative research,* ed 2, Thousand Oaks, Calif, 2000, Sage.

Steward A: *The ethnographer's method*, Thousand Oaks, Calif, 1998, Sage.

Strauss AL: *Qualitative analysis for social scientists*, New York, 1987, Cambridge University Press.

Strauss A and Corbin J: Basics of qualitative research: grounded theory procedures and techniques, Newbury Park, Calif, 1990, Sage.

Strauss A and Corbin J: Grounded theory methodology. In Denzin NK, Lincoln YS, editors: *Handbook of qualitative research*, Thousand Oaks, Calif, 1994, Sage.

Strauss A and Corbin J, editors: *Grounded theory in practice*, Thousand Oaks, Calif, 1997, Sage.

Swanson KM: Research-based practice with women who have had miscarriages, *Image J Nurs Sch* 31(4): 339-345, 1999.

Tarzian AJ: Caring for dying patients who have air hunger, *J Nurs Sch* 32(2):137-143, 2000

Tedlock B: Ethnography and ethnographic representation. In Denzin NK and Lincoln YS, editors: *Handbook of qualitative research*, ed 2, Thousand Oaks, Calif, 2000, Sage.

Torsch VL and Ma GX: Cross-cultural comparisons of health perceptions, concerns, and coping strategies among Asian and Pacific Islander American elders, *Qual Health Res* 10(4):471-489, 2000.

Travisano RV: Alternation and conversion as qualitatively different transformations. In Stone GP and Faberman HA, editors: *Social psychology through symbolic interaction*, Waltham, Mass, 1970, Ginn-Blaisdell.

van Kaam A: *Existential foundations in psychology*, New York, 1969, Doubleday.

Vidick AJ and Lyman SM: Qualitative methods: their history in sociology and anthropology. In Denzin NK and Lincoln YS, editors: *The landscape of qualitative research: theories and issues*, Thousand Oaks, Calif, 1998, Sage.

Volume C: Bridging the gap: a process of weight loss with anorexiant therapy. Unpublished master's thesis, University of Alberta, Edmonton, Canada, 1998.

Volume CI and Farris KB: Hoping to maintain a balance: the concept of hope and the discontinuation of anorexiant medications, *Qual Health Res* 10(2):174-187, 2000.

Waltz CF, Strickland O, and Lenz E: Mesurement in nursing research, ed 3, Philadelphia, 1991, F.A. Davis.

ADDITIONAL READINGS

Cohen MZ, Kahn DL, and Steeves RH: *Hermeneutic phenomenological research*, Thousand Oaks, CA, 2000, Sage Publications.

Morse JM, Swanson J, and Kuzel AJ: *The nature of qualitative research*, Thousand Oaks, CA, 2001, Sage Publications.

Roper JM and Shapira J: *Ethnography in nursing research*, Thousand Oaks, CA, 1999, Sage Publications.

HELEN J. STREUBERT SPEZIALE

Evaluating Qualitative Research

8

Key Terms

auditability
credibility

emic view
fittingness

Learning Outcomes

After reading this chapter, the student should be able to do the following:

- Identify the influence of stylistic considerations on the presentation of a qualitative research report.
- Identify the criteria for critiquing a qualitative research report.
- Evaluate the strengths and weaknesses of a qualitative research report.
- Describe the applicability of the findings of a qualitative research report.
- Construct a critique of a qualitative research report.

Nursing knowledge continues to evolve to meet the increasing demands brought about by accelerated changes in health care. Nurse researchers are called upon to develop, implement, and evaluate scientifically based nursing interventions to meet these changes. Nursing science in the twenty-first century is made up of a combination of quantitative and qualitative research methods. During the last decade, nurse researchers discovered that to study human beings they needed to employ a variety of research approaches to achieve the ultimate goal of improving the nursing care they provide. Today, qualitative and quantitative approaches to nursing research are used to meet the challenges created by complex human interaction in a constantly evolving health care system. Both are used to ensure that nursing interventions are the most appropriate.

Qualitative and quantitative research methods come from strong traditions in the physical and social sciences. Both types of research are different in their approach, format, and conclusions. Therefore the use of each requires an understanding of the traditions upon which the methods are based. The historical development of the methods identified as qualitative or quantitative can be discovered in this and other texts. This chapter aims to demonstrate a set of criteria that can be used to determine the quality of a qualitative research report. To achieve this, a published research report, as well as critiquing criteria, will be presented. The criteria will then be used to demonstrate the process of critiquing a qualitative research report.

STYLISTIC CONSIDERATIONS

Qualitative research reports are generated from a research tradition that is different from the predominant research paradigm of the last century. In a qualitative research report, the reader will usually not find hypotheses; dependent and independent variables; large, random samples; statistical analyses; conceptual frameworks; or scaled instruments. Because the intent of the research is to describe or explain phenomena or culture, the report is generally written in a way that allows the researcher to convey the full meaning and richness of the phenomena or culture being studied. Narrative—including subjective—comments are necessary to convey the depth and richness of the phenomena under study.

The goal of the qualitative research report is to describe in as much detail as possible the "insider's" or emic view of the phenomenon being studied. The **emic view** is the view of the person experiencing the phenomenon that reflects his/ her culture, values, beliefs, and experiences. What the qualitative researcher hopes to produce in the report is an understanding of what it is like to experience a particular phenomenon or be part of a specific culture. One of the most effective ways to help the reader understand the emic view is to use quotes reflecting the phenomenon as experienced. Similar ideas that are shared during the course of observations or interviews are usually clustered together and identified as a theme (see Chapter 7). A theme is a label. Themes represent a way of describing large quantities of data in a condensed format. To clearly demonstrate the application of a theme and how it helps the reader understand the emic view, the following is offered from a report published by Chiu (2000). Chiu reports on the experience of Taiwanese women and their transcendence of breast cancer. One of the themes she identifies is "opening to life and death." The following quote is used by Chiu to demonstrate this theme:

All of my family members hope that when they pass away in the future, they can be like my father, who had a lot of people chanting for him and who did not have to go to the funeral parlor. They all think that this is the luckiest thing one could ever have in their life. For this reason, my aunt thought that we should immediately begin to—and thereafter continue to—cultivate themselves. At that time, I felt that they had brought the topic of death out into the open; by doing so, they had taken the fear out of death and dying. I think this experience had a major effect on me.

The ability to share completely the interview or observation data from a qualitative research study is impossible. It is challenging to convey the depth and richness of the findings in a published research report. Journals generally request that manuscripts not be longer than 15 pages. Despite this limitation, a perusal of the nursing and health care literature will demonstrate a commitment by qualitative researchers and journal editors to publish qualitative research findings.

There are some journals that by virtue of their readership are committed to publication of more lengthy reports. One such journal is *Qualitative Health Research*. Guidelines for publication of research reports are generally listed in each nursing journal. It is important to note that criteria for research publications are not based on a specific type of research method (i.e., quantitative or qualitative). The primary goal of journal editors is to provide their readers with informative, timely, and interesting articles. To meet this goal, regardless of the type of research report, editors prefer to publish articles that have scientific merit, present new knowledge, and engage their readership. The challenge for the qualitative researcher is to meet these editorial requirements, as well as demonstrate the scientific merit of the work and its applicability in the page limit imposed by the journal of interest.

Nursing journals do not generally offer their reviewers specific guidelines for evaluating qualitative and quantitative research reports. The editors make every attempt to see that the reviewers are knowledgeable in the method and subject matter of the study. This determination is often made, however, based on the reviewer's self-identified area of interest. It is important to know that research reports are often evaluated based on the ideas held by the reviewer. The reviewer may have strong feelings about particular types of qualitative or quantitative research methods. Therefore it is important to clearly state the researcher's qualitative tradition and present the study, as well as its findings and implications for practice, within the page limitations set by the specific journal. Box 8-1 provides general guidelines for reviewing qualitative research. Box 8-2 provides guidelines for evaluating grounded theory. For information on specific guidelines for evaluation of phenomenology, ethnography, grounded

theory, historical and action research, see Streubert and Carpenter (1999). If you are interested in additional information on the specifics of qualitative research design, please see Chapter 7.

APPLICATION OF QUALITATIVE RESEARCH FINDINGS IN PRACTICE

The purpose of qualitative research is to describe, understand, or explain phenomena or cultures. Because prediction and control are not the aim of the inquiry, qualitative results are applied differently than the more traditional quantitative research findings. Glesne (1999) offers that the findings of qualitative research can be used to think about the social world in which we live. "A good qualitative research study invites you in. It encourages you to compare its descriptions and analyses to your own experiences." Schepner-Hughes (1992) states that qualitative text can provide the opportunity to give voice to those who are thought to have no history.

Glesne (1999) further relates that qualitative research findings can be used to create solutions to practical problems. For instance, in the development of a grounded theory representing some phenomenon, the theory may provide a profound description of the process a particular group may go through to arrive at a certain point. In their article on the following pages, Schreiber, Stern, and Wilson (2000) demonstrate this when they describe the process West-Indian Canadian women use to manage depression. The study findings can be tested against the experiences of other immigrant women with similar backgrounds to validate its utility in describing the process of managing depression. It is important to view research findings as quantitative or qualitative within context. For instance, a quantitative study of depression in children with chronic disease should not be viewed as having direct application to adults suffering with chronic disease. The findings must be utilized within context or additional studies must be conducted to validate the applicability of the findings across situations.

BOX 8-1 Critiquing Guidelines for Qualitative Research

STATEMENT OF THE PHENOMENON OF INTEREST

1. Is the phenomenon of interest clearly identified?
2. Has the researcher identified why the phenomenon requires a qualitative format?
3. Has the researcher described the philosophic underpinnings of the research?

PURPOSE

1. Has the researcher made explicit the purpose of conducting the research?
2. Does the researcher describe the projected significance of the work to nursing?

METHOD

1. Is the method used to collect data compatible with the purpose of the research?
2. Is the method adequate to address the phenomenon of interest?
3. If a particular approach is used to guide the inquiry, does the researcher complete the study according to the processes described?

SAMPLING

1. Does the researcher describe the selection of participants? Is purposive sampling used?
2. Are the informants who were chosen appropriate to inform the research?

DATA COLLECTION

1. Is data collection focused on human experience?
2. Does the researcher describe data collection strategies (i.e., interview, observation, field notes)?
3. Is protection of human participants addressed?
4. Is saturation of the data described?
5. Has the researcher made explicit the procedures for collecting data?

DATA ANALYSIS

1. Does the researcher describe the strategies used to analyze the data?
2. Has the researcher remained true to the data?

3. Does the reader understand the procedures used to analyze the data?
4. Does the researcher address the credibility, auditability, and fittingness of the data?

   Credibility
   a. Do the participants recognize the experience as their own?

   Auditability
   a. Can the reader follow the researcher's thinking?
   b. Does the researcher document the research process?

   Fittingness
   a. Can the findings be applicable outside of the study situation?
   b. Are the results meaningful to individuals not involved in the research?

5. Is the strategy used for analysis compatible with the purpose of the study?

FINDINGS

1. Are the findings presented within a context?
2. Is the reader able to apprehend the essence of the experience from the report of the findings?
3. Are the researcher's conceptualizations true to the data?
4. Does the researcher place the report in the context of what is already known about the phenomenon?

CONCLUSION, IMPLICATIONS, AND RECOMMENDATIONS

1. Do the conclusions, implications, and recommendations give the reader a context in which to use the findings?
2. Do the conclusions reflect the study findings?
3. Does the researcher offer recommendations for future study?
4. Has the researcher made explicit the significance of the study to nursing?

This is true in qualitative research, as well. Nurses who wish to use the findings of qualitative research in their practice must validate them, either through their own observations or through interaction with groups similar to the study participants, to determine whether the findings accurately reflect the experience.

Morse, Penrod, and Hupcey (2000) offer "qualitative outcome analysis (QOA) [as a] systematic means to confirm the applicability of clinical strategies developed from a single qualitative project, to extend the repertoire of clinical interventions, and evaluate clinical outcomes." Using this process, the researcher employs the findings of a qualitative study to develop interventions and then to test those selected. Qualitative outcome analysis allows the researcher/clinician to implement interventions based on the client's expressed experience of a particular clinical phenomenon. Morse, Penrod, and Hupcey state that "QOA may be considered a form of participant action research." Application of knowledge discovered during qualitative data collection adds to our understanding of clinical phenomena by using interventions that are based on the client's experience. QOA is considered a form of evaluation research.

Another use of qualitative research findings is to initiate examination of important concepts in nursing practice, education, or administration. Caring as a concept has been studied using qualitative approaches. Caring is considered a significant concept in nursing. Therefore studying its multiple dimensions is important. Tarzian (2000) researched nurses' experiences of caring for patients suffering with air hunger. Her study clearly expands the notion of caring to a particular type of caring: caring for dying patients with air hunger. The study adds to the existing body of knowledge on caring and extends the current state of the science by examining a specific type of caring.

Finally, qualitative research can be used to discover information about phenomena of interest that can lead to instrument development. When qualitative methods are used to direct the development of structured research instruments, it is usually part of a larger empirical research project. Instrument development from qualitative research studies is useful to practicing nurses because it is grounded in the reality of human experience with a particular phenomenon.

The study *Being Strong: How Black West-Indian Canadian Women Manage Depression and Its Stigma* by Rita Schreiber, Phyllis Noerager Stern, and Charmaine Wilson, published in *Journal of* *Nursing Scholarship* (2000), is critiqued. The article is presented in its entirety and followed by the critique on p. 179.

BEING STRONG: HOW BLACK WEST-INDIAN CANADIAN WOMEN MANAGE DEPRESSION AND ITS STIGMA

Rita Schreiber, Phyllis Noerager Stern, Charmaine Wilson

Purpose: *To discover how women from a nondominant cultural background (West Indian) experience and manage depression.*

Design: *Explanatory using grounded theory.*

Methods: *Semistructured interviews were conducted with 12 Black West-Indian Canadian women who experienced depression. Between 1994 and 1996, the first author engaged in participant observation.*

Findings: *The women used the basic social process they called "being strong" to manage or ameliorate depression. Being strong included "dwelling on it," "diverting myself," and "regaining my composure." For most of the women, the range of available life choices was limited to the three processes; however, a few engaged in "trying new approaches." These women were less limited in their range of cultural and behavioral boundaries than were the others, and began tentatively to explore other options for themselves.*

Conclusions: *Black West-Indian Canadian women in this study managed their depression in culturally defined ways by being strong and not showing vulnerability. Because being strong was also evident in a previous study of dominant-culture women as a prelude to depression, the process may be widespread in women prone to depression. The findings provide helpful information for intervening in an unfamiliar culture.*

The risk of women developing depression is twice that of men (Coryell, Endicott, & Keller, 1992). Among women, Blacks are more vulnerable than are Whites, and some researchers have found that Black women may be more vulnerable than are other groups (Eaton & Kessler, 1981; Frerichs, Anshensel, & Clark, 1981). In addition to the difference in risk factors, researchers in the United States and Canada suggest that the experiences of depression may be different for Black and White women (Barbee, 1994; Schreiber, 1996). Using a classic grounded-theory design (Glaser, 1978, 1992, 1998; Glaser & Strauss, 1967), we sought to discover the salient problem for Black West-Indian Canadian women who identified themselves as having been depressed and to learn how these women managed the problem.

BACKGROUND

The population of Canada is reported to be 26 million (Wood, 1993). An estimated 265,000 Black women live in Canada, the majority of whom are first- or second-generation immigrants from the former British West Indies (Wood, 1993). These women have unique health concerns, but little is written to guide nurses in caring form them. In a search of Medline, CINAHL, PsychLIT, and Statistics Canada we found no studies on the prevalence of depression among Black Canadian women.

Just the act of immigrating has an effect (Franks & Faux, 1990; Kim & Rew, 1994; Puskar, 1990; Stern, Tilden & Krassen-Maxwell, 1985; Vega, Kolody, Valle, & Weir, 1991), and being a member of a visible minority apparently adds to the stress (Anderson, 1985; Goffman, 1963). For African-American women in the United States, authors suggest that additional jeopardies exist because of minority status, socioeconomic status, and multiple roles (Barbee, 1992; Eaton & Kessler, 1981; Frerichs, Anshensel, & Clark, 1981; Guttiérrez 1990; Jones-Webb & Snowden, 1993; King, 1988; Morris, 1993). Barbee (1992) criticized community surveys for bias. Barbee (1992) and Schreiber (1996) concluded that these surveys, although making important contributions, do not incorporate the rich contextual details of human experience. Despite considerable success treating the symptoms of depression by using a combination of drugs and other therapy (U.S. Department of Health and Human Services, 1993), the root causes of depression remain unclear. Some fundamental origins and human reactions to possible causes were investigated in this study.

Several authors have suggested that culturally specific idioms, different from those of the dominant culture, cause some people not to seek health care for depression. These people might be more likely to somatize their emotional concerns, complaining instead of vague pain, fatigue, headaches, and other problems (Kim & Rew, 1994; Lloyd, 1993, Tabora & Flaskerud, 1994). Although researchers provide some clues about the experiences of Black West-Indian Canadian women with depression, the degree to which any results from American or British studies can be applied to the Canadian situation is unclear. Although some of the challenges faced by visible minority women might be similar, other concerns might differ because of differences in culture and history. Barbee (1992, 1994) and others (Anderson, 1985; Hall, Stevens, & Meleis, 1992) have suggested that research methods that incorporate contextual material would be suitable for understanding depression in Black women and other marginalized people.

METHODS

Using the techniques of classic grounded theory (Glaser, 1978, 1992, 1998; Glaser & Strauss, 1967; Stern, 1980, 1985a, 1985b, 1994), we sought data with variation. All participants in the study either immigrated or were first-born Canadians from English-speaking countries of the West Indies. Many of the participants or their parents took post-secondary education in England. Although this British background gave the women some advantages in becoming acculturated to the Commonwealth society of Canada, a salient difference from their country of origin was that in the West Indies, being Black was the norm; in Canada, the norm is White. Thus, immigration changed their status from being of the dominant race to that of a visible minority.

Data were collected in Southern Ontario. All 12 women referred to themselves as Black West-Indian Canadians. Nine were born in the West Indies; two were born in Canada, and one to West Indian parents in the United Kingdom. All but one of the participants had some post-secondary education, and four held baccalaureate degrees. The terms they used to describe their experiences included "dwelling on it," "private suffering," "life is a struggle," or "depression." The words emphasize the women's own definitions of depression. The basic question we asked them was: "What is it like to go through depression as a Black West-Indian Canadian?" More specific questions were asked to confirm or refute developing hypotheses.

Most of the interview data were collected by the third author, a graduate student in clinical psychology and of West-Indian origin. The first author also conducted interviews and engaged in about 600 hours of participant observation in the community. Each participant was interviewed for approximately 1 hour, from one to four times, and received a transcript of her taped interview to evaluate for accuracy.

In a matrix operation where all research activities from data collection to analysis were performed simultaneously (Stern, 1980), data were subjected to open coding, categorizing, linking, expansion, and reduction until hypotheses were generated. In the constructivist tradition of research, no attempt was made to separate the researcher from the researched. To avoid bias, we relied on the data for accuracy in interpreting the problem and how women managed it. Negative cases were woven into the analysis to create a higher level of abstraction, and to identify limits of the variables. As categories were identified, more data were gathered from certain groups or subgroups to strengthen or refute constructed categories. Collecting data and refining the analysis continued until a basic social process indicated most of the interaction in the phenomenon of study (Stern, 1980). Investigators consulted with selected members of the study group ($n=9$) for verification that the analysis made sense to them. Later, academic colleagues provided comments about the relevancy of the model.

FINDINGS

Black West-Indian Canadian women reported that they managed their depression through a basic social process of "being strong." Being strong happened against a backdrop of visible minority status within a Eurocentric society, and within three contexts: (a) the Black West-Indian Canadian cultural stigma of depression, (b) male-female roles and relationships, and (c) belief in Christian doctrine. The full context in which being strong occurred is explained in more detail elsewhere (Schreiber, Stern, & Wilson, 1998).

Being strong has four sub-processes: "dwelling on it," "diverting myself," "regaining my composure," and "trying new approaches." Three subprocesses overlap as shown in the Figure. The territory for maneuvering was largely limited to the three contexts which defined the boundaries of culturally acceptable behavior. Many of the women hardly questioned these boundaries, but accepted them as a given. A few women used the fourth sub-process, "trying new approaches." These women saw themselves as "more Canadian" and began, albeit tentatively, to explore the wider range of options open to them, thus breaking out of familiar cultural patterns.

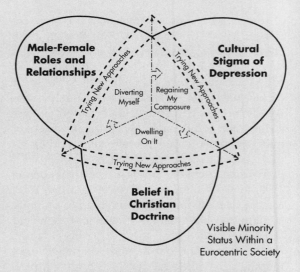

Figure. Being strong: How Black West-Indian Canadian women manage depression and its stigma.

Being Strong: A Cultural Construction

The goal of the women was to be able to manage their depression with grace and to live up to the cultural imperative to be strong. We accepted the women's reported responses to depression as culturally driven because of the way the women spoke of them. The women said that Black women were strong—stronger than White women. One participant said, "I think Black women are stronger [than Whites]. They've been, I mean, I'm talking about going back with generations so you were raised to be, you know, the strength of the home, the mother." One woman spoke of how she thought her friends would respond if she told them she was depressed. She said they would shame her by saying, "Get it together, girl!" or "We're strong, you got to be strong!" Being strong, then, constituted a culturally approved way to manage the culturally stigmatized experience of depression.

Dwelling On It

When women felt controlled by depression, they said they were "dwelling on it." They were aware of their feelings of depression but were unable to do anything about it. Dwelling on it was characterized by four dimensions: "private suffering," "life is a struggle," "showing compassion," and "pinpointing it." Depression for this group was an intensely private experience. A stricken woman was isolated in her misery, suffering in isolation to avoid the culturally defined stigma of depression. The women said that they never let others know about their struggle. "I hid it from the world. I didn't speak about what was happening, because it's like, everything I thought about was private—I withdrew from the world." The women said if they talked to their friends and relatives about their depression, they would be shunned as weak or crazy. They said the stigma of admitting to feelings of depression would reinforce their isolation as well as their private suffering. When comparing themselves to women of the dominant culture, they thought the sentimental order (Glaser & Strauss, 1971) or cultural right way of doing things was to be stronger. One woman's comment was typical, "We might be stronger, because we have to be stronger, you know, to make it in this world. Jamaican women are strong."

Private suffering. In their private suffering, some women took the precaution of walling themselves off from the world. One said, "I feel it coming on, like you know, menstrual cramps" and would stay away from people by going to bed. Another woman said, "I know—like, oh God, here it comes, you know, and there's nothing you can do about it. I would feel that way until I get over it." Others spoke of sleeping more without feeling rested. The women spoke of depression controlling their lives and feelings.

Life is a struggle. The women in this study experienced their world as stressful; many described a variety of life circumstances that were serious and chronic. One single mother had a 5-year-old son who was severely disabled. One university graduate was unable to find employment after several months of searching. An older woman had a major racism lawsuit pending against her former employer. Two women had

grandchildren living with them. One woman's husband was murdered. For many of them, employed in clerical and service positions, finances were a constant source of stress.

Some women compared their lives with the lives of their mothers and other female friends and relatives, and described the struggles these women faced. When they compared their struggles with those of others, they concluded that a normal expectation in life for all women is to struggle: "Certain things in life you have to accept, you know, that you have to live with—that you can't do anything about it." Thinking that life is a struggle for all women they knew reinforced the need for private suffering.

Showing compassion. Showing compassion was another way of being strong. As they reframed their own pain, the women were able to view the actions of others with compassion. Being strong, they were able to forgive what might otherwise have been seen as inconsiderate or insensitive behavior, and assumed primary responsibility for whatever was wrong. Showing compassion was often framed in the context of the woman's own knowledge. As one woman said, "Depending on the person's level of knowledge—those that have a low level of knowledge are very intolerant, and they go around—and with this stigma about people who are depressed—they just—[don't understand]." She could overlook intolerance, implying that if others knew what she knew, they would be more tolerant. Showing compassion enables a woman to feel a sense of competence in being able to transcend "petty" problems. However, by being compassionate she assumes more responsibility for what is happening in her world and thus adds to her already heavy burden.

Pinpointing it. These women began to transcend their depressed feelings when they identified and analyzed them. They recognized a bout of depression for what it was, something familiar: "I know when I'm depressed, sometimes my body tells me, it reacts in a certain way." Pinpointing it is the identification of depression based on past experiences. Pinpointing it allows the woman to take action and move to another sub-process: diverting myself. One woman explained: "Don't let depression enslave you. Get up and get out, and first thing you have to do is recognize that you are depressed and recognize that it is something that you can overcome if you want to."

Diverting Myself: Beginning to Manage

The women spoke about how they diverted themselves as a way of managing their depression by engaging in distracting activities. In diverting themselves, they gave up some of their need to be strong by looking outside themselves for help. Diversionary activities included "seeking help," "getting involved," and "thinking positively."

Seeking help. The most common diversionary activity was seeking help. Seeking help consisted of seeking God's solace and seeking professional help. All the women shared a profound belief in Christian doctrine. Spirituality was a central aspect of their lives—they all prayed routinely, read the Bible, and spoke with God about their pain. One said, "All I can say is you have to have faith. Faith in God is number one." For all the women, religious contemplation provided a diversion that allowed them to direct thoughts in more positive directions. This action is similar to thought blocking recommended by cognitive therapists (Beck, 1967) as a method that can be effective in controlling depressive thoughts. One woman explained that she could turn her troubles over to God, but that God worked through her to give her the strength to do whatever was needed. "God never gives you more trouble than you can bear."

The second way the women sought help was through professionals. However, less than half of the women sought professional counseling for their depression. Those who did found it beneficial to have someone with whom to share their thoughts and feelings, and from whom they could learn. One said:

> The therapists, you know, can really help with insight, give me good insights, help me to have insight into my own problems, right? And then, to sort of interpret for me some of the things, you know—why certain things

are happening to me—maybe certain actions that . . . I've taken, when I should have taken the opposite action, right?

This woman emphasized that friends could never provide this kind of assistance and should not be expected to do so. Another woman described her experience with a psychiatrist as being clarifying.

Guttiérrez (1990), Hooks (1993), and Carter (1995) identified race as important in therapy, emphasizing that ideally, a therapist would present a racial role model, and more importantly, communication and understanding are improved when therapist and client are of the same race. However, in this study, the women who sought counseling went to White therapists. When asked directly about race, the women responded that for them, the race of the therapist was unimportant. In fact, some women preferred a White therapist, feeling that would ensure that their private suffering would remain private in their closely-knit West Indian community, and would provide an "outside" perspective.

Getting involved. The second method of diversion was getting involved. All the women distracted themselves by getting involved, by socializing with friends, exercising, or just getting out of the house. One said:

> What I try to do is just keep myself occupied because it's easy, like if you're not doing anything, you know, for the brain to wander off—that way, you know, I'm not focusing on what the problem is, and I think it helps.

Interestingly, when socializing with friends, the women avoided discussing their problems. They said that simply chatting and being with other people provided the necessary diversion.

Thinking positively. The third type of diversion was thinking positively. Thinking positively is related to seeking God's solace, in that women often referred to faith in God at the same time they talked about positive thought. However, seeking solace occurred before other processes. One woman said:

> I'm in a better position that a lot of people, and um— life is such, you know, just living 1 day at a time, and when I start thinking that way—like I feel you know, in my mind, then I feel lighter.

Thinking positively replaced negative thoughts with positive thoughts to feel better. This approach, like blocking, is a central doctrine of cognitive therapy, and has been demonstrated to be effective. Theoretically, positive thinking works because the individual alters the personal meaning of an event so the new meaning is less threatening (Beck, 1967). Indeed, some of the women emphasized their personal decision making:

> I'm not going to sit down and feel sorry for myself and get bogged down and start thinking about those [depressing] things. Soon [as] it comes into my thought—I, I change it, I replace it with something positive, something good. You know what I mean? I can choose. Now I can choose to be sad or I can choose to be happy. It's not easy, but it's something that, um, can be achieved by continued practicing.

Regaining My Composure

Diverting myself usually leads to the third subprocess, regaining my composure. Regaining my composure, as the women called it, is a process wherein the women gained control of depression and returned to a relatively even mood. Regaining my composure usually consisted of finding God's strength within, and getting on with it.

Finding God's strength within. Finding God's strength within was a consequence of speaking with God. This explanation was typical, "He's my tower of strength. He's where I get my—where I revitalize, you know?" For the women in this study, a framework for understanding depression was grounded in Christian doctrine. Although many were familiar with other possible influences, such as genetic propensity to depression, those factors were seen as being situated within God's plan. That belief provided comfort, understanding, an ability to view others with compassion, and a renewed strength to "carry on." Finding God's strength within was the emotional and spiritual foundation and the necessary antecedent of "regaining my composure."

Getting on with it. Getting on with it was the final dimension of "regaining my composure." When getting on with it, the women became re-engaged with their social and contextual worlds, returning to work, or to their social relationships.

Although they had been physically present within their contextual worlds, before getting on with it, they had not been spiritually and emotionally available. The women were able to reinvolve themselves within their lives, and take a more active part. Getting on with it had much to do with the women accepting some of life's realities. One talked about moving on after the death of her husband, "So sometimes you have to get up and say, well—you shake off your cobwebs and [say], 'Let's go, this is reality, this is life.'" She described how she began to accept the loss, and that she knew she had to move on. Other women told similar stories of how "things happen" in people's lives, and it is important to learn the skills to deal with them.

Trying New Approaches

These first three subprocesses of "being strong" comprise a culturally approved approach Black West-Indian Canadian women use to manage depression. The model constructed from the data illustrates (see Figure) that the pull toward being strong, enacted in three culturally accepted behaviors, is much like the pull of gravity—cultural forces pull the individual toward the cultural center. A few of the women began to pull away from the processes at the center and began to examine their options. In particular, they began to examine other ways of being. This examination was subtle, not requiring serious challenges to the central processes. Nonetheless, through examination the women were able to see other possible behaviors—to understand that depression might well be related to their social condition rather than to their inability to be strong. Realizing this possibility, some of the women were able to change their social atmosphere by challenging it. However, some found such action difficult and disorienting.

Trying new approaches is a strategy in which some women began to understand and interact within their worlds in somewhat different ways, taking advantage of new options that became apparent. Trying new approaches, represented in the model by triangular bands that surround the first three subprocesses, enabled women to extend beyond their traditional behaviors. Women who question and think in ways that are new to them are likely to change their behaviors (Schreiber, Stern, & Wilson, 1998). Changing requires taking risks, and by implication, challenging the existing situation, which is why the women moved tentatively. For some women, engaging in culturally appropriate behavior was more important than challenging and risking.

Some women found that they were able to make certain changes in their lives based on new understandings gained from sources other than their religious faith. Their behavior was based on varied sources including therapists and popular culture. In general, women changed their behavior with some reluctance. For example, one became involved in anti-racist activities because of a situation at work that she thought left her no other option. For her, the choices were to "cave in or fight back," and she chose to fight back. Nonetheless, although she was committed to the struggle, it was clear that she was uncomfortable in her new role. Similarly, another woman who was the primary advocate for the well-being of her disabled child had experiences that convinced her that professionals in the health care and school systems did not understand her child's situation. She learned to manipulate the system (Wuest & Stern, 1991) to get adequate health care and education for her son, but she was uncomfortable doing it because, "I'm not like that." These and some other women were forced into situations that led them to trying new approaches. They changed their behavior because they saw no other option.

Some of the women had been in therapy and spoke about learning relationship skills. One woman talked of learning to handle her anger at the father of her child and developing self-esteem: "I think I'm better now than I was, like a year or two ago, you know—definitely I am better." Better to her meant being able to "communicate more clearly" to others. Another spoke about learning to be more assertive, which she believed had been a particular challenge because she was raised to believe that adults who are older are always right and should be respected. Obeying her mother was still an underlying concern as she struggled with asserting her own wishes:

I don't feel comfortable saying, "Well, I don't like so and so," or whatever, you know [but] I'm now 29 years old, I'm running my own life now, so I can basically do anything I want—we're in Canada now you know, like in a different age and everything.

Her words reveal the conflict between allegiance to her cultural background and her adopted culture. However, she was moving toward a more "Canadian" understanding of her world. For another woman, changing interactions within her world was similar, "I basically have to feel comfortable with myself first—I need to just, to be able to think, work things out with myself." For this woman, being more sure of herself was the precursor to changed behavior. While many of the women in the study seemed locked into old, culturally approved behaviors, some were able to venture into trying new approaches.

THEORETICAL IMPLICATIONS

An extensive search of the literature on depression yielded no references to the concept of "being strong" as antecedent to depression, or as a way to resolve a depressive episode. The theoretical construct of being strong, indicated in our data, is both unique and important in mental health nursing. Being strong is similar to Barbee's (1994) finding that African-American women accept depression as part of living. However, the Black West-Indian Canadian women in our study did not think of depression as a time of "healing" as did the women in Barbee's study. Those in our study viewed depression as something to move away from as quickly as possible by being strong. Hooks (1993) identified being strong as a myth that African-American women accept, share, and perpetuate. According to Hooks, the "assumption that [we] are somehow an earthy mother goddess who has built-in capacities to deal with all manner of hardship without breaking down, physically or mentally" (p. 70) provides a mask that can hide suffering and mental illness. From Hooks' perspective, this assumption results in many Black women suffering periods of suicidal depression that are not noticed or treated.

The women in our study tended to avoid discussing suicide. One woman mentioned it in passing, but when questioned, was not willing to speak of it further. Other women deflected the discussion of suicide with phrases such as "losing my faith" or "needing to find my strength." These women may have experienced severe depression that they were unwilling to discuss because of social and cultural taboos.

In a study by Schreiber (1996, 1998), some women no longer suffered major depressive episodes. Although they experienced some sadness, they were no longer governed by it. The women in Schreiber's study recovered fully from depression only after they realized that they did not need to be totally capable, always "strong," while the Black West-Indian Canadian women in this study continued to experience depression periodically, at the same time, managing it by being strong. Differences in the study groups could be an explanation. Although about a third of the women in Schreiber's 1996 study were immigrants, few were members of a visible minority. The additional factors of racism and cultural conflict might have complicated the situation.

Similarly, many of the women in Schreiber's study seriously challenged what was taken for granted in their lives, raising questions about the relevance of their religious upbringing, relationships, and for some, their sexual orientation. This subgroup in Schreiber's study were the women who made the fullest recoveries, in that they were no longer subject to severe depression. Furthermore, they believed they had the necessary problem-solving and communication skills for dealing with whatever issues might lead to depression. In contrast, the women in our study were less comfortable challenging the "sentimental order" (Glaser & Strauss, 1971), or "right way" of their lives, and thus made less sweeping changes. Their need to maintain the sentimental order might indicate effects of factors such as culture, religion, immigrant, and visible minority status within a Eurocentric society.

CONCLUSIONS

This study of Black West-Indian Canadian women adds to our understanding of the importance of cultural and social contexts within which women construct the meanings of their lives. To provide "culturally competent care" (Davis et al., 1992) clinicians need to be sensitive to the relative importance of cultural background for each woman, seeking guidance from the women themselves about understanding how those might differ from both understandings of women in the dominant culture, and from the nurse's own background. As clinicians acknowledge their own prejudices and assumptions (Capponi, 1992; Carter, 1995) and recognize that social stigma may prevent a woman from talking directly about the pain of depression, they may need to "decode" her messages to find the personal meanings. The women in this study refused to talk about suicide, which may indicate that they considered it culturally inappropriate to do so. Nonetheless, they may have found it helpful to learn more about depression in a way that normalized the experience.

One purpose of grounded theory research is the development of more abstract formal theory, raising questions for further investigation. The concept of "being strong," evident in this study as a strategy for managing depression, was seen as a prelude to depression in a previous study of women of the dominant culture (Schreiber, 1996, 1998). Is it possible that "being strong" prevents Black West-Indian Canadian women from recovering completely from depression? What causes women of the dominant culture to move from being strong to severe depression while Black West-Indian Canadian women apparently do not? What are the effects of contextual factors on these changes? The answers to these and other questions will help researchers and clinicians better understand how women experience and manage depression. We believe "being strong" may be a factor in inducing depression and slowing or preventing recovery for some women, and it warrants further study.   JNS

REFERENCES

Anderson, J.M. (1985). Perspectives on the health of immigrant women: A feminist analysis. *Advances in Nursing Science, 8(1)*, 61-76.

Barbee, E.L. (1994). Healing time: The blues and African-American women. *Health Care for Women International, 15(1)*, 53-60.

Barbee, E.L. (1992). African-American women and depression: A review and critique of the literature. *Archives of Psychiatric Nursing, 6(5)*, 257-265.

Beck, A. (1967). *Depression: Causes and treatment.* Philadelphia: University of Pennsylvania Press.

Capponi, P. (1992). Upstairs at the crazy house. Toronto, Canada: Viking.

Carter, R.T. (1995). *The influence of race and racial identity in psychotherapy: Toward a racially inclusive model.* Toronto, Canada: John Wiley & Sons.

Coryell, W., Endicott, J., & Keller, M. (1992). Major depression in a nonclinical sample. *Archives of General Psychiatry, 49*, 117-125.

Davis, L.H., Dumas, R., Ferketich, S., Flaherty, M.J., Isenber, M., Koener, V.E., Lacey, B., Stern, P.N., Balente, S., & Meleis, A. (1992). AAN expert panel report: Culturally competent health care. *Nursing Outlook, 40*, 277-283.

Eaton, W., & Kessler, G. (1981). Rates of symptoms of depression in a national sample. *American Journal of Epidemiology, 114*, 528-538.

Franks, F., & Faux, S.A. (1990). Depression, stress, mastery, and social resources in four ethnocultural women's groups. *Research in Nursing & Health, 13*, 283-292.

Frerichs, R.R., Anshensel, C.S., & Clark, V.A. (1981). Prevalence of depression in Los Angeles County. *American Journal of Epidemiology, 114*, 691-699.

Glaser, B.G. (1978). *Theoretical sensitivity.* Mill Valley, CA: Sociology Press.

Glaser, B.G. (1992). *Basics of grounded theory analysis.* Mill Valley, CA: Sociology Press.

Glaser, B.G. (1998). *Doing grounded theory: Issues and discussions.* Mill Valley, CA: Sociology Press.

Glaser, B.G., & Strauss, A. (1967). *The discovery of grounded theory.* Chicago: Aldine.

Glaser, B.G., & Strauss, A.L. (1971). *Status passage.* Mill Valley, CA: Sociology Press.

Goffman, I. (1963). *Stigma: Notes on the management of spoiled identity.* Englewood Cliffs, NJ: Prentice-Hall.

Guttiérrez, L.M. (1990). Working with women of color: An empowerment perspective. *Social Work, 35(2)*, 149-153.

Hall, J.M., Stevens, P.E., & Meleis, A.I. (1992). Developing the construct of role integration: A narrative analysis of women clerical workers' daily lives. *Research in Nursing and Health, 15(6)*, 447-457.

Hooks, B. (1993). *Sisters of the yam: Black women and self-recovery.* Boston, MA: South End.

Jones-Webb, R.J., & Snowden, L.R. (1993). Symptoms of depression among Blacks and Whites. *American Journal of Public Health, 83(2)*, 240-244.

Kim, S., & Rew, L. (1994). Ethnic identity, role integration, quality of life and depression Korean-American women. *Archives of Psychiatric Nursing, 8(6)*, 348-356.

King, D.K. (1988). Multiple jeopardy, multiple consciousness: The context of a Black feminist ideology. *Signs: Journal of Women in Culture and Society, 14*, 42-72.

Lloyd, K. (1993). Depression and anxiety among Afri-Caribbean general practice attenders in Britain. *The International Journal of Social Psychiatry, 39(1)*, 1-9.

Puskar, K.R. (1990). International relocation: Women's coping methods. *Health Care for Women International, 11*, 263-276.

Schreiber, R. (1996). (Re)Defining myself: Women's process of recovery from depression. *Qualitative Health Research, 6(4)*, 469-491.

Schreiber, R.S. (1998). Clueing in: How women solve the puzzle of self to recover from depression. *Health Care for Women International, 19(4)*, 101-120.

Schreiber, R.S., Stern, P.N., & Wilson, C. (1998). The contexts for managing depression and its stigma among Black West-Indian Canadian women. *Journal of Advanced Nursing, 27(3)*, 510-517.

Stern, P.N. (1980). Grounded theory methodology: Its uses and processes. *Image, 12*, 20-23.

Stern, P.N. (1985a). Using grounded theory in nursing research. In M.M. Leininger (Ed.), *Qualitative research methods in nursing* (pp. 149-160). New York: Grune & Stratton.

Stern, P.N. (1985b). A comparison of culturally approved behaviors and beliefs between Philippino immigrant women, American-born dominant culture women, and Western female nurses of the San Francisco Bay area: Religiosity of health care. *Health Care for Women International, 6*, 123-124.

Stern, P.N., Tilden, V.P., & Krassen-Maxwell, E. (1985). Culturally induced stress during childbearing: The Philippino-American experience. *Health Care for Women International, 6*, 105-121.

Tabora, B., & Flaskerud, J.H. (1994). Depression among Chinese Americans: A review of the literature. *Issues in Mental Health Nursing, 15*, 569-584.

U.S. Department of Health and Human Services. (1993). *Depression in primary care: Volume 2. Treatment of major depression. Clinical Practice Guideline Number 5.* AHCPR Publication No. 93-0551. Washington, DC: Government Printing Office.

Vega, W.A., Kolody, B., Valle, R., & Weir, J. (1991). Social networks, social support, and their relationship to depression among immigrant Mexican women. *Human Organization, 50(2)*, 154-162.

Wood, J. (Ed.). (1993). *Canada yearbook.* Ottawa, Canada: Statistics Canada, Queen's Printer.

Wuest, J., & Stern, P.N. (1991). Empowerment in primary health care: The challenge for nurses. *Qualitative Health Research, 1*, 80-99.

INTRODUCTION TO THE CRITIQUE

The research report *Being Strong: How Black West-Indian Canadian Women Manage Depression and Its Stigma* (Schreiber, Stern, and Wilson, 2000) is critically examined for its rigor as a grounded theory study, its contribution to nursing, and its usefulness in practice. The criteria identified in Box 8-2 are used to guide the critique. These criteria are specific for grounded theory research.

STATEMENT OF THE PHENOMENON OF INTEREST

Schreiber, Stern, and Wilson (2000) clearly state the phenomenon of interest. They address the risk of depression among all women and then elaborate on the vulnerability of black women.

BOX 8-2 Guidelines for Critiquing Research Using Grounded Theory Method

STATEMENT OF THE PHENOMENON OF INTEREST
1. Is the phenomenon of interest clearly identified?
2. Has the researcher identified why the phenomenon requires a qualitative format?

PURPOSE
1. Has the researcher made explicit the purpose for conducting the research?
2. Does the researcher describe the projected significance of the work to nursing?

METHOD
1. Is the method used to collect data compatible with the purpose of the research?
2. Is the method adequate to address the research topic?
3. What approach is used to guide the inquiry? Does the researcher complete the study according to the processes described?

SAMPLING
1. Does the researcher describe the selection of participants?
2. What major categories emerged?
3. What were some of the events, incidents, or actions that pointed to some of these major categories?
4. What were the categories that led to theoretical sampling?
5. After the theoretical sampling was done, how representative did the categories prove to be?

DATA GENERATION
1. Does the researcher describe data collection strategies?
2. How did theoretical formulations guide data collection?

DATA ANALYSIS
1. Does the researcher describe the strategies used to analyze the data?
2. Does the researcher address the credibility, auditability, and fittingness of the data?
3. Does the researcher clearly describe how and why the core category was selected?

EMPIRICAL GROUNDING OF THE STUDY FINDINGS
1. Are concepts grounded in the data?
2. Are the concepts systematically related?
3. Are conceptual linkages described and are the categories well developed? Do they have conceptual density?
4. Are the theoretical findings significant? If yes, to what extent?
5. Was data collection comprehensive and analytical interpretations conceptual and broad?
6. Is there sufficient variation to allow for applicability in a variety of contexts related to the phenomenon investigated?

CONCLUSIONS, IMPLICATIONS, AND RECOMMENDATIONS
1. Do the conclusions, implications, and recommendations give readers a context in which to use the findings?
2. Do the conclusions reflect the study findings?
3. Are recommendations for future study offered?
4. Is the significance of the study to nursing made explicit?

From Streubert, H. J. (1998). Evaluating the qualitative research report. In G. LoBiondo-Wood & J. Haber (Eds.), *Nursing research: Methods, critical appraisal and utilization* (4th ed., pp. 445–465), St. Louis, MO: C.V. Mosby; Strauss. A., & Corbin, J. (1990). *Basics of qualitative research: Grounded theory procedures and techniques*. Newbury Park, CA: Sage. Adapted with permission.

They tell us that there is a lack of information about black women and their depression experience but do not address why they chose black West-Indian Canadian women.

The authors offer statistics reflecting the total population of Canada and then tell the reader the number of women who are black and of West-Indian descent. A discussion then ensues regarding the effect of immigration on individuals. The introductory material makes a case for studying black women.

Schreiber and associates do not offer a reason for selecting "classic grounded theory design." What they do share is that they are interested in discovering the salient problems for black West-Indian Canadian women who identify themselves as having been depressed and learn to manage the problem. In the literature review, the authors include literature identifying the need to incorporate contextual information on depression in research. Based on what is presented, the reader can conclude that because the authors are examining depression and its management, a process or model is an appropriate outcome. This is an assumption on the part of the reader. Further, the discussion of the need for obtaining contextual data does not in and of itself imply the necessity of using qualitative methodology or more specifically grounded theory. The authors' justification for the method would have been clearer had they stated that they were interested in understanding the participants' experiences and elevating them to the level of a model or theory.

PURPOSE

The purpose of qualitative research studies is often consistent with the identified statement of the problem. In this case Schreiber and associates (2000) do not distinctly state the purpose of the research. They do, however, tell the reader that what they "sought to discover [was] the salient problem for Black West-Indian women who identif[y] themselves as having been depressed and to learn how these women managed the problem."

The authors explain that the significance of the study, which is found in the "Conclusions" section of the report, is to add to clinicians' knowledge of the importance of the cultural and social context that give meaning to each woman's life. They further state that the study is important because it will offer information that will help nurses provide culturally sensitive care.

METHOD

The method used in this study is clearly identified as "classic grounded theory" (Schreiber et al., 2000). The authors do not state why they selected the method. It can be inferred however because of their interest in how black West-Indian women manage depression that a process is occurring. As Carpenter (2000) relates, "grounded theory is a qualitative research approach used to explore the social processes that present within human interaction."

Assuming that the authors are interested in studying depression as a social process, then it is compatible with the purpose of the research and also adequate to address the research topic. Schreiber et al. (2000) could have used phenomenology to explore the experience of depression for the women in the study. When phenomenology is selected, however, the findings would not be reported as a theoretical model. The purpose of phenomenology is to describe, explain, or understand human experience.

For the reader to know whether the research approach was executed fully and properly, it is necessary to return to the original work of two noted grounded theorists, Glaser and Strauss, because little is offered in the text of the manuscript regarding the specifics of the method. The authors do make reference to "matrix operation" (Schreiber, 2000) and offer some elements of the processes required. For the unfamiliar reader, a primary source on grounded theory is necessary to understand the research process.

SAMPLING

Schreiber and associates (2000) report that 12 Black West-Indian Canadian women were the sources for data collection. There is no explanation why or how Black West-Indian Canadian women were selected. In the method section, however, the authors report that "collecting and refining the analysis continued until a basic social process indicated most of the interaction in the phenomenon of study." This, in essence, represents saturation, which is the point at which no new data emerge.

As is appropriate in grounded theory research, additional information was collected from "certain groups and subgroups to strengthen or refute the constructed categories." This is called theoretical sampling and its purpose is to include the insights of additional individuals or groups who can add to or refute developing categories of data. The authors do not address the representative of the categories. They do share that the basic psychological process (BSP) was labeled "being strong." Being strong had four subprocesses, including: "dwelling on it, diverting myself, regaining my composure and trying new approaches."

DATA GENERATION

Schreiber and associates (2000) describe data-collection strategies. They report the question that was asked to solicit the participant's experience: "What is it like to go through depression as a Black West-Indian Canadian?" The first and third author conducted interviews. The third author conducted most of the interviews because she is West Indian herself. In addition, the first author carried out approximately 600 hours of participant observation in the community. In order to demonstrate how data collection guided theoretical formulations, the authors share their use of open coding, categorizing, linking, expansion, and deduction as methods to generate hypothesis. The data resulting from this activity were used to direct additional data collection.

DATA ANALYSIS

Data generation and analysis are iterative processes in grounded theory. Data collection is followed by data analysis, which is followed by more data collection. The analysis leads the researcher to ask other questions of the data in order to build a strong theory. Schreiber and associates (2000) de-

scribe the repeating pattern of their data collection. They tell the reader that the coding and categorizing lead to linking, expansion, and reduction, which at times required the use of persons not in the primary sample.

Generally speaking, the measure of rigor in qualitative research is its **credibility, auditability, and fittingness.** These terms are defined in Chapter 7. In this study, the authors tell the reader that they consulted with nine of the study participants and had them verify that the analysis made sense to them. The model for depression was shared with professional colleagues for comment. These actions represent attention to credibility.

The reader judges auditability. The question to ask is: Did the researcher present enough information for me to see how the raw data lead to the interpretation? Similarly, judging the fittingness of the data rests with the reader. The question to ask is: Is there enough detail here for me to evaluate the relevance and importance of these data for my own practice or for use in research or theory development?

Finally, when judging the quality of data analysis, the reader must ask: Has the researcher shared enough with me so that I can judge why the core variable or BSP was selected? The core category or BSP in this study is "being strong." This is the variable that accounts for the variation in patterns of behavior. In this article, the authors provide readers with a rich contextual narrative. In addition to sharing the core variable and the subconcepts, Schreiber and associates (2000) offer themes that lead them to the subconcepts found to support the core variable. These can be found on pages 172 to 179 of the article.

EMPIRICAL GROUNDINGS OF THE STUDY: FINDINGS

When evaluating the findings, the reader must ask a number of important questions related to the concepts identified. In Schreiber and associates' (2000) study, the subjective comments of the participants are interwoven with the authors' narratives. It is clear from the participant comments that the concepts are grounded in the data. The

Barbara Krainovich-Miller

> ➤ Discuss the similarities and differences between the stylistic considerations of reporting a qualitative vs. a quantitative study in a professional journal.
> ➤ Are critiques of qualitative studies by consumers of research, either in the role of student or practicing nurse, valid? Which type of qualitative study is the most difficult for consumers of research to critique? Discuss what assumptions you made to make this determination.
> ➤ What is essential for the consumer of research to use when critiquing a qualitative research study? Discuss the ways you might use internet resources now or in the future when critiquing studies.

authors offer a clear description of their model and show conceptual linkages. This is most appropriately depicted in the schematic drawing of the model. A discussion of the linkages also can be found in the article's "Findings" section.

The theoretical formulations offered are meaningful within context. Using the proposed model without validation with another cultural group would be inappropriate. Once validated, however, the model may be very useful in directing culturally competent nursing care of women suffering with depression.

CONCLUSIONS, IMPLICATIONS AND RECOMMENDATIONS

The conclusions published are appropriate. The authors offer the reader implications of the theoretical formulations, as well as the overall conclusions of the findings. Schreiber and associates (2000) place the findings in context by sharing their recommendations and comparing what they found with the findings of authors who have studied similar topics. A number of future research questions are offered and the significance of the work is made clear in the opening paragraph of the "Conclusions" section.

Overall, the research is very well-reported and offers the reader an insight into the depression experience of Black West-Indian Canadian women and the process used to cope with it. A rich commentary helps the reader to understand the experience of these women and the process that they go through to manage their depression. In addition, adequate references are included, providing the reader with supplemental materials on the focus of the study.

REFERENCES

Carpenter DR: Grounded theory as method. In Streubert HJ and Carpenter DR: *Qualitative research in nursing: advancing the humanistic imperative*, Philadelphia, 2000, Lippincott.

Chiu L: Transcending breast cancer, transcending death: a Taiwanese population, *Nurs Sci Q* 13(1): 64-72, 2000.

Glesne C: *Becoming qualitative researchers: an introduction*, ed 2, New York, 1999, Longman.

Morse JM, Penrod J and Hupcey JE: Qualitative outcome analysis: Evaluating nursing interventions for complex clinical phenomena, *J Nurs Scholarship* 32(2):125-130, 2000.

Schepner-Hughes N: *Death without weeping: the violence of everyday life in Brazil*, Berkeley, CA, 1992, University of California Press.

Schreiber R, Stern PN, and Wilson C: Being strong: how Black West-Indian Canadian women manage depression and its stigma, *J Nurs Scholarship* 32(1):39-45, 2000.

Streubert HJ and Carpenter DR: *Qualitative research in nursing: advancing the humanistic imperative*, Philadelphia, 1999, Lippincott.

Tarzian AJ: Caring for dying patients who have air hunger, *J Nurs Scholarship* 32(2):137-143, 2000.

Studying Cardiovascular Risk Factors

Studying risk factors with the greatest potential to prevent cardiovascular diseases across the lifespan has been my focus as a nurse researcher. I believe that the future of prevention relies on intervening early in life to modify and compensate for genetic and environmental risk factors.

Studying identical and fraternal twins and their parents provided an opportunity to investigate the role that environment and heredity play in the cardiovascular risk profiles of children and adolescents. We studied blood pressure, lipid profiles, behavior patterns, obesity, and the effect of lifestyle factors (e.g., smoking, physical activity, and diet) on the risk factors. The twins were 6 to 11 years old when enrolled in the study. Funding was obtained from the National Center for Nursing Research (formerly the National Institute of Nursing Research [NINR]) to visit the twins' families and measure the twins' risk factor profiles twice more as they developed during adolescence. In collaboration with nursing, interdisciplinary colleagues and students, five research articles were published between 1988 and 1998 (Hayman et al, 1988a; Hayman et al, 1995; Meininger et al, 1988, 1998; Meininger, Stashinko, and Hayman, 1991) and two articles applying this knowledge to practice were published (Hayman et al, 1988a; 1988b).

Not surprisingly, the twin study confirmed that there is significant genetic influence on risk factors. Importantly, from the standpoint of planning nursing interventions, a considerable non-genetic component was also identified. Body fat was found to play a central role in risk factor development in the transition from childhood to adolescence. The twin study, because it was longitudinal, was able to test the stability of risk factors as children moved through adolescence. Many studies have demonstrated the stability of physiologic

risk factors (e.g., components of the lipid profile and blood pressure), but the twin study demonstrated "tracking" of behavioral risk factors such as anger and hostility over time. That is, as children develop, they tend to maintain their rankings relative to other children on the indices of anger and hostility.

The findings also suggested that something beyond the family environment influenced blood pressure. Our analysis showed that there was variability in blood pressure that could not be explained by genetics or environmental factors shared by family members. This led me to explore the school environment and other environments outside the home as a setting for further research.

Building on the twin study findings, blood pressure and anger became the focus of the next two studies. In collaboration with colleagues, data on 11- to 16-year-olds were collected in middle and high schools. A unique feature of the project is that blood pressure was monitored for a 24-hour period in ethnically diverse samples of healthy adolescents as they went about their usual activities on a school day. This assessment with Spacelab's blood pressure monitors is not usually conducted in non-clinical populations because of its expense. These studies, funded by the NINR, provide much more detailed data on ethnic differences in blood pressure during adolescence than has been available to date.

Another unique feature of this work is attention to the influences of activity, body size, and physical maturation on blood pressure. Activity is monitored electronically with an actigraph device worn on the wrist while the ambulatory blood pressure is monitored. Measurements of body fat, body fat distribution, and physical maturation were collected during a physical exam conducted at school by nurse practitioners. Maturation and anthropometric characteristics (e.g., height and body mass) were measured because they are closely linked with the increases in blood pressure that occur as children grow.

We found that black adolescents had higher blood pressure than their European or Hispanic-American counterparts. Most of these differences, however, were attenuated when other variables such as activity levels, body size, and maturation were taken into account. We found that taking blood pressure for 30 minutes while the adolescents talked about a usual day or an anger-provoking situation predicted blood pressure measured over a 24-hour period (Meininger et al, 1998; Meininger et al, 1999). Because the 30-minute protocol is cost-efficient and practical, it may have potential for screening large populations of adolescents (Meininger et al, 2001). We have also confirmed that physical maturation and measures of body fat are extremely important variables to include in studies of adolescent blood pressure and anger (Liehr et al, 1997; Mueller et al, 1996, 1998).

This research contributes to the knowledge we need for prevention programs. As I continue to review the literature on the effectiveness of school-based interventions to lower cardiovascular risk profiles, studies to date indicate only modest impact of efforts to improve cardiovascular risk profiles of children and adolescents (Meininger, 1997; 2000). Nursing has a prominent role in this area of research. The challenge is to find new ways to reach children and create environments that support cardiovascular health.

Hayman LL et al: Nongenetic influences of obesity on risk factors for cardiovascular disease during two phases of development, *Nurs Res* 44:277-283, 1995.

Hayman LL et al: Type A behavior and other cardiovascular disease risk factors in twin children, *Nurs Res* 37:290-296, 1988a.

Hayman LL et al: Which child is at risk for heart disease? Part I, *Am J Maternal Child Nurs* 13:398-340, 1988b.

Hayman LL et al: Reducing risk for heart disease in children, Part II, *Am J Maternal Child Nurs* 13:442-448, 1988c.

Liehr P et al: Blood pressure reactivity in urban youth during angry and normal talking, *J Cardiovascular Nurs* 11(4): 85-94, 1997.

Meininger JC: Primary prevention of cardiovascular disease risk factors: review and implications for population-based practice, *Adv Pract Nurs Q* 3(2):70-79, 1997.

Meininger JC: School-based interventions for primary prevention of cardiovascular disease: evidence of effects for minority populations. In Fitzpatrick J, editor: *Annual Review of Nursing Research,* New York, 2000, Springer.

Meininger JC et al: Genetics or environment? Type A behavior and physiological cardiovascular disease risk factors in twin children, *Nurs Res* 37:341-346, 1988.

Meininger JC et al: Genetic and environmental influences on cardiovascular disease risk factors in adolescents, *Nurs Res* 47:11-18, 1998.

Meininger JC et al: Predictors of ambulatory blood pressure: identification of high-risk adolescents, *Adv Nurs Sci* 20(3):51-65, 1998.

Meininger JC et al: Identification of high risk adolescents for interventions to lower blood pressure. In Funk S, editor: *Key aspects of managing chronic illness,* New York, 2001, Springer.

Meininger JC et al: Stress-induced alterations and 24-hour ambulatory blood pressure in adolescents, *Blood Pressure Monitoring* 4:115-120, 1999.

Meininger JC, Stashinko EE, and Hayman LL: Components of type A behavior in children: psychometric properties of the Matthews Youth Test for Health, *Nurs Res* 40:221-227, 1991.

Mueller WH et al: Adolescent blood pressure and anger and hostility: possible links with body fat, *Ann Human Biol* 25:295-307, 1998.

Mueller WH et al: Demographic moderation of biological variables: lessons from a pilot program of anger and blood pressure, *Revisita di Antropologia (Roma)* 74:139-146, 1996.

Mueller WH et al: Conicity: a new index of body fat distribution: what does it tell us?, *Am J Human Biol* 8:489-496, 1996.

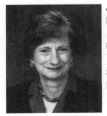

Janet C. Meininger, PhD, RN, FAAN
Lee & Joseph Jamail
 Distinguished Professor,
UT-Houston Health Science
 Center,
School of Nursing,
Houston, Texas

GERI LOBIONDO-WOOD

Introduction to Quantitative Research

9

Key Terms

constancy
control
control group
dependent variable
experimental group
external validity

extraneous or mediating
 variable
history
homogeneity
independent variable
instrumentation
internal validity

maturation
measurement effects
mortality
randomization
reactivity
selection
selection bias

Learning Outcomes

After reading this chapter, the student should be able to do the following:

- Define research design.
- Identify the purpose of the research design.
- Define control as it affects the research design.
- Compare and contrast the elements that affect control.
- Begin to evaluate what degree of control should be exercised in the design.
- Define internal validity.
- Identify the threats to internal validity.
- Define external validity.
- Identify the conditions that affect external validity.
- Evaluate the design using the critiquing questions.

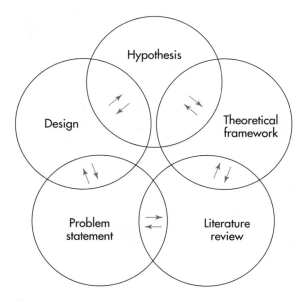

Figure 9-1   Interrelationships of design, problem statement, literature review, theoretical framework, and hypothesis.

The word *design* implies the organization of elements into a masterful work of art. In the world of art and fashion, design conjures up images of processes and techniques that are used to express a total concept. When an individual creates, process and form are employed. The form, process, and degree of adherence to structure depend on the aims of the creator. The same can be said of the research process. The research process does not need to be a sterile procedure, but one where the researcher develops a masterful work within the limits of a problem and the related theoretical basis. The framework that the researcher creates is the design. When reading a study, the research consumer should be able to recognize that the research problem, purpose, literature review, theoretical framework, and hypothesis all interrelate with, complement, and assist in the operationalization of the design (Figure 9-1).

Nursing is concerned with a variety of structures that require varying degrees of process and form, such as the provision of quality, cost-effective patient care, organizational structure, and student education. When patient care is administered, the

nursing process is used. Previous chapters stress the importance of theory and subject matter knowledge. How a researcher structures, implements, or designs a study affects the results of a research project.

For the consumer to understand the implications and the use of research, the central issues in the design of a research project should be understood. This chapter provides an overview of the meaning, purpose, and issues related to quantitative research design, and Chapters 10 and 11 present specific types of quantitative designs.

PURPOSE OF RESEARCH DESIGN

The purpose of the research design is to provide the plan for answering research questions. The design in quantitative research then becomes the vehicle for hypothesis testing or answering research questions. The design involves a plan, as well as structure and strategy. These three design concepts guide a researcher in writing the hypothesis or research questions, conducting the project, and analyzing and evaluating the data. The overall purpose of the research design is twofold: to aid in the solution of research problems and maintain control. All research attempts to solve problems. The design coupled with the methods and procedures are the mechanisms for finding solutions to research problems. *Control* is defined as the measures that the researcher uses to hold the conditions of the study uniform and avoid possible impingement of bias on the **dependent variable** or outcome.

A research example that demonstrates how the design can aid in the solution of a research question and maintain control is the study by Bull, Hansen, and Gross (2000; see Appendix A). The aims of the study were to examine the differences in outcomes for elders hospitalized with heart failure and caregivers who participated in a professional-patient partnership model of discharge planning compared with those who received the usual discharge planning, as well as to examine differences in costs associated with hospital readmission and use of the emergency room following hospital discharge. To maintain control, the investigators collected data at two hospitals that were matched in terms of size, type, and discharge planning practices used in their cardiac units. To further maintain control and be eligible for the study, potential subjects had to meet the eligibility criteria, which included being able to speak and understand English, being an elder (i.e., at least 55 years of age) hospitalized with heart failure, being able to identify a family member or friend who would help with after care following hospitalization, and being able to achieve a score indicating cognitive competence on a mental status questionnaire. By establishing the specific sample criteria, subject eligibility, and the use of a matched, control setting, the researchers were able to maintain control over the study's conditions and suggest an extension of this outcome study with further research. A variety of considerations, including the type of design chosen, affect the accomplishment of the study. These considerations include objectivity in the conceptualization of the problem, accuracy, feasibility, control of the experiment, internal validity, and external validity. There are statistical principles behind the many forms of control, but it is more important that the research consumer have a clear conceptual understanding.

OBJECTIVITY IN THE PROBLEM CONCEPTUALIZATION

Objectivity in the conceptualization of the problem is derived from a review of the literature and development of a theoretical framework (see Figure 9-1). Using the literature, the researcher assesses the depth and breadth of available knowledge on the problem. The literature review and theoretical framework should demonstrate to the reader that the researcher reviewed the literature with a critical and objective eye (see Chapters 4 and 5), because this affects the type of design chosen. For example, a question about the relationship of the length of a breastfeeding teaching program may suggest either a correlational or an experimental design (see Chapters 10 and 11), whereas a question regarding the physical changes in a woman's body during pregnancy and the maternal perception of the unborn child may suggest a survey or correlation study (see Chapter 11). Therefore the literature review should reflect the following:

- When the problem was studied
- What aspects of the problem were studied
- Where it was investigated
- By whom it was investigated
- The gaps or inconsistencies in the literature

HELPFUL HINT A review that incorporates the aspects presented here allows the consumer to judge the objectivity of the problem area and therefore whether the design chosen matches the problem.

ACCURACY

Accuracy in determining the appropriate design is also accomplished through the theoretical framework and review of the literature (see Chapters 4 and 5). Accuracy means that all aspects of a study systematically and logically follow from the research problem. The beginning researcher is wise to answer a question involving few variables that will not require the use of sophisticated designs. The simplicity of a research project does not render it useless or of a lesser value for practice. Although the project is simple, the researcher should not forego accuracy. The consumer should feel that the researcher chose a design that was consistent with the research problem and offered the maximum amount of control. The issues of control are discussed later in this chapter. Also, many clinical problems have not yet been researched. Therefore a preliminary or pilot study would be a wise approach. The key is the accuracy, validity, and objectivity used by the researcher in attempting to answer the question. Accordingly, when reading research one should read various types of studies and assess how and if the criteria for each step of the research process were followed. Research consumers will find that many nursing journals publish not only sophisticated clinical research projects but also smaller clinical studies that can be applied to practice.

Berger and Higginbotham (2000) conducted an example of a preliminary study that investigated a clinical problem. This pilot study was done to examine patterns of and relationships among activity/rest (activity), sleep/wake (sleep), symptoms, health status, and fatigue during and following adjuvant cancer chemotherapy. The goal was to explore the issues related to fatigue in order to help plan future fatigue-intervention studies. The idea for the study grew from clinical observations and the literature suggesting that fatigue in breast cancer survivors following treatment had not received much attention. The researchers felt that if they followed a group of women through their treatment cycle and assessed patterns of fatigue, they could develop and test individualized intervention plans for women receiving chemotherapy as a result of breast cancer. The researchers acknowledge the limitations of the study and although this study does not give nurses all the data needed to decide whether the variables tested are related, it does provide important information for future inquiry.

FEASIBILITY

When critiquing the research design one also needs to be aware of the pragmatic consideration of feasibility. Sometimes the reality of feasibility does not truly sink in until one does research. It is important to consider feasibility when reviewing a study, including availability of the subjects, timing of the research, time required for the subjects to participate, costs, and analysis of the data (Table 9-1). These pragmatic considerations are not presented as a step in the research process as are the theoretical framework or methods, but they do affect every step of the process and as such, should be considered when assessing a study. The student researcher may or may not have monies or accessible services. When critiquing a study, note the credentials of the author and whether the investigation was part of a stu-

dent project or part of a fully funded grant project. If the project was a student project, the standards of critiquing are applied more liberally than for a doctorally prepared, experienced researcher or clinician. Finally, the pragmatic issues raised affect the scope and breadth of an investigation and therefore its generalizability.

CONTROL

A researcher attempts to use a design to maximize the degree of control over the tested variables. **Control** involves holding the conditions of the study constant and establishing specific sampling criteria as described by Bull, Hansen, and Gross (2000) (Appendix A). An efficient design can maximize results, decrease errors, and control preexisting conditions that may affect outcome. To accomplish these tasks, the research design and methods should demonstrate the researcher's efforts at control.

For example, in their study, Mahon, Yarcheski, and Yarcheski (2000) (see Appendix C) attempted to examine symptom patterns and diminished general well-being as negative outcomes, and vigor and change as positive outcomes of state and trait anger via two proposed models. The research hypotheses were as follows:

- Trait anger would have a direct effect on state anger.
- Trait anger and state anger would have a direct effect on vigor and inclination to change.
- Trait anger would have an indirect effect on vigor and inclination to change through state anger.
- Is health status related to illness outcome?

To test these questions/hypotheses and apply control, the investigators calculated a sample size (see Chapter 12) and, based on guidelines of what early adolescence is, chose a sample that consisted of 12- to 14-year-olds who were not in special education courses. The researchers also had teachers review and approve the instrument packets for appropriateness of content and reading level. This study illustrates how the investi-

TABLE **9-1**   Pragmatic Considerations in Determining the Feasibility of a Research Problem

FACTOR	PRAGMATIC CONSIDERATION
Time	The research problem must be one that can be studied within a realistic period of time. All researchers have deadlines for completion of a project. The scope of the problem must be circumscribed enough to provide ample time for the completion of the entire project. Research studies generally take longer than anticipated to complete.
Subject availability	The researcher must determine whether a sufficient number of eligible subjects will be available and willing to participate in the study. If one has a captive audience (e.g., students in a classroom), it may be relatively easy to enlist their cooperation. When a study involves the subjects' independent time and effort, they may be unwilling to participate when there is no apparent reward for doing so. Other potential subjects may have fears about harm or confidentiality and be suspicious of the research process in general. Subjects with unusual characteristics are often difficult to locate. People are generally fairly cooperative about participating, but a researcher must consider needing a larger subject pool than will actually participate. At times, when reading a research report the researcher may note how the procedures were liberalized or the number of subjects was altered—probably as a result of some unforeseen pragmatic consideration.
Facility and equipment availability	All research projects require some kind of equipment. The equipment may be questionnaires, telephones, stationery, stamps, technical equipment, or some other apparatus. Most research projects require the availability of some kind of facility. The facility may be a hospital site for data collection or a laboratory space or computer center for data analysis.
Money	Many research projects require some expenditure of money. Before embarking on a study the researcher probably itemized the expenses and projected the total cost of the project. This provides a clear picture of the budgetary needs for items like books, stationery, postage, printing, technical equipment, telephone and computer charges, and salaries. These expenses can range from about $200 for a small-scale student project to hundreds of thousands of dollars for a large-scale federally funded project.
Researcher experience	The selection of the research problem should be based on the nurse's experience and interest. It is much easier to develop a research study related to a topic that is either theoretically or experientially familiar. Selecting a problem that is of interest to the researcher is essential for maintaining enthusiasm when the project has its inevitable ups and downs.
Ethics	Research problems that place unethical demands on subjects may not be feasible for study. Researchers must take ethical considerations seriously. The consideration of ethics may affect the choice of the design and methodology.

gators in one study planned the design to apply controls. Control is important in all designs. When various research designs are critiqued, the issue of control is always raised but with varying levels of flexibility. The issues discussed here will become clearer as you review the various types of designs discussed in later chapters (see Chapters 10 and 11). Control is accomplished by ruling out extraneous or mediating variables that compete with the independent variables as an explanation for a study's outcome. An **extraneous or mediating variable** is one that interferes with the operations of the phenomena being studied (e.g., age and gender or as in the previous example of chronically ill youth). Means of controlling extraneous variables include the following:

- Use of a homogeneous sample
- Use of consistent data-collection procedures
- Manipulation of the independent variable
- Randomization

The following example illustrates and defines these concepts:

An investigator might be interested in how a new stop-smoking program (independent variable) affects smoking behavior (dependent variable). The independent variable is assumed to affect the outcome or dependent variable. An investigator needs to be relatively sure that the decrease in smoking is truly related to the stop-smoking program rather than to some other variable, such as motivation. The design of the research study alone does not inherently provide control. But an appropriately designed study with the necessary controls can increase an investigator's ability to answer a research question.

HOMOGENEOUS SAMPLING

In the stop-smoking study, extraneous variables may affect the dependent variable. The characteristics of a study's subjects are common extraneous variables. Age, gender, length of time smoked, amount smoked, and even smoking rules may affect the outcome in the stop-smoking example. These variables may therefore affect the outcome, even though they are extraneous or outside of the study's design. As a control for these and other similar problems, the researcher's subjects should demonstrate **homogeneity** or similarity with respect to the extraneous variables relevant to the particular study (see Chapter 12). Extraneous variables are not fixed but must be reviewed and decided on, based on the study's purpose and theoretical base. By using a sample of homogeneous subjects, the researcher has used a straightforward step of control.

For example, in the study described earlier by Mahon, Yarcheski, and Yarcheski (2000), the researchers ensured homogeneity of the sample. The sample was homogenous based on age and demographics. This control step limits the generalizability or application of the outcomes to other populations when analyzing and discussing the outcomes (see Chapter 18). Results can then be generalized only to a similar population of individuals. You may say that this is limiting. This is not necessarily so because no treatment or program may be applicable to all populations, and the consumer of research findings must take the differences in populations into consideration. In the case of Mahon, Yarcheski, and Yarcheski's study (2000), the findings provided information for nursing practice and raised several important questions for practice and future research.

HELPFUL HINT When reviewing studies remember that it is better to have a "clean" study that can be used to make generalizations about a specific population than a "messy" one that can generalize little or nothing.

If the researcher feels that one of the extraneous variables is important, it may be included in the design. In the smoking example, if individuals are working in an area where smoking is not allowed and this is considered to be important, the researcher could build it into the design and set up a control for it. This can be done by comparing two different work areas: one where smoking is allowed and one where it is not. The important idea to keep in mind is that before the data are collected, the researcher should have identified, planned for, or controlled the important extraneous variables.

CONSTANCY IN DATA COLLECTION

Another basic, yet critical, component of control is constancy in data-collection procedures. **Constancy** refers to the notion that the data-collection procedures should reflect to the consumer a cookbook-like recipe of how the researcher controlled the conditions of the study. This means that environmental conditions, timing of data collection, data-collection instruments, and data-collection procedures used to gain the data are the same for each subject (see Chapters 12 and 14). An example of a well-controlled study was done by Defloor and DeSchuijmer (2000). The objective of this study was to assess the effect of the type of operating table mattress and surgical position on interface pressures in healthy adults. The investigators solicited healthy volunteers and tested five types of mattresses and four different positions in which patients are often placed during extensive surgery (i.e., > 2 hours in length). To control conditions, the investigators randomized the order of mattresses and the positions for every subject, and each measurement was performed after 1 minute of immobilization. The system used to measure pressure was standardized prior to every measurement, and with every manipulation of the measuring mat, and the interface measurements were done twice for each subject to test the reliability of the measurement. A review of this study shows that data were collected from each subject in the same manner and under the same conditions. This type of control aided the investigators' ability to draw conclusions, discuss, and cite the need for further research in this area. For the consumer, it demonstrates a clear, consistent, and specific means of data collection.

MANIPULATION OF INDEPENDENT VARIABLE

A third means of control is manipulation of the **independent variable.** This refers to the administration of a program, treatment, or intervention to only one group within the study but not to the other subjects in the study. The first group is known as the **experimental group,** and the other group is known as the **control group.** In a control group, the variables under study are held at a constant or comparison level. For example, suppose a researcher wants to study the ways to improve discharge planning and outcomes for elders as in the Bull, Hensen, and Gross (2000, Appendix A) study. The research team matched two hospitals in terms of size and discharge planning practices. One hospital served as the control site, and the other hospital implemented the experimental discharge planning intervention. Experimental and quasi-experimental designs use manipulation. Nonexperimental designs do not manipulate the independent variable. This does not decrease the usefulness of a nonexperimental design, but the use of a control group in an experimental or quasi-experimental design is related to the level of the problem and, again, its theoretical framework.

HELPFUL HINT Be aware that the lack of manipulation of the independent variable does not mean a weaker study. The level of the problem, the amount of theoretical work, and the research that has preceded the project all affect the researcher's choice of the design. If the problem is amenable to a design that manipulates the independent variable, it increases the power of a researcher to draw conclusions; that is, if all of the considerations of control are equally addressed.

RANDOMIZATION

Researchers may also choose other forms of control, such as randomization. **Randomization** is used when the required number of subjects from the population is obtained in such a manner that each subject in a population has an equal chance of being selected. Randomization eliminates bias, aids in the attainment of a representative sample, and can be used in various designs (see Chapters 10 and 12). In their study, Lenz and Perkins (2000) wanted to examine the effectiveness of a psychoeducational intervention in a sample of coronary artery bypass surgery patient/family member caregiver dyads. After obtaining consent to participate in the study from the patients and family members, the researchers randomly assigned each dyad to the experimental (psychoeducational intervention) or control group (standard discharge care).

Randomization can also be done with paper-and-pencil type of instruments. By randomly ordering items on the instruments, the investigator can assess if there is a difference in responses that can be related to the order of the items. This may be especially important in longitudinal studies where bias from giving the same instrument to the same subjects on a number of occasions can be a problem (see Chapter 11).

QUANTITATIVE CONTROL AND FLEXIBILITY

The same level of control cannot be exercised in all types of designs. At times, when a researcher wants to explore an area in which little or no literature on the concept exists, the researcher will probably use an exploratory design. In this type of study, the researcher is interested in describing or categorizing a phenomenon in a group of individuals. Rubin's (1967a, 1967b) early work on the development of maternal tasks during pregnancy is an example of exploratory research. In this research, she attempted to categorize conceptually the various maternal tasks of pregnancy. Rubin interviewed women throughout their pregnancies and developed a framework of the maternal tasks of pregnancy from these extensive interviews. In critiquing this type of study, the issue of control should be applied in a highly flexible manner because of the preliminary nature of the work.

If it is determined from a review of a study that the researcher intended to conduct a correlational study, or a study that looks at the relationship between or among the variables, then the issue of control takes on more importance (see Chapter 11). Control must be exercised as strictly as possible. At this intermediate level of design, it should be clear to the reviewer that the researcher considered the extraneous variables that may affect the outcomes.

All aspects of control are strictly applied to studies that use an experimental design (see Chapter 10). The reviewer should be able to locate in the research report how the researcher met the following criteria (i.e., the conditions of the research were constant throughout the study, assignment of subjects was random, and experimental and control groups were used). The Defloor and DeSchuijmer (2000) study, which was previously discussed, is an example in which the aspects of control were addressed. Because of the control exercised in the study, the reviewer can see that all issues related to control were considered and the extraneous variables were addressed.

INTERNAL AND EXTERNAL VALIDITY

When reading research, one must feel that the results of a study are valid, based on precision, and faithful to what the researcher wanted to measure. For a study to form the basis of further research, practice, and theory development, it must be credible and dependable. There are two important criteria for evaluating the credibility and dependability of the results: internal validity and external validity. Threats to validity are listed in Box 9-1, and discussion follows.

INTERNAL VALIDITY

Internal validity asks whether the independent variable really made the difference or the change in the dependent variable. To establish internal validity the researcher rules out other factors or threats as rival explanations of the relationship between the variables. There are a number of threats to internal validity, and these are considered by researchers in planning a study and by consumers before implementing the results in practice (Campbell and Stanley, 1966). Research consumers should note that the threats to internal validity are most clearly applicable to experimental designs, but attention to factors that can compromise outcomes should be considered to some degree in all quantitative designs. If these threats are not considered, they could negate the results of the research. How these threats may af-

BOX 9-1 Threats to Validity

INTERNAL VALIDITY
History
Maturation
Testing
Instrumentation
Mortality
Selection bias

EXTERNAL VALIDITY
Selection effects
Reactive effects
Measurement effects

TABLE **9-2** Examples of Internal Validity Threats

THREAT	EXAMPLE
History	Bull, Hansen, and Gross (2000, Appendix A) tested a teaching intervention in one hospital and compared outcomes with those of another hospital in which usual care was given. During the final months of data collection, the control hospital implemented a congestive heart failure critical pathway; as a result, data from the control hospital (cohort four) were not included in the analysis.
Maturation	Wikblad and Anderson (1995) controlled for the possibility of maturation in a study of wound healing processes. Normal wound healing could have been a threat to the findings, but the researchers developed a careful data-collection plan to control for the threat of maturation.
Testing	A researcher measured acute pain with a repeated measures design during a lengthy procedure. The researcher would have to consider the results in light of the possible bias of repeating the pain measurements over a short period of time. The measurements may have primed the patients' responses, and the practice of reporting pain repeatedly on the same instrument during a procedure may have influenced the results.
Instrumentation	Marsh and associates' (2000) study estimated the reliability and validity of an assessment tool developed to improve the prediction of 6-month survival and hospice eligibility of individuals with late-stage Alzheimer's dementia, as well as identify clinical and demographic indicators that contribute to predicting survival and hospice appropriateness. The study was well-developed, but the realities of conducting clinical research lead to the following problems, "some data collectors reported having limited time to conduct adequate medical record reviews and this may have contributed to inaccuracies in recording critical incidents and data collection on weight and food intake was not precise . . ."
Mortality	Clarke and associates (2000) explored the predictive ability of psychological and social variables on functional status in patients with left ventricular dysfunction. At baseline, 4073 subjects completed questionnaires. At 1 year, 2992 subjects completed the follow-up measures; of those who did not, 394 died and 687 did not complete the questionnaires, leaving the mortality rate at 26.5%. The investigators noted the loss and the potential reasons for the loss. Even with the dropout rate, there was an adequate sample size.
Selection bias	Bull, Hansen, and Gross (2000, Appendix A) controlled for selection bias by establishing selection criteria and having an experimental and control site.

fect specific designs are addressed in Chapters 10 and 11. Threats to internal validity include history, maturation, testing, instrumentation, mortality, and selection bias. Table 9-2 provides examples of the threats to internal validity.

History

In addition to the independent variable, another specific event that may have an effect on the dependent variable may occur either inside or outside the experimental setting; this is referred to as **history.** For example, in a study of the effects of a breastfeeding teaching program on the length of time of breastfeeding, an event such as government-sponsored advertisements on the importance of breastfeeding featured on television and newspapers may be a threat of history.

Another example may be that of an investigator testing the effects of a breast self-examination teaching program on the incidence of monthly breast self-examination. Concurrently, a famous movie star or news correspondent is diagnosed as having breast cancer. The occurrence of this diagnosis in a public figure engenders a great deal of media and press attention. In the course of the media attention, medical experts are interviewed widely and the importance of breast self-examination is supported. If the researcher finds that breast self-examination behavior is improved, the researcher may not be able to conclude that the change in behavior is the result of the teaching program because it may be the result of the diagnosis given to the known figure and the resultant media coverage. An example of history from a published study can be found in the Bull, Hansen, and Gross (2000, Appendix A) study (see Table 9-2).

Maturation

Maturation refers to the developmental, biological, or psychological processes that operate within an individual as a function of time and are external to the events of the investigation. For example, suppose one wishes to evaluate the effect of a specific teaching method on baccalaureate students' achievements on a skills test. The investigator would record the students' abilities before and after the teaching method. Between the pretest and posttest, the students have grown older and wiser. The growth or change is unrelated to the investigation and may explain the differences between the two testing periods rather than the experimental treatment.

Maturation could also occur in a study focused on investigating the relationship between two methods of teaching about children's knowledge of self-care measures. Posttests of student learning must be conducted in a relatively short time period after the teaching sessions are completed. A relatively short interval allows the investigator to conclude that the results were the result of the design of the study and not maturation in a population of children who are learning new skills rapidly. It is important to remember that maturation is more than change due to an age-related developmental process but could be related to physical changes, as well (see Table 9-2).

Testing

The effect of taking a pretest on the subject's posttest score is known as testing. The effect of taking a pretest may sensitize an individual and improve the score of the posttest. Individuals generally score higher when they take a test a second time, regardless of the treatment. The differences between posttest and pretest scores may not be a result of the independent variable but rather of the experience gained through testing. Table 9-2 provides an example.

Instrumentation

Instrumentation threats are changes in the measurement of the variables or observational techniques that may account for changes in the obtained measurement. For example, a researcher may wish to study various types of thermometers (e.g., tympanic, digital, electronic, chemical indicator, plastic strip, and mercury) to compare the accuracy of the mercury to the other temperature-taking methods. To prevent instrumentation, a researcher must check the calibration of the thermometers according to the manufacturer's specifications before and after data collection.

Another example that fits into this area is related to techniques of observation or data collection. If a researcher has several raters collecting observational data, all must be trained in a similar manner. If they are not similarly trained, or even if they are similarly trained but unable to conduct the study as planned, a lack of consistency may occur in their ratings and therefore a threat to internal validity will occur. For an example, see Table 9-2. At times, even though the researcher takes steps to prevent problems of instrumentation, this threat may still occur. When a critiquer finds such a threat, it must be evaluated within the total context of the study, as, in fact, the researchers did in this study.

Mortality

Mortality is the loss of study subjects from the first data collection point (pretest) to the second data collection point (posttest). If the subjects who remain in the study are not similar to those who dropped out, the results could be affected. In a study of the ways a media campaign affects the incidence of breastfeeding, if most dropouts were nonbreastfeeding women, the perception given could be that exposure to the media campaign increased the number of breastfeeding women, whereas it was the effect of experimental mortality that led to the observed results. See Table 9-2 for an example of a study in which mortality may have influenced the results.

Selection Bias

If the precautions are not used to gain a representative sample, **selection bias** could result from the way the subjects were chosen. Selection effects are a problem in studies in which the individuals themselves decide whether to participate in a study. Suppose an investigator wishes to assess if a new stop-smoking program contributes to smoking cessation. If the new program is offered to all, chances are, only individuals who are more motivated to learn about how to stop smoking will take part in the program. Assessment of the effectiveness of the program is problematic, because the investigator cannot be sure if the new program encouraged smoking-cessation behaviors or if only highly motivated individuals joined the program. To avoid selection bias, the researcher could randomly assign subjects to either the new teaching method group or a control group that receives a different type of instruction. Table 9-2 provides another example of selection bias.

HELPFUL HINT The list of internal validity threats is not exhaustive. More than one threat can be found in a study, depending on the type of study design. Finding a threat to internal validity in a study does not invalidate the results and is usually acknowledged by the investigator in the "Results" or "Discussion" section of the study.

EXTERNAL VALIDITY

External validity deals with possible problems of generalizability of the investigation's findings to additional populations and to other environmental conditions. External validity questions under what conditions and with what types of subjects the same results can be expected to occur. The goal of the researcher is to select a design that maximizes both internal and external validity. This is not always possible; if this is the case, the

researcher must establish a minimum requirement of meeting the criteria of external validity.

The factors that may affect external validity are related to selection of subjects, study conditions, and type of observations. These factors are termed effects of selection, reactive effects, and effects of testing. The reader will notice the similarity in the names of the factors of selection and testing and those of the threats to internal validity. When considering factors as internal threats, the reader assesses them as they relate to the *independent* and *dependent* variables within the study, and when assessing them as external threats, the reader considers them in terms of the *generalizability* or use outside the study to other populations and settings. The Critical Thinking Decision Path for threats to validity displays the way threats to internal and external validity can interact with each other. It is important to remember that this path is not exhaustive of the type of threats and their interaction. Problems of internal validity are generally easier to control. Generalizability issues are more difficult to deal with because it means that the researcher is assuming that other populations are similar to the one being tested. External validity factors include effect of selection, reactivity effects, and effect of testing.

Selection Effects

Selection refers to the generalizability of the results to other populations. An example of the effects of selection occurs when the researcher can not attain the ideal sample population. At times, numbers of available subjects may be low or not accessible to the researcher; the researcher may then need to choose a nonprobability method of sampling over a probability method (see Chapter 12). Therefore the type of sampling method utilized and how subjects are assigned to research conditions affect the generalizability to other groups or the external validity.

Examples of selection effects are depicted when researchers note any of the following:
• "The sample in this study was too small to generate statistically significant conclusion" (Lee et al, 2000);

CRITICAL THINKING DECISION PATH Potential Threats to a Study's Validity

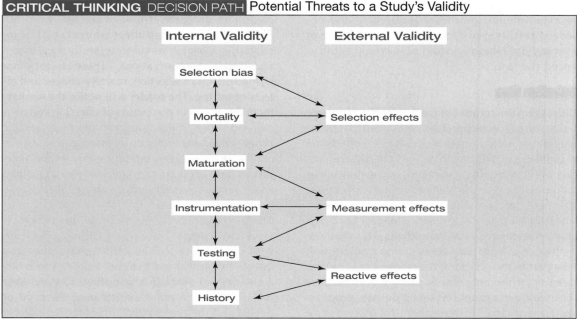

• "Findings from this study can be generalized only to patients receiving liver transplants" (Schmelzer et al, 2000);
• "The small sample size, limited to mothers, does not permit generalization" (LoBiondo-Wood et al, 2000; see Appendix D).

These remarks caution the reader but also point out the usefulness of the findings for practice and future research aimed at building the data in these areas.

Reactive Effects

Reactivity is defined as the subjects' responses to being studied. Subjects may respond to the investigator not because of the study procedures but merely as an independent response to being studied. This is also known as the Hawthorne effect, which is named after Western Electric Corporation's Hawthorne plant, where a study of working conditions was conducted. The researchers developed several different working conditions (i.e., turning up the lights, piping in music loudly or softly, and changing work

hours). They found that no matter what was done, the workers' productivity increased. They concluded that production increased as a result of the workers' knowing that they were being studied rather than because of the experimental conditions. For example, in a study that tested an educational intervention to reduce cardiovascular disease, the subjects may exercise and eat nutritiously during the study but soon afterwards returned to old habits.

Measurement Effects

Administration of a pretest in a study affects the generalizability of the findings to other populations and is known as **measurement effects.** Just as pretesting affects the posttest results within a study, pretesting affects the posttest results and generalizability outside the study. For example, suppose a researcher wants to conduct a study with the aim of changing attitudes toward AIDS. To accomplish this, an education program on the risk factors for AIDS is incorporated. To test whether the education program changes attitudes toward AIDS, tests are given before and after the teaching intervention. The pretest on attitudes allows the subjects to examine their attitudes regarding AIDS. The subjects' responses on follow-up testing may differ from those of individuals who were given the education program and did not see the pretest. Therefore when a study is conducted and a pretest is given, it may prime the subjects and affect their ability to generalize to other situations.

HELPFUL HINT When reviewing a study, be aware of the internal and external threats to validity. These threats do not make a study useless—but

actually more useful—to you. Recognition of the threats allows researchers to build on data and consumers to think through what part of the study can be applied to practice. Specific threats to validity depend on the type of design and generalizations the researcher hopes to make.

There are other threats to external validity that depend on the type of design and methods of sampling utilized by the researcher, but these are beyond the scope of this text. Campbell and Stanley (1966) offer detailed coverage of the issues related to internal and external validity.

CRITIQUING Quantitative Research

Critiquing the design of a study requires one to first have knowledge of the overall implications that the choice of a particular design may have for the study as a whole (Critiquing Criteria Box). The concept of the research design is an all-inclusive one that parallels the concept of the theoretical framework. The research design is similar to the theoretical framework in that it deals with a piece of the research study that affects the whole. For one to knowledgeably critique the design in the light of the entire study, it is important to understand the factors that influence the choice and the implications of the design. In this chapter, the meaning, purpose, and important factors of design choice, as well as the vocabulary that accompanies these factors, have been introduced.

Several criteria for evaluating the design can be drawn from this chapter. One should remember that the criteria are applied differently with various designs. Different application does not mean that the consumer will find a haphazard approach to design. It means that each design has particular criteria that allow the consumer to classify the design by type (e.g., experimental or nonexperimental). These criteria must be met and addressed in conducting an experiment. The particulars of specific designs are addressed in Chapters 10 and 11. The following discussion primarily pertains to the overall evaluation of a quantitative research design.

The research design should reflect that an objective review of the literature and the establishment of a theoretical framework guided the choice of the

---

CRITIQUING CRITERIA

1. Is the type of design employed appropriate?
2. Does the researcher use the various concepts of control that are consistent with the type of design chosen?
3. Does the design used seem to reflect the issues of economy?
4. Does the design used seem to flow from the proposed research problem, theoretical framework, literature review, and hypothesis?
5. What are the threats to internal validity?
6. What are the controls for the threats to internal validity?
7. What are the threats to external validity?
8. What are the controls for the threats to external validity?

design. There is no explicit statement regarding this in a research study. A consumer can evaluate this by critiquing the theoretical framework (see Chapter 5) and literature review (see Chapter 4). Is the problem new and not extensively researched? Has a great deal been done on the problem, or is it a new or different way of looking at an old problem? Depending on the level of the problem, the investigators make certain choices. For example, in their study assessing the pressure-reducing effects of five operating-table mattresses, Defloor and DeSchuijmer (2000) decided to have normal volunteers test the mattresses rather than patients undergoing surgery. This choice allowed the researchers to look for differences in a controlled, comparative manner.

The consumer should be alert for the means investigators use to maintain control (e.g., homogeneity in the sample, consistent data-collection procedures, how or if the independent variable was manipulated, and whether randomization was used). As you can see in Chapter 10, all of these criteria must be met for an experimental design. As you begin to understand the types of designs (i.e., namely, experimental, quasiexperimental, and nonexperimental designs such as survey and relationship designs), you will find that control is applied in varying degrees, or—as in the case of a survey study—the independent variable is not manipulated at all (see Chapter 11). The level of control and its applications presented in Chapters 10 and 11 provide the remaining knowledge to fully critique the aspects of a study's design.

Once it has been established whether the necessary control or uniformity of conditions has been maintained, the consumer must determine whether the study is believable or valid. The consumer should ask whether the findings are the result of the variables tested—and thus internally valid—or whether there could be another explanation. To assess this aspect, the threats to internal validity should be reviewed. If the investigator's study was systematic, well-grounded in theory, and followed the criteria for each of the processes, the consumer will probably conclude that the study is internally valid.

In addition, the consumer must know whether a study has external validity or generalizability to other populations or environmental conditions. External validity can be claimed only after internal validity has been established. If the credibility of a study (internal validity) has not been established, a study could not be generalized (external validity) to other populations. Determination of external validity goes hand in hand with the sampling frame (see Chapter 12). If the study is not representative of any one group or phenomena of interest, external validity may be limited or not present at all. The consumer will find that establishment of internal and external validity requires not only knowledge of the threats to internal and external validity but also knowledge of the phenomena being studied. Knowledge of the phenomena being studied allows critical judgments to be made about the linkage of theories and variables for testing. The consumer should find that the design follows from the theoretical framework, literature review, problem statement, and hypotheses. The consumer should feel, on the basis of clinical knowledge and knowledge of the research process, that the investigators are not comparing apples to oranges.

Critical Thinking Challenges

Barbara Krainovich-Miller

➤ Would you support or refute the following statement: "All research attempts to solve problems"?

➤ As a consumer of research, you recognize that control is an important concept in the issue of research design. You are critiquing an assigned experimental study as part of your "open book" midterm exam. From what is written, you cannot determine how the researchers kept the conditions of the study constant. How would you use the computer or other forms of technology to answer your question?

➤ Box 9-1 lists six major threats to the internal validity of an experimental study. Prioritize them and defend the one that you have made the essential or number one threat to address in a study.

➤ This is your first time as a consumer of research when you will be critiquing the research design of an assigned study. Discuss the process you will use. What must you do first?

Key Points

- The purpose of the design is to provide the format of a masterful and creative piece of research.
- There are many types of designs. No matter which type of design the researcher uses, the purpose always remains the same.
- The research consumer should be able to locate within the study a sense of the question that the researcher wished to answer. The question should be proposed with a plan or scheme for the accomplishment of the investigation. Depending on the question, the consumer should be able to recognize the steps taken by the investigator to ensure control.
- The choice of the specific design depends on the nature of the problem. To specify the nature of the problem requires that the design reflects the investigator's attempts to maintain objectivity, accuracy, pragmatic considerations, and, most important, control.
- Control affects not only the outcome of a study but also its future use. The design should also reflect how the investigator attempted to control threats to both internal and external validity.
- Internal validity must be established before external validity can be. Both are considered within the sampling structure.
- No matter which design the researcher chooses, it should be evident to the reader that the choice was based on a thorough examination of the problem within a theoretical framework.
- The design, problem statement, literature review, theoretical framework, and hypothesis should all interrelate to demonstrate a woven pattern.
- The choice of the design is affected by pragmatic issues. At times, two different designs may be equally valid for the same problem.

REFERENCES

Berger AM and Higginbotham P: Correlates of fatigue during and following adjuvant breast cancer chemotheraphy: a pilot study, *Oncol Nurs Forum* 27:1443-1448, 2000.

Bull MJ, Hansen HE, and Gross CR: A professional-patient partnership model of discharge planning with elders hospitalized with heart failure, *Appl Nurs Res* 13:19-28, 2000.

Campbell D and Stanley J: *Experimental and quasi-experimental designs for research,* Chicago, 1966, Rand-McNally.

Clarke SP et al: Psychocial factors as predictors of functional status at 1 year in patients with left ventricular dysfunction, *Res Nurs Health* 23:290-300, 2000.

Defloor T and DeSchuijmer DS: Preventing pressure ulcers: an evaluation of four operating-table mattresses, *Appl Nurs Res* 13:134-141, 2000.

Lee H et al: Fatigue, mood and hemodynamic patterns after myocardial infarction, *Appl Nurs Res* 13:60-69, 2000.

Lenz ER and Perkins S: Coronary artery bypass graft surgery patients and their family member caregivers: outcomes of a family-focused staged psychoeducational intervention, *Appl Nurs Res* 13:142-150, 2000.

Marsh GW et al: Predicting hospice appropriateness for patients with dementia of the Alzheimer's type, *Appl Nurs Res* 13:187-196, 2000.

Rubin R: Attainment of the maternal role: 1. Processes, *Nurs Res* 16:237-245, 1967a.

Rubin R: Attainment of the maternal role: 2. Models and referents, *Nurs Res* 16:342-346, 1967b.

Schmelzer M, Chappell SM, and Wright KB: Colonic cleansing, fluid absorption, and discomfort following tap water and soapsuds enemas, *Appl Nurs Res* 13:83-91, 2000.

Wikblad K and Anderson B: Comparison of three wound dressings in patients undergoing heart surgery, *Nurs Res* 44:312-316, 1995.

ADDITIONAL READINGS

Cook TD and Campbell DT: Quasi-experimentation: design analysis issues for field settings, Boston, 1979, Houghton-Mifflin.

Creswell JW: *Research design: qualitative and quantitative approaches,* Thousand Oaks, 1994, Sage Publications.

Knapp TS: *Quantitative nursing research,* Thousand Oaks, 1998, Sage Publications.

Lipsey MW: Design sensitivity: statistical power for experimental research, Newbury Park, 1990, Sage Publications.

Myers JL and Well AD: Research design and statistical analysis, Mahwah, NJ, 1995, Lawrence Erlbaum Associates, Inc.

SUSAN SULLIVAN-BOLYAI
MARGARET GREY

10

Experimental and Quasiexperimental Designs

Key Terms

a priori
after-only design
after-only nonequivalent
  control group design
antecedent variable
control
dependent variable
design
evaluation research

experiment
experimental design
independent variable
intervening variable
manipulation
mortality
nonequivalent control group
  design

quasiexperiment
quasiexperimental design
randomization
Solomon four-group design
testing
time series design
true experiment

Learning Outcomes

After reading this chapter, the student should be able to do the following:

- List the criteria necessary for inferring cause-and-effect relationships.
- Distinguish the differences between experimental and quasiexperimental designs.
- Define internal validity problems associated with experimental and quasiexperimental designs.
- Describe the use of experimental and quasiexperimental designs for evaluation research.
- Critically evaluate the findings of selected studies that test cause-and-effect relationships.

RESEARCH PROCESS

One of the fundamental purposes of scientific research in any profession is to determine cause-and-effect relationships. In nursing, for example, we are concerned with developing effective approaches to maintaining and restoring wellness. Testing such nursing interventions to determine how well they actually work—that is, evaluating the outcomes in terms of efficacy and cost-effectiveness—is accomplished by using experimental and quasiexperimental **designs.** These designs differ from nonexperimental designs in one important way: the researcher actively seeks to bring about the desired effect and does not passively observe behaviors or actions. In other words, the researcher is interested in making something happen, not merely observing customary patient care. Experimental and quasiexperimental studies are also important to consider in relation to evidence-based practice. It is the findings of such studies that provide the validation of clinical practice and rationale for changing specific aspects of practice (see Chapter 20).

Experimental designs are particularly suitable for testing cause-and-effect relationships because they help eliminate potential alternative explanations (threats to validity) for the findings. To infer causality requires that the following three criteria be met:

- The causal variable and effect variable must be associated with each other.
- The cause must precede the effect.
- The relationship must not be explainable by another variable.

When you critique studies that use experimental and quasiexperimental designs, the primary focus is on the validity of the conclusion that the experimental treatment, or the **independent variable,** caused the desired effect on the outcome, or **dependent variable.** The validity of the conclusion depends on just how well the researcher has controlled the other variables that may explain the relationship studied. Thus the focus of this chapter is to explain how the var-

BOX 10-1 Summary of Experimental and Quasiexperimental Research Designs

EXPERIMENTAL DESIGNS
True experiment (pretest-posttest control group) design
Solomon four-group design
After-only design

QUASIEXPERIMENTAL DESIGNS
Nonequivalent control group design
After-only nonequivalent control group design
Time series design

ious types of experimental and quasiexperimental designs control extraneous variables.

It should be made clear, however, that most research in nursing is not experimental. This is because nursing, unlike the physical sciences, is still identifying the content and theory that are the exclusive province of nursing science. In addition, an experimental design requires that all of the relevant variables have been defined so that they can be manipulated and studied. In most problem areas in nursing, this requirement has not been met. Therefore nonexperimental designs used in identifying variables and determining their relationship to each other often need to be done before experimental studies are performed.

The purpose of this chapter is to acquaint you with the issues involved in interpreting studies that use **experimental design** and **quasiexperimental design.** These designs are listed in Box 10-1. The Critical Thinking Decision Path shows an algorithm that influences a researcher's choice of experimental or quasiexperimental design.

TRUE EXPERIMENTAL DESIGN

An **experiment** is a scientific investigation that makes observations and collects data according to explicit criteria. A **true experiment** has three identifying properties—randomization, control, and manipulation. These properties allow for other explanations of the phenomenon to be

CRITICAL THINKING DECISION PATH Experimental and Quasiexperimental Design

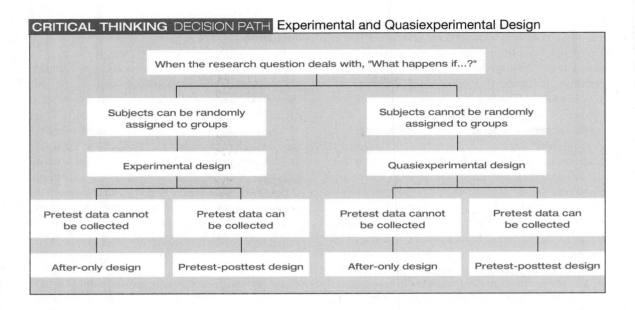

ruled out and thereby provide the strength of the design for testing cause-and-effect relationships.

RANDOMIZATION

Randomization, or random assignment to group, involves the distribution of subjects to either the experimental or control group on a purely random basis. That is, each subject has an equal and known probability of being assigned to any group. Random assignment may be done individually or by groups (Conlon and Anderson, 1990; Rudy et al, 1993). Random assignment to experimental or control groups allows for the elimination of any systematic bias in the groups with respect to attributes that may affect the dependent variable being studied. The procedure for randomization assumes that any important intervening variables will be equally distributed between the groups and, as discussed in Chapter 9, minimizes variance. Note that random assignment to groups is different from random sampling discussed in Chapter 12.

CONTROL

Control means the introduction of one or more constants into the experimental situation. Con-

trol is acquired by manipulating the causal or independent variable, by randomly assigning subjects to a group, by very carefully preparing experimental protocols, and by using comparison groups. In experimental research, the comparison group is the control group, or the group that receives the usual treatment, rather than the innovative experimental one.

MANIPULATION

As discussed previously, experimental designs are characterized by the researcher "doing something" to at least some of the involved subjects. This "something," or the independent variable, is manipulated by giving it (the experimental treatment) to some participants in the study and not to others or by giving different amounts of it to different groups. The independent variable might be a treatment, a teaching plan, or a medication. It is the effect of this **manipulation** that is measured to determine the result of the experimental treatment.

The concepts of control, randomization, and manipulation and their application to experimental design are sometimes confusing for students. To see the way these properties allow researchers to have confidence in the causal inferences they make by allowing them to rule out other potential explanations, the use of these properties is examined in one report. Grey and associates (1999) used a clinical randomized experiment to study if a behavioral intervention (Coping Skills Training [CST]) could improve the quality of life for adolescents with type 1 diabetes. Teenagers 13 to 20 years old who were beginning intensive insulin therapy were randomly assigned (once parent and child consent were obtained) to one of two groups: CST with intensive management or intensive management alone. The use of random assignment means that all the patients who met the study criteria had an equal and known chance of being assigned to the control or the experimental group. The use of random assignment to groups helps ensure that the two study groups are comparable on preexisting factors that might affect the outcome of interest, such as gender, age, length of stay in the intensive care unit, and severity of illness. Note that the researchers checked statistically whether the procedure of random assignment did in fact produce groups that were similar.

Both groups received intensive management that consisted of either multiple daily injections (3 or more daily) or being placed on an external insulin pump, frequent glucose monitoring (at least 4 times daily), monthly outpatient visits, and interim telephone calls to the diabetes team. The control group received intensive management alone. The intervention group received intensive management and CST, which consisted of a series of small group sessions designed to teach problem solving skills, decision making, and communication. CST was designed to assist adolescents to deal better with potential stresses of daily life encountered when following the prescribed intensive therapy. The degree of control exerted over the experimental conditions is illustrated by the detailed description in the report of the CST intervention. This *control* helps ensure that all members of the experimental group receive similar treatment and assists the reader in understanding the nature of the experimental treatment. The control group provides a comparison against which the experimental group can be judged.

In this study, receiving CST was the manipulated treatment. Patient outcomes of diabetes, general and medical self-efficacy, coping, depression, and quality of life were measured for all the participants.

The use of the experimental design allowed the researchers to rule out many of the potential threats to internal validity of the findings, such as selection, history, and maturation (see Chapter 9).By clearly and carefully controlling the experimental CST intervention by the use of standard protocols and recordings, the investigators were able to make the assertion that the CST intervention was effective in improving metabolic control and quality of life.

The strength of the true experimental design lies in its ability to help the researcher control the effects of any extraneous variables that might constitute threats to internal validity. Such extraneous variables can be either antecedent or intervening. The **antecedent variable** occurs before the study but may affect the dependent variable and confuse the results. Factors such as age, gender, socioeconomic status, and health status might be important antecedent variables in nursing research because they may affect dependent variables such as recovery time and ability to integrate health care behaviors. Antecedent variables that might affect the dependent variables in the study by Grey and associates (1999) include gender, ethnicity, age, duration of illness, and treatment regimen. Random assignment to groups helps ensure that groups will be similar on these variables so that differences in the dependent variable may be attributed to the experimental treatment. It should be noted, however, that the researcher should check and report how the groups actually compared on such variables. Grey and associates (1999) clearly stated in their article that these variables at study entry were similar between both the experimental and control groups. An **intervening variable** occurs during the course of the study and is not part of the study, but it affects the dependent variable and could affect the study outcomes. An

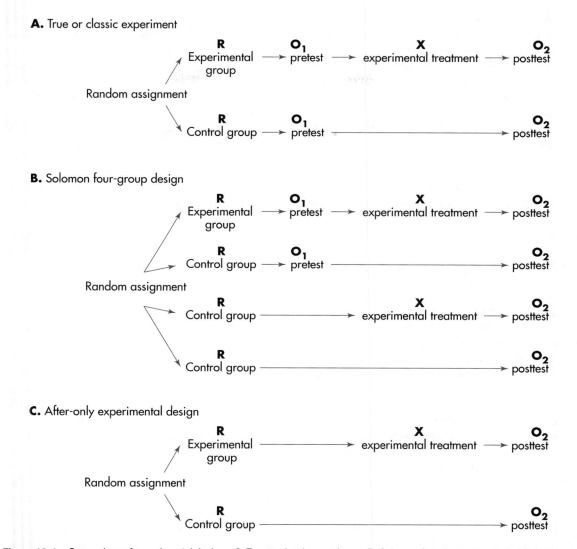

A. True or classic experiment

B. Solomon four-group design

C. After-only experimental design

Figure 10-1 Comparison of experimental designs. **A,** True or classic experiment. **B,** Solomon four-group design. **C,** After-only experimental design.

example of an intervening variable that might affect the outcomes of this study (Grey et al, 1999) is a change in health care status in any of the participants such as a newly diagnosed medical condition or mental illness. Certainly, if care provided to patients changed in any major way while the study was being implemented, the study also would be affected.

TYPES OF EXPERIMENTAL DESIGNS

There are several different experimental designs (Campbell and Stanley, 1966). Each is based on the classic design called the true experiment diagrammed in Figure 10-1, *A.* Above the description diagram, symbolic notations are routinely used. **R** represents random assignment (for both the experimental and control group). **O** signifies observation via data collection on the dependent variable. O_1 signifies pretest data collection whereas O_2 represents posttest data collection. **X** represents the group exposure to the intervention. Therefore, in this figure, you will note that subjects were assigned randomly **(R)** to the experimental or the control group. The experimental treatment **(X)** was given only to those in the experimental group, and the pretests **(O_1)** and posttests **(O_2)** are those measurements of the dependent variables that were made before and after the experimental treatment is performed. All true experimental designs have subjects randomly assigned to groups, have an experimental treatment introduced to some of the subjects, and have the effects of the treatment observed. Designs vary primarily in the number of observations that are made.

As shown in Figure 10-1, *A,* subjects are randomly assigned to the two groups, experimental and control, so that antecedent variables are controlled. Then pretest measures or observations are made so that the researcher has a baseline for determining the effect of the independent variable. The researcher then introduces the experimental variable to one of the groups and measures the dependent variable again to see whether it has changed. The control group gets no experimental treatment but also is measured later for comparison with the experimental group. The degree of difference between the two groups at the end of the study indicates the confidence the researcher has that a causal link exists between the independent and dependent variables. Because random assignment and the control inherent in this design minimize the effects of many threats to internal validity, it is a strong design for testing cause-and-effect relationships. However, the design is not perfect. Some threats cannot be controlled in true experimental studies (see Chapter 9). People tend to drop out of studies that require their participation over an extended period. The influence over the outcome of an experiment of people dropping out or dying is commonly known as **mortality** effects. If there is a difference in the number or type of people who drop out of

the experimental group from that of the control group, a mortality effect might explain the findings. When reading such a work, it is important to examine the sample and the results carefully to see if drop outs or deaths occurred. **Testing** also can be a problem in these studies, because the researcher is usually giving the same measurement twice, and subjects tend to score better the second time just by learning the test. Researchers can get around this problem in one of two ways: they might use different forms of the same test for the two measurements, or they might use a more complex experimental design called the Solomon four-group design.

The **Solomon four-group design,** shown in Figure 10-1, *B,* has two groups that are identical to those used in the classic experimental design, plus two additional groups, an experimental after-group and a control after-group. As the diagram shows, all four groups have randomly assigned **(R)** subjects as in all experimental studies. However, the addition of these last two groups helps rule out testing threats to internal validity that the before and after groups may experience. Suppose a researcher is interested in the effects of some counseling on chronically ill patients' self-esteem, but just taking a measure of self-esteem **(O_1)** may influence how the subjects report themselves. For example, the items might make the subjects think more about how they view themselves so that the next time they fill out the questionnaire **(O_2),** their self-esteem might appear to have improved. In reality, however, their self-esteem may be the same as it was before; it just looks different because they took the test before. The use of this design with the two groups that do not receive the pretest allows for evaluating the effect of the pretest on the posttest in the first two groups. Although this design helps evaluate the effects of testing, the threat of mortality remains a problem as with the classic experimental design.

A less frequently used experimental design is the **after-only design,** shown in Figure 10-1, *C.* This design, which is sometimes called the posttest-only control group design, is composed of two randomly assigned groups **(R),** but unlike the true experimental design, neither group is pretested or measured. Again, the independent variable is introduced to the experimental group **(X)** and not to the control group. The process of randomly assigning the subjects to groups is assumed to be sufficient to ensure a lack of bias so that the researcher can still determine whether the treatment **(X)** created significant differences between the two groups **(O)**. This design is particularly useful when testing effects are expected to be a major problem and the number of available subjects is too limited to use a Solomon four-group design. O'Sullivan and Jacobson (1992) used this design in their study of the impact of a program for adolescent mothers because it was impossible to measure infant outcomes before the birth of the infant. They carefully examined the two groups to ensure that the groups were equivalent at baseline, so that they could be assured that random assignment had yielded equivalent groups. Other interventions, such as postoperative pain management, cannot be measured before surgery and require an after-only design.

FIELD AND LABORATORY EXPERIMENTS

Experiments also can be classified by setting. Field experiments and laboratory experiments share the properties of control, randomization, and manipulation, and they use the same design characteristics, but they are conducted in different environments. Laboratory experiments take place in an artificial setting created specifically for the purpose of research. In the laboratory, the researcher has almost total control over the features of the environment, such as temperature, humidity, noise level, and subject conditions. On the other hand, field experiments are exactly what the name implies—experiments that take place in some real, pre-existing social setting such as a hospital or clinic where the phenomenon of interest usually occurs. Because most experiments in the nursing literature are field experiments and control is such an important element in the conduct of experiments, it should be obvious that studies conducted in the field are subject to treat-ment contamination by factors specific to the setting that the researcher cannot control. However, studies conducted in the laboratory are by nature "artificial," because the setting is created for the purpose of research. Thus laboratory experiments, although stronger with respect to internal validity questions than field work studies, suffer more from problems with external validity. For example, a subject's behavior in the laboratory may be quite different from the person's behavior in the real world—a dichotomy that presents problems in generalizing findings from the laboratory to the real world. When research reports are read, then, it is important to consider the setting of the experiment and what impact it might have on the findings of the study.

Consider the study comparing two different wound dressings for the management of pressure sores (Dealey, 1998). This study could have been done in a laboratory using animals, which would have allowed complete control over the external environment of the study, a variable that might be important in studying wound healing. However, there is no guarantee that the results found in a study in a laboratory would be applicable to patients in hospital settings, so the study would lose some external validity.

ADVANTAGES AND DISADVANTAGES OF THE EXPERIMENTAL DESIGN

As previously discussed, experimental designs are the most appropriate for testing cause-and-effect relationships. This is because of the design's ability to control the experimental situation. Therefore it offers better corroboration than if the independent variable is manipulated in such a way that certain consequences can be expected to ensue. Such studies are important because one of nursing's major research priorities is documenting outcomes to provide a basis for changing or supporting current nursing practice (see Chapter 1). In the study by Grey and associates (1999), the authors were able to conclude from their findings that CST is useful in helping adolescents with type 1 diabetes achieve intensive management and quality of life goals. Their study helps support using CST intervention with other age groups and other chronic conditions. Similarly, in a study by Naylor and associates (1999), the authors were able to conclude that by implementing a transitional discharge planning and home care intervention for high-risk elders, fewer readmissions, lengthened time between discharge and readmission, and reduced health care costs occurred. These studies and others like them allow nurses to anticipate in a scientific manner the outcomes of their actions and provide the basis for effective, high-quality care strategies.

Still, experimental designs are not the ones most commonly used in nursing research for several reasons. First, experimentation assumes that all of the relevant variables involved in a phenomenon have been identified. For many areas of nursing research, this simply is not the case, and descriptive studies need to be completed before experimental interventions can be applied. Second, these designs have some significant disadvantages.

One problem with an experimental design is that many variables important in predicting outcomes of nursing care are not amenable to experimental manipulation. It is well known that health status varies with age and socioeconomic status. No matter how careful a researcher is, no one can assign subjects randomly by age or a certain level of income. In addition, some variables may be technically manipulable, but their nature may preclude actually doing so. For example, the ethics of a researcher who tried to randomly assign groups for the study of the effects of cigarette smoking and asked the experimental group to smoke two packs of cigarettes a day would be seriously questioned. It is also potentially true that such a study would not work because nonsmokers randomly assigned to the smoking group would be unlikely to comply with the research task. Thus, sometimes, even when a researcher plans to conduct a true experiment, subjects dropping out of the study or other factors may, in effect, make the study a quasiexperiment. For instance, in the study by Bull,

Hansen, and Gross (2000) (see Appendix A) that provided a transitional discharge planning program for elderly patients hospitalized with heart failure, subjects were recruited from two hospitals matched by similar size, type, and discharge planning practices used for cardiac patients. Using two hospitals may sometimes be necessary to ensure a large enough sample. The goal of the intervention was to promote safer, more cost-effective transitions to home for both the elderly patients and their caregivers. The subjects were not randomly assigned, although there were control groups; thus the study is considered a quasiexperimental study.

Another problem with experimental designs is that they may be difficult or impractical to perform in field settings. It may be quite difficult to randomly assign patients on a hospital floor to different groups when they might talk to each other about the different treatments. Experimental procedures also may be disruptive to the usual routine of the setting. If several nurses are involved in administering the experimental program, it may be impossible to ensure that the program is administered in the same way to each subject.

Finally, just the act of being studied may influence the results of a study. This is called the Hawthorne effect. As discussed in Chapter 9, this effect means that merely because subjects know that they are subjects in a study, they may answer questions or perform differently.

HELPFUL HINT Remember that the Hawthorne effect is nearly always a problem in research situations, simply because of the attention being paid to the subjects. The difficulty is in determining when the findings of the study may be applicable to real clinical situations.

Because of these problems in carrying out true experiments, researchers frequently turn to another type of research design to evaluate cause-and-effect relationships. Such designs, because they look like experiments but lack some of the control of the true experimental design, are called quasiexperiments.

QUASIEXPERIMENTAL DESIGNS

In a quasiexperimental design, full experimental control is not possible. **Quasiexperiments** are research designs in which the researcher initiates an experimental treatment but some characteristic of a true experiment is lacking. Control may not be possible because of the nature of the independent variable or the nature of the available subjects. Usually what is lacking in a quasiexperimental design is the element of randomization as described earlier with the Bull, Hansen, and Gross (2000) study. In other cases the control group may be missing. However, like experiments, quasiexperiments involve the introduction of an experimental treatment.

Compared with the true experimental design, quasiexperiments are similar in their utilization. Both types of designs are used when the researcher is interested in testing cause-and-effect relationships. However, the basic problem with the quasiexperimental approach is a weakened confidence in making causal assertions. Because of the lack of some controls in the research situation, quasiexperimental designs are subject to contamination by many, if not all, of the threats to internal validity discussed in Chapter 9.

HELPFUL HINT Remember that researchers often make trade-offs and sometimes use a quasiexperimental design instead of an experimental design because it may be pragmatically impossible to randomly assign subjects to groups. Not using the "purest" design does not decrease the value of the study even though it may decrease the utility of the findings.

TYPES OF QUASIEXPERIMENTAL DESIGNS

There are many different quasiexperimental designs. Only the ones most commonly used in nursing research are discussed in this book. Again, the symbols and notations introduced earlier in the chapter are used. Refer back to the true experimental design shown in Figure 10-1, *A,* and compare it with the **nonequivalent control group design** shown in Figure 10-2, *A.* Note that this design looks exactly like the true experiment except that subjects are not randomly assigned to groups. Suppose a researcher is interested in the effects of a new diabetes education program on the physical and psychosocial outcomes of patients newly diagnosed with diabetes. If conditions were right, the researcher might be able to randomly assign subjects to either the group receiving the new program or the group receiving the usual program, but for any number of reasons, that design might not be possible. For example, nurses on the unit where patients are admitted might be so excited about the new program that they cannot help but include the new information for all patients. So the researcher has two choices—to abandon the experiment or to conduct a quasiexperiment. To conduct a quasiexperiment the researcher might find a similar unit that has not been introduced to the new program and study the newly diagnosed patients with diabetes who are admitted to that unit as a comparison group. The study would then involve this type of design.

Bull, Hansen, and Gross (2000) (see Appendix A) used the nonequivalent control group design to study the effectiveness of a transitional discharge planning program for promoting safer and more cost-effective discharges for elderly patients hospitalized with heart failure and their caregivers. There were two hospitals from which patients were recruited. Hospital I had two control groups without any interventions and Hospital II had one intervention group and one control group. The researchers collected a variety of data (see Appendix A) from the patients and their caregivers before and after the intervention was introduced. They demonstrated that the intervention program led to the patients and caregivers feeling more prepared to manage home care and perceiving they had received more information about home care services. Further, when the patients were readmitted to the hospital they spent less time in the hospital than the control groups. The caregivers receiving the intervention also had more positive feelings about the care management at 2 weeks and 2 months post-discharge. In

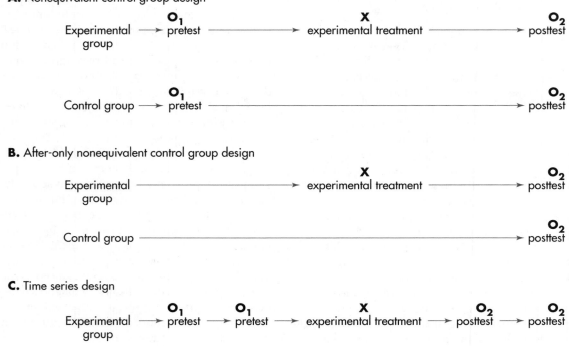

A. Nonequivalent control group design

$$O_1 \qquad\qquad X \qquad\qquad O_2$$

Experimental ⟶ pretest ⟶ experimental treatment ⟶ posttest
group

$$O_1 \qquad\qquad\qquad O_2$$

Control group ⟶ pretest ⟶ posttest

B. After-only nonequivalent control group design

$$X \qquad O_2$$

Experimental ⟶ experimental treatment ⟶ posttest
group

$$O_2$$

Control group ⟶ posttest

C. Time series design

$$O_1 \qquad O_1 \qquad X \qquad O_2 \qquad O_2$$

Experimental ⟶ pretest ⟶ pretest ⟶ experimental treatment ⟶ posttest ⟶ posttest
group

Figure 10-2   Comparison of quasiexperimental designs. **A,** Nonequivalent control group design. **B,** After-only nonequivalent control group design. **C,** Time series design.

discussing their findings, the authors noted that there were differences among the control caregiver groups between the two hospitals. These differences required separate comparisons of the control caregiver groups with the intervention group, thus weakening the findings.

The nonequivalent control group design is commonly used in nursing research studies conducted in field settings. The basic problem with the design is the weakened confidence the researcher can have in assuming that the experimental and comparison groups are similar at the beginning of the study. Threats to internal validity, such as selection, maturation, testing, and mortality, are possible with this design. However, the design is relatively strong because the gathering of the data at the time of pretest allows the researcher to compare the equivalence of the two groups on important antecedent variables

before the independent variable is introduced. In the previous example, the motivation of the patients to learn about their medical condition might be important in determining the effect of the discharge teaching program. The researcher could include in the measures taken at the outset of the study some measure of motivation to learn. Then differences between the two groups on this variable could be tested, and if significant differences existed, they could be controlled statistically in the analysis. Nonetheless the strength of the causal assertions that can be made on the basis of such designs depends on the ability of the researcher to identify and measure or control possible threats to internal validity.

Now suppose that the researcher did not think to measure the subjects before the introduction of the new treatment (or she or he was hired after the new program began) but later decided that it would be useful to have data demonstrating the effect of the program. Perhaps, for example, a third party asks for such data to determine whether they should pay the extra cost of the new teaching program. Sometimes, the outcomes simply cannot be measured before the intervention, as with prenatal interventions that are expected to impact birth outcomes. The study that could be conducted would look like the **after-only nonequivalent control group design,** shown in Figure 10-2, *B*.

This design is similar to the after-only experimental design, but randomization is not used to assign subjects to groups. This design makes the assumption that the two groups are equivalent and comparable before the introduction of the independent variable **(X).** Thus the soundness of the design and the confidence that we can put in the findings depend on the soundness of this assumption of preintervention comparability. Often it is difficult to support the assertion that the two nonrandomly assigned groups are comparable at the outset of the study because there is no way of assessing its validity.

In the example of the teaching program for patients with newly diagnosed diabetes, measuring the subjects' motivation after the teaching program would not tell us whether their motivations differed before they received the program, and it is possible that the teaching program would motivate individuals to learn more about their health problem. Therefore the researcher's conclusion that the teaching program improved physical status and psychosocial outcome would be subject to the alternative conclusion that the results were an effect of preexisting motivations (selection effect) in combination with greater learning in those so motivated (selection-maturation interaction). Nonetheless this design is frequently used in nursing research because opportunities for data collection are often limited and because it is particularly useful when testing effects may be problematic. Consider again the example of the experiment conducted by Grey and associates (1999). Suppose that they had not randomly assigned the patients to the CST, but rather took all

patients before a certain point and assigned them to the control group and then assigned all new patients to the experimental treatment. The study would then be an example of an after-only nonequivalent control group design. If the authors had chosen to conduct the study with this design and had found the same results, they would have been less confident of the results because selection and effects may have been more problematic.

A study by Maxey (1997) used an after-only quasiexperimental design to test the time effectiveness of using a case map (clinical pathway) for emergency administration of thrombolytic therapy for patients with acute myocardial infarctions (AMI). Because of the standardized clinical protocol used for patients admitted to the emergency department (ED) with an AMI, randomization was not appropriate, so a quasiexperimental approach was used instead. Further, data could not be collected regarding the amount of time it took to administer the drug regimen until after the patient entered the ED, so an after-only design was used. The researcher was still able to demonstrate the case map's effectiveness in improving patient outcomes in the ED.

One approach used by researchers when only one group is available is to study that group over a longer period. This quasiexperimental design is called a **time series design,** and it is illustrated in Figure 10-2, *C*. Time series designs are useful for determining trends. Goldberg and associates (2000) studied the effects of a computer-generated preventive reminder for a large group of patients in need of mammograms, colorectal cancer screening, and cholesterol testing using a nonrandomized controlled trial. Although mammography performance increased for the experimental group, cholesterol offering decreased for both groups over time. This trend was attributed to the change in national guidelines to retreat from recommending cholesterol screening for healthy young adults.

To rule out some alternative explanations for the findings of a one-group pretest-posttest design, researchers can measure the phenomenon of interest over a longer period and introduce the experimental treatment sometime during the course of the data collection period. Even with the absence of a control group, the broader range of data-collection points helps rule out such threats to validity as history effects. Obviously our problem related to the earlier example of teaching patients with diabetes does not lend itself to this design because we do not have access to the patients before the diagnosis.

An example of how a time series design can strengthen causal conclusions is provided again by Goldberg and associates (2000). The time series design allowed the researchers to look at the effects of the reminder system over time and also to look at the changing national preventive health recommendations. During the time series study, the recommendations for cholesterol screening had changed significantly. Thus differences were seen in the ordering of these tests. Also, if a control group had not been used, the decrease in cholesterol screening may have been attributed to the reminder system. The use of a time series design without a control group would have weakened the alternative explanation that the changes occurred because of something else that happened during the study period. However, the testing threat to validity looms large in these designs because measures are repeated so many times (see Chapters 9 and 11).

HELPFUL HINT One of the reasons replication is so important in nursing research is that so many problems cannot be subjected to experimental methods. Therefore the consistency of findings across many populations helps support a cause-and-effect relationship even when an experiment cannot be conducted.

ADVANTAGES AND DISADVANTAGES OF QUASIEXPERIMENTAL DESIGNS

Given the problems inherent in interpreting the results of studies using quasiexperimental designs, you may be wondering why anyone would use them. Quasiexperimental designs are used frequently because they are practical, feasible, and generalizable. These designs are more adaptable to the real-world practice setting than the controlled experimental designs. In addition, for some hypotheses, these designs may be the only way to evaluate the effect of the independent variable of interest.

The weaknesses of the quasiexperimental approach involve mainly the inability to make clear cause-and-effect statements. However, if the researcher can rule out any plausible alternative explanations for the findings, such studies can lead to increased knowledge about causal relationships. Researchers have several options for ruling out these alternative explanations. They may control extraneous variables (alternative events that could explain the findings) **a priori** (before initiating the intervention) by design. For example, Bull, Hansen, and Gross (2000) could have requested written assurance from the hospital administration that no new programs would be started during the course of their study that could affect the intervention findings. Such assurance would have made the introduction of the critical pathway that the control group received less likely. There are also methods to control extraneous variables statistically. In some cases, common sense knowledge of the problem and the population can suggest that a particular explanation is not plausible. Nonetheless it is important to replicate such studies to support the causal assertions developed through the use of quasiexperimental designs.

The literature on cigarette smoking is an excellent example of how findings from many studies, experimental and quasiexperimental, can be linked to establish a causal relationship. A large number of well-controlled experiments with laboratory animals randomly assigned to smoking and nonsmoking conditions have documented that lung disease will develop in smoking animals. Although such evidence is suggestive of a link between smoking and lung disease in humans, it is not directly transferable because animals and humans are different. But we cannot randomly assign humans to smoking and nonsmoking groups for ethical and other reasons. So researchers interested in this problem have to use quasiexperimental data to test their hypotheses about smoking and lung disease. Several different quasiexperimental designs have been used to study this problem, and all had similar results—a causal relationship does exist between cigarette smoking and lung disease. Note that the combination of results from both experimental and quasiexperimental studies led to the conclusion that smoking causes cancer because the studies together meet the causal criteria of relationship, timing, and lack of an alternative explanation. Nonetheless, the tobacco industry has taken the stand that because the studies on humans are not true experiments, there may be another explanation for the relationships that have been found. For example, they suggest that the tendency to smoke is linked to the tendency for lung disease to develop and smoking is merely an unimportant intervening variable. The reader needs to study the evidence from studies to determine whether the cause-and-effect relationship postulated is believable.

EVALUATION RESEARCH AND EXPERIMENTATION

As the science of nursing expands and the cost of health care rises, nurses and others have become increasingly concerned with the ability to document the costs and the benefits of nursing care (see Chapter 1). This is a complex process, but at its heart is the ability to evaluate or measure the outcomes of nursing care. Such studies usually are associated with quality assurance, quality improvement, and evaluation. Studies of evaluation or quality assurance do exactly what the name implies—such studies are concerned with the determination of the quality of nursing and health care and with assurance that the public is receiving high-quality care.

Quality assurance and quality improvement in nursing are a present and important topic for nursing care. Experimentation techniques are just beginning to be applied to the study of the delivery of nursing care. Many early quality as-

surance studies documented whether nursing care met predetermined standards. The goal of quality improvement studies is to evaluate the effectiveness of nursing interventions and to provide direction for further improvement in the achievement of quality clinical outcomes and cost effectiveness.

Evaluation research is the utilization of scientific research methods and procedures to evaluate a program, treatment, practice, or policy; it uses analytical means to document the worth of an activity. Such research is not a different design. Evaluation research uses both experimental and quasiexperimental designs (as well as nonexperimental designs) for the purpose of determining the effect or outcomes of a program. Bigman (1961) listed the following purposes and uses of evaluation research:

1. To discover whether and how well the objectives are being fulfilled
2. To determine the reasons for specific successes and failures
3. To direct the course of experiment with techniques for increasing effectiveness
4. To uncover principles underlying a successful program
5. To base further research on the reasons for the relative success of alternative techniques
6. To redefine the means to be used for attaining objectives and to redefine subgoals, in light of research findings

Evaluation studies may be either formative or summative. Formative evaluation refers to assessment of a program as it is being implemented; usually the focus is on evaluation of the process of a program rather than the outcomes. Summative evaluation refers to the assessment of the outcomes of a program that is conducted after completion of the program. One example of a study using both formative and summative evaluation with experimental design is a study by McCain and associates (1996). The authors studied the effects of a 6-week stress-management training program with standard outpatient care for 45 men with the human immunodeficiency virus (HIV) disease. In addition to the summative evaluation, they described the evaluation of the stress-management program as it developed. Data were collected before the interventions and at 6 weeks and 6 months after the intervention. The study by Rudy and associates (1995) that evaluated the effectiveness of the nurse special care unit is another example of the experimental design applied to summative evaluation.

The use of experimental and quasiexperimental designs in quality improvement and evaluation studies allows for the determination of not only whether care is adequate but also which method of care is best under certain conditions. Furthermore, such studies can be used to determine whether a particular type of nursing care is cost effective, that is, that the care not only does what it is intended to do but that it also does it at less or equivalent cost. The classic study by Brooten and associates (1986) was very important to nursing, as well as health care in general, because the authors were able to demonstrate

that the intervention was safe and efficacious and that there was a significant cost savings because of early discharge from the hospital with follow-up care by clinical nurse specialists. That model has now been expanded to other clinical areas, such as gerontological nursing (Bull, Hansen, and Gross, 2000; see Appendix A). In an era of health care reform and cost containment for health expenditures, it has become increasingly important to evaluate the relative costs and benefits of new programs of care. Relatively few studies in nursing and medicine have done so, but in terms of outcomes, nursing costs and cost savings will be important to future studies.

HELPFUL HINT Think of quality assurance and quality improvement projects as research-related activities that enhance the ability of nurses to generate cost and quality outcome data. These outcome data contribute to documenting the way nursing practice makes a difference.

CRITIQUING Experimental and Quasiexperimental Designs

As discussed earlier in the chapter, various designs for research studies differ in the amount of control the researcher has over the antecedent and intervening variables that may impact the results of the study. True experimental designs offer the most possibility for control, and preexperimental designs offer the least. Quasiexperimental designs fall somewhere in between. Research designs must balance the needs for internal validity and external validity to produce useful results. In addition, judicious use of design requires that the chosen design be appropriate to the problem, free of bias, and capable of answering the research question.

Questions that the reader should pose when reading studies that test cause-and-effect relationships are listed in the Critiquing Criteria box. All of these questions should help the reader judge whether it can be confidently believed that a causal relationship exists.

For studies in which either experimental or quasiexperimental designs are used, first try to determine the type of design that was used. Often a statement describing the design of the study appears in the abstract and in the methods sections of the paper. If such a statement is not present, the reader should examine the paper for evidence of the following three characteristics: control, randomization, and manipulation. If all are discussed, the design is probably experimental. On the other hand, if the study involves the administration of an experimental treatment but does not involve the random assignment of subjects to groups, the design is quasiexperimental. Next, try to identify which of the various designs within these two types of designs was used. Determining the answer to these questions gives you a head start, because each design has its inherent threats to validity and this step makes it a bit easier to critically evaluate the study. The next question to ask is whether the researcher required a

CRITIQUING CRITERIA

1. What design is used in the study?
2. Is the design experimental or quasiexperimental?
3. Is the problem one of a cause-and-effect relationship?
4. Is the method used appropriate to the problem?
5. Is the design suited to the setting of the study?

Experimental Designs

1. What experimental design is used in the study, and is it appropriate?
2. How are randomization, control, and manipulation applied?
3. Are there any reasons to believe that there are alternative explanations for the findings?
4. Are all threats to validity, including mortality, addressed in the report?
5. Whether the experiment was conducted in the laboratory or a clinical setting, are the findings generalizable to the larger population of interest?

Quasiexperimental Designs

1. What quasiexperimental design is used in the study, and is it appropriate?
2. What are the most common threats to the validity of the findings of this design?
3. What are the plausible alternative explanations, and have they been addressed?
4. Are the author's explanations of threats to validity acceptable?
5. What does the author say about the limitations of the study?
6. Are there other limitations related to the design that are not mentioned?

Evaluation Research

1. Does the study identify a specific problem, practice, policy, or treatment that it will evaluate?
2. Are the outcomes to be evaluated identified?
3. Is the problem analyzed and described?
4. Is the program to be analyzed described and standardized?
5. Is measurement of the degree of change (outcome) that occurs identified?
6. Is there a determination of whether the observed outcome is related to the activity or to some other cause(s)?

solution to a cause-and-effect problem. If so, the study is suited to these designs. Finally, think about the conduct of the study in the setting. Is it realistic to think that the study could be conducted in a clinical setting without some contamination?

The most important question to ask yourself as you read experimental studies is, "What else could have happened to explain the findings?" Thus it is important that the author provide adequate accounts of how the procedures for randomization, control, and manipulation were carried out. The paper should include a description of the procedures for random assignment to such a degree that the reader could determine just how likely it was for any one subject to be assigned to a particular group. The description of the independent variable also should be detailed. The inclusion of this information helps the reader decide if it is possible that the treatment given to some subjects in the experimental group might be different from what was given to others in the same group. In addition, threats to validity, such as testing and mortality, should be addressed. Otherwise there is the potential for the findings of the study to be in error and less believable to the reader.

HELPFUL HINT Remember that mortality is a problem in most experimental studies because data are usually collected more than once. The researcher should demonstrate that the groups are equivalent when they enter the study and at the final analysis.

This question of potential alternative explanations or threats to internal validity for the findings is even more important when critically evaluating a quasiexperimental study because quasiexperimental designs cannot possibly control many plausible alternative explanations. A well-written report of a quasiexperimental study systematically reviews potential threats to the validity of the findings. Then the reader's work is to decide if the author's explanations make sense.

When critiquing evaluation research, the reader should look for a careful description of the program, policy, procedure, or treatment being evaluated. In addition, the reader may need to determine the design used to evaluate the program and assess the appropriateness of the design for the evaluation. Once the design has been determined, the reader assesses threats to validity for the appropriate design in determining the appropriateness of the author's conclusions related to the outcomes. As with all research, studies using these designs need to be generalizable to a larger population of people than those actually studied. Thus it is important to decide whether the experimental protocol eliminated some potential subjects and whether this affected not only internal validity but also external validity.

Critical Thinking Challenges

Barbara Krainovich-Miller

➢ Discuss the barriers to nurse researchers meeting the three criteria of a true experimental design.
➢ How is it possible to have a research design that includes an experimental treatment intervention and a control group yet is not considered a true experimental study?
➢ Argue your case for supporting or not supporting the following claim, including examples with your reasons: A study that does not use the "purest" design (i.e., true experimental design) does not decrease the value of the study even though it may decrease the utility of the findings.
➢ How would you use the internet to determine if your critique of an assigned study is accurate and fair?
➢ Respond to the following question. Are experimental studies still considered the best evidence for an evidence-based practice? Justify your answer.

Key Points

- Two types of design commonly used in nursing research to test hypotheses about cause-and-effect relationships are experimental and quasiexperimental designs. Both are useful for the development of nursing knowledge because they test the effects of nursing actions and lead to the development of prescriptive theory.
- True experiments are characterized by the ability of the researcher to control extraneous variation, to manipulate the independent variable, and to randomly assign subjects to research groups.
- Experiments conducted either in clinical settings or in the laboratory provide the best evidence in support of a causal relationship because the following three criteria can be met: (1) the independent and dependent variables are related to each other, (2) the independent variable chronologically precedes the dependent variable, and (3) the relationship cannot be explained by the presence of a third variable.
- Researchers frequently turn to quasiexperimental designs to test cause-and-effect relationships because experimental designs often are impractical or unethical.
- Quasiexperiments may lack either the randomization or comparison group characteristics of true experiments or both of these factors. Their usefulness in studying causal relationships depends on the ability of the researcher to rule out plausible threats to the validity of the findings, such as history, selection, maturation, and testing effects.
- The overall purpose of critiquing such studies is to assess the validity of the findings and to determine whether these findings are worth incorporating into the nurse's personal practice.

REFERENCES

Bigman SK: Evaluating the effectiveness of religious programs, *Rev Relig Res* 2:99-110, 1961.

Brooten D et al: A randomized clinical trial of early hospital discharge and home follow-up of very-low-birth-weight infants, *N Engl J Med* 315:934-939, 1986.

Bull MJ, Hansen HE, and Gross CR: A professional-patient partnership model of discharge planning with elders hospitalized with heart failure, *Appl Nurs Res* 13:19-28, 2000

Campbell D and Stanley J: *Experimental and quasiexperimental designs for research,* Chicago, 1966, Rand-McNally.

Conlon M and Anderson GC: Three methods of random assignment: comparison of balance achieved on potentially confounding variables, *Nurs Res* 39(6):376-378, 1990.

Dealey C: Obtaining the evidence for clinically effective wound care, *Br J Nurs* 7(20):1236-1238, 1240, 1242, 1998.

Goldberg HI et al: A controlled time series trial of clinical reminders, *Health Serv Res* 34:1519-1534, 2000.

Grey M et al: Coping skills training for youths with diabetes on intensive therapy, *Appl Nurs Res* 12:3-12, 1999.

Maxey C: A case map reduces time to administration of thrombolytic therapy in patients experiencing an acute myocardial infarction, *Nurse Case Management* 2:229-237, 1997.

McCain NL et al: The influence of stress management training in HIV disease, *Nurs Res* 45:246-253, 1996.

Naylor M et al: Comprehensive discharge planning and home follow-up of hospitalized elders, *JAMA* 281:613-620, 1999.

O'Sullivan AO and Jacobson BJ: A randomized trial of a health care program for first-time adolescent mothers and their infants, *Nurs Res* 41(4):210-215, 1992.

Rudy EB et al: Permuted block design for randomization in a clinical nursing trial, *Nurs Res* 42:287-289, 1993.

Rudy EB et al: Patient outcomes for the chronically critically ill: special care unit versus intensive care unit, *Nurs Res* 44:324-331, 1995.

ADDITIONAL READINGS

Atwood JR and Taylor W: Regression discontinuity design: alternative for nursing research, *Nurs Res* 40(5):312-315, 1991.

Cook TD: The generalization of causal connections: multiple theories in search of clear practice. In Sechrest L, Perrin E, and Bunker J, editors: *AHCPR conference proceedings: research methodology: strengthening causal interpretations of nonexperimental data,* Rockville, MD, 1990, Agency for Health Care Policy and Research.

Cook TD and Campbell DT: *Quasi-experimentation: design and analysis issues for field settings,* Chicago, 1979, Rand-McNally.

Given BA et al: Strategies to minimize attrition in longitudinal studies, *Nurs Res* 39(3):184-186, 1990.

Jacobson BS and Meininger JC: Seeing the importance of blindness, *Nurs Res* 39:54-57, 1990.

Polivka BJ and Nickel JT: Case-control design: an appropriate strategy for nursing research, *Nurs Res* 41:250-253, 1992.

Weinert C and Burman M: Nurturing longitudinal samples, *West J Nurs Res* 18:360-364, 1996.

GERI LOBIONDO-WOOD
JUDITH HABER

11

Nonexperimental Designs

Key Terms

cohort
correlational study
cross-sectional studies
developmental studies
ex post facto studies
longitudinal studies

metaanalysis
methodological research
nonexperimental research
  designs
prospective studies
psychometrics

relationship/difference
  studies
retrospective studies
secondary analysis
survey studies

Learning Outcomes

After reading this chapter, the student should be able to do the following:

- Describe the overall purpose of nonexperimental designs.
- Describe the characteristics of survey, relationship, and difference designs.
- Define the differences between survey, relationship, and difference designs.
- List the advantages and disadvantages of surveys and each type of relationship and difference designs.
- Identify methodological, secondary analysis, and metaanalysis types of research.
- Identify the purposes of methodological, secondary analysis, and metaanalysis types of research.
- Discuss relational inferences versus causal inferences as they relate to nonexperimental designs.
- Identify the criteria used to critique nonexperimental research designs.
- Apply the critiquing criteria to the evaluation of nonexperimental research designs as they appear in research reports.

Nonexperimental ——————→ Quasiexperimental ——————→ Experimental

Figure 11-1   Continuum of quantitative research design.

Many phenomena of interest and relevant to nursing do not lend themselves to an experimental design. For example, nurses studying pain may be interested in the amount of pain, variations in the amount of pain, and patient responses to postoperative pain. The investigator would not design an experimental study that would potentially intensify a patient's pain just to study the pain experience. Instead, the researcher would examine the factors that contribute to the variability in a patient's postoperative pain experience using a nonexperimental design. **Nonexperimental research designs** are used in studies in which the researcher wishes to construct a picture of a phenomenon; explore events, people, or situations as they naturally occur; or test relationships and differences among variables. Nonexperimental designs may construct a picture of a phenomenon at one point or over a period of time.

In experimental research, the independent variable is manipulated; in nonexperimental research, it is not. In nonexperimental research, the independent variable(s) have naturally occurred, so to speak, and the investigator cannot directly control them by manipulation. In contrast, in an experimental design the researcher actively manipulates one or more variables, and in a nonexperimental design the researcher explores relationships or differences among the variables. Nonexperimental research requires a clear, concise research problem or hypothesis that is based on a theoretical framework. Even though the researcher does not actively manipulate the variables, the concepts of control (see Chapter 9) should be considered as much as possible.

Researchers are not in agreement on how to classify nonexperimental studies. A continuum of quantitative research design is presented in Figure 11-1. Nonexperimental studies explore the re-

BOX 11-1   Summary of Nonexperimental Research Designs

I. Survey studies
   A. Descriptive
   B. Exploratory
   C. Comparative
II. Relationship/difference studies
   A. Correlational studies
   B. Developmental studies
      1. Cross-sectional
      2. Longitudinal and prospective studies
      3. Retrospective and ex post facto studies

lationships or the differences between variables. This chapter divides nonexperimental designs into survey studies and relationship/difference studies as illustrated in Box 11-1. These categories are somewhat flexible, and other sources may classify nonexperimental studies in a different way. Some studies fall exclusively within one of these categories, whereas other studies have characteristics of more than one category (see Table 11-1). As you read the research literature you will often find that researchers who are conducting a nonexperimental study use several design classifications. This chapter introduces the various types of nonexperimental designs, their advantages and disadvantages, the use of nonexperimental research, the issues of causality, and the critiquing process as it relates to nonexperimental research. The Critical Thinking Decision Path outlines the path to the choice of a nonexperimental design.

SURVEY STUDIES

The broadest category of nonexperimental designs is the survey study. **Survey studies** are further classified as descriptive, exploratory, or com-

CRITICAL THINKING DECISION PATH Nonexperimental Design Choice

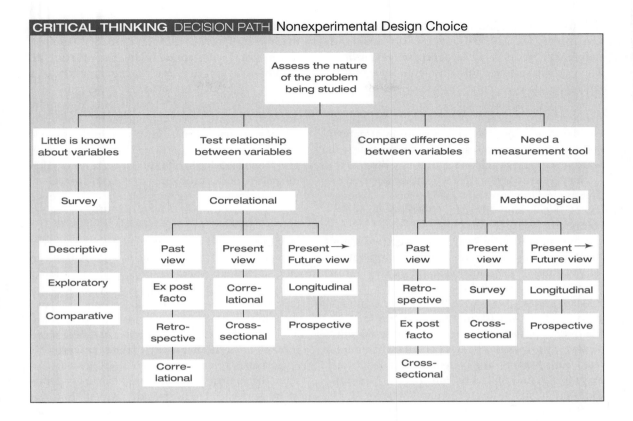

parative. *Descriptive, exploratory,* or *comparative surveys* collect detailed descriptions of existing variables and use the data to justify and assess current conditions and practices or to make more plans for improving health care practices. The reader of research will find that the terms *exploratory, descriptive, comparative* and *survey* are used either alone, interchangeably, or together to describe the design of a study (see Table 11-1). Investigators may use a descriptive or exploratory survey design to search for accurate information about the characteristics of particular subjects, groups, institutions, or situations or about the frequency of a phenomenon's occurrence, particularly when little is known about the phenomenon. The types of variables of interest can be classified as opinions, attitudes, or facts. Thimbault-Prevost, Jensen, and Hodgins (2000) conducted a survey study to explore the perceptions of nurses regard-

ing do-not-resuscitate (DNR) decisions in the critical care setting. Studies such as this provide the basis for the development of educational programs that help health care professionals understand issues regarding DNR decisions.

Fact variables include attributes of individuals that are a function of their membership in society, such as gender, income level, political and religious affiliations, ethnicity, occupation, and educational level. Burns, Camaione, and Chatterton (2000) conducted a survey study that explored facts. The overall purpose of their study was to determine whether adult nurse practitioners (ANPs) met the objective of routinely counseling clients about physical activity. To accomplish this aim, the researchers conducted a national survey of 1000 ANPs. They asked the ANPs if they counseled people about physical activity, and if so, the ANPs were asked to describe the methods and guidelines they used to access and counsel clients about physical activity. The ANPs also were asked about the perceived barriers to physical activity counseling. The researchers noted that the significance of this study was to assess if nurse practitioners, who provide a significant amount of primary care, were meeting the national objective of promoting health. The results provide useful information about how nurses in advance roles are working toward improving health and preventing disease.

Surveys are comparative when they are used to determine differences between variables. Anderson, Higgins, and Rozmus (1999) conducted a comparative survey study that addressed an important dimension of health care—cost containment. They conducted a descriptive, comparative survey study to examine the length of stay in the intensive care unit (ICU) after coronary bypass (CABG) surgery relative to the number of hours postoperation, when ambulation occurred, and the overall postoperative length of hospital stay. This study assessed whether patients who ambulated earlier after surgery had shorter length of stays in the intensive care unit (ICU). The study did find a significant difference between ICU length of stay and the time when ambulation began. This study, like the two previously discussed, does not manipulate variables but assesses data in order to provide data for future nursing intervention studies.

Data in survey research can be collected through a questionnaire or an interview (see Chapter 14). For example, Cole and Ramirez (2000) knew that nurse practitioners (NPs) had been practicing in emergency care settings for 25 years, but little was known about the activities and procedures they perform. They sent questionnaires to NPs by mail and email to collect information. Survey researchers study either small or large samples of subjects drawn from defined populations. The sample can be either broad or narrow and can be made up of people or institutions. For example, if a primary care rehabilitation unit based on a case management model were to be established in a hospital, a survey might be done on the prospective applicants' attitudes with regard to case management before the unit staff are selected. In a broader example, if a hospital were contemplating converting all patient care units to a case management model, a survey might be conducted to determine attitudes of a representative sample of nurses in the hospital toward case management. The data might provide the basis for projecting in-service needs of nursing regarding case management. The scope and depth of a survey are a function of the nature of the problem.

In surveys, investigators attempt only to relate one variable to another, or assess differences between variables, but they do not attempt to determine causation. The two major advantages of surveys are that a great deal of information can be obtained from a large population in a fairly economical manner and that survey research information can be surprisingly accurate. If a sample is representative of the population (see Chapter 12), a relatively small number of subjects can provide an accurate picture of the population.

Survey studies have several disadvantages. First, the information obtained in a survey tends to be superficial. The breadth rather than the depth of the information is emphasized. Second, conducting a survey requires a great deal of expertise in various research areas. The survey investigator must know sampling techniques, questionnaire construction, interviewing, and data analysis to produce a reliable and valid study. Third, large-scale surveys can be time-consuming and costly, although the use of on-site personnel can reduce costs.

HELPFUL HINT Research consumers should recognize that a well-constructed survey can provide a wealth of data about a particular phenomenon of interest, even though causation is not being examined.

RELATIONSHIP AND DIFFERENCE STUDIES

Investigators also endeavor to trace the relationships or differences between variables that can provide a deeper insight into a phenomenon. These studies can be classified as relationship or difference studies. The following types of **relationship/difference studies** are discussed: correlational studies and developmental studies.

CORRELATIONAL STUDIES

In a **correlational study**, an investigator examines the relationship between two or more variables. The researcher is not testing whether one variable causes another variable or how different one variable is from another variable. The researcher is testing whether the variables covary; that is, as one variable changes, does a related change occur in the other variable? The researcher using this design is interested in quantifying the strength of the relationship between the variables or in testing a hypothesis about a specific relationship. The positive or negative direction of the relationship is also a central concern (see Chapter 17 for an explanation of the correlation coefficient). For example, in their correlational study of families in which a child is to undergo organ transplantation, LoBiondo-Wood and associates (2000) (see Appendix D) explored if there was a relationship between family stress, coping, social support, perception of stress, and family adaptation during the pretransplantation evaluation period from the mother's perspective. The researchers noted that the process of seeking a transplant for a child is very stressful and before interventions can be developed, clinicians need to understand how aspects of family life are affected. They also noted the need to extend knowledge not only about the child who will be the recipient of a transplant but also the family. Each step of this study was consistent with the aims of exploring a relationship among the variables.

It should be remembered that the researchers were not testing a cause-and-effect relationship. All that is known is that the researchers found a relationship and that one variable (family stress) varied in a consistent way with another variable (family adaptation) for the particular sample studied. When reviewing a correlational study, remember what relationship the researcher

tested and notice whether the researcher implied a relationship that is consistent with the theoretical framework and hypotheses being tested. Correlational studies offer researchers and research consumers the following advantages:

- An increased flexibility when investigating complex relationships among variables
- An efficient and effective method of collecting a large amount of data about a problem
- A potential for practical application in clinical settings
- A potential foundation for future, experimental research studies
- A framework for exploring the relationship between variables that cannot be inherently manipulated

The reader will find that the correlational design has a quality of realism and is particularly appealing because it suggests the potential for practical solutions to clinical problems. The following are disadvantages of correlational studies:

- The researcher is unable to manipulate the variables of interest
- The researcher does not employ randomization in the sampling procedures because of dealing with preexisting groups, and therefore generalizability is decreased
- The researcher is unable to determine a causal relationship between the variables because of the lack of manipulation, control, and randomization

One of the most common misuses of a correlational design is the researcher's conclusion that a causal relationship exists between the variables. In their study, LoBiondo-Wood and associates (2000) appropriately concluded that a relationship existed between the variables, not that patient's concerns caused the family member's level of concern. The investigators also appropriately concluded that the ability to generalize from this study is limited by the small, homogeneous sample. The study concludes with some very thoughtful recommendations for future studies in this area. This study is a good example of a clinical study that uses a correlational design

TABLE **11-1** Examples of Studies with More than One Design Label

DESIGN TYPE	STUDY'S PURPOSE
Descriptive with repeated measures	To describe fatigue, mood, and hemodynamic patterns after myocardial infarction (from 5 to 21 days postadmission) (Lee et al, 2000)
Descriptive, correlational	To determine the types and intensity of sensations that patients experience when chest tubes and Jackson-Pratt abdominal tubes are removed (Mimnaugh et al, 1999)
Correlational, cross-sectional	To describe the extent to which decentralization and expertise are related to decision-making participation among different groups of nurses (Anthony, 1999)
Comparative, longitudinal	To determine differences in caregiver fatigue between two groups of mothers of preterm infants over a period of 1 month (Williams et al, 1999)
Prospective, descriptive	To examine to effect of gender (female) on early recovery from cardiac surgery at 1, 6, and 12 months (King, 2000)
Cross-sectional, descriptive, comparative	To identify factors that predict nurses' spiritual care perspectives and practices and compare these perspectives and practices between different nursing subspecialties (Taylor, Highfield, and Amenta, 1999)

well. The inability to draw causal statements should not lead the research consumer to conclude that a nonexperimental correlational study uses a weak design. It is a very useful design for clinical research studies because many of the phenomena of clinical interest are beyond the researcher's ability to manipulate, control, and randomize.

DEVELOPMENTAL STUDIES

There are also classifications of nonexperimental designs that use a time perspective. Investigators who use **developmental studies** are concerned not only with the existing status and the relationship and differences among phenomena at one point in time but also with changes that result from elapsed time. The following three types of developmental study designs are discussed: cross-sectional, longitudinal or prospective, and retrospective or ex post facto. Remember that in the literature, however, studies may be designated by more than one design name. This practice is accepted because many studies have elements of several nonexperimental designs. Table 11-1 provides examples of studies classified with more than one design label.

Cross-Sectional Studies

Cross-sectional studies examine data at one point in time, that is, the data collected on only one occasion with the same subjects rather than on the same subjects at several time points. For example, Nyamathi and associates (2000) studied the type of social support reported by homeless women and examined the characteristics of homeless women with different types of support. The data were collected from 1302 sheltered homeless women. Each woman (subject) met with an investigator on one occasion when the questionnaires were administered. The goal was to explore what types of support were associated with poor psychological profile, health behaviors, and positive use of medical care.

Another cross-sectional study approach is to simultaneously collect data on the study's variables from different **cohort** (subjects) groups. An example of a cross-sectional study with different cohort groups is one conducted by Anthony (1999). This study focused on the extent of nurses' participation in decision making within two different types of hospital nursing administration. The cohorts were nurses from different hospitals in the same city. Nurses from the hospitals completed the study's instruments on one occasion and responses were compared between the different types of administrations.

Cross-sectional studies can explore relationships and correlations, or differences and comparisons, or both. For instance, Nyamathi and associates' (2000) study posed research questions that allowed them to explore both differences and relationships among and between variables.

Longitudinal/Prospective Studies

In contrast to the cross-sectional design, **longitudinal** or **prospective studies** collect data from the same group at different points in time. Prospective or longitudinal studies also explore differences and relationships. Longitudinal studies also are referred to as a *repeated measures* study. For instance, the investigator conducting a study with diabetic children could elect to use a longitudinal design. In that case, the investigator could collect yearly data or follow the same children over a number of years to compare changes in the variables at different ages. By collecting data from each subject at yearly intervals, a longitudinal perspective of the diabetic process is accomplished. As another example of a longitudinal study, Anderson (2000) collected data from a sample of 98 men and women infected with HIV on two occasions, 18 months apart. The purpose of the study was to examine the relationship of self-esteem and optimism to appraisal, outcomes of well-being, and other selected variables over the 18-month period.

Williams and associates (1999) conducted a comparative, longitudinal study whose purpose was to determine if there were differences in caregiver fatigue between two groups of mothers of preterm infants from hospitalization through 1 month postdischarage. Data were collected on three occasions over a period of a month to look for differences that may have existed among the subjects at each time period.

Cross-sectional and longitudinal designs have many advantages and disadvantages. When assessing the appropriateness of a cross-sectional study versus a longitudinal study, the research consumer should first assess what the researcher's goal is in light of the theoretical framework. For example, in a study of infant colic, the researchers are exploring a developmental process; therefore, a longitudinal design seems more appropriate. However, the disadvantages inherent in a longitudinal design also must be considered. Data collection may be of long duration because of the time it takes for the subjects to progress to each data-collection point. In the infant colic study, it took the researchers between 12 months and 18 months to collect the data from the total sample. Internal validity threats such as testing and mortality also are ever present and unavoidable in a longitudinal study.

These realities make a longitudinal design costly in terms of time, effort, and money. There is also a chance of confounding variables that could affect the interpretation of the results. Subjects in such a study may respond in a socially desirable way that they believe is congruent with the investigators' expectations (see Hawthorne Effect in Chapters 9 and 10). However, despite the pragmatic constraints imposed by a longitudinal study, the researcher should proceed with this design if the theoretical framework supports a longitudinal developmental perspective.

The advantages of a longitudinal study are that each subject is followed separately and thereby serves as his or her own control, increased depth of responses can be obtained, and early trends in the data can be analyzed. The researcher can assess changes in the variables of interest over time, and both relationships and differences can be explored between variables.

Cross-sectional studies, when compared with longitudinal studies, are less time-consuming, less expensive, and thus more manageable for the researcher. Because large amounts of data can be collected at one point, the results are more readily available. In addition, the confounding variable of maturation, resulting from the elapsed time, is not present. However, the investigator's ability to establish an in-depth developmental assessment of the interrelationships of the phenomena being studied is lessened. Thus the researcher is unable

TABLE **11-2**   Paradigm for the Ex Post Facto Design

GROUPS (NOT RANDOMLY ASSIGNED)	INDEPENDENT VARIABLE (NOT MANIPULATED BY INVESTIGATOR)	DEPENDENT VARIABLE
Exposed group: Cigarette smokers	X Cigarette smoking	Y_E Lung cancer
Control group: Nonsmokers		Y_C No lung cancer

to determine whether the change that occurred is related to the change that was predicted because the same subjects were not followed over a period of time. In other words, the subjects are unable to serve as their own controls (see Chapter 9). In summary, longitudinal studies begin in the present and end in the future and cross-sectional studies look at a broader perspective of a cross section of the population at a specific point in time.

Retrospective/Ex Post Facto Studies

Retrospective studies are essentially the same as **ex post facto studies.** Epidemiologists primarily use the term *retrospective*, whereas social scientists prefer the term *ex post facto*. In either case, the dependent variable already has been affected by the independent variable, and the investigator attempts to link present events to events that have occurred in the past. When scientists wish to explain causality or the factors that determine the occurrence of events or conditions, they prefer to employ an experimental design. However, they cannot always manipulate the independent variable X or use random assignments. In cases in which experimental designs cannot be employed, ex post facto studies may be used. Ex post facto literally means "from after the fact." Ex post facto or retrospective studies also are known as *causal-comparative* studies or *comparative* studies. As we discuss this design further, you will see that many elements of ex post facto research are similar to quasiexperimental designs because they explore differences between variables (Campbell and Stanley, 1963).

In retrospective/ex post facto studies, a researcher hypothesizes, for instance, that X (ciga-

rette smoking) is related to and a determinant of Y (lung cancer), but X, the presumed cause, is not manipulated and subjects are not randomly assigned to groups. Rather, a group of subjects who have experienced X (cigarette smoking) in a normal situation is located and a control group of subjects who have not experienced X is chosen. The behavior, performance, or condition (lung tissue) of the two groups is compared to determine whether the exposure to X had the effect predicted by the hypothesis. Table 11-2 illustrates this example. Examination of Table 11-2 reveals that although cigarette smoking appears to be a determinant of lung cancer, the researcher is still not able to conclude a causal relationship exists between the variables because the independent variable has not been manipulated and subjects were not randomly assigned to groups.

Tolle and associates (2000) conducted a retrospective study in which they identified family barriers to optimal care by querying a sample of families 2 to 5 months after they experienced the death of a family member. They conducted telephone interviews with 475 family informants who had been involved in caring for a dying family member in the last month of life. From the data they gathered about family views of health services and clinician care, they identified several barriers that families experienced.

A study by Bernardo and associates (2000) is another example of a retrospective study. The researchers noted that the leading cause of disability and death among young children is unintentional injury. One preventable injury is dog bites. The purpose of the investigation was to examine the characteristics of dog bite injuries to assist in providing healthy environments for children. The researchers reviewed 204 charts of children who were seen in an emergency department within 24 hours of the bite. They collected data on the demographic characteristics of the children, treatment information, the environment in which the injury occurred, information on the dog who did the biting, and costs of the emergency visit. The researchers presented conclusions and educational recommendations for dog and children interaction that would promote childhood safety.

The advantages of the retrospective/ex post facto design are similar to those in the correlational design. The additional benefit of the ex post facto design is that it offers a higher level of control than a correlational study. For example, in the cigarette smoking study, a group of nonsmokers' lung tissue samples are compared with samples of smokers' lung tissue. This comparison enables the researcher to establish the existence of a differential effect of cigarette smoking on lung tissue. However, the researcher remains unable to draw a causal linkage between the two variables, and this inability is the major disadvantage of the retrospective/ex post facto design.

Another disadvantage of retrospective research is the problem of an alternative hypothesis being the reason for the documented relationship. If the researcher obtains data from two existing groups of subjects, such as one that has been exposed to X and one that has not, and the data support the hypothesis that X is related to Y, the researcher cannot be sure whether X or some extraneous variable is the real cause of the occurrence of Y. Finding naturally occurring groups of subjects who are similar in all respects except for their exposure to the variable of interest is very difficult. There is always the possibility that the groups differ in some other way, such as exposure to some other lung irritants such as asbestos, which can affect the findings of the study and produce spurious results. Consequently, the reader of such a study needs to cautiously evaluate the conclusions drawn by the investigator.

HELPFUL HINT When reading research reports, the reader will note that at times researchers classify a study's design with more than one design type label. This is correct because research studies often reflect aspects of more than one design label.

Longitudinal/prospective studies are less common than retrospective studies. This may be explained by the fact that it can take a long time for the phenomenon of interest to become evident in a prospective study. For example, if researchers were studying pregnant women who regularly consume alcohol, it would take 9 months for the effect of low–birth-weight in the subjects' infants to become evident. The problems inherent in a prospective study are therefore similar to those of a longitudinal study. However, longitudinal/prospective studies are considered to be stronger than retrospective studies because of the degree of control that can be imposed on extraneous variables that might confound the data.

HELPFUL HINT Remember that nonexperimental designs can test relationships, differences, comparisons, or predictions, depending on the purpose of the study.

PREDICTION AND CAUSALITY IN NONEXPERIMENTAL RESEARCH

A concern of researchers and research consumers are the issues of prediction and causality. Researchers are interested in explaining cause-and-effect relationships. Historically, researchers have said that only experimental research can support the concept of causality. For example, nurses are interested in discovering what causes anxiety in many settings. If we can uncover the causes, we could perhaps develop interventions that would prevent or decrease the anxiety. Causality makes it necessary to order events chronologically; that is, if we find in a randomly assigned experiment that event 1 (stress) occurs before event 2 (anxiety) and that those in the stressed group were anxious while those in the unstressed group were not, we can say that the hypothesis of stress caus-ing anxiety is supported by these empirical obser-vations. If these results were found in a nonexper-imental study where some subjects underwent the stress of surgery and were anxious and others did not have surgery and were not anxious, we would say that there is an association or relation-ship between stress (surgery) and anxiety. But on the basis of the results of a nonexperimental study we could say that the stress of surgery caused the anxiety.

Many variables (e.g., anxiety) that nurse re-searchers wish to study cannot be manipulated, nor would it be wise to try to manipulate them. Yet there is a need to have studies that can assert a predictive or causal sequence; in light of this need, many nurse researchers are using several analytical techniques that can explain the rela-tionships among variables to establish predic-tive or causal links. These techniques are called *causal modeling, model testing,* and *associated causal analysis techniques* (Hoyle, 1995; Kaplan, 2000; Schumacker and Lomax, 1996). The reader of research also will find the terms *path analysis, LISREL, analysis of covariance structures,* and *structural equation modeling (SEM)* used to de-scribe the statistical techniques (see Chapter 17) used in these studies. Dilorio and associates (2000) used causal modeling in their study test-ing a social cognitive-based model of condom use behaviors among college students. The re-searchers tested Bandura's model of Social Cog-nitive Theory. To accomplish a test of the model, the researchers asked the subjects to respond to questionnaires that corresponded to the vari-ables in the model. The study results have led to an increased understanding of condom use based on social cognitive theory and will assist in the development of interventions that can de-crease anxiety about condom use and have im-plications for HIV prevention. The researchers' recommendations for further research also point to the fact that no matter which type of design or which statistical procedure is used, there is a need for future testing and refinement of the principles that guide nursing care.

Researchers at times want to make a forecast or prediction about how patients will respond to an intervention or a disease process or how suc-cessful individuals will be in a particular setting or field of specialty. In this case, a model may be tested to assess which independent variables can best explain the dependent variable(s). For exam-ple, Poss (2000) wanted to analyze the relation-ship between variables such as susceptibility, severity, and barriers among others of the Health Belief Model and the Theory of Reasoned Action and participation by Mexican migrant workers in a tuberculosis (TB) screening program. The re-searcher recruited subjects who had participated in a tuberculosis education program and inter-viewed them to assess which of the independent variables predicted their intention and behavior to participate in the TB screening program.

In another example, Stuifbergen, Seraphine, and Roberts (2000) tested an explanatory model of variables influencing health promotion and quality of life in persons living with multiple sclerosis (MS). The variables of the model were developed from previous systematic study and further tested in this study. The researchers ex-plained the development of the model and the premise of the study. The explanation provided by the researchers allows the reader of the study to clearly understand the purpose and aim of the research and the test of the model using SEM. Although the research does not test a cause-and-effect relationship between the chosen independ-ent predictor variables and the dependent crite-rion variable, it does demonstrate a theoretically meaningful model of how variables work to-gether in a group in a particular situation.

As nurse researchers develop their programs of research in a specific area, more studies that test models will be available. The statistics used in model-testing studies are advanced, but the beginning reader should be able to read the arti-cle and understand the purpose of the study and if the model generated was logical and devel-oped with a solid basis from the literature and past research. This section cites several studies that conducted sound tests of theoretical models.

A full description of the techniques and principles of causal modeling is beyond the scope of this text. A review of the additional references provides the reader with the basic assumptions and principles of these techniques.

HELPFUL HINT Nonexperimental clinical research studies have progressed to the point where prediction models are used to explore or test relationships between independent and dependent variables.

ADDITIONAL TYPES OF QUANTITATIVE STUDIES

Other types of quantitative studies complement the science of research. These additional types of designs provide a means of viewing and interpreting phenomena that gives further breadth and knowledge to nursing science and practice. The additional types are methodological, meta-analysis, and secondary analysis.

METHODOLOGICAL RESEARCH

Methodological research is the development and evaluation of data-collection instruments, scales, or techniques. As you will find in succeeding chapters (see Chapters 14 and 15), methodology influences research strongly.

The most significant and critically important aspect of methodological research addressed in measurement development is called **psychometrics.** Psychometrics deals with the theory and development of measurement instruments (such as questionnaires) or measurement techniques (such as observational techniques) through the research process. Psychometrics thus deals with the measurement of a concept, such as anxiety or interpersonal conflict, with reliable and valid tools (see Chapter 15 for a discussion of reliability and validity). Psychometrics is a critical issue for nurse researchers. Nurse researchers have used the principles of psychometrics to develop and test measurement instruments that focus on nursing phenomena. Nurse researchers also use instruments developed by other disciplines such as

psychology and sociology. Sound measurement tools are critical to the reliability and validity of a study. Although a study's purpose, problems, and procedures may be clear and the data analysis correct and consistent, if the measurement tool that was used by the researcher has inherent psychometric problems, the findings are rendered questionable or limited.

The main problem for nurse researchers is locating appropriate measurement tools. Many of the phenomena of interest to nursing practice and research are intangible, such as interpersonal conflict, caring, coping, and maternal-fetal attachment. The intangible nature of various phenomena, yet the recognition of the need to measure them, places methodological research in an important position. Methodological research differs from other designs of research. First, it does not include all of the research process steps as discussed in Chapter 2. Second, to implement its techniques the researcher must have a sound knowledge of psychometrics or must consult with a researcher knowledgeable in psychometric techniques. The methodological researcher is not interested in the relationship of the independent variable and dependent variable or in the effect of an independent variable on a dependent variable. The methodological researcher is interested in identifying an intangible construct (concept) and making it tangible with a paper-and-pencil instrument or observation protocol.

A methodological study basically includes the following steps:
- Defining the construct/concept or behavior to be measured
- Formulating the tool's items
- Developing instructions for users and respondents
- Testing the tool's reliability and validity

These steps require a sound, specific, and exhaustive literature review to identify the theories underlying the construct. The literature review provides the basis of item formulation. Once the items have been developed, the researcher assesses the tool's reliability and validity (see Chapter 15). Various aspects of these procedures

TABLE **11-3** Common Considerations in the Development of Measurement Tools

CONSIDERATION	EXAMPLE
The well-constructed scale, test, interview schedule, or other form of index should consist of an objective, standardized measure of samples of a behavior that has been clearly defined. Observations should be made on a small but carefully chosen sampling of the behavior of interest, thus permitting us to feel confident that the samples are representative.	In their study of continuity of care, Bull et al (2000) developed the scales items by reviewing qualitative data collected from several previous studies of hospitalized elders and their family caregivers. The tool also was based on a thorough review of previous theoretical and research literature.
The tool should be standardized, that is, a set of uniform items and response possibilities that are uniformly administered and scored.	In the study by Bull et al (2000) the evaluation of the continuity of care scale consisted of objective assessment by the research team and community dwelling elders. Without specific criteria and rating procedures the evaluations of the items would be based on the subjective impressions, which may have varied significantly between observers and conditions.
The items of a measurement tool should be unambiguous; they should be clear-cut, concise, exact statements with only one idea per item. Negative stems or items with negatively phrased response possibilities result in a double negative and ambiguity in meaning and scoring.	In constructing a tool to measure job satisfaction, a nurse scientist writes the following items, "I never feel that I don't have time to provide good nursing care." The response format consists of "Agree," "Undecided," and "Disagree." It is very likely that a response of "Disagree" will not reflect the respondent's true intent because of the confusion that is created by the double negatives.
The type of items used in any one test or scale should be restricted to a limited number of variations. Subjects who are expected to shift from one kind of item to another may fail to provide a true response as a result of the distraction of making such a change.	Mixing true-or-false items with questions that require a yes-or-no response and items that provide a response format of five possible answers is conducive to a high level of measurement error.
Items should not provide irrelevant clues. Unless carefully constructed, an item may furnish an indication of the expected response or answer. Furthermore, the correct answer or expected response to one item should not be given by another item.	An item that provides a clue to the expected answer may contain value words that convey cultural expectations, such as, "A good wife enjoys caring for her home and family."

may differ according to the tool's use, purpose, and stage of development.

As an example of methodological research, Bull, Luo, and Maruyama (2000) identified the construct of continuity of care that incorporates the perspectives of elders and their family caregivers. The researchers defined the concept conceptually and operationally. Common considerations that researchers incorporate into methodological research are outlined in Table 11-3. Many more examples of methodological research can be found in nursing research literature (Frank-Stromberg and Olsen, 1997; Strickland and Waltz, 1988; Waltz and Strickland, 1988) and many nursing journals. Psychometric or methodological studies are found primarily in journals that report research. The *Journal of Nursing Measurement* is devoted to the publication of information on instruments, tools, and approaches for measurement of variables. The specific procedures of methodological research are beyond the scope of this book, but the reader is urged to look closely at the tools used in studies.

TABLE **11-3** Common Considerations in the Development of Measurement Tools—cont'd

CONSIDERATION	EXAMPLE
The items of a measurement tool should not be made difficult by requiring unnecessarily complex or exact operations. Furthermore, the difficulty of an item should be appropriate to the level of the subjects being assessed. Limiting each item to one concept or idea helps accomplish this objective.	A test constructed to evaluate learning in an introductory course in research methods may contain an item that is inappropriate for the designated group, such as, "A nonlinear transformation of data to linear data is a useful procedure before testing a hypothesis of curvilinearity."
The diagnostic, predictive, or measurement value of a tool depends on the degree to which it serves as an indicator of a relatively broad and significant area of behavior known as the universe of content for the behavior. As already emphasized, a behavior must be clearly defined before it can be measured. The definition is developed from the universe of content, that is, the information and research findings that are available for the behavior of interest. The items should reflect that definition. To what extent the test items appear to accomplish this objective is an indication of the validity of the instrument.	Two nurse researchers, A and B, are studying the construct of quality of life. Each has defined this construct in a different way. Consequently, the measurement tool that each nurse devises will include different questions. The questions on each tool will reflect the universe of content for quality of life as defined by each researcher.
The instrument also should adequately cover the defined behavior. The primary consideration is whether the number and nature of items in the sample are adequate. If there are too few items, the accuracy or reliability of the measure must be questioned. In general, there should be a minimum of 10 items for each independent aspect of the behavior of interest.	Very few people would be satisfied with an assessment of such traits as intelligence if the scales were limited to three items.
The measure must prove its worth empirically through tests of reliability and validity.	A researcher should demonstrate to the reader that the scale is accurate and measures what it purports to measure (see Chapter 15).

References of psychometric and methodological research are provided in the Additional Readings list in this chapter.

METAANALYSIS

Metaanalysis is not a design per se but a research method that takes the results of many studies in a specific area and synthesizes their findings to draw conclusions regarding the state of the art in the area of focus. The synthesis of the data can be accomplished in several different ways (Cooper,

1998; Lipsey and Wilson, 2000; Rosenthal, 1991). The consumer of research should note that a researcher who conducts a metaanalysis does not conduct the original analysis of data in the area but rather takes the data from already published studies and synthesizes the information by following a set of controlled and systematic steps. Metaanalysis can be used to synthesize both nonexperimental and experimental research studies. Studies of this nature have become more prevalent in nursing research. For example, Floyd and associates (2000) conducted a metaanalysis to determine the magnitude of change over the adult life span in key sleep characteristics and to explore research design features that may account for the variability in age-related sleep changes. The researchers analyzed the data using metaanalysis techniques from 41 studies that dealt with sleep and age to address the research purpose. Metaanalysis studies provide nurses with a synthesis and integration of research findings in an area and provide indicators of future research needs.

SECONDARY ANALYSIS

Secondary analysis also is not a design but rather a form of research in which the researcher takes previously collected and analyzed data from *one* study and reanalyzes the data for a *secondary* purpose. The original study may be either an experimental or nonexperimental design. For example Morin, Gennaro, and Fehder (1999) conducted a secondary analysis of a longitudinal study. The original study collected data from postpartum

mothers over a 4-month period. The purpose of the original study was to compare stress and immune response in mothers of low-birth-weight infants and term infants. Data from the healthy mothers of the term infants were used for the secondary analysis to describe whether nutrition and physical activity differ in postpartum women according to four weight categories: underweight, normal weight, overweight, and obese. The data from the original study served the purpose of answering two clinical questions.

HELPFUL HINT As you read the literature you will find labels such as outcomes research, needs assessments, evaluation research, and quality assurance. These studies are not designs per se. These studies use either experimental or nonexperimental designs. Studies with these labels are designed to test effectiveness of health care techniques, programs, or interventions. When reading such a research study, the reader should assess which design was used and if the principles of the design, sampling strategy, and analysis are consistent with the study's purpose.

CRITIQUING Nonexperimental Designs

Criteria for critiquing nonexperimental designs are presented in the accompanying box. When critiquing nonexperimental research designs, the consumer should keep in mind that such designs offer the researcher the least amount of control. The first step in critiquing nonexperimental research is to determine which type of design was used in the study. Often a statement describing the design of the study appears in the abstract and in the methods section of the report. If such a statement is not present, the reader should closely examine the paper for evidence of which type of design was employed. The reader should be able to discern that either a survey or relationship design was used, as well as the specific subtype. For example, the reader would expect an investigation of self-concept development in children from birth to 5 years of age to be a relationship study using a longitudinal design.

Next, the reader should evaluate the theoretical framework and underpinnings of the study to deter-

mine if a nonexperimental design was the most appropriate approach to the problem. For example, many of the studies on pain discussed throughout this text are suggestive of a nonmanipulable relationship between pain and any of the independent variables under consideration. As such, these studies suggest a nonexperimental correlational, longitudinal, or cross-sectional design. Investigators will use one of these designs to examine the relationship between the variables in naturally occurring groups. Sometimes the reader may think that it would have been more appropriate if the investigators had used an experimental or quasiexperimental design. However, the reader must recognize that pragmatic or ethical considerations also may have guided the researchers in their choice of design (see Chapters 9 and 13).

Then the evaluator should assess whether the problem is at a level of experimental manipulation. Many times researchers merely wish to examine if

CRITIQUING CRITERIA

1. Which nonexperimental design is used in the study?
2. Based on the theoretical framework, is the rationale for the type of design evident?
3. How is the design congruent with the purpose of the study?
4. Is the design appropriate for the research problem?
5. Is the design suited to the data-collection methods?
6. Does the researcher present the findings in a manner congruent with the design used?
7. Does the research go beyond the relational parameters of the findings and erroneously infer cause-and-effect relationships between the variables?
8. Are there any reasons to believe that there are alternative explanations for the findings?
9. Where appropriate, how does the researcher discuss the threats to internal and external validity?
10. How does the author deal with the limitations of the study?

relationships exist between variables. Therefore when one critiques such studies, the purpose of the study should be determined. If the purpose of the study does not include describing a cause-and-effect relationship, the researcher should not be criticized for not looking for one. However, the evaluator should be wary of a nonexperimental study in which the researcher suggests a cause-and-effect relationship in the findings.

Finally, the factor or factors that actually influence changes in the dependent variable are often ambiguous in nonexperimental designs. As with all complex phenomena, multiple factors can contribute to variability in the subjects' responses. When an experimental design is not used for controlling some of these extraneous variables that can influence results, the researcher must strive to provide as much control of them as possible within the context of a nonexperimental design. For example, when it has not been possible to randomly assign subjects to treatment groups as an approach to controlling an independent variable, the researcher may use a strategy of matching subjects for identified variables. For example, in a study of infant birth weight, pregnant women could be matched on variables such as weight, height, smoking habits, drug use, and other factors that might influence birth weight. The independent variable of interest, such as the type of prenatal care, would then be the ma-

jor difference in the groups. The reader would then feel more confident that the only real difference between the two groups was the differential effect of the independent variable because the other factors in the two groups were theoretically the same. However, the consumer should remember also that there might be other influential variables that were not matched, such as income, education, and diet. Threats to internal and external validity represent a major influence on the interpretation of a nonexperimental study because they impose limitations on the generalizability of the results.

If the consumer is critiquing one of the additional types of research discussed, it is important first to identify the type of research used. Once the type of research is identified, its specific purpose and format need to be understood. The format and methods of secondary analysis, methodological research, and metaanalysis vary; knowing how they vary allows a consumer to assess whether the process was applied appropriately. Some of the basic principles of these methods were presented in this chapter. The specific criteria for evaluating these designs are beyond the scope of this text, but the references provided will assist in this process. Even though the format and methods vary, it is important to remember that all research has a central goal: to answer questions scientifically.

| Critical Thinking Challenges | *Barbara Krainovich-Miller* |

➤ Discuss which type of nonexperimental design might help validate the defining characteristics of a particular nursing diagnosis you use in practice. Do you think it is possible to use nurses and patients/clients, as the subjects in this type of study?

➤ The midterm group (five students) assignment for your research class is to critique an assigned quantitative study. To proceed you must first decide what the study's overall type is. You think it is an ex post facto nonexperimental design; the others think it is an experimental design because it has several explicit hypotheses. How would you convince them that you are correct?

➤ You are completing your senior practicum on a surgical step-down unit. The nurses completed an evidence-based practice protocol for patient-controlled analgesics (PCAs). Some of the nurses want to implement it immediately, while others want to implement it with only some of the patients. You think that it should be implemented as a research study. Discuss if either of the ways the nurses chose to implement the protocol could be considered a research study.

➤ Discuss the reasons for conducting a methodological study and how the researcher's use of the internet might contribute to implementing such a study.

Key Points

• Nonexperimental research designs are used in studies that construct a picture or make an account of events as they naturally occur. The major difference between nonexperimental and experimental research is that in nonexperimental designs the independent variable is not actively manipulated by the investigator.

• Nonexperimental designs can be classified as either survey studies or relationship/difference studies.

• Survey studies and relationship/difference studies are both descriptive and exploratory in nature.

• Survey research collects detailed descriptions of existing phenomena and uses the data either to justify current conditions and practices or to make more intelligent plans for improving them.

• Relationship studies endeavor to explore the relationships between variables that provide deeper insight into the phenomena of interest.

• Correlational studies examine relationships.

• Developmental studies are further broken down into categories of cross-sectional, longitudinal, prospective, retrospective, and ex post facto studies.

• Methodological research, secondary analysis, and metaanalysis are examples of other means of adding to the body of nursing research. Both the researcher and the reader must consider the advantages and disadvantages of each design.

• Nonexperimental research designs do not enable the investigator to establish cause-and-effect relationships between the variables. Consumers must be wary of nonexperimental studies that make causal claims about the findings unless a causal modeling technique is used.

• Nonexperimental designs also offer the researcher the least amount of control. Threats to validity represent a major influence on the interpretation of a nonexperimental study because they impose limitations on the generalizability of the results and as such should be fully assessed by the critical reader.

• The critiquing process is directed toward evaluating the appropriateness of the selected nonexperimental design in relation to factors such as the research problem, theoretical framework, hypothesis, methodology, and data analysis and interpretation.

REFERENCES

Anderson B, Higgins L, and Rozmus C: Critical pathways: application to selected patient outcomes following coronary bypass graft, *Appl Nurs Res* 12(4): 168-174, 1999.

Anderson EH: Self-esteem and optimism in men and women infected with HIV, *Nurs Res* 49(5):262-271, 2000.

Anthony MK: The relationship of authority to decision-making behavior: implications for redesign, *Res Nurs Health* 22(22):388-398, 1999.

Bernardo LM et al: *J Soc Pediatr Nurs* 5(20):87-95, 2000.

Bull MJ, Luo D, and Maruyama GM: Measuring continuity of elders' posthospital care, *J Nurs Meas* 8(1):41-60, 2000.

Burns KJ, Camaione DN, and Chatterton CT: Prescription of physical activity by adult nurse practitioners: a national survey, *Nurs Outlook* 48(1):28-33, 2000.

Campbell DT and Stanley JC: *Experimental and quasi-experimental designs for research*, Chicago, 1963, Rand-McNally.

Cole FL and Ramirez E: Activities and procedures performed by nurse practitioners in emergency care, *J Emerg Nurs* 26(5):455-463, 2000.

Cooper H: *Applied social science research methods*, vol 2, 1998, Newbury Park, 1998, Sage Publications.

Dilorio C et al: A social cognitive-based model for condom use among college strudents, *Nurs Res* 49(4):208-214, 2000.

Floyd JA et al: Age-related changes in initiation and maintenance of sleep: a meta-analysis, *Res Nurs Health* 23(2):106-117, 2000.

Frank-Stromberg MF and Olsen SJ, editors: *Instruments for clinical nursing research*, Boston, 1997, Jones and Bartlett.

Hoyle R, editor: *Structural equation modeling*, Newbury Park, CA, 1995, Sage Publications.

Kaplan D: *Structure equation modeling: foundations and extensions*, Thousand Oaks, CA, 2000, Sage Publications.

Kerlinger FH: *Foundations of behavioral research*, ed 3, New York, 1986, Holt, Rinehart & Winston.

King KK: Gender and short-term recovery from cardiac surgery, *Appl Nurs Res* 49(6):29-36, 2000.

Lee H et al: Fatigue, mood, and hemodynamic patterns after myocardial infarction, *Appl Nurs Res* 13(2):60-69, 2000.

Lipsey MW and Wilson DB: *Practice meta-analysis*, Thousand Oaks, CA, 2000, Sage Publications.

Morin K, Gennaro S, and Fehder W: Nutrition and exercise in overweight and obese postpartum women, *Appl Nurs Res* 12(1):13-21, 1999.

Mimnaugh L et al: Sensations experienced during removal of tubes in acute postoperative patients, *Appl Nurs Res* 12(2):78-85, 1999.

Nyamathi A et al: Type of social support among homeless women: its impact on psychological resources, health and health behaviors, and use of health services, *Nurs Res* 49(6):318-326, 2000.

Pedhazur EJ and Schmelkin LP: *Measurement, design, and analysis*, Hillsdale, NJ, 1991, Lawrence Erlbaum Associates.

Poss JE: Factors associated with participation by Mexican migrant farmworkers in a tuberculosis screening program, *Nurs Res* 49(1):20-28, 2000.

Rosenthal R: *Meta-analysis procedures for social research* (rev ed), Newbury Park, CA, 1991, Sage Publications.

Schumacker RE and Lomax RC: *A beginner's guide to structural equation modeling*, New Jersey, 1996, Lawrence Erlbaum Associates.

Strickland OL and Waltz CF: *Measurement of nursing outcomes: measuring client outcomes*, vol 1, New York, 1988, Springer.

Stuifbergen AK, Seraphine A, and Roberts G: An explanatory model of health promotion and quality of life in chronic disabling conditions, *Nurs Res* 49(3):122-129, 2000.

Taylor EJ, Highfield MF, and Amenta M: Predictors of oncology and hospice nurses' spiritual care perspectives and practices, *Appl Nurs Res* 12(1):30-37, 1999.

Thimbault-Prevost J, Jensen LA, and Hodgins M: Critical care nurses' perceptions of DNR status, *J Nurs Scholarship* 32(3):259-266, 2000.

Waltz CF and Strickland OL: *Measurement of nursing outcomes: measuring client outcomes*, vol 2, New York, 1988, Springer.

Williams PD et al: Fatigue in mothers of infants discharged to the home on apnea moniters, *Appl Nurs Res* 12(2):69-77, 1999.

ADDITIONAL READINGS

Anastasi A: *Psychological testing*, ed 6, New York, 1988, Macmillan.

Cooper H: *Synthesizing research*, ed 3, Thousand Oaks, CA, 1998, Sage Publications.

Creswell JW: *Research design: qualitative & quantitative approaches*, Thousand Oaks, CA, 1994, Sage Publications.

Fox J: *Applied regression analysis, linear models and related methods*, Thousand Oaks, CA, 1997, Sage Publications.

Miller D: *Handbook of research design and social measurement*, ed 5, Newbury Park, CA, 1991, Sage Publications.

Waltz CF and Bausell RB: *Nursing research, design, statistics and computer analysis*, Philadelphia, 1991, FA Davis.

JUDITH HABER

Sampling

12

Key Terms

accessible population
convenience sampling
data saturation
delimitations
element
eligibility criteria
matching
multistage (cluster) sampling
network (snowball effect)
  sampling

nonprobability sampling
pilot study
population
probability sampling
purposive sampling
quota sampling
random selection
representative sample
sample

sampling
sampling frame
sampling interval
sampling unit
simple random sampling
snowball effect
stratified random sampling
systematic sampling
target population

Learning Outcomes

After reading this chapter, the student should be able to do the following:

- Identify the purpose of sampling.
- Define population, sample, and sampling.
- Compare and contrast a population and a sample.
- Discuss the eligibility criteria for sample selection.
- Define nonprobability and probability sampling.
- Identify the types of nonprobability and probability sampling strategies.
- Compare the advantages and disadvantages of specific nonprobability and probability sampling strategies.
- Discuss the factors that influence determination of sample size.
- Discuss the procedure for drawing a sample.
- Identify the criteria for critiquing a sampling plan.
- Use the critiquing criteria to evaluate the *Sample* section of a research report.

Sampling is the process of selecting representative units of a population for study in a research investigation. Although sampling is a complex process, it is a familiar one. In our daily lives, we gather knowledge, make decisions, and formulate predictions based on sampling procedures. For example, nursing students may make generalizations about the overall quality of nursing professors as a result of their exposure to a sample of nursing professors during their undergraduate programs. Patients may make generalizations about a hospital's food or quality of nursing care during a 1-week hospital stay. It is apparent that limited exposure to a limited portion of these phenomena forms the basis of our conclusions, and so much of our knowledge and decisions are based on our experience with samples.

Scientists also derive knowledge from samples. Many problems in scientific research cannot be solved without employing sampling procedures. For example, when testing the effectiveness of a medication for patients with cancer, the drug is administered to a sample of the population for whom the drug is potentially appropriate. The scientist must come to some conclusions without administering the drug to every known patient with cancer or every laboratory animal in the world. But because human lives are at stake, the scientist cannot afford to arrive casually at conclusions that are based on the first dozen patients available for study. The consequences of arriving at erroneous conclusions or making generalizations from a small nonrepresentative sample are much more severe in scientific investigations than in everyday life. Consequently, research methodologists have expended considerable effort to develop sampling theories and procedures that produce accurate and meaningful information. Essentially, researchers sample representative segments of the population because it is rarely feasible or necessary to sample the entire population of interest to obtain relevant information.

This chapter will familiarize the research consumer with the basic concepts of sampling as they primarily pertain to the principles of quantitative research design, nonprobability and probability sampling, sample size, and the related critiquing process. Sampling issues that relate to qualitative research designs are mainly discussed in Chapter 7.

SAMPLING CONCEPTS

POPULATION

A **population** is a well-defined set that has certain specified properties. A population can be composed of people, animals, objects, or events. For example, if a researcher is studying undergraduate nursing students, the type of educational preparation of the population must be specified. In this instance, the population consists of undergraduate students enrolled in a generic baccalaureate nursing program. Examples of other possible populations might be all of the female patients admitted to a certain hospital for lumpectomies for treatment of breast cancer during the year 2001, all of the children with asthma in the state of New York, or all of the men and women with a diagnosis of schizophrenia in the United States. These examples illustrate that a population may be broadly defined and potentially involve millions of people or narrowly specified to include only several hundred people.

The reader of a research report should consider whether the researcher has identified the population descriptors that form the basis for the inclusion (eligibility) or exclusion (**delimitations**) criteria that are used to select the sample from the array of all possible units—whether people, objects, or events. These four terms, inclusion or **eligibility criteria** and exclusion criteria or delimitations, are used synonomously when considering subject attributes that would lead a researcher to specify inclusion or exclusion criteria. Consider the population previously defined as undergraduate nursing students enrolled in a generic baccalaureate program. Would this population include both part-time and full-time students? Would it include students who had previously attended another nursing program? What about foreign students? Would freshmen through seniors qualify? Insofar as it is possible, the researcher must demonstrate that the exact criteria used to decide whether an individual would be classified as a member of a given population have been specifically delineated. The population descriptors that provide the basis for inclusion (eligibility) criteria should be evident in the sample; that is, the characteristics of the population and the sample should be congruent. The degree of congruence is evaluated to assess the representativeness of the sample. For example, if a population is defined as full-time, American-born, senior nursing students enrolled in a generic baccalaureate nursing program, the sample would be expected to reflect these characteristics.

Think about the concept of inclusion or eligibility criteria applied to a research study where the subjects are patients. For example, participants in a study investigating how coping skills training as a behavioral intervention, combined with intensive diabetes management, improved the metabolic control and quality of life in adolescents with diabetes (Grey et al, 1999) had to meet the following inclusion (eligibility) criteria:

1. Age—between 12.5 and 20 years of age
2. Health status—no other existing health problems except for treated hypothyroidism
3. Status—no severe hypoglycemic events had occurred in the past 6 months
4. Medications—treatment with insulin for at least 1 year
5. Laboratory values—a recent HbA1c between 7.0% and 14% (normal range is 4.0% to 6.3%)
6. Education—subjects were in a school grade that was appropriate to their age within 1 year

Inclusion or eligibility criteria may also be viewed as exclusion criteria or delimitations, those characteristics that restrict the population to a homogeneous group of subjects. Examples of exclusion criteria or delimitations include the following: gender, age, marital status, socioeconomic status, religion, ethnicity, level of education, age of children, health status, and diagnosis.

In a study evaluating the effect of caring-based counseling, and measurement of time on the impact of miscarriage and womens' emotional well-being (Swanson, 1999), the researcher established the following exclusion criteria:

- Women under 18 years of age
- Women miscarrying after the twentieth week of pregnancy
- Women miscarrying more than 5 weeks after the time of their potential enrollment in the study

These exclusion criteria or delimitations were selected because of their potential effect on the accurate evaluation of the effect of caring-based counseling, and measurement of the passage of time on the impact of miscarriage and women's emotional well-being (self-esteem and moods) in the first year subsequent to miscarrying. Let us consider the passage of time. If women who had recently experienced pregnancy loss and women who were 6 months post-miscarriage were both included and grouped together in the sample, the researchers would have two groups for whom the passage of time following pregnancy loss may be very different because of the natural therapeutic effect associated with passage of time since the miscarriage. Heterogeneity of this sample group would inhibit the researchers' ability to interpret the findings meaningfully and make generalizations. It is much wiser to study only one homogeneous group or include specific groups as distinct subsets of the sample and study the groups comparatively, as was the case in the Swanson (1999) study.

For example, in a study investigating the length of stay in the intensive care unit (ICU) after coronary artery bypass graft (CABG) surgery relative to patient outcomes (i.e., the number of hours postoperatively when ambulation occurred and the overall postoperative length of stay) (Anderson, Higgins, and Rozmus, 1999), the sample consisted of 152 charts of individuals who had been admitted to a large teaching hospital over a 2-year period and had undergone CABG surgery. The sample was divided equally into two groups that were studied comparatively.

Group I (n=76) consisted of patients admitted to the ICU after CABG surgery who remained 24 hours or less. Group II (n=76) consisted of patients whose stay in the ICU after CABG surgery lasted more than 24 hours, up to a maximum of 48 hours. Remember that exclusion criteria or delimitations are not established in a casual or meaningless way but are established to control for extraneous variability or bias. Each exclusion criterion should have a rationale, presumably related to a potential contaminating effect on the dependent variable. The careful establishment of sample exclusion criteria or delimitations will increase the precision of the study and contribute to the accuracy and generalizability of the findings (see Chapter 9).

The population criteria establish the **target population;** that is, the entire set of cases about which the researcher would like to make generalizations. A target population might include all undergraduate nursing students enrolled in generic baccalaureate programs in the United States. Because of time, money, and personnel, however, it is often not feasible to pursue using a target population. An **accessible population,** one that meets the population criteria and that is available, is used instead. For example, an accessible population might include all full-time generic baccalaureate students attending school in Indiana. Pragmatic factors must also be considered when identifying a potential population of interest.

It is important to know that a population is not restricted to human subjects. It may consist of hospital records; blood, urine, or other specimens taken from patients at a clinic; historical documents; or laboratory animals. For example, a population might consist of all the urine specimens collected from patients in the Crestview Hospital antepartum clinic or all of the patient charts on file at the Day Surgery Center. It is apparent that a population can be defined in a variety of ways. The important point to remember is that the basic unit of the population must be clearly defined because the generalizability of the findings will be a function of the population criteria.

> **HELPFUL HINT** Often, researchers do not clearly identify the population under study, or the population is not clarified until the "Discussion" section when the effort is made to discuss the group (population) to which the study findings can be generalized.

SAMPLES AND SAMPLING

Sampling is a process of selecting a portion or subset of the designated population to represent the entire population. A **sample** is a set of elements that make up the population; an **element** is the most basic unit about which information is collected. The most common element in nursing research is individuals, but other elements (e.g., places or objects) can form the basis of a sample or population. For example, a researcher was planning a study that compared the effectiveness of different nursing interventions on reducing the use of restraints. Four hospitals, each using a different treatment protocol, were identified as the sampling units rather than the nurses themselves or the treatment alone.

The purpose of sampling is to increase the efficiency of a research study. The novice reviewer of research reports must realize that it would not be feasible to examine every element or unit in the population. When sampling is done properly, the researcher can draw inferences and make generalizations about the population without examining each unit in the population. Sampling procedures that entail the formulation of specific criteria for selection ensure that the characteristics of the phenomena of interest will be, or are likely to be, present in all of the units being studied. The researcher's efforts to ensure that the sample is representative of the target population puts the researcher in a stronger position to draw conclusions from the sample findings that are generalizable to the population (see Chapter 9).

After having reviewed a number of research studies, you will recognize that samples and sampling procedures vary in terms of merit. The foremost criterion in evaluating a sample is its representativeness. A **representative sample** is one whose key characteristics closely approximate those of the population. If 70% of the population in a study of child-rearing practices consisted of women and 40% were full-time employees, a representative sample should reflect these characteristics in the same proportions.

It must be understood that there is no way to guarantee that a sample is representative without obtaining a database about the entire population. Because it is difficult and inefficient to assess a population, the researcher must employ sampling strategies that minimize or control for sample bias. If an appropriate sampling strategy is used, it almost always is possible to obtain a reasonably accurate understanding of the phenomena under investigation by obtaining data from a sample.

TYPES OF SAMPLES

Sampling strategies are generally grouped into two categories: nonprobability sampling and probability sampling. In **nonprobability sampling,** elements are chosen by nonrandom methods. The drawback of this strategy is that there is no way of estimating each element's probability of being included in the samples. Essentially, there is no way of ensuring that every element has a chance for inclusion in the nonprobability sample. **Probability sampling** uses some form of random selection when the sample units are chosen. This type of sample enables the researcher to estimate the probability that each element of the population will be included in the sample. Probability sampling is the more rigorous type of sampling strategy and is more likely to result in a representative sample. The remainder of this section is devoted to a discussion of different types of nonprobability and probability sampling strategies. A summary of sampling strategies appears in Table 12-1. You may wish to refer to this table as the various nonprobability and probability strategies are discussed in the following sections.

HELPFUL HINT Research articles are not always explicit about the type of sampling strategy that was used. If the sampling strategy is not specified, assume that a convenience sample was used for a quantitative study and a purposive sample was used for a qualitative study.

NONPROBABILITY SAMPLING

Due to lack of randomization, the nonprobability sampling strategy is less generalizable than the probability sampling strategy, and it tends to produce less representative samples. Such samples are more feasible for the researcher to obtain, however, and most samples—not only in nursing research but also in other disciplines—are nonprobability samples. When a nonprobability sample is carefully chosen to reflect the target population, through the careful use of inclusion and exclusion criteria, the research consumer can have more confidence in the representativeness of the sample and the external validity of the findings. The three major types of nonprobability sampling are the following: convenience, quota, and purposive sampling strategies.

Convenience Sampling

Convenience sampling is the use of the most readily accessible persons or objects as subjects in a study. The subjects may include volunteers, the first 25 patients admitted to hospital X with a particular diagnosis, all of the people who enrolled in program Y during the month of September, or all of the students enrolled in course Z at a particular university during 2001. The subjects are convenient and accessible to the researcher and are thus called a convenience sample. For example, a researcher studying women's concerns about having coronary artery bypass graft (CABG) surgery and living with coronary artery disease used a convenience sample of 116 women ranging in age from 39 to 85 years of age admitted over a 20-month period to one university hospital for CABG surgery who met the eligibility criteria and who volunteered to participate in the study (King, Rowe, and Zerwic, 2000). Another researcher studying the effect of a nursing intervention intended to diminish the anxiety level of parents of children being transferred from a pediatric intensive care unit (PICU) to a general pediatric floor used all biological parents of children hospitalized

TABLE **12-1** Summary of Sampling Strategies

SAMPLING STRATEGY	EASE OF DRAWING SAMPLE	RISK OF BIAS	REPRESENTATIVENESS OF SAMPLE
NONPROBABILITY			
Convenience	Very easy	Greater than any other sampling strategy	Because samples tend to be self-selecting, representativeness is questionable
Quota	Relatively easy	Contains unknown source of bias that affects external validity	Builds in some representativeness by using knowledge about the population of interest
Purposive	Relatively easy	Bias increases with greater heterogeneity of the population; conscious bias is also a danger	Very limited ability to generalize because sample is handpicked
PROBABILITY			
Simple random	Laborious	Low	Maximized; probability of nonrepresentativeness decreases with increased sample size
Stratified random	Time-consuming	Low	Enhanced
Cluster	Less time-consuming than simple or stratified	Subject to more sampling errors than simple or stratified	Less representative than simple or stratified
Systematic	More convenient and efficient than simple, stratified, or cluster sampling	Bias in the form of nonrandomness can be inadvertently introduced	Less representative if bias occurs as a result of coincidental nonrandomness

in a PICU in hospital X in the southeastern United States and who met the eligibility criteria (Bouve, Rozmus, and Giordano, 1999).

The advantage of a convenience sample is that it is easier for the researcher to obtain subjects. The researcher may have to be concerned only with obtaining a sufficient number of subjects who meet the same criteria.

The major disadvantage of a convenience sample is that the risk of bias is greater than in any other type of sample (see Table 12-1). The problem of bias is related to the fact that convenience samples tend to be self-selecting; that is, the researcher ends up obtaining information only from the people who volunteer to participate. In this case, the following questions must be raised: What motivated some of the people to participate and others to not participate? What kind of data would have been obtained if nonparticipants had also responded? How representative are the people who did participate in relation to the population? For example, a researcher may stop people on a street corner to ask their opinion on some issue; place advertisements in the newspaper; or place signs in local churches, community centers, or supermarkets indicating that volunteers are needed for a particular study. In a study examining psychological distress and gastrointestinal symptoms in women with irritable bowel syndrome, for example, subjects were recruited from local advertisements in a large metropolitan community and posters placed on two military bases in an adjoining community (Jarrett et al, 1998). Because acquiring research

TABLE **12-2** Numbers and Percentages of Students in Strata of a Quota Sample
of 5000 Graduates of Nursing Programs in City X

	DIPLOMA GRADUATES	ASSOCIATE DEGREE GRADUATES	BACCALAUREATE GRADUATES
Population	1000 (20%)	2000 (40%)	2000 (40%)
Strata	100	200	200

subjects is a problem that confronts many nurse researchers, innovative recruitment strategies may be used. For example, a researcher may even offer to pay the participants for their time. A unique method of accessing and recruiting subjects is the use of on-line computer networks (e.g., disease-specific chat rooms and bulletin boards).

The evaluator of a research report should recognize that the convenience sample strategy, although the most common, is the weakest form of sampling strategy with regard to generalizability. The use of this strategy should be avoided whenever possible. When a convenience sample is used, caution should be exercised in analyzing and interpreting the data. When critiquing a research study that has employed this sampling strategy, the reviewer will be justifiably skeptical about the external validity of the findings (see Chapter 9).

Quota Sampling

Quota sampling refers to a form of nonprobability sampling in which knowledge about the population of interest is used to build some representativeness into the sample (see Table 12-1). A quota sample identifies the strata of the population and proportionally represents the strata in the sample. For example, the data in Table 12-2 reveal that 20% of the 5000 nurses in city X are diploma graduates, 40% are associate degree students, and 40% are baccalaureate graduates. Each stratum of the population should be proportionately represented in the sample. In this case, the researcher used a proportional quota sampling strategy and decided to sample 10% of a population of 5000 (i.e., 500 nurses). Based on the proportion of each stratum in the popula-

tion, 100 diploma graduates, 200 associate degree graduates, and 200 baccalaureate graduates were the quotas established for the three strata. The researcher recruited subjects who met the eligibility criteria of the study until the quota for each stratum was filled. In other words, once the researcher obtained the necessary 100 diploma graduates, 200 associate degree graduates, and 200 baccalaureate graduates, the sample was complete in light of the research design, as well as other pragmatic matters, such as economy.

The researcher systematically ensures that proportional segments of the population are included in the sample. The quota sample is not randomly selected (i.e., once the proportional strata have been identified, the researcher obtains subjects until the quota for each stratum has been filled) but does increase the representativeness of the sample. This sampling strategy addresses the problem of overrepresentation or underrepresentation of certain segments of a population in a sample.

The characteristics chosen to form the strata are selected according to a researcher's judgment based on knowledge of the population and the literature review. The criterion for selection should be a variable that reflects important differences in the dependent variables under investigation. Age, gender, religion, ethnicity, medical diagnosis, socioeconomic status, level of completed education, and occupational rank are among the variables that are likely to be important stratifying variables in nursing research investigations.

The critiquer of a research study seeks to determine whether the sample strata appropriately reflect the population under consideration and whether the stratifying variables are homogeneous enough to ensure a meaningful comparison of differences among strata. Even when the preceding factors have been addressed by the researcher, the evaluator must remember that as a nonprobability sample, the quota strategy contains an unknown source of bias that affects external validity.

The problem is that those who choose to participate may not be typical of the population with regard to the variables being measured. There is no way to assess the biases that may be operating. In cases where the phenomena under investigation are relatively homogeneous within the population, the risk of bias may be minimal. In heterogeneous populations, however, the risk of bias is great.

Purposive Sampling

Purposive sampling is an increasingly common strategy in which the researcher's knowledge of the population and its elements is used to hand-pick the cases to be included in the sample. The researcher usually selects subjects who are considered to be typical of the population. For example, in a qualitative research study by Cohen and Ley (2000) examining the experience of bone marrow transplantation, a purposive sample of cancer patients who had undergone an autologous bone marrow transplant following a cancer diagnosis (e.g., leukemia, Hodgkins disease, breast cancer, lymphoma, myeloma) were used because they were typical of the population under consideration and could illuminate the phenomenon being studied (see Chapters 7 and 8 and Appendix B).

A purposive sample is used also when a highly unusual group is being studied such as a population with a rare genetic disease (e.g., Tay-Sachs disease). In this case, the researcher would describe the sample characteristics precisely to ensure that the reader will have an accurate picture of the subjects in the sample. This type of sample can also be used to study the differential effect of risk factors in a specific population longitudinally. For example, participant families in the longitudinal Delaware Valley Twin Study examining the differential effect of cardiovascular risk factors that have a potential to respond to en-

vironmental and lifestyle modification were recruited from Mothers of Twins Clubs and schools in the Philadelphia metropolitan area. Same-sex monozygotic and dizygotic twin pairs who met the eligibility criteria were recruited into this study (Meininger et al, 1998).

In another situation, the researcher may wish to interview individuals who reflect different ends of the range of a particular characteristic. For example, LoBiondo-Wood and associates (2000) explored the relationship between family stress, family coping, and social support and family adaptation from the mother's perspective during her child's pre-liver transplant screening phase. Twenty-nine mothers whose children were being evaluated for a liver transplant constituted the sample.

Today, computer networks (e.g., on-line services) can be of great value in helping researchers access and recruit subjects for purposive samples. One researcher used the Prodigy Cancer Support Group Bulletin Board and personal mailbox to help access and acquire subjects when testing the psychometric properties of the Sexual Behaviors Questionnaire (Wilmoth, 1995). A posting was placed on the Cancer Support Group Bulletin Board, and 11 replies were received within 24 hours. Several respondents were participants in breast cancer support groups and offered to distribute copies of the questionnaires to support group members. This method contributed 4% of the sample in an inexpensive and timely way. Other on-line support group bulletin boards exist for people with rheumatoid arthritis, systemic lupus erythematosus, HIV/AIDS, bipolar disorder, Lyme disease, and many others.

The researcher who uses a purposive sample assumes that errors of judgment in overrepresenting or underrepresenting elements of the population in the sample will tend to balance out. There is no objective method, however, for determining the validity of this assumption. The evaluator must be aware of the fact that the more heterogeneous the population, the greater the chance of bias being introduced in the selection of a purposive sample. As indicated in Table 12-1, conscious bias in the selection of subjects remains a constant danger. Therefore the findings from a study using a purposive sample should be regarded with caution. As with any nonprobability sample, the ability to generalize is very limited. The following are several instances when a purposive sample may be appropriate:

- The effective pretesting of newly developed instruments with a purposive sample of divergent types of people
- The validation of a scale or test with a known-groups technique
- The collection of exploratory data in relation to an unusual or highly specific population, particularly when the total target population remains an unknown to the researcher
- The collection of descriptive data (e.g., as in qualitative studies) that seek to describe the lived experience of a particular phenomenon (e.g., postpartum depression, caring, hope, or surviving childhood sexual abuse)
- The focus of the study population relates to a specific diagnosis (e.g., type I diabetes, multiple sclerosis) or condition (e.g., legal blindness, terminal illness) or demographic characteristic (e.g., same-sex twin pairs)

Even when the use of a purposive sample is appropriate, the researcher, as well as the critiquer, should be cognizant of the limitations of this sampling strategy.

PROBABILITY SAMPLING

The primary characteristic of probability sampling is the random selection of elements from the population. **Random selection** occurs when each element of the population has an equal and independent chance of being included in the sample. Four commonly used probability sampling strategies are simple random sampling, stratified random sampling, cluster sampling, and systematic sampling.

Random selection of sample subjects should not be confused with random assignment of subjects. The latter, as discussed in Chapter 10, refers to the assignment of subjects to either an experimental or a control group on a purely random basis.

Simple Random Sampling

Simple random sampling is a laborious and carefully controlled process. Because more complex probability designs incorporate the principles of simple random sampling in their procedures, the principles of this strategy are presented.

The researcher defines the population (a set), lists all of the units of the population (a **sampling frame**), and selects a sample of units (a subset) from which the sample will be chosen. For example, if American hospitals specializing in the treatment of cancer were the sampling unit, a list of all such hospitals would be the sampling frame. If certified adult nurse practitioners (NP) constituted the accessible population, a list of those nurses would be the sampling frame.

Once a list of the population elements has been developed, the best method of selecting a sample is to employ a table of random numbers containing columns of digits, such as the one appearing in Figure 12-1. Such tables can be generated by computer programs. After assigning consecutive numbers to units of the population, the researcher starts at any point on the table of random numbers and reads consecutive numbers in any direction (i.e., horizontally, vertically, or diagonally). When a number is read that corresponds with the written unit on a card, that unit is chosen for the sample. The investigator continues to read until a sample of the desired size is drawn. The advantages of simple random sampling are as follows:

- The sample selection is not subject to the conscious biases of the researcher.
- The representativeness of the sample in relation to the population characteristics is maximized.
- The differences in the characteristics of the sample and the population are purely a function of chance.
- The probability of choosing a nonrepresentative sample decreases as the size of the sample increases.

Simple random sampling was used in a study examining the relationship between nursing care requirements and nursing resource consumption in home health care using both an intensity index

1000 random integers between 0 and 99

40	23	0	29	10	94	17	58	12	85	13	25	80	84	72	74	54	63	55	31
32	98	49	23	74	97	51	42	21	87	48	64	54	38	84	68	14	17	35	48
84	34	84	14	53	65	67	37	2	45	84	21	71	34	10	80	72	27	11	13
86	37	24	89	23	4	44	40	72	81	44	69	25	44	34	34	34	75	50	50
50	58	85	8	22	24	73	20	63	35	60	87	91	92	96	80	19	22	87	24
1	87	43	82	9	31	40	88	33	28	82	73	18	6	48	64	59	45	34	3
21	19	42	76	84	67	29	68	8	66	93	89	96	28	12	14	38	47	52	65
32	66	33	21	81	97	39	76	67	27	97	22	76	89	41	11	91	29	6	66
16	82	42	75	35	42	92	90	77	24	21	8	36	16	5	54	89	51	57	85
74	32	63	65	93	96	18	36	82	72	39	69	37	97	51	17	36	71	38	30
50	94	4	66	17	37	10	53	8	29	67	74	88	38	11	59	60	91	56	17
71	47	81	18	53	98	7	87	29	37	22	93	13	6	95	7	95	71	14	6
71	93	48	16	33	19	46	21	60	44	52	91	52	58	10	9	41	31	35	18
20	94	13	99	45	6	53	54	1	25	79	28	1	48	36	26	68	37	59	7
75	22	69	56	62	40	64	45	40	99	94	14	98	84	22	38	24	87	43	71
16	87	41	0	88	83	11	37	71	78	22	39	43	37	75	84	84	11	55	58
92	90	80	2	30	37	85	55	56	50	3	71	24	13	62	74	82	44	90	32
96	89	31	32	37	45	70	67	80	55	58	9	55	60	61	55	86	44	27	77
38	29	36	94	65	39	56	29	29	65	88	13	71	38	71	8	81	66	31	44
20	6	61	66	90	13	70	60	92	53	87	49	34	42	14	47	75	33	26	9
63	44	94	21	14	13	41	80	39	72	29	3	25	89	44	88	13	49	18	58
13	32	93	90	31	75	86	95	18	51	61	59	84	95	67	54	40	30	29	63
26	35	48	81	19	24	36	36	76	16	46	5	93	41	97	46	79	54	95	49
89	74	96	95	94	69	31	60	16	69	76	42	28	71	69	34	46	55	20	42
50	39	28	64	20	68	60	33	92	82	61	70	5	68	95	88	12	85	18	94
55	86	5	96	87	69	75	93	54	79	0	57	45	8	86	59	25	21	9	29
75	35	1	2	86	62	70	83	85	13	97	37	13	73	16	38	36	23	54	11
74	50	1	77	87	92	68	87	57	36	17	47	0	97	78	72	72	45	54	51
34	24	35	13	26	42	22	75	47	2	34	87	15	50	65	27	5	72	28	68
73	33	42	65	91	24	44	84	71	55	70	1	27	30	8	61	65	61	18	92
7	55	12	6	61	17	23	95	91	58	60	30	35	61	34	27	75	44	35	64
10	94	18	4	3	19	21	37	28	55	76	25	10	29	80	64	8	81	20	32
20	48	92	87	95	58	57	73	42	1	12	81	94	85	63	97	24	19	93	51
81	10	92	49	70	15	76	4	36	92	62	99	78	32	86	74	43	22	98	46
66	67	82	94	67	75	16	88	84	98	0	52	37	0	43	9	0	51	2	62
64	92	36	11	3	52	44	65	45	67	97	86	92	2	50	5	93	66	73	40
36	29	98	46	88	23	28	44	8	71	69	43	53	16	87	21	56	23	37	24
15	11	82	30	59	94	23	30	40	25	87	26	24	30	44	53	33	65	72	55
89	57	49	79	83	88	42	45	41	93	38	24	15	80	97	18	61	12	13	42
23	36	65	9	64	26	93	37	26	44	42	17	45	68	27	77	74	56	49	34
9	93	90	61	45	40	75	85	64	66	36	89	72	43	99	90	92	10	10	85
53	94	30	31	62	92	82	30	94	56	40	4	50	53	9	74	87	2	36	36
18	69	77	38	89	78	30	68	71	92	22	93	91	74	52	1	97	69	71	42
50	20	76	36	6	20	75	56	36	5	14	70	9	78	23	33	91	33	25	72
30	46	1	10	16	72	69	26	94	39	80	36	36	68	92	74	22	74	41	42
59	47	7	92	77	55	2	12	5	24	0	30	25	62	83	36	92	96	36	75
93	22	3	20	82	44	16	69	98	72	30	57	77	15	90	29	32	38	3	48
9	55	27	41	40	94	77	14	54	10	25	75	1	74	72	15	69	80	33	58
70	8	3	5	46	89	28	86	40	6	25	40	81	26	63	97	87	48	26	41
19	6	89	31	80	60	13	89	17	69	38	93	58	55	54	69	74	33	8	55

Figure 12-1   A table of random numbers.

and nursing diagnoses. Using a table of random numbers, a random sample of 306 patient records was drawn from patients discharged during a 6-month period who received at least three nursing visits at home from a specific home health care agency.

Consumers must remember that despite the utilization of a carefully controlled sampling procedure that minimizes error, there is no guarantee that the sample will be representative. Factors such as sample heterogeneity and subject dropout may jeopardize the representativeness of the sample despite the most stringent random sampling procedure. In a study examining family perspectives about the final month of life for Oregon decedents dying in hospitals, nursing homes, and private homes, all death certificates for all Oregon deaths occurring in the 14 months between November 1996 and December 1997 were systematically randomly sampled, excluding decedents under age 18 years and deaths attributable to sucicide, homicide, accident, or those undergoing medical examiner review. Out of a sampling frame of n = 24,074, the systematic random sample yielded 1458 death certificates. A potential factor jeopardizing representativeness of this sample is due to the fact that although the name of a family contact is listed on each death certificate, Oregon death certificates do not list an address or telephone number for family contacts. As a result, case finding for family contacts was unsuccessful for 44% of the sample (Tolle et al, 2000).

The major disadvantage of simple random sampling is that it is a time-consuming and inefficient method of obtaining a random sample. (Consider the task of listing all of the baccalaureate nursing students in the United States.) With random sampling, it may also be impossible to obtain an accurate or complete listing of every element in the population. Imagine trying to obtain a list of all completed suicides in New York City for the year 2001. It often is the case that although suicide may have been the cause of death, another cause (e.g., cardiac failure) appears on the death certificate. It would be difficult to estimate how many elements

of the target population would be eliminated from consideration. The issue of bias would definitely enter the picture despite the researcher's best efforts. Thus the evaluator of a research paper must exercise caution in generalizing from reported findings, even when random sampling is the stated strategy, if the target population has been difficult or impossible to list completely.

Stratified Random Sampling

Stratified random sampling requires that the population be divided into strata or subgroups. The subgroups or subsets that the population is divided into are homogeneous. An appropriate number of elements from each subset are randomly selected on the basis of their proportion in the population. The goal of this strategy is to achieve a greater degree of representativeness. Stratified random sampling is similar to the proportional stratified quota sampling strategy discussed earlier in the chapter. The major difference is that stratified random sampling uses a random selection procedure for obtaining sample subjects. Figure 12-2 illustrates the use of stratified random sampling.

The population is stratified according to any number of attributes, such as age, gender, ethnicity, religion, socioeconomic status, or level of education completed. The variables selected to make up the strata should be adaptable to homogeneous subsets with regard to the attributes being studied. The following criteria can be used in the selection of a stratified sample:

- Is there a critical variable or attribute that provides a logical basis for stratifying the sample?
- Does the population list contain sufficient information about the attributes that will be used to divide the sample into subsets?
- Is it appropriate for each subset to be equal in size, or is it more appropriate for each subset to be proportionally stratified based on the proportion of each subset in the population?
- If proportional sampling is being used, is there a sufficient number of subjects in each subset for basing meaningful comparisons?

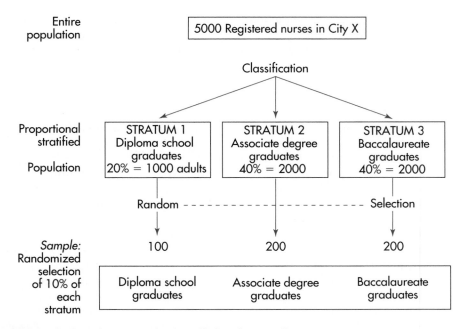

Entire
population

5000 Registered nurses in City X

Classification

Proportional
stratified

Population

| STRATUM 1 Diploma school graduates 20% = 1000 adults | STRATUM 2 Associate degree graduates 40% = 2000 | STRATUM 3 Baccalaureate graduates 40% = 2000 |

Random ─ ─ ─ ─ ─ ─ ─ ─ ─ ─ ─ ─ ─ ─ ─ ─ ─ Selection

Sample:
Randomized
selection
of 10% of
each
stratum

| 100 | 200 | 200 |
| Diploma school graduates | Associate degree graduates | Baccalaureate graduates |

Figure 12-2   Subject selection using a proportional stratified random sampling strategy.

• Once the subset comparison has been determined, are random procedures used for selection of the sample?

As illustrated in Table 12-1, there are several advantages to a stratified sampling strategy, as follows: (1) the representativeness of the sample is enhanced; (2) the researcher has a valid basis for making comparisons among subsets if information on the critical variables has been available; and (3) the researcher is able to oversample a disproportionately small stratum to adjust for their underrepresentation, statistically weigh the data accordingly, and continue to make legitimate comparisons.

The obstacles encountered by a researcher using this strategy include the following: (1) the difficulty of obtaining a population list containing complete critical variable information; (2) the time-consuming effort of obtaining multiple enumerated lists; (3) the challenge of enrolling proportional strata; and (4) the time and money involved in carrying out a large-scale study using a stratified sampling strategy. The critiquer must

question the appropriateness of this sampling strategy to the problem under investigation. For example, in an intervention study testing the effect of a support-boosting intervention on levels of stress, coping, and social support among caregivers of children with HIV/AIDS, caregivers were stratified a priori according to caregiver type (e.g., biological parent, extended family member, or foster parent) using computer-generated random numbers and then randomly assigning caregivers to study groups (Hansell et al, 1998). Stratification of the sample by caregiver type was conducted to achieve equal distribution of caregiver type between the experimental and control groups in proportion to the study population. It is appropriate for the researcher to strive to represent all strata proportionately in the study sample.

Multistage Sampling (Cluster Sampling)

Multistage (cluster) sampling involves a successive random sampling of units (clusters) that progress from large to small and meet sample eligibility criteria. The first-stage **sampling unit**

consists of large units or clusters. The second-stage sampling unit consists of smaller units or clusters. Third-stage sampling units are even smaller. For example, if a sample of nurse practitioners (NP) is desired, the first sampling unit would be a random sample of hospitals, obtained from an American Hospital Association list, that meet the eligibility criteria (e.g., size, type). The second-stage sampling unit would consist of a list of acute care nurse practitioners (ACNP) practicing at each hospital selected in the first stage (i.e., the list obtained from the vice president for nursing at each hospital). The criteria for inclusion in the list of ACNPs were as follows: (1) certified ACNP with at least 2 years experience as an ACNP; (2) at least 75% of the ACNP's time must be spent in providing direct patient care in acute or critical care practices; and (3) full-time employment at the hospital. The second-stage sampling strategy called for random selection of two ACNPs from each hospital who met the previously mentioned eligibility criteria.

When multistage sampling is used in relation to large national surveys, states are used as the first-stage sampling unit, followed by successively smaller units like counties, cities, districts, and blocks as the second-stage sampling unit, and then households as the third-stage sampling unit.

Sampling units or clusters can be selected by simple random or stratified random sampling methods. Suppose that the hospitals, described in the example above, were grouped into four strata according to size (i.e., number of beds), as follows: (1) 200 to 299; (2) 300 to 399; (3) 400 to 499; and (4) 500 or more. Stratum 1 comprised 25% of the population; stratum 2 comprised 30% of the population; stratum 3 comprised 20% of the population; and stratum 4 comprised 25% of the population. This means that either a simple random or a proportional, stratified sampling strategy is used to randomly select hospitals that would proportionately represent the population of hospitals in the American Hospital Association list.

The main advantage of cluster sampling, as illustrated in Table 12-1, is that it is considerably more economical in terms of time and money than other types of probability sampling, particularly when the population is large and geographically dispersed or a sampling frame of the elements is not available. There are two major disadvantages, as follows: (1) more sampling errors tend to occur than with simple random or stratified random sampling; and (2) the appropriate handling of the statistical data from cluster samples is very complex.

The critiquer of a research report will need to consider whether the use of cluster sampling is justified in light of the research design, as well as other pragmatic matters, such as economy. For example, using data from the 1994 Canadian National Population Health Survey, a study by Wolff and Ratner (1999) focused on sense of social coherence (SOC), the foundational concept of the Salutogenic Model of health maintenance, to explore the effects of stress, social support, and traumatic life events experienced during childhood and adulthood on SOC. A multistage stratified cluster design was used as the primary sampling method in all 10 Canadian provinces. Within the provinces, each sample was further stratified between major urban centers, urban towns, and rural areas; each area formed a separate geographic and/or socioeconomic stratum that reflected household responses. The target population included almost all residents of Canada, residents of Indian reserves, and Canadian Forces Bases. Because Canadians did not have an equal opportunity of participating within this complex sampling strategy, however, use of sampling weights permits generalization to the Canadian population.

Systematic Sampling

Systematic sampling refers to a sampling strategy that involves the selection of every "kth" case drawn from a population list at fixed intervals, such as every tenth member listed in the directory of the American Psychiatric Nurses Association. Systematic sampling might be used to sample every "kth" person to enter a hospital lobby or be hospitalized with a diagnosis of AIDS in 2002. When systematic sampling is used, the population must be narrowly defined as consisting, for example, of all those people entering or leaving for the sample to be considered as a probability sample. If senior citizens were sampled systematically upon entering a hospital lobby, the resulting sample would not be called a probability sample, because not every senior citizen would have a chance of being selected. As such, systematic sampling can sometimes represent a nonprobability sampling strategy.

Systematic sampling strategies can be designed, however, to fulfill the requirements of a probability sample. First, the listing of the population (sampling frame) must be random in relation to the variable of interest. For example, subjects were being selected from every tenth hospital room for a study on patient satisfaction with nursing care. Every tenth room happens to be a private room in the hospital where the study is being conducted. It is possible that the responses of patients in private rooms with regard to patient satisfaction might be different from those of patients in semiprivate rooms. Because of the nonrandom arrangement of the rooms, bias may have been introduced.

Second, the first element or member of the sample must be selected randomly. In this case, the researcher—who has a population list or sampling frame—first divides the population (N) by the size of the desired sample (n) to obtain the sampling interval width (k). The **sampling interval** is the standard distance between the elements chosen for the sample. For example, to select a sample of 50 family nurse practitioners from a population of 500 family nurse practitioners, the sampling interval would be as follows:

$$k = \frac{500}{50} = 100$$

Essentially, every tenth case on the family nurse practitioner list would be sampled. Once the sampling interval has been determined, the researcher uses a table of random numbers (see Figure 12-1) to obtain a starting point for the selection of the 50 subjects. If the population size is 500 and a sample size of 50 is desired, a number between 1 and 500 is randomly selected as the starting point. In this instance, if the first number is 51, the family nurse practitioners corresponding to numbers 51, 61, 71, and so forth, would be included in the sample of 50. Another procedure recommended in many texts is to randomly select the first element from within the first sampling interval. If the sampling interval is 5, a number between 1 and 5 is selected as the random starting point. For example, the number 3 is randomly chosen. Keeping in mind the sampling interval of 5, the next elements selected would correspond to the numbers 8, 13, 18, and so on, until the sample was obtained. Although this procedure is technically correct, choosing a random starting point from across the total population of elements is more attractive because every element has a chance to be chosen for the sample during the first selection step.

Systematic sampling and simple random sampling are essentially the same type of procedure. The advantage of systematic sampling is that the results are obtained in a more convenient and efficient manner (see Table 12-1). The disadvantage of systematic sampling is that bias in the form of nonrandomness can inadvertently be introduced to the procedure. This problem may occur if the population list is arranged so that a certain type of element is listed at intervals that coincide with the sampling interval. Let us say that if every tenth nursing student on a population list of all types of nursing students in Illinois were a baccalaureate student and the sampling interval was 10, baccalaureate students would be overrepresented in the sample. Cyclical fluctuations are also a factor. For example, if a list of nursing students using the college library each day to do computer literature searches is kept, a biased sample will probably be obtained if every seventh day is chosen as the sampling interval because fewer and perhaps different nursing students probably use the library on Sundays than on weekdays. Therefore caution must be exercised about departures from randomness as they affect the representativeness of the sample and, as a result, affect the external validity of the study.

The critiquer will want to note whether a satisfactory random selection procedure was carried out. If randomization was not used, the systematic sampling may have become a nonprobability quota sample. It is important to be cognizant of this issue because the implications related to interpretation and generalizability are drastically altered if the evaluator is dealing with a nonprobability sample. For example, in their study, Boyer, Wade, and Madigan (2000) sought to determine whether patients in need of postacute services after cardiothoracic surgery could be identified during preadmission testing and included the records of all patients who had been seen in a cardiothoracic preadmission testing area before cardiothoracic surgery during a 3-month pilot program. A variety of cardiothoracic procedures was included in this sample, and all subjects were stratified by procedure (e.g., coronary artery bypass graft [CABG], valve surgery with or without CABG, or other cardiac surgery). Because randomization was not used at any phase of the sampling procedure, the evaluator would consider this to be a non-probability stratified sample with the external validity limitations of that sampling strategy (see Chapter 9).

In contrast, in a study investigating the effect of comprehensive, multidisciplinary maternity care (Genesis Program) on maternity outcomes in a matched sample of pregnant women of low socioeconomic class, a systematic sampling procedure was used (Lowry and Beikirch, 1998). Data on Genesis clients were retrieved by a retrospective chart review in which the sample was randomly selected from 1200 charts of the women who presented for prenatal care during the first fully operational year of the Genesis program and who delivered between July 1, 1991 and July 1, 1992. Every sixth chart was reviewed for a total of 200 Genesis records and a similar number of matched subject charts for subjects who had received care from county public health units and one of the local migrant clinics. Because random selection was used in this example of systematic sampling, the critiquer could have more confidence in the generalizability of the findings to a similar target population.

SPECIAL SAMPLING STRATEGIES

Several special sampling strategies are used in nonprobability sampling. **Matching** is a special strategy used to construct an equivalent comparison sample group by filling it with subjects who are similar to each subject in another sample group in relation to preestablished variables such as age, gender, level of education, medical diagnosis, or socioeconomic status. Theoretically, any variable other than the independent variable that could affect the dependent variable should be matched. In reality, the more variables matched, the more difficult it is to obtain an adequate sample size. For example, matching was used in a study that sought to identify the factors (e.g., mother and father's perception of parenting stress, child's prematurity status, socioeconomic status) or combination of factors that predicted the development of healthy pre-term and full-term children at 18 months (adjusted age). In this sample, pre-term infants were matched with full-term infants by gender, expected due date (within 1 week) and hospital of birth (Magill-Evans and Harrison, 1999). When an organization or institution composes the sampling unit, matching may also be an important consideration. In the study by Bull, Hansen, and Gross (2000), which studied the effect of the professional-patient partnership model of discharge planning on health outcomes for elders hospitalized with heart failure, two hospitals were matched in terms of size, type, and discharge-planning practices used in cardiac units. One hospital was randomly selected for implementation of the partnership model intervention, and the other hospital was the control site.

Networking sampling, sometimes referred to as snowballing, is a strategy used for locating samples that are difficult or impossible to locate in other ways. This sampling strategy takes advantage of social networks and the fact that friends tend to have characteristics in common. When a few subjects with the necessary eligibility criteria are found, the researcher asks for their assistance in getting in touch with others with similar criteria. For example, Thomas (2000) used networking and snowballing to obtain participants

Assessing the Relationship between the Type of Sampling Strategy and the Appropriate Generalizability

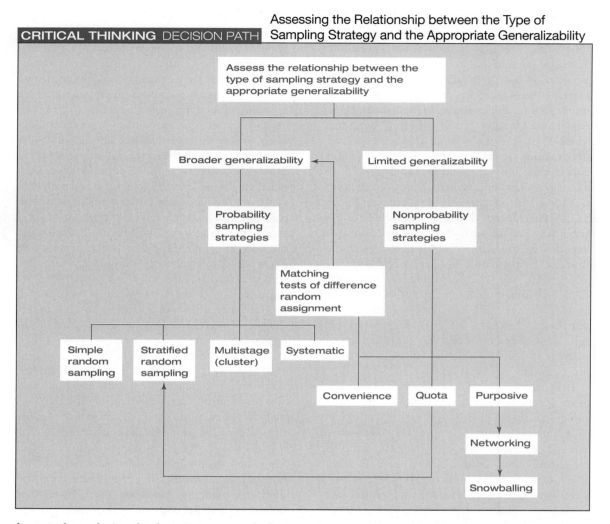

for a study exploring the deeper meaning of what it is like to live with chronic pain. Individuals were recruited for the study via a newspaper article and network sampling techniques (i.e., contacts with colleagues, friends, and community members), as well as word-of-mouth referrals by interview participants—all of which capture the essence of the network **(snowball effect)** sampling strategy that resulted in a diverse sample of 13 individuals experiencing chronic pain. Today, on-line computer networks, as described in the section on purposive sampling, can be used to assist researchers in acquiring otherwise difficult to

locate subjects, thereby taking advantage of the networking or snowball effect. The Critical Thinking Decision Path illustrates the relationship between the type of sampling strategy and the appropriate generalizability.

HELPFUL HINT Look for a brief discussion of a study's sampling strategy in the "Methods" section of a research article. Sometimes there is a separate subsection with the heading "Sample, Subjects, or Study Participants." A statistical description of the characteristics of the actual sample often does not appear until the "Results" section of a research article.

SAMPLE SIZE

There is no single rule that can be applied to the determination of a sample's size. When arriving at an estimate of sample size, many factors, such as the following, must be considered:

- The type of design used
- The type of sampling procedure used
- The type of formula used for estimating optimum sample size
- The degree of precision required
- The heterogeneity of the attributes under investigation
- The relative frequency that the phenomenon of interest occurs in the population (i.e., a common vs. a rare health problem)
- The projected cost of using a particular sampling strategy

The sample size should be determined before the study is conducted. A general rule of thumb is always to use the largest sample possible. The larger the sample, the more representative of the population it is likely to be; smaller samples produce less accurate results.

One exception to this principle occurs when using certain qualitative designs. In this case, sample size is not predetermined. Sample sizes in qualitative research tend to be small because of the large volume of verbal data that must be analyzed and because this type of design tends to emphasize intensive and prolonged contact with subjects (Streubert and Carpenter, 1999). Subjects are added to the sample until **data saturation** is reached (i.e., new data no longer emerge during the data-collection process). Fittingness of the data is a more important concern than representativeness of subjects (see Chapter 7).

Another exception is in the case of a **pilot study,** which is defined as a small sample study, conducted as a prelude to a larger-scale study that is often called the "parent study." The pilot study is typically a smaller scale of the parent study with similar methods and procedures that yield preliminary data that determine the feasibility of conducting a larger scale study and establish that sufficient scientific evidence exists to justify sub-

sequent, more extensive research (Jaireth, Hogerney, and Parsons, 2000). For example, Hoskins and associates (in press) conducted a pilot study, "Breast Cancer: Education, Counseling and Adjustment," using a small sample (n = 12) to determine the feasibility of and analyze preliminary data about the differential effect of a standardized phase-specific educational and telephone counseling intervention for women with breast cancer and their partners prior to conducting the parent study, a randomized clinical trial that would have a sample size of n = 240.

The principle of "larger is better" holds true for both probability and nonprobability samples. Results based on small samples (under 10) tend to be unstable—the values fluctuate from one sample to the next. Small samples tend to increase the probability of obtaining a markedly nonrepresentative sample. As the sample size increases, the mean more closely approximates the population values, thus introducing fewer sampling errors.

An example of this concept is illustrated by a study in which the average monthly sleeping pill consumption is being investigated for patients on a rehabilitation unit after a cerebrovascular accident. The data in Table 12-3 indicate that the population consists of 20 patients whose average consumption of sleeping pills is 15.15 per month. Two simple random samples with sample sizes of 2, 4, 6, and 10 have been drawn from the population of 20 patients. Each sample average in the right-hand column represents an estimate of the population average, which is known to be 15.15. In most cases, the population value is unknown to the researchers, but because the population is so small, it could be calculated. As we examine the data in Table 12-3, we note that with a sample size of 2, the estimate might have been wrong by as much as 8 sleeping pills in sample 1B. As the sample size increases, the averages get closer to the population value, and the differences in the estimates between samples A and B also get smaller. Large samples permit the principles of randomization to work effectively (i.e., to counterbalance atypical values in the long run).

TABLE **12-3** Comparison of Population and Sample Values and Averages in Study of Sleeping Pill Consumption

NUMBER IN GROUP	GROUP	NUMBER OF SLEEPING PILLS CONSUMED (VALUES EXPRESSED MONTHLY)	AVERAGE
20	Population	1, 3, 4, 5, 6, 7, 9, 11, 13, 15, 16, 17, 19, 21, 22, 23, 25, 27, 29, 30	15.15
2	Sample 1A	6, 9	7.5
2	Sample 1B	21, 25	23.0
4	Sample 2A	1, 7, 15, 25	12.0
4	Sample 2B	5, 13, 23, 29	17.5
6	Sample 3A	3, 4, 11, 15, 21, 25	13.3
6	Sample 3B	5, 7, 11, 19, 27, 30	16.5
10	Sample 4A	3, 4, 7, 9, 11, 13, 17, 21, 23, 30	13.8
10	Sample 4B	1, 4, 6, 11, 15, 17, 19, 23, 25, 27	14.8

It is possible to estimate the sample size with the use of a statistical procedure known as power analysis (Cohen, 1977). It is beyond the scope of this chapter to describe this complex procedure in great detail, but a simple example will illustrate its use. A researcher wants to determine the effect of nurse preoperative teaching on patient postoperative anxiety. Patients are randomly assigned to an experimental group or a control group. How many patients should be used in the study? When using power analysis, the researcher must estimate how large of a difference will be observed between the groups (i.e., the difference in the mean amount of postoperative anxiety after the experimental preoperative teaching program). If a small difference is expected, the sample must be large (in this case, 196 patients in each group) to ensure that the differences will actually be revealed in a statistical analysis. If a medium-size difference is expected, the total sample size would be 128—64 in each group. When expected differences are large, it does not take a very large sample to ensure that differences will be revealed through statistical analysis. Power analysis is an advanced statistical technique that is commonly used by researchers and is a requirement for external funding. When it is not used, research studies may be

based on samples that are too small. When samples are too small, the researcher may have unsupported hypotheses and commit a type I error of rejecting a null hypothesis when it should have been accepted (see Chapter 17). A researcher may also commit a type II error of accepting a null hypothesis when it should have been rejected if the sample is too small (see Chapter 17).

Despite the principles related to determining sample size that have been identified, the consumer should be aware that large samples do not ensure representativeness or accuracy. A large sample cannot compensate for a faulty research design. The proportion of the population that is sampled does not provide a guarantee of accurate results. It is often possible to obtain accurate results from only a small fraction of a large population. For example, a 10% probability sample of a population containing 1500 elements will yield more precise results than a nonprobability 0.01% sample of a population with 100,000 elements.

The critiquer should evaluate the sample size in terms of the following: (1) how representative the sample is relative to the target population, and (2) to whom the researcher wishes to generalize the results of the study. The goal of sampling is to have a sample as representative as possible with as little sampling error as possible. Unless representativeness is ensured, all the data in the world become inconsequential.

HELPFUL HINT Remember to look for some rationale about the sample size and those strategies the researcher has used (e.g., matching, test of differences on demographic variables) to ascertain or build in sample representativeness.

SAMPLING PROCEDURES

The criteria for drawing a sample vary according to the sampling strategy. Regardless of which strategy is used, it is important that the procedure be systematically organized. This organization will eliminate the bias that occurs when sample selection is carried out inconsistently. Bias in sample representativeness and generalizability of findings are important sampling issues that have generated national concern. Many of the landmark adult health studies (e.g., the Framingham heart study and the Baltimore longitudinal study on aging) historically excluded women as subjects. Despite the all-male samples, the findings of these studies were generalized from males to all adults despite the lack of female representation in the samples. Similarly, the use of largely Euro-American subjects in medication clinical trials limits the identification of variant responses to drugs in ethnic or racially distinct groups (Campinha-Bacote, 1997). Findings based on Euro-American data cannot be generalized to African-Americans, Asians, Hispanics, or any other cultural group. Consequently, careful identification of the target population is a crucial step in the process. If a researcher wants to be able to draw conclusions about psychosocial stressors related to all patients with a first-time myocardial infarction, then both males and females must be included in the target population. When a researcher wants to be able to draw conclusions about the incidence of extrapyramidal side effects of haloperidol (Haldol) in African-American psychiatric patients compared to Euro-Americans, the target population must be diverse. Sometimes the target population has to be gender-

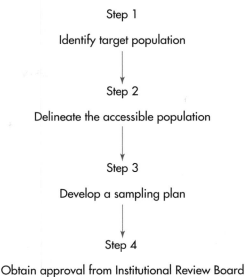

Step 1

Identify target population

Step 2

Delineate the accessible population

Step 3

Develop a sampling plan

Step 4

Obtain approval from Institutional Review Board

Figure 12-3 Summary of general sampling procedure.

specific, as when breast or prostate cancer or aspects of pregnancy or menopause are studied.

Several general steps, as illustrated in Figure 12-3, that will ensure a consistent approach by the researcher can be identified. Initially, the target population (i.e., the entire group of people or objects about whom the researcher wants to draw conclusions or make generalizations) must be identified. The target population may consist of all female patients with a first-time diagnosis of breast cancer, all children with asthma, all pregnant teenagers, or all doctoral students in the United States. Next, the accessible portion of the target population must be delineated. An accessible population might consist of all of the NPs in the state of California, all of the male patients with AIDS admitted to hospital X during 2001, all of the pregnant teenagers in a specific prenatal clinic, or all of the children with rheumatoid arthritis under care at a specific hospital specializing in treatment of autoimmune diseases. Then a sampling plan or a protocol for actually selecting the sample from the accessible population is formulated. The researcher makes decisions about how subjects will be approached, how the study will be explained, and who will select the sample—the researcher or a research assistant. Regardless of who implements the sampling plan, consistency in how it is done is paramount. The reader of a research study will want to find a description of the sample, as well as the sampling procedure, in the report. On the basis of the appropriateness of what has been reported, the critiquer can make judgments about the soundness of the sampling protocol, which of course will affect the interpretations made about the findings. Finally, once the accessible population and sampling plan have been established, permission is obtained from the institution's research board, which is commonly referred to as the Institutional Review Board. This permission provides free access to the desired population.

When an appropriate sample size and sampling strategy have been used, the researcher can feel more confident that the sample is representative of the accessible population; however, it is more difficult to feel confident that the accessible population is representative of the target population. Are NPs in California representative of all NPs in the United States? It is impossible to be sure about this. Researchers must exercise judgment when assessing typicality. Unfortunately there are no guidelines for making such judgments, and there is even less basis for the critiquer to make such decisions. The best rule of thumb to use when evaluating the representativeness of a sample and its generalizability to the target population is to be realistic and conservative about making sweeping claims relative to the findings.

HELPFUL HINT Remember to evaluate the appropriateness of the generalizations made about the study findings in light of the target population, the accessible population, the type of sampling strategy, and the sample size.

CRITIQUING the Sample

The criteria for critiquing the sampling technique of a study are presented in the Critiquing Criteria box. The research consumer approaches the "Sample" section of a research report with a different perspective than the researcher. The consumer must raise two questions: "If this study were to be replicated, would there be enough information presented about the nature of the population, the sample, the sampling strategy, and sample size of another investigator to carry out the study?" and "Are the previously mentioned factors appropriate in light of the particular research design, and if not, which factors require modification, especially if the study is to be replicated?"

Sampling is considered to be one important aspect of the methodology of a research study. As such, data pertaining to the sample usually appear in the "Methodology" section of the research report. The sampling content presented should reflect the outcome of a series of decisions based on sampling criteria appropriate to the design of the study, as well as the options and limitations inherent in the context of the investigation. The following discussion will highlight several sampling criteria that the research consumer will want to consider when evaluating the merit of a sampling strategy as it relates to a specific research study.

Initially, the parameters or attributes of the study population should clearly specify to what population the findings may be generalized. In general, the target population of the study is not specifically identified by the researcher, but the nature of it is implied in the description of the accessible population and/or the sample. For example, if a researcher states that 100 subjects were randomly drawn from a population of men and women over 65 years of age diagnosed with chronic obstructive pulmonary disease who were treated in a respiratory rehabilitation program at hospital X during 2001, the critiquer can specifically evaluate the parameters of the population. Demographic characteristics of the sample (e.g., age, gender, diagnosis, ethnicity, religion, and marital status) should also be presented in either a tabled or a narrative summary because they provide further explication about the nature of the sample and enable the cri-

---

CRITIQUING CRITERIA

1. Have the sample characteristics been completely described?
2. Can the parameters of the study population be inferred from the description of the sample?
3. To what extent is the sample representative of the population as defined?
4. Are criteria for eligibility in the sample specifically identified?
5. Have sample delimitations been established?
6. Would it be possible to replicate the study population?
7. How was the sample selected? Is the method of sample selection appropriate?
8. What kind of bias, if any, is introduced by this method?
9. Is the sample size appropriate? How is it substantiated?
10. Are there indications that rights of subjects have been ensured?
11. Does the researcher identify the limitations in generalizability of the findings from the sample to the population? Are they appropriate?
12. Does the researcher indicate how replication of the study with other samples would provide increased support for the findings?

---

tiquer to evaluate the sampling procedure more accurately. For example, in their study titled "A Professional-Patient Partnership Model of Discharge Planning with Elders Hospitalized with Heart Failure," Bull, Hansen, and Gross (2000) present detailed data summarizing demographic variables of importance. These data are reproduced as follows:

The average age of the patients was 73.7 years (SD = 8.8; range is 55 to 94), and their education level ranged from seventh grade through graduate school, with a mean of 12 years of schooling (SD = 2.5). The majority of the patients were white (93.6%). Caregivers ranged in age from 20 to 86 years, with a mean of 58.5 years (SD = 14.9), and their mean level of education was 12.9 years of schooling (SD = 2.2). The majority of the caregivers were white (93.6%) and female (73%). Half of the caregivers were spouses of the patient, 28.6% were daughters, 9.8% were sons, 7.1% were siblings or grandchildren, and 4.5% were friends. The patients had been hospitalized for either a primary (67.2%) or secondary (32.8%) diagnosis of congestive heart failure (see Appendix A).

This example illustrates how a detailed description of the sample both provides the critiquer with a frame of reference for the study population and sample and generates questions to be raised. For instance, the critiquer will note the variability in the range of age of both the elder subjects (55 to 94 years) and their caregivers (20 to 86 years). The evaluator who has this demographic sample information available is able to question a sampling strategy that does not

also consider the differential effect of age or type of relationship on the professional-patient partnership model of discharge planning. It would seem logical that there might be a difference in the caregiver's response to caregiving in a 20- to 40-year-old cohort vs. a 60- to 80-year-old cohort, as well as whether the caregiver was a spouse, adult child, or grandchild.

It is also helpful if the researcher has presented a rationale for having elected to study one type of population vs. another. For example, why did the previously cited study focus only on elders who had a diagnosis of primary or secondary heart failure as opposed to including elders with a diverse array of cardiac diagnoses (e.g., myocardial infarction, angina, coronary artery bypass graft surgery, cardiac valve replacement)? In a research study that uses a nonprobability sampling strategy, it is particularly important to fully describe the population and the sample in terms of who the study subjects are, the way they were chosen, and the reason they were chosen. If these criteria are adhered to, the degree of heterogeneity or homogeneity of the sample can be determined. The use of a homogeneous sample minimizes the amount of sampling error introduced, a problem particularly common in nonprobability sampling.

Next, the defined representativeness of the population should be examined. Probability sampling is clearly the ideal sampling procedure for ensuring the representativeness of a study population. Use of random selection procedures (e.g., simple random, stratified, cluster, or systematic sampling strategies) minimizes the occurrence of conscious and unconscious biases, which affect the researcher's ability to generalize about the findings from the sample to the population. The critiquer should be able to identify the type of probability strategy used and determine whether the researcher adhered to the criteria for a particular sampling plan. In experimental and quasiexperimental studies, the evaluator must also know whether or how the subjects were assigned to groups. If the criteria have not been followed, the reader has a valid basis for being cautious about the proposed conclusions of the study.

Although random selection is the ideal in establishing the representativeness of a study population, more often realistic barriers (e.g., institutional policy, inaccessibility of subjects, lack of time or money, and current state of knowledge in the field) necessitate the use of nonprobability sampling strategies. Many important research problems that are of interest to nursing do not lend themselves to experimental design and probability sampling. This is particularly true with qualitative research designs. A well-designed, carefully controlled study using a nonprobability sampling strategy can yield accurate and meaningful findings that make a significant contribution to nursing's scientific body of knowledge. As the critiquer, you must ask a philosophical question: "If it is not possible or appropriate to conduct an experimental or quasiexperimental investigation that uses probability sampling, should the study be abandoned?" The answer usually suggests that it is better to carry out the investigation and be fully aware of the limitations of the methodology than to lose the knowledge that can be gained. The researcher is always able to move on to subsequent studies that either replicate the study or use more stringent design and sampling strategies to refine the knowledge derived from a nonexperimental study.

The greatest difficulty in nonprobability sampling stems from the fact that not every element in the population has an equal chance of being represented in the sample. Therefore it is likely that some segment of the population will be systematically underrepresented. If the population is homogeneous on critical characteristics, systematic bias will not be very important. Few of the attributes that researchers are interested in, however, are sufficiently homogeneous to render sampling bias an irrelevant consideration.

Next, the sampling plan's suitability to the research design should be evaluated. Experimental and quasiexperimental designs use some form of random selection or random assignment of subjects to groups (see Chapter 10). The critiquer evaluates whether the researcher adhered to the principles of random selection and assignment. Lack of adherence to such principles compromises the representativeness of the sample and the external validity of the study. The following are questions the evaluator might pose relative to this issue:

- Has a random selection procedure (e.g., a table of random numbers) been identified?
- Has the appropriate random sampling plan been selected; that is, has a proportional stratified sampling plan been selected instead of a simple random sampling plan in a study where there are three distinct occupational levels that appear to be critical variables for stratification?
- Has the particular random sampling plan been carried out appropriately; that is, if a cluster sampling strategy was used, did the sampling units logically progress from the largest to the smallest?

Random sampling should not be looked on as a cure-all. Sometimes bias is inadvertently introduced even when the principle of random selection is used.

Nonexperimental designs often use nonprobability sampling strategies. In this instance, the question that can be raised by the critiquer is whether a nonexperimental design and a related nonprobability sampling plan were most appropriate for this study. It is sometimes true that if the researcher had used another type of design or sampling plan, he or she could have constructed a stronger study that would have allowed more generalizability and greater confidence to be placed in the findings. The critiquer, however, is rarely in a position to know what factors entered into the decision to plan one type of study vs. another.

When critiquing qualitative research designs, the evaluator applies criteria related to sampling strategies that are relevant for a particular type of qualitative study. In general, sampling strategies are purposive because the study of specific phenomenon in their natural setting is emphasized; any subject belonging to a specified group is considered to represent that group. For example, when a qualitative study such as "Bone Marrow Transplantation: the Battle for Hope in the Face of Fear" (Cohen and Ley, 2000) is conducted, the specified group is people with cancer who are autologous bone marrow transplant survivors. The researcher's goal is to establish the meaning of their slices of life; that is, the typicality or atypicality of the observed events, behaviors, or responses in the lives of the bone marrow transplant survivors in order to better understand the effect of this treatment on peoples' lives and how nursing can best meet their needs (see Chapters 6 and 7 and Appendix B).

The evaluator should then determine whether the sample size is appropriate and its size is justifiable. It is common for the researcher to indicate in a research article how the sample size was determined; this is also seen commonly in doctoral dissertations. The method of arriving at the sample size and the rationale should be briefly mentioned. For example, a researcher may state in a very detailed way:

Based on a power analysis (Cohen, 1977), it was estimated that if the sample size diminished to 40 per group, there would remain a 60% chance of detecting a treatment effect of ½ standard deviation and a 90% chance of detecting a treatment effect of ¾ standard deviation (two-tailed alpha = 0.05). Allowing for a 25% attrition rate, target sample size was set for 60 subjects per group (Swanson, 1999).

The importance of this example lies not in understanding every technical word cited, but in understanding that this type of statement or some abbreviated form of it meets the criteria stated at the beginning of the paragraph and should be evident on the research report.

Other considerations with respect to sample size, especially when the sample size appears to be small or inadequate and there is no stated rationale for the size, are as follows:

- How will the sample size affect the accuracy of the results?
- Are any subsets or cells of the sample overrepresented or underrepresented?
- Are any of the subsets so small as to limit meaningful comparisons?

- Has the researcher examined the effect of attrition or dropouts on the results?
- Has the researcher recognized and identified any limitations posed by the size of the sample?

Essentially, these criteria demand that the critiquer carefully scrutinize several important elements pertaining to sample size that have implications for the generalizability of the findings. Keep in mind that qualitative studies will not discuss predetermining sample size or method of arriving at sample size. Rather, sample size will tend to be small and a function of data saturation (see Chapter 7).

Finally, evidence that the rights of human subjects have been protected should appear in the "Sample" section of the research report. The critiquer will evaluate whether permission was obtained from an institutional review board that reviewed the study relative to the maintenance of ethical research standards (see Chapter 13). For example, the review board examines the research proposal to determine whether the introduction of an experimental procedure may be potentially harmful and therefore undesirable. The critiquer also examines the report for evidence of the subjects' informed consent, as well as protection of their confidentiality or anonymity. It is highly unusual for research studies not to demonstrate evidence of having met these criteria. Nevertheless, the careful critiquer will want to be certain that ethical standards that protect sample subjects have been maintained.

It is evident that there are many factors to consider when critiquing the "Sample" section of a research report. The type and appropriateness of the sampling strategy become crucial elements in the analysis and interpetation of data, in the conclusions derived from the findings, and in the generalizability of the findings from the sample to the population. As stated earlier in this chapter, the major purpose of sampling is to increase the efficiency of a research study by using a sample that is representative of the particular population so that every element need not be studied, and yet generalizing the findings from the sample to the population. The critiquer must justify that the sampling strategy used provided a valid basis for the findings and their generalizability in order to feel confident.

| Critical Thinking Challenges | *Barbara Krainovich-Miller* |

➤ A research classmate asks the instructor the following question: "Why isn't it better to study an entire population of patients with lung cancer instead of using the research technique of sampling?" How would you answer this question? Include examples that will help the student see it from your point of view.

➤ A quasiexperimental study indicates that it used a convenience sample with random assignment. How is this possible? Would this be a nonprobability or probability sample? If you agree that this is a legitimate sampling technique, present both the advantages and the disadvantages; if you disagree, indicate your rationale.

➤ Your research class is having a debate on probability vs. nonprobability sampling in regard to desirability and feasibility. You are assigned to present the pros of nonprobability sampling in nursing research. What arguments would you use?

➤ Discuss the principle of "larger is better" and its relationship to "networking" sampling and the sample size of qualitative studies. Include in your discussion the concept of "data saturation," as well as the use of computer technology.

➤ Your research classmate is arguing that a random sample is always better, even if it is small and represents only one site. Another student is arguing that a very large convenience sample representing multiple sites can be very significant. Which classmate would you defend and why?

Key Points

- Sampling is a process that selects representative units of a population for study. Researchers sample representative segments of the population because it is rarely feasible or necessary to sample entire populations of interest to obtain accurate and meaningful information.

- Researchers establish eligibility criteria; these are descriptors of the population and provide the basis for selection into a sample. Eligibility criteria, which are also referred to as delimitations, include the following: age, gender, socioeconomic status, level of education, religion, and ethnicity.

- The researcher must identify the target population (i.e., the entire set of cases about which the researcher would like to make generalizations). Because of the pragmatic constraints, however, the researcher usually utilizes an accessible population (i.e., one that meets the population criteria and is available).

- A sample is a set of elements that makes up the population.

- A sampling unit is the element or set of elements used for selecting the sample. The foremost criterion in evaluating a sample is the representativeness or congruence of characteristics with the population.

- Sampling strategies consist of nonprobability and probability sampling.

- In nonprobability sampling, the elements are chosen by nonrandom methods. Types of nonprobability sampling include convenience, quota, and purposive sampling.

- Probability sampling is characterized by the random selection of elements from the population. In random selection, each element in the population has an equal and independent chance of being included in the sample. Types of probability sampling include simple random, stratified random, cluster, and systematic sampling.

- Sample size is a function of the type of sampling procedure being used, the degree of precision required, the type of sample estimation formula being used, the heterogeneity of the study attributes, the relative frequency of occurrence of the phenomena under consideration, and cost.

- Criteria for drawing a sample vary according to the sampling strategy. Systematic organization of the sampling procedure minimizes bias. The target population is identified, the accessible portion of the target population is delineated, permission to conduct the research study is obtained, and a sampling plan is formulated.

- The critiquer of a research report evaluates the sampling plan for its appropriateness in relation to the particular research design. Completeness of the sampling plan is examined in light of potential replicability of the study. The critiquer evaluates whether the sampling strategy is the strongest plan for the particular study under consideration.
- An appropriate systematic sampling plan will maximize the efficiency of a research study. It will increase the accuracy and meaningfulness of the findings and enhance the generalizability of the findings from the sample to the population.

REFERENCES

Anderson B, Higgins L, and Rozmus C: Critical pathways: application to selected patient outcomes following coronary artery bypass graft, *Appl Nurs Res* 12(4):168-174, 1999.

Bouve LR, Rozmus CL, and Giordano P: Preparing parents for their child's transfer from the PICU to the pediatric floor, *Appl Nurs Res* 12(3):114-120, 1999.

Boyer CL, Wade DC, and Madigan EA: Prescreening cardiothoracic surgical patient population for post acute care services, *Outcomes Management Nurs Pract* 4(4):167-171, 2000.

Bull MJ, Hansen HE, and Gross CR: A professional-patient partnership model of discharge planning with elders hospitalized with heart failure, *Appl Nurs Res* 13(1):19-28, 2000.

Campinha-Bacote J: Understanding the influence of culture. In Haber J et al, editors: *Comprehensive psychiatric nursing,* ed 5, St Louis, 1997, Mosby.

Cohen J: *Statistical power analysis for the behavioral sciences,* New York, 1977, Academic Press.

Cohen MZ and Ley CD: Bone marrow transplantation: the battle for hope in the face of fear, *Oncol Nurs Forum* 27(3):473-480, 2000.

Grey M et al: Coping skills training for youths with diabetes on intensive therapy, *Appl Nurs Res* 12(1):3-12, 1999.

Hansell PS et al: The effect of a social support boosting intervention on stress, coping, and social support in caregivers of children with HIV/AIDs, *Nurs Res* 47(2):79-86, 1998.

Hoskins CN et al: Breast cancer: education, counseling and adjustment: a pilot study, *Psychologic Reports,* in press.

Jaireth N, Hogerney M, and Parsons C: The role of the pilot study: a case illustration from cardiac nursing research, *Appl Nurs Res* 13(2):92-96, 2000.

Jarrett M et al: The relationship between psychological distress and gastrointestinal symptoms in women with irritable bowel syndrome, *Nurs Res* 47(3):154-161, 1998.

King KB, Rowe MA, and Zerwic JJ: Concerns and risk factor modification in women during the year after coronary artery surgery, *Appl Nurs Res* 49(3):167-172, 2000.

LoBiondo-Wood G et al: Family adaptation to a child's transplant: pretransplant phase, *Progress in Transplantation* 16(2):1-5, 2000.

Lowry LW and Beikirch P: Effect of comprehensive care on pregnancy outcomes, *Appl Nurs Res* 11(2):55-61, 1998.

Magill-Evans J and Harrison MJ: Parent-child interactions and development of toddlers born preterm, *West J Nurs Res* 21(3):292-312, 1999.

Meininger JC et al: Genetic and environmental influences on cardiovascular disease risk factors in adolescents, *Nurs Res* 47(1):11-18, 1998.

Streubert HJ and Carpenter DR: *Qualitative research in nursing,* ed 2, Philadelphia, 1999, JB Lippincott.

Swanson KM: Effects of caring, measurement, and time on miscarriage impact and women's well-being, *Nurs Res* 48(6):288-298, 1999.

Tolle SW et al: Family reports of barriers to optimal care of the dying, *Nurs Res* 49(6):310-317, 2000.

Thomas SP: A phenomenologic study of chronic pain, *West J Nurs Res* 22(6):683-705, 2000.

Wilmoth MC: Computer networks as a source of research subjects, *West J Nurs Res* 17(3):335-338, 1995.

Wolff AC and Ratner PA: Stress, social support, and sense of coherence, *West J Nurs Res* 21(2):182-197, 1999.

ADDITIONAL READINGS

Demi AS and Warren NA: Issues in conducting research with vulnerable families, *West J Nurs Res* 17(2):188-202, 1995.

Nield-Anderson L, Dixon JK, and Lee K: Random assignment and patient choice in a study of alternative pain relief for sickle cell disease, *West J Nurs Res* 21(2):266-274, 1999.

Orsi AJ et al: Conceptual and technical considerations when combining large data sets, *West J Nurs Res* 21(2):130-142, 1999.

Porter EJ: Defining the eligible accessible population for a phenomenological study, *West J Nurs Res* 21(6):796-803, 1999.

Salyer J et al: Commitment and communication: keys to minimizing attrition in multisite longitudinal organizational studies, *Nurs Res* 47(2):123-125, 1998.

Timmerman GM: The art of advertising for research subjects, *Nurs Res* 45(6):339-340, 1996.

JUDITH HABER

Legal and Ethical Issues

13

Key Terms

animal rights
anonymity
assent
beneficence
benefits
confidentiality

consent
ethics
informed consent
institutional review boards
 (IRBs)
justice

product testing
respect for persons
risk-benefit ratio
risks

Learning Outcomes

After reading this chapter, the student should be able to do the following:

- Describe the historical background that led to the development of ethical guidelines for the use of human subjects in research.
- Identify the essential elements of an informed consent form.
- Evaluate the adequacy of an informed consent form.
- Describe the institutional review board's role in the research review process.
- Identify populations of subjects who require special legal and ethical research considerations.
- Appreciate the nurse researcher's obligations to conduct and report research in an ethical manner.
- Describe the nurse's role as patient advocate in research situations.
- Discuss the nurse's role in ensuring that FDA guidelines for testing of medical devices are followed.
- Discuss animal rights in research situations.
- Critique the ethical aspects of a research study.

"In the 'court of imagination,' where Americans often play out their racial politics, a ceremony, starring a southern white President of the United States offering an apology and asking for forgiveness from a 94-year-old African-American man, seemed like a fitting close worthy in its tableaux quality of a William Faulkner or Toni Morrison novel. The reason for this drama was the federal government's May 16th formal ceremony of repentance tendered to the aging and ailing survivors of the infamous Tuskegee Syphilis Study. The study is a morality play for many among the African-American public and the scientific research community, serving as our most horrific example of a racist "scandalous story . . . when government doctors played God and science went mad. At the formal White House gathering, when President William J. Clinton apologized on behalf of the American government to the eight remaining survivors of the study, their families, and heirs seemingly a sordid chapter in American research history was closed 25 years after the study itself was forced to end. As the room filled with members of the Black Congressional Caucus, cabinet members, civil rights leaders, members of the Legacy Committee, the Centers for Disease Control (CDC), and five of the survivors, the sense of a dramatic restitution was upon us" (Reverby, 2000).

Nurses are in an ideal position to promote patients' awareness of the role played by research in the advancement of science and improvement in patient care. Embedded in our professional Code of Ethics (ANA, in press) is the charge to protect patients from harm; the codes are not only rules and regulations regarding the involvement of human research subjects to ensure that research is conducted legally and ethically, but also they address the conduct of the people who are supposed to be governed by the rules. Researchers themselves and caregivers providing care to patients, who also happen to be research subjects, must be fully committed to the tenets of informed consent and patients' rights. The principle "the ends justify the means" must never be tolerated. Researchers and caregivers of research subjects must take every precaution to protect people being studied from physical or mental harm or discomfort. It is not always clear what constitutes harm or discomfort.

The focus of this chapter is the legal and ethical considerations that must be addressed before, during, and after the conduct of research. Informed consent, institutional review boards, and research involving vulnerable populations—the elderly, pregnant women, children, prisoners, persons with AIDS, and animals—are discussed. The nurse's role as patient advocate, whether functioning as researcher, caregiver, or research consumer, is addressed.

ETHICAL AND LEGAL CONSIDERATIONS IN RESEARCH: A HISTORICAL PERSPECTIVE

PAST ETHICAL DILEMMAS IN RESEARCH

Ethical and legal considerations with regard to research first received attention after World War II. When the then U.S. Secretary of State and Secretary of War learned that the trials for war criminals would focus on justifying the atrocities committed by Nazi physicians as "medical research," the American Medical Association was asked to appoint a group to develop a code of ethics for research that would serve as a standard for judging the medical atrocities committed by physicians on concentration camp prisoners.

The 10 rules included in what was called the Nuremberg Code appear in Box 13-1. Its definitions of the terms *voluntary, legal capacity, sufficient understanding,* and *enlightened decision* have been the subject of numerous court cases and presidential commissions involved in setting ethical standards in research (Creighton, 1977). The code that was developed requires informed consent in all cases but makes no provisions for any special treatment of children, the elderly, or the mentally incompetent. Several other international standards have followed, the most notable of which was the Declaration of Helsinki, which was adopted in 1964 by the World Medical Assembly and then later revised in 1975 (Levine, 1979).

In the United States, federal guidelines for the ethical conduct of research involving human subjects were not developed until the 1970s. Despite the supposed safeguards provided by the federal guidelines, some of the most atrocious, and hence memorable, examples of unethical re-

BOX **13-1** Articles of the Nuremberg Code

1. The voluntary consent of the human subject is absolutely essential.
2. The study should be such as to yield fruitful results for the good of society, unprocurable by other means of study, and not random and unnecessary in nature.
3. The experiment should be so designed and based on the results of animal experimentation and knowledge of the natural history of the disease or other problems under study that the anticipated results will justify the performance of the experiment.
4. The experiment should be conducted to avoid all unnecessary physical and mental suffering and injury.
5. No experiment should be conducted where there is a prior reason to believe that death or disabling injury will occur.
6. The degree of risk to be taken should never exceed that determined by the humanitarian importance of the problem to be solved by the experiment.
7. Proper preparations should be made and adequate facilities provided to protect the subject against . . . injury, disability, or death.
8. The experiment should be conducted only by scientifically qualified persons.
9. The human subject should be at liberty to bring the experiment to an end.
10. During the experiment, the scientist . . . if he or she has probable cause to believe that a continuation of the experiment is likely to result in injury, disability, or death to the experimental subject . . . will bring it to a close.

Modified from Katz J: *Experimentation with human beings,* New York, 1972, Russell Sage Foundation.

search studies took place in the United States as recently as the 1990s. These examples are highlighted in Table 13-1. They are sad reminders of our own tarnished research heritage and illustrate the human consequences of not adhering to ethical research standards.

The conduct of harmful, illegal research made additional controls necessary. In 1973, the Department of Health, Education, and Welfare published the first set of proposed regulations on the protection of human subjects. The most important provision was a regulation mandating that an institutional review board (IRB) functioning in accordance with specifications of the department must review and approve all studies. The National Research Act, passed in 1974 (Public Law 93-348), created the National Commission for the Protection of Human Subjects of Biomedical and Behavioral Research. A major charge of the Commission was to identify the basic principles that should underlie the conduct of biomedical and behavioral research involving human subjects and to develop guidelines to ensure that research is conducted in accordance with those principles (Levine, 1986). Three ethical principles were identified as relevant to the conduct of research involving human subjects: the principles of **respect for persons, benefi-**

cence, and **justice.** They are defined in Box 13-2. Included in a report issued in 1979, called the Belmont Report, these principles provided the basis for regulations affecting research sponsored by the federal government. The Belmont Report also served as a model for many of the ethical codes developed by scientific disciplines (National Commission, 1978).

In 1980, the Department of Health and Human Services (DHHS) developed a set of regulations in response to the Commission's recommendations. These regulations were published in 1981 and revised in 1983 (DHHS, 1983). These regulations include the following:

- General requirements for informed consent
- Documentation of informed consent
- IRB review of research proposals
- Exempt and expedited review procedures for certain kinds of research
- Criteria for IRB approval of research

These regulations are discussed in the sections on informed consent and institutional review later in this chapter.

In 1992, the National Institutes of Health (NIH) Office of Research Integrity was established to set standards for dealing with allegations of scientific misconduct. In 1993, Congress passed the NIH Revitalization Act, which, among other provisions,

TABLE **13-1** Highlights of Unethical Research Studies Conducted in the United States

RESEARCH STUDY	YEAR(S)	FOCUS OF STUDY	ETHICAL PRINCIPLE VIOLATED
Hyman vs. Jewish Chronic Disease Hospital case	1965	Doctors injected aged and senile patients with their cancer cells to study their rejection response.	Informed consent was not obtained, and there was no indication that the study had been reviewed and approved by an ethics committee. The two physicians claimed that they did not wish to evoke emotional reactions or refusals to participate by informing the subjects of the nature of the study (Hershey and Miller, 1976).
Ivory Coast, Africa, AIDS/AZT case	1994	In clinical trials supported by the U.S. government and conducted in the Ivory Coast, Dominican Republic, and Thailand, some pregnant women infected with the HIV virus were given placebo pills rather than AZT, a drug known to prevent mothers from passing on the virus to their babies. Babies born to these mothers were in danger of contracting a fatal disease unnecessarily.	Subjects who consented to participate and who were randomized to the control group, were denied access to a medication regimen with a known benefit. This violates the subjects' right to fair treatment and protection (French, 1997; Wheeler, 1997).
Midgeville, Georgia, case	1969	Investigational drugs were used on mentally disabled children without first obtaining the opinion of a psychiatrist.	There was no review of the study protocol or institutional approval of the program before implementation (Levine, 1986).
Tuskegee, Alabama, syphilis study	1932-1973	For 40 years the United States Public Health Service conducted a study using two groups of poor black male sharecroppers. One group consisted of those who had untreated syphilis; the other group was judged to be free of the disease. Treatment was withheld from the group having syphilis even after penicillin became generally available and accepted as effective treatment in the 1950s. Steps were taken to prevent the subjects from obtaining it. The researcher wanted to study the untreated disease.	Many of the subjects who consented to participate in the study were not informed about the purpose and procedures of the research. Others were unaware that they were subjects. The degree of risk outweighed the potential benefit. Withholding of known effective treatment violates the subjects' right to fair treatment and protection from harm (Levine, 1986).

created a 12-member Commission on Research Integrity to propose new procedures for addressing scientific misconduct. A report, "Integrity and Misconduct in Research," issued by the Commission in 1995, proposed a new definition of scientific misconduct, additional protection for "whistle blowers," and a set of guidelines for handling allegations of scientific misconduct (Commission on Research Integrity, 1995; National Bioethics Advisory Commission, 1998; Ryan, 1996). In 1996,

TABLE **13-1**   Highlights of Unethical Research Studies Conducted in the United States—cont'd

RESEARCH STUDY	YEAR(S)	FOCUS OF STUDY	ETHICAL PRINCIPLE VIOLATED
San Antonio contraceptive study	1969	In a study examining the side effects of oral contraceptives, 76 impoverished Mexican-American women were randomly assigned to an experimental group receiving birth control pills or a control group receiving placebos. Subjects were not informed about the placebo and attendant risk of pregnancy. Eleven subjects became pregnant, 10 of whom were in the placebo control group.	Principles of informed consent were violated; full disclosure of potential risk, harm, results, or side effects was not evident in the informed consent document. The potential risk outweighed the benefits of the study. The subjects' right to fair treatment and protection from harm was violated (Levine, 1986).
Willowbrook Hospital	1972	Mentally incompetent children ($n = 350$) were not admitted to Willowbrook Hospital, a residential treatment facility, unless parents consented to their children being subjects in a study examining the natural history of infectious hepatitis and the effect of gamma globulin. The children were deliberately infected with the hepatitis virus under various conditions; some received gamma globulin; others did not.	Principle of voluntary consent was violated. Parents were coerced to consent to their children's participation as research subjects. Subjects or their guardians have a right to self-determination; that is, they should be free of constraint, coercion, or undue influence of any kind. Many subjects feel pressured to participate in studies if they are in powerless, dependent positions (Rothman, 1982).
UCLA Schizophrenia Medication Study	1983 to present	In a study examining the effects of withdrawing psychotropic medications of 50 patients under treatment for schizophrenia, 23 subjects suffered severe relapses after their medication was stopped. The goal of the study was to determine if some schizophrenics might do better without medications that had deleterious side effects.	Although all subjects signed informed consent documents, they were not informed about how severe their relapses might be, or that they could suffer worsening symptoms with each recurrence. Principles of informed consent were violated; full disclosure of potential risk, harm, results, or side effects was not evident in the informed consent document. The potential risk outweighed the benefits of the study. The subjects' right to fair treatment and protection from harm was violated (Hilts, 1995).

President Clinton appointed members of the National Bioethics Advisory Commission, which provides guidance to federal agencies on the ethical conduct of current and future human biological and behavioral research.

CURRENT AND FUTURE ETHICAL DILEMMAS IN RESEARCH

On a national level, the ethical dilemmas in research for the twenty-first century concern biotechnology, use of animals for research, and the

13-2 Basic Ethical Principles Relevant to the Conduct of Research

Respect for Persons

People have the right to self-determination and to treatment as autonomous agents. Thus they have the freedom to participate or not participate in research. Persons with diminished autonomy are entitled to protection.

Beneficence

Beneficence is an obligation to do no harm and maximize possible benefits. Persons are treated in an ethical manner when their decisions are respected, they are protected from harm, and efforts are made to secure their well-being.

Justice

Human subjects should be treated fairly. An injustice occurs when benefit to which a person is entitled is denied without good reason or when a burden is imposed unduly.

---

creation of an organizational culture that values and nurtures research ethics and the rights of people who engage in research either as investigators or subjects (Pranulis, 1996). For example, the Human Genome Project, an international research project launched by Congress in 1988, in only 12 years has provided a vast amount of DNA data, including the molecular details about the DNA of more than 26 organisms. In a postgenomic world, the focus is on studying (1) groups of genes, rather than single genes; (2) functions of genes, rather than structures of genes; and (3) protcomes, the proteins based on genes (Wheeler, 1999). A new scientific frontier, nanoscience and its related nanotechnology, makes materials by manipulating materials at the atomic level. In the year 2000, Congress allocated $423 million dollars to nanoscience research, which promises radically improved health care treatments (Monaghan, 2000).

In 1993, the U.S. Government ended a 5-year moratorium and began approving animal patents. Patents have been issued to organizations for the development of "transgenic" or genetically engineered animals suited to research in humans (Andrews, 1993). Another use of animals for research is in the area of xenograft transplantation. In 1992 three liver transplants were done using two baboons and one pig (Appel, Alwayn, and Cooper, 2000). Several centers have obtained approval from their IRBs to perform xenograft transplants and several preliminary trials that employ the transplantation of animal cells or the ex vivo perfusion of animal tissue are underway (Cooper and Lanza, 2000). The **ethics,** as well as the **risks** and **benefits** of this type of human/animal research, are still in question; the issue is very controversial.

Other areas of research that engender much discussion and controversy are fetal tissue research and use of women who are of childbearing potential as subjects in drug/therapeutic studies. In 1993, an executive order lifted the government's ban on fetal tissue research. This allows the resumption of research into the testing of fetal tissue for use in the treatment of such diseases as Parkinson's. More recently, federal lawyers opined that support of stem-cell research would not violate the federal ban on support of embryo research if researchers use stem cells that have already been isolated. The National Institutes of Health (NIH) has developed guidelines for stem-cell research that include protection for couples whose in vitro embryos may be used in research (Andrews, 1999; Kiernan, 1999).

In the past, women of childbearing potential were denied access to participation as subjects in drug or potentially therapeutic studies because of the unknown potentially harmful effects of drugs and other therapies that were in various stages of testing on fetuses. Guidelines related to the inclusion of pregnant women as research subjects have been even more stringent. This policy has led to the exclusion of women from many important drug and research studies over the years. Currently researchers seeking funds from the NIH have to justify excluding women from such studies. Similarly, inclusion of ethnic minorities in federally funded research studies also is a priority (Campbell, 1999a; Julion, Gross, and Barclay-McLaughlin, 2000).

In 1993, the NIH issued guidelines requiring grantees to include enough women in clinical trials to determine whether and how experimental drugs affect them differently from men (McDonald, 1999). And, in 1994, the Food and Drug Administration (FDA) allowed researchers to include AIDS-infected pregnant women, without the father's consent, in studies to determine whether the drug AZT would prevent transmission of the virus from mother to fetus (Wheeler, 1997).

Over the next decade many questions and controversies will arise in relation to the risks and benefits of the just-mentioned areas of research and as a result of ever-increasing technology in health care in areas that have not been defined as yet. Although these areas of research may seem far removed from nursing research and patient care, they will affect the type of patients nurses will care for and the type of clinical research nurses will conduct.

EVOLUTION OF ETHICS IN NURSING RESEARCH

The evolution of ethics in nursing research can be traced back to 1897 and the constitution of the Nurses' Associated Alumnae Organization. One of the first purposes of this organization was to establish a code of ethics for the nursing profession. In 1900, Isabel Hampton Robb wrote *Nursing Ethics: For Hospital and Private Use*. In describing moral laws by which people must abide, she states:

Etiquette, speaking broadly, means a form of behavior or manners expressly or tacitly required on particular occasions. It makes up the code of polite life and includes forms of ceremony to be observed, so that we invariably find in societies that a certain etiquette is required and observed either tacitly or by expressed agreement.

Clearly, Hampton Robb's comments reflect the norms of Victorian society. However, they also highlight an historical concern for ethical actions by nurses as health care providers (Robb, 1900).

In 1967, the American Nurses Association (ANA) charged its Committee on Research Studies with the task of developing guidelines for the nurse researcher in clinical research. In 1968, the Board of Directors approved the statement titled "The Nurse in Research: ANA Guidelines on Ethical Values." Not only were basic principles regarding the use of human subjects endorsed, but the role of the nurse as investigator, as well as practitioner, also was described.

The ANA established the Commission on Nursing Research in 1970. By doing so, it publicly affirmed nursing's obligation to support the advancement of scientific knowledge and reflected a commitment to support two sets of human rights: (1) the rights of qualified nurses to engage in research and have access to resources necessary for implementing scientific investigation and (2) the rights of all persons who are participants in research performed by investigators whose studies impinge on the patient care provided by nurses. The ANA emphasized human rights in terms of three domains: (1) right to freedom from intrinsic risk or injury, (2) right to privacy and dignity, and (3) right to anonymity.

The ANA's Human Rights Guidelines for Nursing in Clinical and Other Research, published in 1975, reflects the nursing profession's code of ethics for research. Box 13-3 provides a summary of this document, one that helps ensure that research maintains ethical and scientific rigor. This document is relevant for all nurses; the nurse as a researcher or caregiver must assure patients that their human rights will be safeguarded. In fact, nurses, when interviewing for potential employment, should ask what is expected of them in terms of research responsibilities. For example, nurses might ask the following:

- Are nurses required to collect data or administer medications or treatments in double-blind clinical trials?
- Are written research protocols available as references?

- Has the IRB ruled on each protocol?
- Are nurses free to decline to participate without jeopardizing their position?
- What channels exist for addressing ethical concerns with regard to research being conducted?

Clearly, ignorance and naiveté vis-a-vis ethical and legal guidelines for the conduct of research must never be an excuse for a nurse's failure to be familiar with and act on behalf of the patients whose human rights must, at all times, be safeguarded. Nurse researchers are often among the most responsible and conscientious investigators when it comes to respecting the rights of human subjects. All nurses should be aware that the tenets of the ANA's Code for Nurses (in press) are integral with the ANA Human Rights Guidelines for Nursing in Clinical and Other Research mentioned earlier.

Fowler (1988), a nurse ethicist, calls for an international code of ethics for nursing research. She raises many ethical questions that nurses around the world need to address now and in the future. Davis (1990) supports the concept of shared values among all nurses, stating that many of nursing's shared values are found in their professional codes. Some countries have their own code; others use the International Council of Nurses (ICN) Code for Nurses.

BOX 13-3

American Nurses Association Human Rights Guidelines for Nurses in Clinical and Other Research

GUIDELINE I: RIGHT TO SELF-DETERMINATION
Implementation

Where research participation is a condition of employment, nurses must be informed in writing of the nature of the activity involved in advance of employment. If nurses are not so informed, they must be given the opportunity of not participating in the research.

Potential of risk to others must be clarified in relation to the types of risk involved, the ways of recognizing when risk is present, and the ways in which to counteract potential and unnecessary danger.

GUIDELINE 2: RIGHT TO FREEDOM FROM RISK OR HARM
Implementation

Investigators must ensure freedom of risk from harm by estimating the potential physical or emotional risk and benefit involved. Vulnerable and captive subjects, such as students, patients, prisoners, the mentally incompetent, children, the elderly, and the poor, must be carefully monitored for sources of potential risk of injury so they can be protected.

GUIDELINE 3: SCOPE OF APPLICATION
Implementation

Guidelines for protection of human rights apply to all individuals, that is, subjects involved in research activities. The use of subjects with limited civil freedom usually can be justified only when there is benefit to them or others in similar circumstances.

GUIDELINE 4: RESPONSIBILITIES TO SUPPORT KNOWLEDGE DEVELOPMENT
Implementation

Nurses have an obligation to support the development of knowledge that expands the depth and breadth of the scientific knowledge or base of nursing practice.

GUIDELINE 5: INFORMED CONSENT
Implementation

The right to self-determination is protected when informed consent is obtained from the prospective subject or legal guardian.

GUIDELINE 6: PARTICIPATION ON INSTITUTIONAL REVIEW BOARDS
Implementation

As professionals accountable to the public who are the consumers of health care, nurses have an obligation to support the inclusion of nurses on institutional review boards (IRBs). Nurses also have an obligation to serve on IRBs to review ethical implications of proposed and ongoing research. All studies involving data collection from humans, animals, or records should be reviewed by a review board of health professionals and community representatives who ensure the protection of subjects' rights.

From American Nurses Association: *Guidelines for nurses in clinical and other research,* Kansas City, Mo, 1975, ANA.

PROTECTION OF HUMAN RIGHTS

Human rights are the claims and demands that have been justified in the eyes of an individual or by a group of individuals. The term refers to the following five rights outlined in the ANA (in press) guidelines:

1. Right to self-determination
2. Right to privacy and dignity
3. Right to anonymity and confidentiality
4. Right to fair treatment
5. Right to protection from discomfort and harm

These rights apply to everyone involved in a research project, including research team members who may be involved in data collection, practicing nurses involved in the research setting, and subjects participating in the study. As consumers of research read a research article, they must realize any issues highlighted in Table 13-2 should have been addressed and resolved before a research study is approved for implementation.

HELPFUL HINT Recognize that the right to personal privacy may be more difficult to protect when carrying out qualitative studies because of the small sample size and because the subjects' verbatim quotes are often used in the results/findings section of the research report to highlight the findings.

PROCEDURES FOR PROTECTING BASIC HUMAN RIGHTS

Informed Consent

Informed consent illustrated by the ethical principles of respect and its related right to self-determination are outlined in Box 13-4 and Table 13-2. Nurses need to understand elements of informed consent so that they are knowledgeable participants in obtaining informed consents from patients and/or in critiquing this process as it is presented in research articles.

Informed consent is the legal principle that, at least in theory, governs the patient's ability to accept or reject individual medical interventions designed to diagnose or treat an illness. It is also

TABLE **13-2**   Protection of Human Rights

BASIC HUMAN RIGHT	DEFINITION
Right to self-determination	Based on the ethical principle of respect for persons; people should be treated as autonomous agents who have the freedom to choose without external controls. An autonomous agent is one who is informed about a proposed study and is allowed to choose to participate or not to participate (Brink, 1992); subjects have the right to withdraw from a study without penalty.
	Subjects with diminished autonomy are entitled to protection. They are more vulnerable because of age, legal or mental incompetence, terminal illness, or confinement to an institution. Justification for use of vulnerable subjects must be provided.
Right to privacy and dignity	Based on the principle of respect, privacy is the freedom of a person to determine the time, extent, and circumstances under which private information is shared or withheld from others.
Right to anonymity and confidentiality	Based on the principle of respect, anonymity exists when the subject's identity cannot be linked, even by the researcher, with his or her individual responses (ANA, 1985).
	Confidentiality means that individual identities of subjects will not be linked to the information they provide and will not be publicly divulged.

Continued

TABLE **13-2** Protection of Human Rights—cont'd

VIOLATION OF BASIC HUMAN RIGHT	EXAMPLE
A subject's right to self-determination is violated through the use of coercion, covert data collection, and deception. • Coercion occurs when an overt threat of harm or excessive reward is presented to ensure compliance. • Covert data collection occurs when people become research subjects and are exposed to research treatments without knowing it. • Deception occurs when subjects are actually misinformed about the purpose of the research. • Potential for violation of the right to self-determination is greater for subjects with diminished autonomy; they have decreased ability to give informed consent and are vulnerable.	Subjects may feel that their care will be adversely affected if they refuse to participate in research. The Jewish Chronic Disease Hospital Study (see Table 13-1) is an example of a study in which patients and their doctors did not know that cancer cells were being injected. In the Milgrim (1963) Study, subjects were deceived when asked to administer electric shocks to another person; the person was really an actor who pretended to feel the shocks. Subjects administering the shocks were very stressed by participating in this study although they were not administering shocks at all. The Willowbrook Study (see Table 13-1) is an example of how coercion was used to obtain parental consent of vulnerable mentally retarded children who would not be admitted to the institution unless the children participated in a study in which they were deliberately injected with the hepatitis virus.
The Privacy Act of 1974 was instituted to protect subjects from such violations. These occur most frequently during data collection when invasive questions are asked that might result in loss of job, friendships, or dignity or might create embarrassment and mental distress. It also may occur when subjects are unaware that information is being shared with others.	Subjects may be asked personal questions such as "Were you sexually abused as a child?" "Do you use drugs?" "What are your sexual preferences?" When questions are asked using hidden microphones or hidden tape recorders, the subjects' privacy is invaded because they have no knowledge that the data are being shared with others. Subjects also have a right to control access of others to their records.
Anonymity is violated when the subjects' responses can be linked with their identity.	Subjects are given a code number instead of using names for identification purposes. Subjects' names are never used when reporting findings.
Confidentiality is breached when a researcher, by accident or by direct action, allows an unauthorized person to gain access to study data that contain information about subject identity or responses that create a potentially harmful situation for subjects.	Breaches of confidentiality with regard to sexual preference, income, drug use, prejudice, or personality variables can be harmful to subjects. Data are analyzed as group data so that individuals cannot be identified by their responses.

BASIC HUMAN RIGHT	DEFINITION
Right to fair treatment	Based on the ethical principle of justice, people should be treated fairly and should receive what they are due or owed. Fair treatment is equitable selection of subjects and their treatment during the research study. This includes selection of subjects for reasons directly related to the problem studied versus convenience, compromised position, or vulnerability. It also includes fair treatment of subjects during the study, including fair distribution of risks and benefits regardless of age, race, or socioeconomic status.

TABLE **13-2**   Protection of Human Rights—cont'd

BASIC HUMAN RIGHT—cont'd	DEFINITION
Right to protection from discomfort and harm	Based on the ethical principle of beneficence, people must take an active role in promoting good and preventing harm in the world around them, as well as in research studies. Discomfort and harm can be physical, psychological, social, or economic in nature. There are five categories of studies based on levels of harm and discomfort: 1. No anticipated effects 2. Temporary discomfort 3. Unusual level of temporary discomfort 4. Risk of permanent damage 5. Certainty of permanent damage

VIOLATION OF BASIC HUMAN RIGHT	EXAMPLE
Injustices with regard to subject selection have occurred as a result of social, cultural, racial, and gender biases in society.	The Tuskegee Syphilis Study (1973), the Jewish Chronic Disease Study (1965), the San Antonio Contraceptive Study (1969), and the Willowbrook Study (1972) (see Table 13-1) all provide examples related to unfair subject selection.
Historically, research subjects often have been obtained from groups of people who were regarded as having less "social value," the poor, prisoners, slaves, the mentally incompetent, and the dying. Often subjects were treated carelessly, without consideration of physical or psychological harm.	Investigators should not be late for data-collection appointments, should terminate data collection on time, should not change agreed upon procedures or activities without consent, and should provide agreed upon benefits such as a copy of the study findings or a participation fee.
Subjects' right to be protected is violated when researchers know in advance that harm, death, or disabling injury will occur and thus the benefits do not outweigh the risk.	Temporary physical discomfort involving minimal risk includes fatigue or headache; emotional discomfort includes the expense involved in traveling to and from the data-collection site. Studies examining sensitive issues, such as rape, incest, or spouse abuse, might cause unusual levels of temporary discomfort by opening up current and/or past traumatic experiences. In these situations, researchers assess distress levels and provide debriefing sessions during which the subject may express feelings and ask questions. The researcher has the opportunity to make referrals for professional intervention. Studies having the potential to cause permanent damage are more likely to be medical rather than nursing in nature. A recent clinical trial of a new drug, a recombinant activated protein C (rAPC) (Zovan) for treatment of sepsis, was halted when interim findings from the Phase III clinical trials revealed a reduced mortality rate for the treatment group versus the placebo group. Evaluation of the data led to termination of the trial to make available a known beneficial treatment to all patients. In some research, such as the Tuskegee Syphilis Study or the Nazi medical experiments, subjects experienced permanent damage or death.

a doctrine that determines and regulates participation in research (Dubler and Post, 1998; Pranulis, 1996). The Code of Federal Regulations (1983) defines the meaning of informed consent:

The knowing consent of an individual or his/her legally authorized representative, under circumstances that provide the prospective subject or representative sufficient opportunity to consider whether or not to participate without undue inducement or any element of force, fraud, deceit, duress, or other forms of constraint or coercion.

No investigator may involve a human as a research subject before obtaining the legally effective informed consent of a subject or legally authorized representative. Prospective subjects must have time to decide whether to participate in a study. The researcher must not coerce the subject into participating. Nor may researchers collect data on subjects who have explicitly refused to participate in a study. An ethical violation of this principle is illustrated by the halting of eight experiments by the Food and Drug Administration (FDA) at the University of Pennsylvania's Institute for Human Gene Therapy four months after the death of an 18-year-old male, Jesse Gelsinger, who received experimental treatment as part of the institute's research. The Institute could not document that all patients had been informed of the risks and benefits of the procedures. Furthermore, some patients who received the therapy should have been considered ineligible because their illnesses were more severe than allowed by the clinical protocols. Mr. Gelsinger had a non–life-threatening genetic disorder that permits toxic amounts of ammonia to build up in the liver. Nevertheless, he volunteered for an experimental treatment in which normal genes were implanted directly into his liver and he subsequently died of multiple organ failure. The Institute failed to report to the FDA that two patients in Mr. Gelsinger's trial had suffered severe side effects, including inflammation of the liver, as a result of their treatment; this should have triggered a halt to the trial (Brainard and Miller, 2000).

The language of the consent form must be understandable. For example, the reading level should be no greater than eighth grade for adults and the use of technical research language should be avoided (Rempusheski, 1991). According to the Code of Federal Regulations, subjects should in no way be asked to waive their rights or release the investigator from liability for negligence.

The elements that need to be contained in an informed consent are listed in Box 13-4. It is important to note that many institutions require additional elements. A sample of an informed consent form is presented in Figure 13-1.

HELPFUL HINT Remember that research reports rarely provide readers with detailed information regarding the degree to which the researcher adhered to ethical principles, such as informed consent, because of space limitations in journals that make it impossible to describe all aspects of a study. Failure to mention procedures to safeguard subjects' rights does not necessarily mean that such precautions were not taken.

Most investigators obtain **consent** through personal discussion with potential subjects. This process allows the person to obtain immediate answers to questions. However, consent forms, written in narrative or outline form, highlight elements that both inform and remind subjects of the nature of the study and their participation (Dubler and Post, 1998; Haggerty and Hawkins, 2000).

Assurance of **anonymity** and **confidentiality** (defined in Table 13-2) is usually conveyed in writing. This is sometimes difficult in unique research situations that capture the public's attention, for example, when physicians at Loma Linda University Hospital in California transplanted a baboon's heart into a 2-week old infant, the identity of the infant was protected; she was known only as Baby Fae.

The consent form must be signed and dated by the subject. The presence of witnesses is not always necessary but does constitute evidence that the subject concerned actually signed the form.

BOX **13-4**   Elements of Informed Consent

1. A statement that the study involves research.
2. An explanation of the purposes of the research, delineating the expected duration of the subject's participation.
3. A description of the procedures to be followed and identification of any procedures that are experimental.
4. A description of any reasonably foreseeable risks or discomforts to the subject.
5. A description of any benefits to the subject or to others that may reasonably be expected from the research.
6. A disclosure of appropriate alternative procedures or course of treatment, if any, that might be advantageous to the subject.
7. A statement describing the extent to which anonymity and confidentiality of the records identifying the subject will be maintained.

8. For research involving more than minimal risk, an explanation as to whether any medical treatments are available if injury occurs and, if so, what they consist of, or where further information may be obtained.
9. An explanation about who to contact for answers to questions about the research and researcher subjects' rights, and who to contact in the event of a research-related injury to the subject.
10. A statement that participation is voluntary, that refusal to participate will not involve any penalty or less benefit to which the subject is otherwise entitled, and the subject may discontinue participation at any time without penalty or loss of otherwise entitled benefits.

From Code of Federal Regulations: Protection of human subjects, 45 CFR 46, *OPRR Reports*, Revised March 8, 1983.

In cases in which the subject is a minor or is physically or mentally incapable of signing the consent, the legal guardian or representative must sign. The investigator also signs the form to indicate commitment to the agreement.

Generally the signed informed consent form is given to the subject. The researcher should keep a copy also. Some research, such as a retrospective chart audit, may not require informed consent—only institutional approval. Or in some cases when minimal risk is involved, the investigator may have to provide the subject only with an information sheet and verbal explanation. In other cases, such as a volunteer convenience sample, completion and return of research instruments provide evidence of consent. The IRB will help advise on exceptions to these guidelines, cases in which the IRB might grant waivers or amend its guidelines in other ways. The IRB makes the final determination regarding the most appropriate documentation format. Research consumers should note whether and what kind of evidence of informed consent has been provided in a research article.

HELPFUL HINT   Note that researchers often do not obtain written, informed consent when the major means of data collection is through self-administered questionnaires. The researcher usually assumes applied consent in such cases; that is, the return of the completed questionnaire reflects the respondent's voluntary consent to participate.

Institutional Review Board

Institutional review boards (IRBs) are boards that review research projects to assess that ethical standards are met in relation to the protection of the rights of human subjects. The National Research Act (1974) requires that such agencies as universities, hospitals, and other health agencies applying for a grant or contract for any project or program that involves the conduct of biomedical or behavioral research involving human subjects must submit with their application assurances that they have established an IRB, sometimes called a human subjects committee, which reviews the research projects and protects the rights of the human subjects (Code of Federal

---

Informed Consent

The Caldwell Medical Center

Code No. _____

    I understand that I am being treated with the drug *cis*-platin, which may cause the unpleasant side effects of nausea and vomiting. Treatment to control these side effects includes using various medications, reducing the intake of food and fluids before chemotherapy, maintaining a quiet environment, and accepting support from others. In addition, I understand that using various coping strategies is helpful to persons in similar situations.

    I understand that the purpose of this study is to help clients learn some coping techniques and evaluate how their use affects the occurrence of nausea and vomiting after *cis*-platin is administered. If I agree to participate in this research study, I understand that I will be randomly assigned to one of the following three nursing treatment programs:

1. I will meet with one of the investigators before I receive my chemotherapy. We will discuss my experience and the methods that other clients and I have found helpful.

or

2. I will meet with one of the investigators before I receive my chemotherapy. I will follow directions for practicing a technique that produces, under my own control, a state of altered consciousness called *self-hypnosis*. I will be asked to practice this technique during and after receiving my chemotherapy. I will be expected to practice this technique daily so that I may learn to use it without being directed by another person.

or

3. I will be given the customary nursing care that is rendered to every client taking the drugs that I am receiving.

    In addition, if necessary, I will receive only the medication Reglan to control nausea and vomiting.

    I understand that in no case will I receive less than the usual standard and expected level of nursing care that I am already receiving.

    I understand that if I am selected to be in Group 2, a simple test to determine my susceptibility to this technique will be performed. Most people are susceptible, but if I am not and I wish to continue in the study, I will be randomly assigned to one of the two remaining groups.

    I understand that this research study has been discussed with my physician and that he or she is aware of my participation. The treatments prescribed to control the side effects of nausea and vomiting will not be altered if I participate in this study.

Figure 13-1 Example of an informed consent form.

Informed Consent—cont'd

I understand that a nurse investigator will be in my room while my chemotherapy is ending and for 4 hours after the treatment. I understand that nursing care will be provided by the nurses on the unit and not by the nurse-investigator. The research nurse will be taking notes on my reactions to the chemotherapy. Once an hour she will ask me to rate my nausea. I can expect that this will take only a few minutes of my time and that, if I am sleeping, I will not be awakened.

I have been told that this routine will be followed for three courses of chemotherapy, during three separate hospitalizations.

I understand that the benefits from this treatment are that I may experience less nausea and vomiting or fewer of the feelings of being sick to my stomach that often occur with *cis*-platin. There are no side effects or risks from my participation.

My participation is voluntary and I may choose to not participate or to withdraw at any time without jeopardizing my future treatment.

My identity will not be revealed in any way. My name will be encoded so that I will remain anonymous.

I also understand that if I believe I have sustained an injury as a result of participating in this research study, I may contact the investigators, Ms. B. J. Simon at 608-0011 or B. A. Smith at 124-6142, or the Office of the Institutional Review Board at 124-2500 so that I can review the matter and identify the medical resources that may be available to me.

I understand the following statements:
1. The Caldwell Medical Center will furnish whatever emergency medical care that the medical staff of this hospital determine to be necessary.
2. I will be responsible for the cost of such emergency care personally, through my medical insurance, or by another form of coverage.
3. No monetary compensation for wages lost as a result of an injury will be paid to me by The Caldwell Medical Center.
4. I will receive a copy of this consent form.

_____   _____
Date   Patient

_____   _____
Witness   Investigator

The Institutional Review Board of the Caldwell Medical Center has approved the solicitation of subjects for participation in this research proposal.

Figure 13-1, cont'd

13-5 Code of Federal Regulations for IRB Approval of Research Studies

To approve research, the IRB must determine that the following Code of Federal Regulations has been satisfied:
1. The risks to subjects are minimized.
2. The risks to subjects are reasonable in relation to anticipated benefits.
3. The selection of the subjects is equitable.
4. Informed consent, in one of several possible forms, must be and will be sought from each prospective subject or the subject's legally authorized representative.
5. The informed consent form must be properly documented.

6. Where appropriate, the research plan makes adequate provision for monitoring the data collected to ensure subject safety.
7. Where appropriate, there are adequate provisions to protect the privacy of subjects and the confidentiality of data.
8. Where some or all of the subjects are likely to be vulnerable to coercion or undue influence, such as persons with acute or severe physical or mental illness or persons who are economically or educationally disadvantaged, appropriate additional safeguards are included.

Regulations, 1983). At agencies where no federal grants or contracts are awarded, there is usually a review mechanism similar to an IRB process, such as a research advisory committee.

The National Research Act requires that the IRB have at least five members of various backgrounds to promote complete and adequate project review. The members must be qualified by virtue of their expertise and experience and reflect professional, gender, racial, and cultural diversity. Membership must include one member whose concerns are primarily nonscientific (lawyer, clergy, ethicist) and at least one member from outside the agency. Members of IRBs often have mandatory training in scientific integrity and prevention of scientific misconduct as does the principal investigator of a research study and his or her research team members.

The IRB is responsible for protecting subjects from undue risk and loss of personal rights and dignity. For a research proposal to be eligible for consideration by an IRB, it must already have been approved by a departmental review group such as a nursing research committee that attests to the proposal's scientific merit and congruence with institutional policies, procedures, and mission. The IRB reviews the study's protocol to ensure that it meets the requirements of ethical research that appear in Box 13-5. Most boards provide guidelines or instructions for researchers that include steps to be taken to receive IRB approval. For example, guidelines for writing a

standard consent form or criteria for qualifying for an expedited rather than a full IRB review may be made available. The IRB has the authority to approve research, require modifications, or disapprove a research study. A researcher must receive IRB approval before beginning to conduct research. Institutional review boards have the authority to suspend or terminate approval of research that is not conducted in accordance with IRB requirements or that has been associated with unexpected serious harm to subjects (Pallikkathayll, Crighton, and Aaronson, 1998).

IRBs also have mechanisms for reviewing research in an expedited manner when the risk to research subjects is minimal (Code of Federal Regulations, 1983). An expedited review usually shortens the length of the review process. Keep in mind that although a researcher may determine that a project involves minimal risk, the IRB makes the final determination, and the research may not be undertaken until then. A full list of research categories eligible for expedited review is available from any IRB office. It includes the following:

- Collection of hair and nail clippings in a nondisfiguring manner
- Collection of excreta and external secretions including sweat
- Recording of data on subjects 18 years or older, using noninvasive procedures routinely employed in clinical practice
- Voice recordings

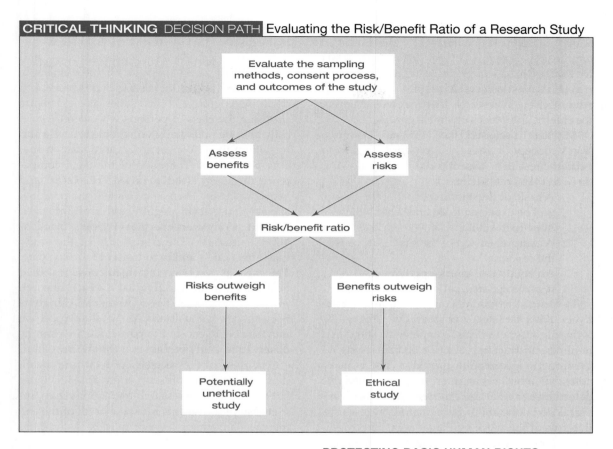

CRITICAL THINKING DECISION PATH | Evaluating the Risk/Benefit Ratio of a Research Study

- Study of existing data, documents, records, pathological specimens, or diagnostic data

An expedited review does not automatically exempt the researcher from obtaining informed consent.

The Federal Register is a publication that contains updated information about federal guidelines for research involving human subjects. Every researcher should consult an agency's research office to ensure that the application being prepared for IRB approval adheres to the most current requirements. Nurses who are critiquing published research should be conversant with current regulations to determine whether ethical standards have been met. The Critical Thinking Decision Path illustrates the ethical decision-making process an IRB might use in evaluating the risk/benefit ratio of a research study.

PROTECTING BASIC HUMAN RIGHTS OF VULNERABLE GROUPS

Researchers are advised to consult their agency's IRB for the most recent federal and state rules and guidelines when considering research involving vulnerable groups such as the elderly, children, pregnant women, the unborn, those who are emotionally or physically disabled, prisoners, the deceased, students, and persons with AIDS (Baskin et al, 1998; Campbell,1999a; Campbell, 1999b; Haggerty and Hawkins, 2000; Lutz, 1999; National Bioethics Advisory Commission, 1998). In addition, researchers should consult the IRB before planning research that potentially involves an oversubscribed research population, such as organ transplantation patients, AIDS patients, or "captive" and convenient populations, such as prisoners. It should be emphasized that use of special populations does not preclude undertaking research; extra precautions must be taken, however, to protect their rights (Levine, 1995). Davis (1981) reminds us that a society can be judged by the way it treats its most vulnerable people—a point worth remembering in research that involves children, the elderly, and other vulnerable groups.

Mitchell discussed the National Commission's concept of assent vs. consent in regard to pediatric research. **Assent** contains the following three fundamental elements:

1. A basic understanding of what the child will be expected to do and what will be done to the child
2. A comprehension of the basic purpose of the research
3. An ability to express a preference regarding participation

In contrast to assent, consent requires a relatively advanced level of cognitive ability. Informed consent reflects competency standards requiring abstract appreciation and reasoning regarding the information provided. The issue of assent vs. consent is an interesting one when one determines at what age children can make meaningful decisions about participating in research. In terms of the work by Piaget regarding cognitive ability, children at age 6 and older can participate in giving assent. Children at age 14 and older, although not legally authorized to give sole consent unless they are emancipated minors, can make such decisions as capably as adults (Mitchell, 1984).

Federal regulations require parental permission whenever a child is involved in research unless otherwise specified, for example, in cases of child abuse or mature minors at minimal risk (Flaskerud and Winslow, 1998). If the research involves more than minimal risk and does not offer direct benefit to the individual child, both parents must give permission. When individuals reach maturity, usually at 18 years of age in cases of research, they may render their own consent. They may do so at a younger age if they have been legally declared emancipated minors. Questions regarding this should be addressed by the IRB and/or research administration office and not left to the discretion of the researcher to answer.

The American Geriatrics Society Ethics Committee (1998), as an advocate for the vulnerable elderly who are of increasing dependence and declining cognitive ability, states that elders are precisely the class of persons who were historically and are potentially vulnerable to abuse and for whom the law must struggle to fashion specific protections. The issue of the legal competence of elders is often raised (Flaskerud and Winslow, 1998). There is no issue if the potential subject can supply legally effective informed consent. Competence is not a clear "black or white" situation. The complexity of the study may affect one's ability to consent to participate. The capacity to obtain informed consent should be assessed in each individual for each research protocol being considered (American Geriatrics Society, 1998). For example, an elderly person may be able to consent to participate in a simple observation study but not in a clinical drug trial.

The issue of the necessity of requiring the elderly to provide consent often arises. Dubler (1993) refers to the research regulations that provide that requirements for some or all of the elements of informed consent may be waived for the following:

1. The research involves no more than minimal risk to the subjects.
2. The waiver or alteration will not adversely affect the rights and welfare of the subjects.
3. The research could not feasibly be carried out without the waiver or alteration.
4. Whenever appropriate, the subjects will be provided with additional pertinent information after participation.

No vulnerable population may be singled out for study because it is simply convenient. For example, neither people with mental illness nor prisoners may be studied simply because they are an available and convenient group. Prisoners may be studied if the study pertains to them, that is, studies concerning the effects and processes of incarceration. Similarly, people with mental illness may participate in studies that focus on expanding knowledge about psychiatric disorders and treatments. Students also are often a convenient group. They must not be singled out as research subjects because of convenience; the research questions must have some bearing on their status as students.

Researchers and patient caregivers involved in research with vulnerable people are well advised to seek advice from appropriate IRBs, clinicians, lawyers, ethicists, and others. In all cases, the burden should be on the investigator to show the IRB that it is appropriate to involve vulnerable subjects in research.

> **HELPFUL HINT**   Keep in mind that researchers rarely mention explicitly that the study participants were vulnerable subjects or that special precautions were taken to appropriately safeguard the human rights of this vulnerable group. Research consumers need to be attentive to the special needs of groups who may be unable to act as their own advocates or are unable to adequately assess the risk/benefit ratio of a research study.

SCIENTIFIC FRAUD AND MISCONDUCT

FRAUD

Periodically articles reporting unethical actions of researchers appear in the professional and lay literature. Data may have been falsified or fabricated or subjects may have been coerced to participate in a research study (Kevles, 1996; Office of Research Integrity website, 2000; Tilden, 2000). In a climate of "publish or perish" in academic and scientific settings and declining research dollars, there is increasing pressure on academics and scientists to produce significant research findings. Job security and professional recognition are coveted, essential, and often predicated on being a productive scientist and prolific writer. These pressures have been known to overpower some people, who then take shortcuts, fabricate data, and falsify findings to advance their positions (Rankin and Esteves, 1997; Tilden, 2000).

The risks are many, including harming research subjects or basing clinical practice on false data. Nurses, as advocates of patient welfare and professional practice, should be aware that, albeit ideally rare, there are occasions when misconduct of the researcher is observed or suspected. In such cases, nurses must be advised to contact the appropriate group, such as the IRB, to ensure that this matter receives appropriate attention and review.

MISCONDUCT

Of equal importance is the issue of basing practice on reports that appear in journals, where subsequent research and reports on those subjects change the scientific basis for practice. Journals may print corrections or further research in follow-up reports that are buried, obscure, or underreported. A physician, Lawrence K. Altman (1988), stated, "Such shortcomings are critically important because the thousands of journals that cover a range of specialties are the central reservoir of scientific knowledge. They are the standard references for crediting discoveries and determining treatments." It is incumbent on nurses as patient advocates and research consumers to keep up to date on scientific reports related to nursing practice and adjust practice as directed by ever-evolving evidence-based research findings. In addition, it is the responsibility of the researcher to make sure that she or he keeps current with federal compliance regulations on prevention, detection, and inquiry into and adjudication of scientific misconduct. For example, the federal government is proposing to change the definition of misconduct, a change that will appear in the Federal Register when the change is approved by the Office of Research Integrity (ORI). How many researchers or research consumers regularly check the Federal Register or other government documents or websites to maintain their currency in legal and ethical research issues?

UNAUTHORIZED RESEARCH

At times, ad hoc or informal and unauthorized research does go on, including **product testing.** Although the testing may seem harmless, again it is not the purview of the investigator to make that determination. Nurses must carefully avoid being involved in unauthorized research for a number of reasons, including the following (Raybuck, 1997):

- These treatments or methods of care are usually not monitored as closely for untoward effects, hence exposing the client to unwarranted risk.
- Clients' rights to informed consent in clinical trials are not protected.
- The success or failure of these unrecorded trials contributes nothing to the organized scientific knowledge of the efficacy or complications of the treatment.
- The lack of independent quality supervision allows deviations from the adopted experimental program that may eliminate the program's effectiveness.

Sometimes the nurse plays the dual role of researcher and caregiver. In that situation, the nurse must question whether risks may be inherent in the research that do not exist in the care. Even when these risks are clearly identified—and they must be—the caregiver must be comfortable that the level of risk is acceptable and that the benefits outweigh the risks. Patients must feel comfortable in refusing to participate in the caregiver's research while continuing to require the nurse's care. It must be made clear to patients that they may refuse to participate or withdraw from the study at any time without consequence or compromise to their care or relationship to the institution. The nurse in this dual role must consider whether the research will incur additional expense for the patient, whether that is warranted, and whether the subject has been apprised of such expenses (Sailer, 1999).

PRODUCT TESTING

Nurses are often approached by manufacturers to test products on patients. They often assume the role of research coordinator in clinical drug or product trials (Raybuck, 1997). Nurses should be aware of the FDA guidelines and regulations for testing of medical devices before they initiate any form of clinical testing. Medical devices are classified under Section 513 in the Federal Food, Drug and Cosmetic Act according to the extent of control necessary to ensure safety and effectiveness of each device. Classes related to product testing are defined in Table 13-3.

It is important that nurses be aware of their own institution's policies for product testing. The class of the product will obviously make a difference to the institution's position. If a nurse suspects that, for example, a Class II device is being tested in an ad hoc or unauthorized manner and without patient consent, this should be discussed with a supervisor or other appropriate authorities.

LEGAL AND ETHICAL ASPECTS OF ANIMAL EXPERIMENTATION

The federal laws that have been written to protect **animal rights** in research emanate from an interesting history of attitudes toward animals and the value people place on them. Animal activists (e.g., the Animal Liberation Front) and antivivisectionist societies began to gain considerable public attention in the 1970s. Of interest, however, is the fact that the oldest piece of legislation controlling animal experimentation goes back to 1876 in the United Kingdom. With the increase in the use of animals in research after World War II, a number of states passed legislation called "pound seizure laws" that allowed and even mandated the release of unclaimed animals from pounds to laboratories. The first pound seizure law was enacted in 1949; not until 1972 was the first law of that type repealed. In 1966 in the United States, the first Laboratory Animal Welfare Act was passed. The act did not deal with what we consider today to be some of the most salient issues related to animal experimentation (e.g., pain management), and amendments continued to be passed to address these concerns. The 1970 Act provided for the establishment of an institutional Animal Care and Use Committee (ACUC), one member of which must be a veterinarian. The United States Department of Agricul-

TABLE **13-3**   Classes Related to Product Testing

CLASSES	EXAMPLES
CLASS I: GENERAL CONTROLS Included in Class I are devices whose safety and effectiveness can be guaranteed reasonably by the general controls of the Good Manufacturing Practices Regulations. The Regulations part of the act ensures that manufacturers will follow specific guidelines for packaging, storing, and providing specific product instructions.	Ostomy supplies
CLASS II: PERFORMANCE STANDARDS General controls are insufficient in this case to ensure safety and efficacy of the product, and the manufacturer must provide this assurance in the form of information.	Cardiac pacemakers, sutures, surgical metallic mesh, and biopsy needles
CLASS III: PREMARKET APPROVAL This class includes devices whose safety and effectiveness are insufficiently ensured by general controls and for which performance standards are insufficient to ensure safety and effectiveness. These products are represented to be life sustaining or life supporting, are implanted into the body, or present a potential, unreasonable risk of illness or injury to the patient. Devices in this class are required to have approved applications for premarket approval. Extensive laboratory, animal, and human studies, which often require 2 to 3 years to complete, are required for Class III devices.	Heart valves, bone cements, contact lenses, and implantable devices left in the body for 30 days or longer

ture (USDA) oversees compliance with animal welfare acts and holds institutions' administration accountable for such compliance.

In 1985, President Reagan signed PL 99-108, which contains the Improved Standards for the Laboratory Animals' Act. Provisions in the series of acts and amendments to acts pertaining to animal experimentation include, but are by no means limited to, the list that appears in Box 13-6 (PHS Policy on Humane Care, 1985).

This section serves only as an introduction to the concept of legal and ethical issues related to animal experimentation. Principles of protection of animal rights in research have evolved over time. Animals, unlike humans, cannot give informed consent, but other conditions related to their welfare must not be ignored. Nurses who encounter the use of animals in research should be alert to their rights.

BOX 13-6 Basic Provisions of Acts Pertaining to Animal Experimentation

1. The transportation, care, and use of animals should be in accordance with the Animal Welfare Act and other applicable federal laws, guidelines, and policies.

2. Procedures involving animals should be designed and performed with consideration of their relevance to human or animal health, the advancement of knowledge, or the good of society.

3. The animals selected for a procedure should be of an appropriate species and quality and the minimum number required to obtain valid results. Methods such as mathematical models, computer simulation, and in vitro biological systems should be considered.

4. Proper use of animals, including the avoidance or minimization of discomfort, distress, and pain when consistent with sound scientific practices, is imperative. Unless the contrary is established, investigators should consider that the procedures that cause pain or distress in human beings may cause pain or distress in other animals.

5. Procedures with animals that may cause more than temporary or slight pain or distress should be performed with appropriate sedation, analgesia, or anesthesia. Surgical or other painful procedures should not be performed on anaesthetized animals paralyzed by chemical agents.

6. Animals that would otherwise suffer severe or chronic pain or distress that cannot be relieved should be painlessly killed at the end of the procedure or, if appropriate, during the procedure.

7. The living conditions of animals should be appropriate for their species and contribute to their health and comfort. Normally the housing, feeding, and care of all animals used for biomedical purposes must be directed by a veterinarian or other scientist trained and experienced in the proper care, handling, and use of the species being maintained or studied. In any case, veterinary care shall be provided as indicated.

8. Investigators and other personnel shall be appropriately qualified and experienced for conducting procedures on living animals. Adequate arrangements shall be made for their in-service training, including the proper and humane care and use of laboratory animals.

9. Where exceptions are required in relation to the provision of these principles, the decisions should not rest with the investigators directly concerned but should be made, with regard to principle 2, by an appropriate review group, such as an institutional animal research committee. Such exceptions should not be made solely for the purposes of teaching or demonstration.

CRITIQUING the Legal and Ethical Aspects of a Research Study

Research articles and reports often do not contain detailed information regarding the degree to which or all of the ways in which the investigator adhered to the legal and ethical principles presented in this chapter. Space considerations in articles preclude extensive documentation of all legal and ethical aspects of a research study. Lack of written evidence regarding the protection of human rights does not imply that appropriate steps were not taken.

The Critiquing Criteria box provides guidelines for evaluating the legal and ethical aspects of a research report. Although research consumers reading a research report will not see all areas explicitly addressed in the research article, they should be aware of them and should determine that the researcher has addressed them before gaining IRB

approval to conduct the study. A nurse who is asked to serve as a member of an IRB will find the critiquing criteria useful in evaluating the legal and ethical aspects of the research proposal.

Information about the legal and ethical considerations of a study is usually presented in the Methods section of a research report. The subsection on the sample or data collection methods is the most likely place for this information. The author most often indicates in a few sentences that informed consent was obtained and that approval from an IRB or similar committee was granted. It is likely that a paper will not be accepted for publication without such a discussion. This also makes it almost impossible for unauthorized research to be published. Therefore when a research article provides evidence of having been approved by an external review committee, the reader

CRITIQUING CRITERIA

1. Was the study approved by an IRB or other agency committee members?
2. Is there evidence that informed consent was obtained from all subjects or their representatives? How was it obtained?
3. Were the subjects protected from physical or emotional harm?
4. Were the subjects or their representatives informed about the purpose and nature of the study?
5. Were the subjects or their representatives informed about any potential risks that might result from participation in the study?
6. Is the research study designed to maximize the benefit(s) to human subjects and minimize the risks?
7. Were subjects coerced or unduly influenced to participate in this study? Did they have the right to refuse to participate or withdraw without penalty? Were vulnerable subjects used?
8. Were appropriate steps taken to safeguard the privacy of subjects? How have data been kept anonymous and/or confidential?

can feel confident that the ethical issues raised by the study have been thoroughly reviewed and resolved.

To protect subject and institutional privacy, the locale of the study frequently is described in general terms in the sample subsection of the report. For example, the article might state that data were collected at a 1000-bed tertiary care center in the Southwest, without mentioning its name. Protection of subject privacy may be explicitly addressed by statements indicating that anonymity or confidentiality of data was maintained or that grouped data were used in the data analysis.

Determining whether participants were subjected to physical or emotional risk is often accomplished indirectly by evaluating the study's methods section. The reader evaluates the **risk-benefit ratio,** that is, the extent to which the benefits of the study are maximized and the risks are minimized such that subjects are protected from harm during the study (Dubler and Post, 1998; Pruchino and Hayden, 2000).

For example, the study by Grey and associates (1999) compared the effect of a behavioral intervention, coping skills training (CST) combined with intensive diabetes management or intensive therapy only on quality of life and improved metabolic control in adolescents with type I diabetes mellitus. Results from this clinical trial demonstrate that adolescents who participated in the CST plus intensive management had better psychosocial and metabolic outcomes as measured by self-efficacy, coping, impact of diabetes, satisfaction, worry, depression, and decreased HbA1c levels to below 8%.

The findings related to the outcomes of this low-cost intervention have implications for significant cost savings, at no risk and potential significant benefit to both patients and health care institutions that treat diabetic adolescents.

In another example, the study by LoBiondo-Wood and associates (2000) investigated the relationship between family stress, family coping, social support, perception of stress, and family adaptation in families of children undergoing liver transplants. The benefits to the participants were increased knowledge about the family stressors, strains, and resources needed by families during the long-term process of seeking a transplant for a chronically ill child. Risk is minimized because subjects were mothers of children being evaluated for a liver transplant; the children's usual regimen was not being altered in any way. LoBiondo-Wood and colleagues (2000) state that before interventions can be developed to assist such families during this crisis, clinicians need to understand how aspects of family life are affected. The evaluator could infer from a description of the method that the benefits were greater than the risks and subjects were protected from harm. The findings of the study highlighted the need to understand the impact of transplantation on the family as a whole. As health care providers move to cost containment and documentation of outcomes that affect the child's family and that family's ability to cope and care for a member with chronic health care needs, research needs to focus on what aspects of the child's care are compromised if the family's needs are not addressed. The obligation to balance the risks and benefits of a study is the responsibility of the researcher. However, the research consumer reading a research report also should be confident that subjects have been protected from harm (see Appendix B).

When considering the special needs of vulnerable subjects, research consumers should be sensitive to whether the special needs of groups, unable to act on their own behalf, have been addressed. For instance, has the right of self-determination been addressed by the informed consent protocol identified in the research report? For example, in a study by Koenes and Karshmer (2000) comparing whether the incidence of depression was greater among blind adolescents than a sighted comparison group, the study was approved by the institutional committee for review of research involving human subjects, as well as the school administrators and parents or guardians who had to provide written consent for subject participation. Actual student participation was entirely voluntary, they were invited to participate in a study designed to "explore stress and its impact on adolescence." All students were individually recruited, and 22 adolescents who had been legally blind since birth and 29 sighted adolescents participated in the study.

When qualitative studies are reported, verbatim quotes from informants often are incorporated into the findings section of the article. In such cases, the reader will evaluate how effectively the author protected the informant's identity, either by using a fictitious name or withholding information such as age, gender, occupation, or other potentially identifying data (see Chapter 7 for special ethical issues related to qualitative research).

It should be apparent from the preceding sections that although the need for guidelines for the use of human and animal subjects in research is evident and the principles themselves are clear, there are many instances when the nurse must use best judgment both as a patient advocate and as a researcher when evaluating the ethical nature of a research project. In any research situation, the basic guiding principle of protecting the patient's human rights must always apply. When conflicts arise, the nurse must feel free to raise suitable questions with appropriate resources and personnel. In an institution these may include contacting the researcher first and then, if there is no resolution, the director of nursing research and the chairperson of the IRB. In cases when ethical considerations in a research article are in question, clarification from a colleague, agency, or IRB is indicated. The nurse should pursue his or her concerns until satisfied that the patient's rights and his or her rights as a professional nurse are protected.

Critical Thinking Challenges

Barbara Krainovich-Miller

➤ Your state government is interested in determining the number of babies infected with the human immunodeficiency virus (HIV) as needs assessment for future health care delivery planning. A state-wide study is funded that will include the testing of all newborns for HIV, but the mothers will not be told that the test is being done, nor will they be told the results. Using the basic ethical principles found in Box 13-2, defend or refute this practice.

➤ The IRB of your health care agency does not include a nurse and you think it should. You discuss this with your supervisor and she states that it really isn't necessary because the IRB uses strict guidelines. What essential arguments and explanations should you include in your proposal for including a nurse on your institution's IRB?

➤ A qualitative researcher intends to conduct a phenomenological study on caring and use informants who are severely and persistently mentally ill who attend an outpatient clinic. The IRB denies the study indicating that informed consent cannot be obtained and that these patients will not be able to tolerate an interview. What assumptions have the members of this IRB made? If you were the researcher and you were given the opportunity to address their concerns, what would you say? Include information from Table 13-2.

➤ How do you see computer electronic databases and websites assisting researchers in conducting ethical studies? Do you think that IRBs can use this technology to assist them in their goals?

Key Points

- Ethical and legal considerations in research first received attention after World War II during the Nuremberg Trials, from which developed the Nuremberg Code. This became the standard for research guidelines protecting the human rights of research subjects.
- The National Research Act, passed in 1974, created the National Commission for the Protection of Human Subjects of Biomedical and Behavioral Research. The findings, contained in the Belmont Report, discuss three basic ethical principles (respect for persons, beneficence, and justice), which underlie the conduct of research involving human subjects. Federal regulations developed in response to the Commission's report provide guidelines for informed consent and IRB protocols.
- The American Nurses Association's Commission on Nursing Research published Human Rights Guidelines for Nursing in Clinical and Other Research in 1975, for protection of human rights of research subjects. It is relevant to nurses as researchers, as well as caregivers. The ANA Code for Nurses is integral with the Research Guidelines.
- Protection of human rights includes (1) right to self-determination, (2) right to privacy and dignity, (3) right to anonymity and confidentiality, (4) right to fair treatment, and (5) right to protection from discomfort and harm.
- Procedures for protecting basic human rights include gaining informed consent, which illustrates the ethical principle of respect, and obtaining IRB approval, which illustrates the ethical principles of respect, beneficence, and justice.
- Special consideration should be given to studies involving vulnerable populations, such as children, the elderly, prisoners, and those who are mentally or physically disabled.
- Scientific fraud or misconduct represents unethical conduct and must be monitored as part of professional responsibility. Informal, ad hoc, or unauthorized research may expose patients to unwarranted risk and may not protect subject rights adequately.
- Nurses who are asked to be involved in product testing should be aware of FDA guidelines and regulations for testing medical devices before becoming involved in product testing and, perhaps, violating guidelines for ethical research.
- Animal rights need to be protected, and regulations for animal research have evolved over time.

- Nurses who encounter the use of animals in research should be alert to their rights.
- Nurses as consumers of research must be knowledgeable about the legal and ethical components of a research study so they can evaluate whether a researcher has ensured appropriate protection of human or animal rights.

REFERENCES

Altman LK: A flaw in the research process: uncorrected errors in journals. Medical science, *New York Times*, May 31, 1988.

American Geriatrics Society Ethics Committee: Informed consent for research on human subjects with dementia, *J Am Geriatric Soc* 46(10):1308-1310, 1998.

American Nurses Association (ANA): *Guidelines for nurses in clinical and other research*, Kansas City, Mo, 1975, ANA.

American Nurses Association (ANA): *Code for nurses with interpretive statements*, Kansas City, Mo, 1985, ANA.

American Nurses Association (ANA): *Code for nurses*, Washington, DC: American Nurses Publishing, in press.

Andrews EL: U.S. resumes granting patents on genetically altered animals, *New York Times*, C1, February 3, 1993.

Andrews LB: Legal, ethical, and social concerns in the debate over stem-cell research, *Chronicle of Higher Education*, B4-5, January 29, 1999.

Appel JZ, Alwayn IPJ, and Cooper DKC: Xenotransplantation: The challenge in current psychosocial attitudes, *Progress in Transplantation* 10(4):217-225, 2000.

Baskin SA, et al: Barriers to obtaining consent in dementia research: implications for surrogate decision-making, *J Am Geriatric Soc* 46(3):287-290, 1998.

Brainard J and Miller DW: U.S. regulators suspend medical studies at two universities, *Chronicle of Higher Education*, A30, February 4, 2000.

Brink PJ: Antonomy versus do no harm, *West J Nurs Res* 14(3):264-266, 1992.

Campbell PW: Report urges protections for the mentally ill who serve as research subjects, *Chronicle of Higher Education*, A28, July 31, 1998.

Campbell PW: Lawmakers push NIH to focus research on minority populations and cancer, *Chronicle of Higher Education*, A32-33, March 5, 1999a.

Campbell PW: Federal officials fault two New York institutions for research risks to children, *Chronicle of Higher Education*, A43, June 25, 1999b.

Code of Federal Regulations: Protection of human subjects, 45 CFR 46, OPRR Reports, Revised March 8, 1983.

Commission on Research Integrity: Integrity and misconduct in research, Washington, DC, 1995, USDHHS.

Cooper DKC and Lanza RP: *Xeno: the promise of transplanting animal organs into humans,* New York, 2000, Oxford University Press, 2000.

Creighton H: Legal concerns of nursing research, *Nurs Res* 26(4):337-340, 1977.

Davis A: Ethical issues in gerontological nursing research, *Geriatr Nurs* 2:267-272, 1981.

Davis A: Ethical similarities internationally, *West J Nurs Res* 12(5):685-688, 1990.

Department of Health and Human Services: Department of Health and Human Services rules and regulations, 45CF46, Title 45, Pt 46, *Fed Regul* March 8, 1983.

Dubler NN: Personal communication, 1993.

Dubler NN and Post LF: Truth telling and informed consent. In Holland JC, editor: *Textbook of psycho-oncology,* New York, 1998, Oxford Press.

Flaskerud JH and Winslow BJ: Conceptualizing vulnerable populations health-related research, *Nurs Res* 47(2):69-78, 1998.

Fowler MDM: Ethical issues in nursing research: a call for an international code of ethics for nursing research, *West J Nurs Res* 3(10):352-355, 1988.

French HW: AIDS research in Africa: Juggling risks and hopes, *New York Times,* A1 and A12, October 9, 1997.

Grey M et al: Coping skills training for youths with diabetes on intensive therapy, *Appl Nurs Res* 12(1):3-12, 1999.

Haggerty LA and Hawkins J: Informed consent and the limits of confidentiality, *West J Nurs Res* 22(4):508-514, 2000.

Hershey N and Miller RD: *Human experimentation and the law,* Germantown, Md, 1976, Aspen.

Hilts PJ: Agency faults a UCLA study for suffering of mental patients, *New York Times,* A1, 11, March 9, 1995.

Julion W, Gross D, and Barclay-McLaughlin: Recruiting families of color from the inner city: Insights from the recruiters, *Nurs Outlook* 48(5):230-237, 2000.

Katz J: Experimentation with human beings, New York, 1972, Russell Sage Foundation.

Kevles DJ: An injustice to a scientist is reversed, and we learn some lessons, *Chronicle of Higher Education,* B1-2, July 5, 1996.

Kiernan V: The growing conflict over producing stem cells, *Chronicle of Higher Education,* A21-22, September 10, 1999.

Koenes SG and Karshmer JF: Depression: a comparison study between blind and sighted adolescents, *Iss Mental Health Nurs* 21: 269-279, 2000.

Levine RJ: Clarifying the concepts of research ethics, *Hastings Cent Rep* 93(3):21-26, 1979.

Levine RJ: *Ethics and regulation of clinical research,* ed 2, Baltimore-Munich, 1986, Urban and Schwartzenberg.

Levine RJ: Consent for research on children, *Chronicle of Higher Education,* B1-2, November 10, 1995.

LoBiondo-Wood G et al: Family adaptation to a child's transplant: Pretransplant phase, *Progress in Transplantation* 10(2):1-6, 2000.

Lutz KF: Maintaining client safety and scientific integrity in research with battered women, *Image J Nurs Schol* 31(1):89-93, 1999.

McDonald KA: Studies on women's health produce a wealth of knowledge on the biology of gender differences, *Chronicle of Higher Education,* A19-22, June 25, 1999.

Mitchell K: Protecting children's rights during research, *Pediatr Nurs* 10:9-10, 1984.

Monaghan P: The Gods of very small things, *Chronicle of Higher Education,* A19-21, December 15, 2000.

National Bioethics Advisory Commission: Report and recommendations on research involving persons with mental disorders that may affect decisional capacity, 1998.

National Commission for the Protection of Human Subjects of Biomedical and Behavioral Research: *Belmont report: ethical principles and guidelines for research involving human subjects,* DHEW Pub No 05, Washington, DC, 1978, US Government Printing Office, 78-0012.

Office of Research Integrity Website: *http://ori.dhhs.gov,* 2000.

Pallikkathayll L, Crighton F, and Aaronson LS: Balancing ethical quandries with scientific rigor: Part I, *West J Nurs Res* 20(3):388-393, 1998.

Pranulis MF: Protecting rights of human subjects, *West J Nurs Res* 18(4):474-478, 1996.

Pruchino RA and Hayden JM: Interview modality: Effects on costs and data quality in a sample of older women, *J Aging Health* 12(1):3-24, 2000.

Public Health Service Policy on Humane Care in Use of Lab Animals by Awardee Institution: NIH guidelines for grants and contracts, 14(8), 1985.

Rankin M and Esteves MD: Perceptions of scientific misconduct in nursing, Nursing Research 46:270-276, 1997.

Raybuck JA: The clinical nurse specialist as research coordinator in clinical drug trials, *Clin Nurse Specialist* 11(1):15-19, 1997.

Rempusheski VF: Elements, perceptions, and issues of informed consent, *Appl Nurs Res* 4(4):201-204, 1991.

Reverby, SM: History of an apology: From Tuskegee to the White House, *Res Pract* (8):1-12, 2000.

Robb IH: *Nursing ethics: for hospital and private use,* Milwaukee, Wi, 1900, GN Gaspar.

Rothman DJ: Were Tuskegee and Willowbrook studies in nature? *Hastings Cent Rep* 12(2):5-7, 1982.

Ryan K: Scientific misconduct in perspective: the need to improve accountability, *Chronicle of Higher Education,* B1-2, July 19, 1996.

Sailer GR et al: Nurses' unique roles in randomized clinical trials, *J Prof Nurs* 15(6):106-115, 1999.

Tilden VP: Preventing scientific misconduct—times have changed, *Nurs Res* 49(5):243, 2000.

Wheeler DL: Three medical organizations embroiled in controversy over use of placebos in AIDS studies abroad, *Chronicle of Higher Education,* A15-16, August 13, 1997.

Wheeler DL: For biologists, the postgenomic world promises vast and thrilling new knowledge, *Chronicle of Higher Education,* A17-18, August 13, 1999.

ADDITIONAL READINGS

Blancett SS, Flanagan A, and Young RK: Duplicate publication in the nursing literature, *Image J Nurs Schol* 27(1):51-56, 1995.

Cooper C: Principle-oriented ethics and the ethic of care: a creative tension, *Adv Nurs Sci* 14(2):22-31, 1991.

Levine RJ: Research involving children: an interpretation of the new regulations, *IRB Rev Human Subj Res* 5:1-5, 1983.

Orlans FB, Simmonds RC, and Dodds WJ: Effective animal care use committees, *Lab Animal Sci* 1987 (special issue).

Rothman D: Ethics and human experimentation: Henry Beecher revisited, *N Engl J Med* 317:1195-1199, 1987.

Rothman D: *Strangers at the bedside,* New York, 1991, Basic Books.

Rowen AH: *Of mice, models and men: a critical evaluation of animal research,* Albany, NY, 1984, State University of New York Press.

Wheeler DL: Making amends to radiation victims, *Chronicle of Higher Education,* A10-11, October 13, 1995.

Wheeler DL: Three medical organizations embroiled in controversy over use of placebos in AIDS studies abroad, *Chron Higher Ed* A15, December 12, 1997.

SUSAN SULLIVAN-BOLYAI
MARGARET GREY

14

Data-Collection Methods

Key Terms

close-ended items
concealment
consistency
content analysis
debriefing
external criticism
internal criticism
interrater reliability

intervention
interviews
Likert-type scales
objective
open-ended items
operational definition
operationalization
physiological measurement

questionnaires
reactivity
records or available data
scale
scientific observation
social desirability
systematic

Learning Outcomes

After reading this chapter, the student should be able to do the following:

- Define the types of data-collection methods used in nursing research.
- List the advantages and disadvantages of each of these methods.
- Critically evaluate the data-collection methods used in published nursing research studies.

As nurses, we use all of our senses when collecting data from the patients to whom we provide care. Nurse researchers also have available many ways to collect information about their research subjects. The major difference between the data collected when performing patient care and the data collected for the purpose of research is that the data-collection methods employed by researchers need to be objective and systematic. By **objective,** we mean that the data must not be influenced by another who collects the information; by **systematic,** we mean that the data must be collected in the same way by everyone who is involved in the collection procedure.

The methods that researchers use to collect information about subjects are the identifiable and repeatable operations that define the major variables being studied.

Operationalization is the process of translating the concepts of interest to a researcher into observable and measurable phenomena. There may be a number of ways to collect the same information. For example, a researcher interested in measuring anxiety physiologically could do so by measuring sweat gland activity or by administering an anxiety scale, such as the State-Trait Anxiety Scale for Children (Speilberger, 1973). The researcher could also observe children to see whether they displayed anxious behavior. The method chosen by the researcher would depend on a number of decisions regarding the problem being studied, the nature of the subjects, and the relative costs and benefits of each method.

This chapter's purpose is to familiarize you with the various ways that researchers collect information from and about subjects. The chapter provides nursing research consumers with the tools for evaluating the selection, utilization, and practicality of the various ways of collecting data.

MEASURING VARIABLES OF INTEREST

To a large extent, the success of a study depends on the quality of the data-collection methods chosen and employed. Researchers have many types of methods available for collecting information from subjects in research studies. Determining what measurement to use in a particular investigation may be the most difficult and time-consuming step in study design. In addition, as nursing research develops, researchers are beginning to have an array of quality instruments with adequate reliability and validity (see Chapter 15) from which to choose. This aspect of the research process demands painstaking effort from the researcher. Thus the process of evaluating and selecting the available tools to measure variables of interest is of critical importance to the potential success of the study. In this section, the selection of measures and the implementation of the data-collection process are discussed. An algorithm that influences a researcher's choice of data-collection methods is diagrammed in the Critical Thinking Decision Path.

There are many different ways to collect information about phenomena of interest to nurses. Nurses are interested in biological and physical indicators of health (e.g., blood pressure and heart rates) but are also interested in complex psychosocial questions presented by patients. Psychosocial variables, such as anxiety, hope, social support, and self-concept, may be measured by several different techniques, such as observation of behavior or self-reports of feelings or attitudes by means of interviews or questionnaires. Researchers also may use data that have already been collected for another purpose, such as records, diaries, or other media, to study variables of interest.

As you can surmise, choosing the most appropriate method and instrument is difficult. The method must be appropriate to the problem, the hypothesis, the setting, and the population. For example, if a researcher is interested in studying the behavior of 3-year-old children in day care, it would not be sensible to provide the children with some kind of paper-and-pencil test. Although the children might be able to draw on the paper, they would not be likely to answer written questions appropriately.

CRITICAL THINKING DECISION PATH Data-Collection Methods

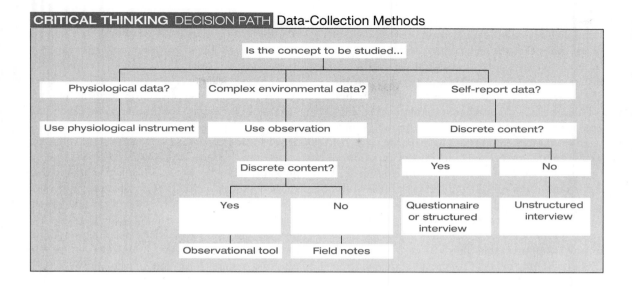

Selection of the data-collection method begins during the literature review. In Chapter 4, it was noted that one purpose of the literature review is to provide clues to instrumentation. As the literature review is conducted, the researcher begins to explore how previous investigators defined and operationalized variables similar to those of interest in the current study. The researcher uses this information to define conceptually the variables to be studied. Once a variable has been defined conceptually, the researcher returns to the literature to define the variable operationally. This **operational definition** translates the conceptual definition into behaviors or verbalizations that can be measured for the study. In this second literature review the researcher searches for measuring instruments that might be used "as is" or adapted for use in the study. If instruments are available, the researcher needs to obtain permission for their use from the author.

An example may illustrate the relationship of the conceptual and operational definitions. Stress research is popular with researchers from many disciplines, including nursing. Definitions of stressors may be psychological, social, or physiological. If a researcher is interested in studying stressors, the researcher needs first to define

what he or she means by the concept of stressor. For example, Holmes and Rahe (1967) defined a stressful life event as any occurrence that required change or adaptation. This definition implies that it is the event that is stressful, not how the individual appraises the event. According to this conceptual definition, the researcher could use a life-event checklist (operational definition) to determine the degree of stress encountered by subjects in the study. If the researcher disagreed with this definition and supported the definition that events are stressful only when individuals appraise them as such (Lazarus and Folkman, 1984), another approach to measurement would be consistent with that view. McCain and associates (1996) used a cognitive appraisal framework in developing their stress management program for men with the human immunodeficiency virus (HIV), so they measured stress levels and coping in a method consistent with that view.

It is sometimes the case that no suitable measuring device exists, so the researcher needs to decide whether the variable is important to the study and whether a new device should be constructed. The construction of new instruments for data collection that have reasonable reliability and validity (see Chapter 15) is a most difficult task. Sometimes researchers decide not to study a variable if no suitable measuring device exists; at other times the researcher may decide to invest time and energy into instrument development. Either decision is acceptable, depending on the goals of the study and the goals of the researcher.

Whether the researcher uses available methods or creates new ones, once the variables have been operationally defined in a manner consistent with the aims of the study, the population to be studied, and the setting, the researcher will determine how the data-collection phase of the study will be implemented. This decision deals with how the instruments for data collection will be given to the subjects. Consistency is the most important issue in this phase.

Consistency means that the data are collected from each subject in the study in exactly the same way or as close to the same way as possible. Consistency can minimize the bias introduced when more than one person collects the data. Thus the researcher must consider ways to minimize subjects' anxiety and to maintain their motivation to complete the data-collection process (Weinert and Burman, 1996), and data collectors must be carefully trained and supervised. To ensure consistency in data collection, researchers must rehearse data collectors in the methods to be used in the study so that each person collects the information in the same way. Information about how to observe, ask questions, and collect data often is included in a kind of "cookbook" protocol for the research project. A researcher may spend several months developing the protocol and training research assistants to collect data systematically and reliably. If data collectors are used, the reader should expect to see some comment about their training and the consistency with which they collected the data for the study. For example, in a study by Rudy and colleagues (1995), the procedure by which consistency of measurement was ensured is clearly presented. Nurses were trained in the scoring of some instruments, such as the Acute Physiological and Chronic Health Evaluation II instrument so that they could accurately extract data from patients'

charts. Another example of the importance of training data collectors is provided by Wikblad and Anderson (1995) in their study comparing three wound dressings in patients undergoing heart surgery. These researchers needed to be accurate in their assessment of surgical wound healing and used a photograph of the wound as the data. Observers rated wounds in several categories such as redness, healing, and blisters. Agreement between raters was calculated using the kappa statistic. The index of agreement in this study was 0.81, and the percent agreement between rates was 91%. These demonstrate a high level of interrater agreement between the two observers. **Interrater reliability** (see Chapter 15) is the consistency of observations between two or more observers; it is often expressed as a percentage of agreement among raters or observers or as a coefficient of agreement that considers the element of chance (coefficient kappa).

HELPFUL HINT Remember that the researcher may not always present complete information about the way the data were collected, especially when established tools were used. To learn about the tool that was used, the reader may need to consult the original article describing the tool.

DATA-COLLECTION METHODS

In general, data-collection methods can be divided into the following five types: physiological, observational, interviews, questionnaires, and records or available data. Each of these methods has a specific purpose, as well as certain pros and cons inherent in its use. Each type of data-collection method is discussed, and then its respective uses and problems are discussed.

PHYSIOLOGICAL OR BIOLOGICAL MEASUREMENTS

In everyday practice, nurses collect physiological data about patients such as their temperature, pulse rate, blood pressure, blood glucose, urine specific gravity, and pH of bodily fluids. Such data are frequently useful to nurse researchers as well, as in the study by Fulton Picot, Zauszniewski, and Debanne (1999). The purpose of the study was to examine the relationship between psychological and blood pressure variables with black female caregivers of elders and noncaregivers. To study this problem, it was important for the researchers to measure the physiological variables at similar intervals and in similar ways for all subjects. The authors chose to measure blood pressure using automated portable monitors, which data collectors were trained to use.

The study by Fulton Picot and associates (1999) is an excellent example of the use of a particular type of data-collection method—physiological. **Physiological measurement** and biological measurement involve the use of specialized equipment to determine physical and biological status of subjects. Frequently such measures also require specialized training. Such measures can be *physical*, such as weight or temperature; *chemical*, such as blood glucose level; *microbiological*, as with cultures; or *anatomical*, as in radiological examinations. What separates these measurements from others used in research is that they require the use of special equipment to make the observation. We can say, "This subject feels warm," but to determine how warm the subject is requires the use of a sensitive instrument, a thermometer.

Erickson, Meyer, and Woo (1996) did a study to determine the clinical accuracy of clinical dot thermometers. They compared temperature measurements with chemical dot thermometers and electronic thermometers at the oral site in 27 adults and the axillary site in 44 adults and 34 young children in critical care units. They found that the chemical dot thermometers provided good temperature estimates, although there were variations by site and by age of the subjects. The study required careful standardization of the procedures so that the instruments were all used in the same way, which is reported in the article.

Physiological or biological measurement is particularly suited to the study of several types of nursing problems. The aforementioned example is typical of studies dealing with ways to improve the performance of certain nursing actions, such

as measuring and recording of patients' physiological data. Physiological measures may yield important criteria for determining the effectiveness of certain nursing actions. A study by Metheny and colleagues (1999) determined nasogastric tube location by testing gastrointestinal samples for pH and bilirubin on acutely ill adults. It is estimated that over 1 million patients in the United States receive tube feedings. The usual air ausulatory nursing action to ensure correct tube placement has been reported as unreliable (Dobranowski et al, 1992). Confirming with an x-ray is the preferred method but is very costly. This study using physiological evidence suggests the measurement of bilirubin and pH in nasogastric tube aspirates as a potentially cheaper and less invasive method to ensure proper tube placement. The study by Fulton Picot and associates (1999) illustrates a type of research that is a priority for the National Institute for Nursing Research: studies of the interface between biology and behavior (termed *biobehavioral interface*).

The advantages of using physiological data-collection methods include their objectivity, precision, and sensitivity. Such methods are generally quite objective because unless there is a technical malfunction, two readings of the same instrument taken at the same time by two different nurses are likely to yield the same result. Because such instruments are intended to measure the variable being studied, they offer the advantage of being precise and sensitive enough to pick up subtle variations in the variable of interest. It is also unlikely that a subject in a study can deliberately distort physiological information.

Physiological measurements are not without inherent disadvantages, however. Some instruments, if they are not available through a hospital, may be quite expensive to obtain. In addition, such instruments often require specialized knowledge and training to be used accurately. Another problem with such measurements is that simply by using them, the variable of interest may be changed. Although some researchers think of these instruments as being nonintrusive, the presence of some types of devices might change the measurement. For example, the presence of a heart rate monitoring device might make some patients anxious and increase their heart rate. In addition, nearly all types of measuring devices are affected in some way by the environment. Even a simple thermometer can be affected by the subject drinking something hot immediately before the temperature is taken. Thus it is important to consider whether the researcher controlled such environmental variables in the study. Finally, there may not be a physiological way to measure the variable of interest. Occasionally researchers try to force a physiological parameter into a study in an effort to increase the precision of measurement. If the device does not really measure the variable of interest, however, the validity of its use is suspect.

OBSERVATIONAL METHODS

Sometimes nurse researchers are interested in determining how subjects behave under certain conditions. For example, the researcher might be interested in how children respond to painful situations. We might ask children how painful an experience was, but they may not be able to answer the question or to quantify the amount of pain, or they may distort their responses to please the researcher. Therefore sometimes observing the subject may give a more accurate picture of the behavior in question than asking the patient.

Although observing the environment is a normal part of living, **scientific observation** places a great deal of emphasis on the objective and systematic nature of the observation. The researcher is not merely looking at what is happening, but rather is watching with a trained eye for certain specific events. To be scientific, observations must fulfill the following four conditions:

1. The observations undertaken are consistent with the study's specific objectives.
2. There is a standardized and systematic plan for the observation and the recording of data.
3. All of the observations are checked and controlled.

4. The observations are related to scientific concepts and theories.

Observation is particularly suitable as a data-collection method in complex research situations that are best viewed as total entities and that are difficult to measure in parts, such as studies dealing with the nursing process, parent-child interactions, or group processes. In addition, observational methods can be the best way to operationalize some variables of interest in nursing research studies, particularly individual characteristics and conditions, such as traits and symptoms, verbal and nonverbal communication behaviors, activities and skill attainment, and environmental characteristics.

Russell and Champion (1996) conducted a study of health beliefs and social influences on the home-safety practices of mothers of preschool children. Because asking mothers to describe the safety precautions they had taken at home would likely miss some important information and thus the data would not be reliable or valid, the researchers used two observational tools to measure the presence of home-safety hazards. The observational tools were adapted from an observation instrument and measured the presence or absence of several observable categories of potential injury situations. The researchers note that there was consistency of recording of these observations between observers because the interrater reliability ranged from 90% to 96.7%.

Observational methods can be distinguished also by the role of the observer. This role is determined by the amount of interaction between the observer and those being observed. Each of the following four basic types of observational roles is distinguishable by the amount of concealment or intervention implemented by the observer:

1. Concealment without intervention
2. Concealment with intervention
3. No concealment without intervention
4. No concealment with intervention

These methods are illustrated in Figure 14-1, and examples are given later. **Concealment** refers to whether the subjects know they are being observed, and **intervention** deals with whether the

Concealment

	Yes	No
Yes Intervention	Researcher hidden An intervention	Researcher open An intervention
No	Researcher hidden No intervention	Researcher open No intervention

Figure 14-1   Types of observational roles in research.

observer provokes actions from those who are being observed. The study of the effect of parent-child interaction education prenatally with expectant couples to promote transition to parenthood by Bryan (2000) is an excellent example of no concealment with intervention. The researcher was not concealed in postnatal observations of parent-child teaching interactions and, if necessary, provided information on how to better interact with the infant after the observations. When a researcher is concerned that the subjects' behavior will change as a result of being observed **(reactivity),** the type of observation most commonly employed is that of concealment without intervention. In this case, the researcher watches the subjects without their knowledge of the observation and he or she does not provoke them into action. Often such concealed observations use hidden television cameras, audiotapes, or one-way mirrors. Concealment without intervention is often used in observational studies of children. You may be familiar with rooms with one-way mirrors in which a researcher can observe the behavior of the occupants of the room without being observed by them. Such studies allow for the observation of children's natural behavior and are often used in developmental research. No concealment without intervention also is commonly used for observational studies. In this case, the researcher obtains informed consent from the subject to be observed and then simply observes his or her behavior. This is the type of observation

done in the Byrne (1998) study in which she observed the feeding interactions of HIV-exposed infants and their caregivers.

Observing subjects without their knowledge may violate assumptions of informed consent, and therefore researchers face ethical problems with this type of approach. However, sometimes there is no other way to collect such data, and the data collected are unlikely to have negative consequences for the subject; in these cases, the disadvantages of the study are outweighed by the advantages. Further, the problem is often handled by informing subjects after the observation and allowing them the opportunity to refuse to have their data included in the study and to discuss any questions they might have. This process is called **debriefing.**

When the observer is neither concealed nor intervening, the ethical question is not a problem. Here the observer makes no attempt to change the subjects' behavior and informs them that they are to be observed. Because the observer is present, this type of observation allows a greater depth of material to be studied than if the observer is separated from the subjects by an artificial barrier, such as a one-way mirror. Participant observation is a commonly used observational technique in which the researcher functions as a part of a social group to study the group in question. The problem with this type of observation is reactivity (also referred to as the Hawthorne effect), or the distortion created when the subjects change behavior because they are being observed.

In the study by Bryan (2000), the researchers used unconcealed observation, because the parents had given full consent for participation in the study. No concealment with intervention is employed when the researcher is observing the effects of some intervention introduced for scientific purposes. Because the subjects know they are participating in a research study, there are few problems with ethical concerns, but reactivity is a problem with this type of study.

Concealed observation with intervention involves staging a situation and observing the behaviors that are evoked in the subjects as a result of the intervention. Because the subjects are un-aware of their participation in a research study, this type of observation has fallen into disfavor and rarely is used in nursing research.

Observations may be structured or unstructured. Unstructured observational methods, such as those suggested by West, Bondy, and Hutchinson (1991) for working with the elderly, are not characterized by a total absence of structure but usually involve collecting descriptive information about the topic of interest. In participant observation, the observer keeps field notes that record the activities, as well as the observer's interpretations of these activities. *Field notes* usually are not restricted to any particular type of action or behavior; rather, they intend to paint a picture of a social situation in a more general sense. Another type of unstructured observation is the use of anecdotes. *Anecdotes* are not necessarily funny but usually focus on the behaviors of interest and frequently add to the richness of research reports by illustrating a particular point. On the other hand, structured observations, such as the standardized tools used to observe feeding interactions in the Byrne (1998) study, require formal training and certification. The use of structured observations without a standardized tool involve specifying in advance what behaviors or events are to be observed and preparing forms for record keeping, such as categorization systems, checklists, and rating scales. Whichever system is employed, the observer watches the subject and then marks on the recording form what was seen. In any case, the observations must be similar among the observers (see earlier discussion and Chapter 15 for an explanation of interrater reliability). Thus it is important that observers be trained to be consistent in their observations and ratings of behavior.

Scientific observation has several advantages as a data-collection method, the main one being that observation may be the only way for the researcher to study the variable of interest. For example, what people say they do often is not what they really do. Therefore if the study is designed to obtain substantive findings about human be-havior, observation may be the only way to ensure the validity of the findings. In addition, no other data-collection method can match the depth and variety of information that can be collected when using these techniques. Such techniques also are quite flexible in that they may be used in both experimental and nonexperimental designs and in laboratory and field studies.

HELPFUL HINT Sometimes a researcher may carefully train observers or data collectors, but the research report does not address this. Often the length of research reports dictates that certain information cannot be included. Readers can often assume that if reliability data are provided, then appropriate training occurred.

As with all data-collection methods, observation also has its disadvantages. We mentioned the problems of reactivity and ethical concerns when we discussed the concealment and intervention dimensions. In addition, data obtained by observational techniques are vulnerable to the bias of the observer. Emotions, prejudices, and values all can influence the way that behaviors and events are observed. In general, the more the observer needs to make inferences and judgments about what is being observed, the more likely it is that distortions will occur. Thus in judging the adequacy of observational methods, it is important to consider how observational tools were constructed and how observers were trained and evaluated.

INTERVIEWS AND QUESTIONNAIRES

Subjects in a research study often have information that is important to the study and that can be obtained only by asking the subject. Such questions may be asked orally by a researcher in person or over the telephone in an interview, or they may be asked in the form of a paper-and-pencil test. Both interviews and questionnaires have the purpose of asking subjects to report data for themselves, but each has unique advantages and disadvantages. **Interviews** are a method of data collection where a data collector questions a subject verbally. Interviews may be face-to-face or performed over the telephone, and they may consist of open-ended or close-ended questions. On the other hand, **questionnaires** are paper-and-pencil instruments designed to gather data from individuals about knowledge, attitudes, beliefs, and feelings. Survey research relies almost entirely on questioning subjects with either interviews or questionnaires, but these methods of data collection also can be used in other types of research.

No matter what type of study is conducted, the purpose of questioning subjects is to seek information. This information may be of either direct interest, such as the subject's age, or indirect interest, such as when the researcher uses a combination of items to estimate to what degree the respondent has some trait or characteristic. An intelligence test is an example of how individual items are combined with several others to develop an overall scale of intelligence. When items of indirect interest are combined to obtain an overall score, the measurement tool is called a **scale.** The investigator determines the content of an interview or questionnaire from the literature review (see Chapter 4). When evaluating these methods, the reader should consider the content of the scale, the individual items, and the order of the items. The basic standard for evaluating the individual items in an interview or questionnaire is that the item must be clearly written so that the intent of the question and the nature of the information sought are clear to the respondent. The only way to know whether the questions are understandable to the respondents is to pilot test them in a similar population. It is also critical not to rely just on the instrument developer's reports of reliability and validity (see Chapter 15). A pilot test allows the researcher to test the reliability and validity for their unique sample rather than rely on the previously reported results. Although items must ask only one question, be free of suggestions, and use correct grammar they may be either open-ended or close-ended. **Open-ended items** are used when the researcher wants the subjects to respond in their own words or when the researcher does not know all of the possible

alternative responses. **Close-ended items** are used when there is a fixed number of alternative responses. Many scales use a fixed-response format called a Likert-type scale.

Likert-type scales are lists of statements on which respondents indicate, for example, whether they "strongly agree," "agree," "disagree," or "strongly disagree." Sometimes finer distinctions are given or there may be a neutral category. The use of the neutral category, however, sometimes creates problems because it often is the most frequent response and this response is difficult to interpret. Fixed-response items also can be used for questions requiring a "yes" or "no" response or when there are categories, as with income. Structured, fixed-response items are best used when the question has a finite number of responses and the respondent is to choose the one closest to the right one. Fixed-response items have the advantage of simplifying the respondent's task and the researcher's analysis, but they may miss some important information about the subject. Unstructured response formats allow such information to be included but require a special technique to analyze the responses. This technique is called **content analysis** and is a method for the objective, systematic, and quantitative description of communications and documentary evidence.

Figure 14-2 shows a few items from a survey of pediatric nurse practitioners (Grey and Flint, 1989). The first items are taken from a list of similar items, and they are both closed and of a Likert-type format. Note that respondents are asked to choose how strongly they agree with each item. In using these questions in the survey, respondents are forced to choose from only these answers because it is thought that these will be the only responses. The only possible alternative response is to skip the item and leave it blank. On the other hand, sometimes researchers have no idea or have only a limited idea of what the respondent will say, or researchers want the answer in the respondent's own words, as with the second set of items. Here, respondents may also leave the item blank but are not forced to make a particular response.

Close-Ended (Likert-Type Scale)

A. How satisfied are you with your current position?
1. Very satisfied
2. Moderately satisfied
3. Undecided
4. Moderately dissatisfied
5. Very dissatisfied

B. To what extent do the following factors contribute to your current level of positive satisfaction?

	Not at all	Very little	Somewhat	Moderate amount	A great deal
1. % of time in patient care	1	2	3	4	5
2. Types of patients	1	2	3	4	5
3. % of time in educational activity	1	2	3	4	5
4. % of time in administration	1	2	3	4	5

Close-Ended

A. On an average, how many clients do you see in one day?
1. 1 to 3
2. 4 to 6
3. 7 to 9
4. 10 to 12
5. 13 to 15
6. 16 to 18
7. 19 to 20
8. More than 20

B. How would you characterize your practice?
1. Too slow
2. Slow
3. About right
4. Busy
5. Too busy

Open-Ended

A. Are there incentives that the National Association of Pediatric Nurse Associates and Practitioners ought to provide for members that are currently not being done?

_____
_____
_____
_____

Figure 14-2   Examples of close-ended and open-ended questions.

Interviews and questionnaires are used commonly in nursing research. Both are strong approaches to gathering information for research, because they approach the task directly. In addition, both have the ability to obtain certain kinds of information, such as the subjects' attitudes and beliefs, which would be difficult to obtain without asking the subject directly. All methods that involve verbal reports, however, share a problem with accuracy. There is often no way to know whether what the researcher is told is indeed true. For example, people are known to respond to questions in a way that makes a favorable impression. This response style is known as **social desirability.** Because there is no way to tell whether the respondent is telling the truth or responding in a socially desirable way, the researcher usually is forced to assume that the respondent is telling the truth.

Questionnaires and interviews also have some specific purposes, advantages, and disadvantages. Questionnaires and paper-and-pencil tests are most useful when there is a finite set of questions to be asked and the researcher can be assured of the clarity and specificity of the items. Questionnaires are desirable tools when the purpose is to collect information. If questionnaires are too long, they are not likely to be completed. Face-to-face techniques or interviews are best used when the researcher may need to clarify the task for the respondent or is interested in obtaining more personal information from the respondent. Telephone interviews allow the researcher to reach more respondents than face-to-face interviews, and they allow for more clarity than questionnaires.

HELPFUL HINT Remember, sometimes researchers make trade-offs when determining the measures to be used. For example, a researcher may want to learn about an individual's attitudes regarding practice; practicalities may preclude using an interview, so a questionnaire may be used instead.

Grey and associates (1995) used a combination of interview and questionnaires to study psychological, social, and physiological adaptation in children and adolescents with diabetes over the first 2 years after diagnosis. One of the measures of social adaptation was the Child and Adolescent Adjustment Profile, which is a parent interview measuring the social role performance of children and adolescents in the areas of productivity, peer relations, dependency, hostility, and withdrawal. Obtaining a more complete evaluation of the adaptation of the children, however, required that the children also report on their own feelings. This was accomplished by using the Self-Perception Profile for Children, which is a questionnaire dealing with children's feelings of competence in several areas. Thus the researchers were able to report both the children's and their parents' accounts of the child's overall adaptation. This use of multiple measures gives a more complete picture than the use of just one measure.

Researchers face difficult choices when determining whether to use interviews or questionnaires. The final decision is often based on what instruments are available and their relative costs and benefits.

Both face-to-face and telephone interviews offer some advantages over questionnaires. All things being equal, interviews are better than questionnaires because the response rate is almost always higher and this helps eliminate bias in the sample (see Chapter 12). Respondents seem to be less likely to hang up the telephone or to close the door in an interviewer's face than to throw away a questionnaire. Another advantage of the interview is that some people, such as children, the blind, and the illiterate, could not fill out a questionnaire, but they could participate in an interview. With an interview, the data collector knows who is giving the answers. When questionnaires are mailed, for example, anyone in the household could be the person who supplies the answers.

Interviews also allow for some safeguards to be built into the interview situation. Interviewers can clarify misunderstood questions and observe the level of the respondent's understanding and cooperativeness. In addition, the researcher has strict control over the order of the questions. With questionnaires, the respondent can answer questions in any order. Sometimes changing the order of the questions can change the response.

Finally, interviews allow for richer and more complex data to be collected. This is particularly so when open-ended responses are sought. Even when close-ended response items are used, interviews can probe to understand why a respondent answered in a particular way. Questionnaires also have certain advantages. They are much less expensive to administer than interviews because interviews may require the hiring and training of interviewers. Thus if a researcher has a fixed amount of time and money, a larger and more diverse sample can be obtained with questionnaires. Questionnaires also allow for complete anonymity, which may be important if the study deals with sensitive issues. Finally, the fact that no interviewer is present assures the researcher and the reader that there will be no interviewer bias. Interviewer bias occurs when the interviewer unwittingly leads the respondent to answer in a certain way. This problem is especially pronounced in studies that use unstructured interview formats. A subtle nod of the head, for example, could lead a respondent to change an answer to correspond with what the researcher wants to hear.

Wilson, Pittman, and Wold (2000) used an unstructured focus group interview method to study Hispanic migrant children's health experiences. These unstructured interviews occurred in small groups (4 to 8 in each group) with children 8 to 14 years of age. These small groups allow the participants to freely participate and explain and share information in an unstructured interview, allowing the researchers to obtain a more complete picture of the experiences of the subjects than would be provided by either a more structured interview or a questionnaire.

RECORDS OR AVAILABLE DATA

All of the data-collection methods discussed thus far concern the ways that nurse researchers gather new data to study phenomena of interest. Not all studies, though, require a researcher to acquire new information. Sometimes existing information can be examined in a new way to study a problem. The use of records and available data sometimes is considered to be primarily the province of historical research, but hospital records, care plans, and existing data sources, such as the census, are frequently used for collecting information. What sets these studies apart from a literature review is that these available data are examined in a new way, are not merely summarized, and answer specific research questions. **Records or available data,** then, are forms of information that are collected from existing materials, such as hospital records, historical documents, or videotapes, and are used to answer research questions in a new manner. Much of the data analyzed in the study by Rudy and associates (1995) consisted of available data, such as mortality and length of stay statistics and hospital charges and costs.

The use of available data has certain advantages. Because the data-collection step of the research process often is the most difficult and time-consuming, the use of available records often allows for a significant savings of time. If the records have been kept in a similar manner over time, as with the National Health and Examination Surveys, analysis of these records allows for the examination of trends over time. In addition, the use of available data decreases problems of reactivity and response set bias. The researcher also does not have to ask individuals to participate in the study.

On the other hand, institutions are sometimes reluctant to allow researchers to have access to their records. If the records are kept so that an individual cannot be identified, this is usually not a problem. However, the Privacy Act, a federal law, protects the rights of individuals who may be identified in records. Another problem that affects the quality of available data is that the researcher has access only to those records that have survived. If the records available are not representative of all of the possible records, the researcher may have a problem with bias. Often there is no way to tell whether the records have been saved in a biased manner, and the researcher has to make an intelligent guess as to their accuracy. For example, a researcher might be interested in studying socioeconomic factors associated with the suicide rate. These data frequently are underreported because of the stigma attached to suicide, and so the records would be biased. Recent interest in computerization of health records has led to an increase in discussion about the desirability of access to such records for research. At this point, it is not clear how much of such data will continue to be readily available for research without consent.

Another problem is related to the authenticity of the records. The distinction of primary and secondary sources is as relevant here as it was in discussing the literature review (see Chapter 4). A book, for example, may have been ghostwritten but credit accorded to the known author. It may be difficult for the researcher to ferret out these types of subtle biases.

Nonetheless, records and available data constitute a rich source of data for study. Cooper (1999) provides an interesting example of using available data to study suicide. Cooper (1999) used coroner's reports, interviews done with key informants (family, friends) and medical records to explore the phenomenon of suicide. She refers to this process as a psychological autopsy. Future health service provisions were recommended from using this unique approach to a very sensitive topic.

CONSTRUCTION OF NEW INSTRUMENTS

As already mentioned in this chapter, researchers sometimes cannot locate an instrument or method with acceptable reliability and validity to measure the variable of interest. This often is the case when testing a part of a nursing theory or when evaluating the effect of a clinical intervention. An example is provided by the work of Gilmer and associates (1993), who were interested in assessing functional status of the elderly for a series of studies of nursing interventions. They developed and tested the Iowa Self-Assessment Inventory to measure seven functional characteristics of the elderly: economic resources, cognitive status, mobility, physical health, emotional balance, social support, and trusting others. Then the items were tested for readability and the items were combined into a test that could be tested and piloted.

Instrument development is complex and time consuming. It consists of the following steps:
- Define the construct to be measured
- Formulate the items
- Assess the items for content validity
- Develop instructions for respondents and users
- Pretest and pilot test the items
- Estimate reliability and validity

To define the construct to be measured requires that the researcher develop an expertise in the construct. This requires an extensive review of the literature and of all tests and measurements that deal with related constructs. The researcher will use all of this information to synthesize the available knowledge so that the construct can be defined.

Once defined, the individual items measuring the construct can be developed. The researcher will develop many more items than are needed to address each aspect of the construct or subconstruct. The items are evaluated by a panel of experts in the field so that the researcher is assured that the items measure what they are intended to measure (content validity; see Chapter 15). Eventually the number of items will be decreased because some items will not work as they were intended and they will be dropped. In this phase, the researcher needs to ensure consistency among the items, as well as consistency in testing and scoring procedures.

Finally, the researcher administers or pilot tests the new instrument by giving it to a group of people who are similar to those who will be studied in the larger investigation. The purpose of this analysis is to determine the quality of the instrument as a whole (reliability and validity), as well as the ability of each item to discriminate individual respondents (variance in item response). The researcher also may administer a related instrument to see if the new instrument is sufficiently different from the older one.

It is important that researchers who invest significant amounts of time in tool development publish those results. This type of research serves not only to introduce other researchers to the tool but also to ultimately enhance the field because our ability to conduct meaningful research is limited only by our ability to measure important phenomena.

HELPFUL HINT Determine whether a newly developed paper-and-pencil test was pilot tested to obtain preliminary evidence of reliability and validity.

Savedra and associates (1995) developed the Adolescent Pediatric Pain Tool (APPT; Savedra and associates, 1993) to measure pain in children and adolescents but found that they needed to add a temporal dimension to the measurement. To do so, they conducted a study in two phases. First, they tested the usefulness of a dot matrix format to assist children and adolescents to communicate the change in their pain over time. They also generated a list of words related to onset, duration, and changing pattern of pain. Then they examined the validity of the list of words and the representation by the dot matrix format by asking children to rate pain experiences associated with short- and long-term painful events.

CRITIQUING Data-Collection Methods

Evaluating the adequacy of data-collection methods from written research reports is often problematic for new nursing research consumers. This is because the tool itself is not available for inspection and the reader may not feel comfortable judging the adequacy of the method without seeing it. However, a number of questions can be asked to judge the method chosen by the researcher. These questions are listed in the Critiquing Criteria box.

All studies should have clearly identified data-collection methods. The conceptual and operational definitions of each important variable should be present in the report. Sometimes it is useful for the researcher to explain why a particular method was chosen. For example, if the study dealt with young children, the researcher may explain that a questionnaire was deemed to be an unreasonable task, so an interview was chosen.

Once you have identified the method chosen to measure each variable of interest, you should decide if the method used was the best way to measure the variable. If a questionnaire was used, for example, you might wonder why the decision was made not to use an interview. In addition, consider whether the method was appropriate to the clinical

situation. Does it make sense to interview patients in the recovery room, for example?

Once you have decided whether all relevant variables are operationalized appropriately, you can begin to determine how well the method was carried out. For studies using physiological measurement, it is important to determine whether the instrument was appropriate to the problem and not forced to fit it. The rationale for selecting a particular instrument should be given. For example, it may be important to know that the study was conducted under the auspices of a manufacturing firm that provided the measuring instrument. In addition, provision should be made to evaluate the accuracy of the instrument and those who use it.

Several considerations are important when reading studies that use observational methods. Who were the observers, and how were they trained? Is there any reason to believe that different observers saw events or behaviors differently? Remember that the more inferences the observers are required to make, the more likely there will be problems with biased observations. Also consider the problem of reactivity; in any observational situation, the possibility exists that the mere presence of the observer

CRITIQUING CRITERIA

1. Are all of the data-collection instruments clearly identified and described?
2. Is the rationale for their selection given?
3. Is the method used appropriate to the problem being studied?
4. Were the methods used appropriate to the clinical situation?
5. Are the data-collection procedures similar for all subjects?

Physiological Measurement

1. Is the instrument used appropriate to the research problem and not forced to fit it?
2. Is a rationale given for why a particular instrument was selected?
3. Is there a provision for evaluating the accuracy of the instrument and those who use it?

Observational Methods

1. Who did the observing?
2. Were the observers trained to minimize any bias?
3. Was there an observational guide?
4. Were the observers required to make inferences about what they saw?
5. Is there any reason to believe that the presence of the observers affected the behavior of the subjects?
6. Were the observations performed using the principles of informed consent?

Interviews

1. Is the interview schedule described adequately enough to know whether it covers the subject?
2. Is there clear indication that the subjects understood the task and the questions?
3. Who were the interviewers, and how were they trained?
4. Is there evidence of any interviewer bias?

Questionnaires

1. Is the questionnaire described well enough to know whether it covers the subject?
2. Is there evidence that subjects were able to perform the task?
3. Is there clear indication that the subjects understood the questionnaire?
4. Are the majority of the items appropriately close- or open-ended?

Available Data and Records

1. Are the records used appropriate to the problem being studied?
2. Are the data examined in such a way as to provide new information and not summarize the records?
3. Has the author addressed questions of internal and external criticism?
4. Is there any indication of selection bias in the available records?

could change the behavior in question. What is important here is not that reactivity could occur, but rather how much reactivity could affect the data. Finally, consider whether the observational procedure was ethical. The reader needs to consider whether subjects were informed that they were being observed, whether any intervention was performed, and whether subjects had agreed to be observed.

Interviews and questionnaires should be clearly described to allow the reader to decide whether the variables were adequately operationalized. Sometimes the researcher will reference the original report about the tool, and the reader may wish to read this study before deciding if the method was appropriate for the present study. The respondents' task should be clear. Thus provision should be made for the subjects to understand both their overall responsibilities and the individual items. Who were the interviewers in the interview situation? Does the researcher explain how they were trained to decrease any interviewer bias?

Available data are subject to internal and external criticism. **Internal criticism** deals with the evaluation of the worth of the records. Internal criticism primarily refers to the accuracy of the data. The researcher should present evidence that the records are genuine. **External criticism** is concerned with the authenticity of the records. Are the records really written by the first author? Finally, the reader should be aware of the problems with selective survival. The researcher may not have an unbiased sample of all of the possible records in the problem area, and this may have a profound effect on the validity of the results.

Finally, the reader should consider the data-collection procedure. Is any assurance provided that all of the subjects received the same information? In addition, it is important to try to determine whether all of the information was collected in the same way for all of the subjects in the study.

Once you have decided that the data collection method used was appropriate to the problem and the procedures were appropriate to the population studied, the reliability and validity of the instruments themselves need to be considered. These characteristics are discussed in the next chapter.

Critical Thinking Challenges

Barbara Krainovich-Miller

➤ Physiological measurements are objective, precise, and sensitive. Discuss factors that might impact on their validity and feasibility.

➤ A student in research class asks why nurses who participate in a clinical research study in the role of a data collector or perform a "treatment intervention" need to be trained. What important factors or rationale would you offer to support the establishment of interrater reliability?

➤ Observational methods are a frequent data-collection method in nursing research. Discuss what makes nurses perfect potential candidates for this role and what are the disadvantages of using this method.

➤ Discuss how the internet can play a role in critiquing and refining data-collection methods. Include any ethical implications you might anticipate.

➤ Studies often use a survey to collect data. How can researchers increase their return rate of the survey, and how is it determined if the survey return is adequate?

Key Points

- Data-collection methods are described as being both objective and systematic. The data-collection methods of a study provide the operational definitions of the relevant variables.

- Types of data-collection methods include physiological, observational, interviews, questionnaires, and available data or records. Each method has advantages and disadvantages.

- Physiological measurements are those methods that use technical instruments to collect data about patients' physical, chemical, microbiological, or anatomical status. They are suited to studying how to improve the effectiveness of nursing care. Physiological measurements are objective, precise, and sensitive, but they may be very expensive and may distort the variable of interest.

- Observational methods are used in nursing research when the variables of interest deal with events or behaviors. Scientific observation requires preplanning, systematic recording, controlling the observations, and relationship to scientific theory. This method is best suited to research problems that are difficult to view as a part of a whole. Observers may be passive or active and concealed or obvious. Observational methods have several advantages: they provide flexibility to measure many types of situations and they allow for a great depth and breadth of information to be collected. Observation has disadvantages as well: (1) data may be distorted as a result of the observer's presence (reactivity), (2) concealment requires the consideration of ethical issues, and (3) observations may be biased by the person who is doing the observing.

- Interviews are commonly used data-collection methods in nursing research. Items on interview schedules may be of direct or indirect interest. Either open-ended or close-ended questions may be used when asking subjects questions. The form of the question should be clear to the respondent, free of suggestion, and grammatically correct.

- Questionnaires, or paper-and-pencil tests, are useful when there are a finite number of questions to be asked. Questions need to be clear and specific. Questionnaires are less costly in time and money to administer to large groups of subjects, particularly if the subjects are geographically widespread. Questionnaires also can be completely anonymous and prevent interviewer bias.

- Interviews are best used when a large response rate and an unbiased sample are important because the refusal rate for interviews is much less than that for questionnaires. Interviews allow for portions of the population such as children and the illiterate who would otherwise be omitted by the use of a questionnaire to participate in the study. An interviewer can clarify and maintain the order of the questions for all participants.

- Records and available data also are an important source for research data. The use of available data may save the researcher considerable time and money when conducting a study. This method reduces problems with both reactivity and ethical concerns. However, records and available data are subject to problems of availability, authenticity, and accuracy.

- A critical evaluation of data-collection methods should emphasize the appropriateness, objectivity, and consistency of the method employed.

REFERENCES

Bryan AA: Enhancing parent-child interaction with a prenatal couple intervention *MCN* 25(3):139-144, 2000.

Byrne MW: Feeding interactions in a cross section of HIV-exposed infants, *West J Nurs Res* 20:409-430, 1998.

Cooper J: Ethical issues and their practical application in a psychological autopsy study of suicide, *J Clin Nurs* 8(4):467-475, 1999.

Dobranowski J et al: Incorrect positioning of nasogastric feeding tubes and the development of pneumothorax, *Can Assoc Radiol J* 43:35-39, 1992.

Erickson RS, Meyer LT, and Woo TM: Accuracy of chemical dot thermometers in critically ill adults and young children, *Image J Nurs Sch* 28:23-28, 1996.

Fulton Picot SJ, Zauszniewski JA, and Debanne SM: Mood and blood pressure responses in black female caregivers and noncaregivers, *Nurs Res* 48:150-161, 1999.

Gilmer JS et al: Instrument format issues in assessing the elderly: the Iowa Self-Assessment Inventory, *Nurs Res* 42:297-299, 1993.

Grey M and Flint S: 1988 NAPNAP membership survey: characteristics of members' practice, *J Pediatr Health Care* 3:336-341, 1989.

Grey M et al: Psychosocial status of children with diabetes over the first two years, *Diabetes Care* 18:1330-1336, 1995.

Holmes TH and Rahe RH: The social readjustment rating scale, *J Psychosom Res* 11:213-218, 1967.

Lazarus RS and Folkman S: Coping and adaptation. In Gentry WD, ed: *The handbook of behavioral medicine,* New York, 1984, Guildford.

McCain NL et al: The influence of stress management training in HIV disease, *Nurs Res* 45:246-253, 1996.

Metheny NA et al: pH and concentration of bilirubin in feeding tube aspirates as predictors of tube placement, *Nurs Res* 48:189-197, 1999.

Rudy EB et al: Patient outcomes for the chronically critically ill: special care unit versus intensive care unit, *Nurs Res* 44:324-331, 1995.

Russell KM and Champion VL: Health beliefs and social influence in home safety practices of mothers with preschool children, *Image J Nurs Sch* 28: 59-64, 1996.

Savedra MC et al: Assessment of postoperative pain in children and adolescents using the Adolescent Pediatric Pain Tool, *Nurs Res* 42:5-9, 1993.

Savedra MC et al: A strategy to assess the temporal dimension of pain in children and adolescents, *Nurs Res* 44:272-276, 1995.

Speilberger CD: *Manual for the state-trait anxiety inventory for children,* Palo Alto, CA, 1973, Consulting Psychologists.

Weinert C and Burman M: Nurturing longitudinal samples, *West J Nurs Res* 18:360-364, 1996.

West M, Bondy E, and Hutchinson S: Interviewing institutionalized elders: threats to validity, *Image J Nurs Sch* 23:171-176, 1991.

Wikblad K and Anderson B: A comparison of three wound dressings in patients undergoing heart surgery, *Nurs Res* 44(5):312-316, 1995.

Wilson AH, Pittman K, and Lupo Wold J: Listening to the quiet voices of Hispanic migrant children about health, *J Pediatr Nurs* 15:137-147, 2000.

ADDITIONAL READINGS

Buros OK: *Tests in print II,* Highland Park, NJ, 1994, Gryphon Press.

Butz AM and Alexander C: Use of health diaries with children, *Nurs Res* 40:59-61, 1991.

Collins C et al: Interviewer training and supervision, *Nurs Res* 37:122-124, 1988.

Cowan MJ: Measurement of heart rate variability, *West J Nurs Res* 17:32-48, 1995.

DeKeyser FG and Puch LC: Assessment of the reliability and validity of biochemical measures, *Nurs Res* 39:314-317, 1990.

Frank-Stromberg M and Olsen S: *Instruments for clinical health research,* Boston, 1997, Jones & Bartlett.

Hutchinson S and Wilson HS: Validity threats in scheduled semistructured research interviews, *Nurs Res* 41:117-119, 1992.

Jones EJ, Kay M: Instrumentation in cross-cultural research, *Nurs Res* 41:186-188, 1992.

Knapp TR and Brown JK: Ten measurement commandments that often should be broken, *Res Nurs Health* 18:465-469, 1995.

Morse JM: Approaches to qualitative-quantitative methodological triangulation, *Nurs Res* 40:120-123, 1991.

Nield M and Kim MJ: The reliability of magnitude estimation for dyspnea measurement, *Nurs Res* 40:17-19, 1991.

Strickland OL and Waltz CF: *Measurement of nursing outcomes: measuring client outcomes,* vol 1, New York, 1988, Springer.

Waltz CF and Strickland OL: *Measurement of nursing outcomes: measuring client outcomes,* vol 2, New York, 1988, Springer.

GERI LOBIONDO-WOOD
JUDITH HABER

Reliability and Validity

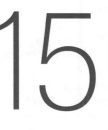

Key Terms

chance (random) errors
concurrent validity
construct validity
content validity
contrasted-groups (known-groups) approach
convergent validity
criterion-related validity
Cronbach's alpha
divergent validity
equivalence

error variance
face validity
factor analysis
homogeneity
hypothesis-testing
internal consistency
interrater reliability
item to total correlations
Kuder-Richardson coefficient
multitrait-multimethod approach

observed test score
parallel or alternate form reliability
predictive validity
reliability
reliability coefficient
split-half reliability
stability
systematic (constant) error
test-retest reliability
validity

Learning Outcomes

After reading this chapter, the student should be able to do the following:

- Discuss how measurement error can affect the outcomes of a research study.
- Discuss the purposes of reliability and validity.
- Define reliability.
- Discuss the concepts of stability, equivalence, and homogeneity as they relate to reliability.
- Compare and contrast the estimates of reliability.
- Define validity.
- Compare and contrast content, criterion-related, and construct validity.
- Identify the criteria for critiquing the reliability and validity of measurement tools.
- Use the critiquing criteria to evaluate the reliability and validity of measurement tools.

Measurement of nursing phenomena is a major concern of nursing researchers. Unless measurement instruments validly and reliably reflect the concepts of the theory being tested, conclusions drawn from a study will be invalid and will not advance the development of nursing theory and evidence-based practice. Issues of reliability and validity are of central concern to the researcher, as well as the critiquer of research. From either perspective, the measurement instruments that are used in a research study must be evaluated. Many new constructs are relevant to nursing theory, and a growing number of established measurement instruments are available to researchers. Researchers often face the challenge of developing new instruments, however, and as part of that process, establishing the reliability and validity of those tools. The growing importance of measurement issues, tool development, and related issues (e.g., reliability and validity) is evident in the issues of the *Journal of Nursing Measurement* and other nursing research journals.

Nurse investigators use instruments that have been developed by researchers in nursing and other disciplines. The critiquer of research, when reading research studies and reports, must assess the reliability and validity of the instruments used in the study to determine the soundness of these selections in relation to the concepts or variables under investigation. The appropriateness of the instruments and the extent to which reliability and validity are demonstrated have a profound influence on the findings and the internal and external validity of the study. Invalid measures produce invalid estimates of the relationships between variables, thus affecting internal validity. The use of invalid measures produces inaccurate generalizations to the populations being studied, thus affecting external validity and the ability to apply or not apply research findings in clinical practice. As such, the assessment of reliability and validity is an extremely important skill for critiquers of nursing research to develop.

Regardless of whether a new or already developed measurement tool is used in a research study, evidence of reliability and validity is of crucial importance. Box 15-1 identifies several

---

BOX 15-1 Computer Resources for Accessing and Evaluating the Validity and Reliability of Measurement Instruments*

- Health and Psychosocial Instruments (HaPI)
  Behavioral Measurement Database Services
  P.O. Box 110287
  Pittsburgh, PA 15232-0787
  412-687-6850
  bmdshapi@aol.com
  A CD-ROM database of measurement instruments in the areas of health and behavioral sciences
- 1997 Guide to Behavioral Resources on the Internet
  Faulkner and Gray, Inc.
  11 Penn Plaza
  New York, NY 10001
  1-800-535-8403
  http://www.faulknergray.com
  A print guide to more than 500 internet resources devoted to mental health and behavioral research, including research tools.
- On-line Journal of Knowledge Synthesis for Nursing
  To subscribe, visit *www.nursingsociety.org*
  Provides full-text articles and searches, hypertext navigation, links to CINAHL and MEDLINE, tables and figures.
- Virginia Henderson International Nursing Library
  To subscribe, visit *www.nursingsociety.org*
  Includes the following databases: registry of nurse researchers, registry of research projects, and registry of research results.
- Sigma Theta Tau International Nursing Honor Society
  550 West North Street
  Indianapolis, IN 46202
  317-634-8171
  www.nursingsociety.org
- CINAHL CD-ROM or On-line Services
  Access to searches in nursing and 17 allied health disciplines
  CINAHL Information Systems
  1509 Wilson Terrace
  Glendale, CA 91206
  1-800-959-7167
  http://www.cinahl.com/

*See Chapter 4 for detailed information about computer resources.

computer resources that research consumers can use to access and evaluate the reliability and validity of the measurement instruments used in research studies. This chapter examines the major types of reliability and validity and demonstrates

$$\text{Observed score } (X_O) = \text{True variance } (X_T) + \text{Error variance } (X_E)$$

Actual score obtained	Consistent, hypothetical stable or true score	CHANCE/RANDOM ERROR — Transient subject factors — Instrumentation variations — Transient environmental factors SYSTEMATIC ERROR — Consistent instrument, subject or environmental factors

Figure 15-1   Components of observed scores.

the applicability of these concepts to the development, selection, and evaluation of measurement tools in nursing research.

RELIABILITY, VALIDITY, AND MEASUREMENT ERROR

Researchers may be concerned about whether the scores that were obtained for a sample of subjects were consistent, true measures of the behaviors and thus an accurate reflection of the differences between individuals. The extent of variability in test scores that is attributable to error rather than a true measure of the behaviors is the **error variance.**

An **observed test score** that is derived from a set of items actually consists of the true score plus error (Figure 15-1). The error may be either chance error or random error, or it may be systematic error. Validity is concerned with systematic error, whereas reliability is concerned with random error. **Chance** or **random errors** are errors that are difficult to control (e.g., a respondent's anxiety level at the time of testing). Random errors are unsystematic in nature. Random errors are a result of a transient state in the subject, the context of the study, or the administration of the instrument (Hoskins, 1998). For example, perceptions or behaviors that occur at a specific point in time (e.g.,

anxiety) are known as a state or transient characteristic and are often beyond the awareness and control of the examiner. Another example of random error is in a study that measures blood pressure. Random error could occur by misplacement of the cuff, not waiting for a specific time period before taking the blood pressure, or placing the arm randomly in relationship to the heart while measuring blood pressure.

Systematic or **constant error** is measurement error that is attributable to relatively stable characteristics of the study population that may bias their behavior and/or cause incorrect instrument calibration. Such error has a systematic biasing influence on the subjects' responses and thereby influences the validity of the instruments. For instance, level of education, socioeconomic status, social desirability, response set, or other characteristics may influence the validity of the instrument by altering measurement of the "true" responses in a systematic way.

For example, a subject who wants to please the investigator may constantly answer items in a socially desirable way, thus making the estimate of validity inaccurate. Systematic error occurs also when an instrument is improperly calibrated. Consider a scale that consistently gives a person's weight at 2 pounds less than the actual body weight. The scale could be quite reliable (i.e., capable of reproducing the precise measurement), but the result is consistently invalid.

HELPFUL HINT Research articles vary considerably in the amount of detail included about reliability and validity. When the focus of a study is tool development, psychometric evaluation—including extensive reliability and validity data—is carefully documented and appears throughout the article rather than briefly in the "Instruments" section, as in other research studies.

VALIDITY

Validity refers to whether a measurement instrument accurately measures what it is supposed to measure. When an instrument is valid, it truly reflects the concept it is supposed to measure.

A valid instrument that is supposed to measure anxiety does so; it does not measure some other construct, such as stress. A reliable measure can consistently rank participants on a given construct (e.g., anxiety), but a valid measure correctly measures the construct of interest. A measure can be reliable but not valid. Let us say that a researcher wanted to measure anxiety in patients by measuring their body temperatures. The researcher could obtain highly accurate, consistent, and precise temperature recordings, but such a measure could not be a valid indicator of anxiety. Thus the high reliability of an instrument is not necessarily congruent with evidence of validity. A valid instrument, however, is reliable. An instrument cannot validly measure the attribute of interest if it is erratic, inconsistent, and inaccurate.

There are three major kinds of validity that vary according to the kind of information provided and the purpose of the investigator (i.e., *content, criterion-related,* and *construct validity*). A critiquer of research articles will want to evaluate whether sufficient evidence of validity is present and whether the type of validity is appropriate to the design of the study and instruments used in the study.

CONTENT VALIDITY

Content validity represents the universe of content, or the domain of a given construct. The universe of content provides the framework and basis for formulating the items that will adequately represent the content. When an investigator is developing a tool and issues of content validity arise, the concern is whether the measurement tool and the items it contains are representative of the content domain that the researcher intends to measure. The researcher begins by defining the concept and identifying the dimensions that are the components of the concept. The items that reflect the concept and its dimensions are formulated.

When the researcher has completed this task, the items are submitted to a panel of judges considered to be experts about this concept. Researchers typically request that the judges indicate their agreement with the scope of the items and the extent to which the items reflect the concept under consideration.

Bakas and Champion (1999) developed the Bakas Caregiving Outcomes Scale (BCOS), a tool for measuring changes in family caregiving outcomes in the stroke population. Based on the conceptual framework including Lazarus's definitions of social functioning (32 items), subjective well-being (6 items), and somatic health (10 items), 48 context-specific items were developed to reflect the important linkage between the conceptualization and operationalization of adaptational outcomes in family caregivers. Content validity was assessed by a doctorally prepared psychologist and a doctorally prepared nurse who were experts in the area of stress and coping, as well as a doctorally prepared sociologist, a doctorally prepared nurse, and a master's prepared nurse who were experts in the area of family caregiving. The criterion for retaining an item was 100% agreement among the experts at the agree or strongly agree level of relevance of the construct. Initial content validity was undertaken with 48 items; 27 were retained measuring social functioning (19 items), subjective well-being (5 items), and somatic health (3 items). Minor changes in wording were made in the remaining

27 items based on comments about clarity, grammar, and issues of gender neutrality. A subtype of content validity is **face validity,** which is a rudimentary type of validity that basically verifies that the instrument gives the appearance of measuring the concept. It is an intuitive type of validity in which colleagues or subjects are asked to read the instrument and evaluate the content in terms of whether it appears to reflect the concept the researcher intends to measure. This procedure may be useful in the tool-development process in relation to determining readability and clarity of content. It should in no way, however, be considered a satisfactory alternative to other types of validity. Bull, Luo, and Maruyama (2000) developed a 12-item questionnaire designed to measure continuity of care. The conceptualization of care continuity was derived from qualitative interviews with elders and family caregivers and focused on continuity of information. The scale comprises two subscales, information on care management and information on continuity of services. Face validity was developed by having elders and their family caregivers review the items for clarity and relevance.

CRITERION-RELATED VALIDITY

Criterion-related validity indicates to what degree the subject's performance on the measurement tool and the subject's actual behavior are related. The criterion is usually the second measure, which assesses the same concept under study.

Two forms of criterion-related validity are concurrent and predictive. **Concurrent validity** refers to the degree of correlation of two measures of the same concept administered at the same time. A high correlation coefficient indicates agreement between the two measures. **Predictive validity** refers to the degree of correlation between the measure of the concept and some future measure of the same concept. Because of the passage of time, the correlation coefficients are likely to be lower for predictive validity studies.

Stuppy (1998) assessed concurrent validity of the Wong-Baker FACES Pain Scale, widely used in clinical pediatric practice, for use in black and white mature adults (over 55 years of age) who are hospitalized after surgery or trauma by correlating scores on the FACES scale with those from highly regarded valid and reliable pain-assessment tools including the Faces Pain Scale (FPS), the Pain Intensity Numbers Scale (PINS), the Verbal Descriptors Scale, and the Visual Analog Scale (VAS). The FACES Pain Scale had a strong positive correlation with each of the other pain scales when rating current level of pain ($r = .81$ to $.95$; $p < .001$). These correlations are similar to those found by others, suggesting that the FACES Pain Scale is sufficiently valid for clinical use by mature adults.

Lyden and associates (1999) evaluated the predictive validity of the Braden Scale, one of the most widely used tools for predicting pressure ulcer risk. It is one of only two existing pressure ulcer prediction tools recognized by the U.S. Agency for Health Care Policy and Research (USDHHS, 1992). To date, little data support the use of the Braden Scale in either black or Latino/Hispanic elder populations. Therefore a study was undertaken to evaluate the predictive validity of the Braden Scale in predicting pressure ulcers in black and Latino/Hispanic elders. A prospective repeated measures design was used, allowing the researchers to develop the criteria and methods for rating pressure ulcer risk in advance to predict which ethnic minority elders were at risk. The subjects were at least 60 years of age; self-reported as either black or Latino/Hispanic; free of pressure ulcers on admission; and had an expected length of stay in the inpatient setting of 5 days or more. Among the 74 subjects, 24 patients (32%) developed either a stage 1 or stage 2 pressure ulcer. Black elders had a higher incidence rate (21%) than Latino/Hispanic elders (11%). A two-tailed Fisher's exact test revealed that the Braden Scale was highly significant ($p < .011$) for predicting pressure ulcers in black elders at least 75 years of age using the optimal cutoff score of 18. Sensitivity was 81%, and specificity was 100%. The female gender was also a highly significant factor in the development of pressure ulcers ($X [N = 49]) = 6.4$, $p < .011$). The Braden Scale was not predictive for black elders up to 74 years of age or for Latino/Hispanic elders up to 74 years of age when the optimal cutoff score of 16, as suggested by Braden and Bergstom (1994), was used. Overall, the Braden Scale was found to be a valid tool in predicting pressure ulcers in black elders at least 75 years of age when a cutoff score of 18 is used.

CONSTRUCT VALIDITY

Construct validity is based on the extent to which a test measures a theoretical construct or trait. It attempts to validate a body of theory underlying the measurement and testing of the hypothesized relationships. Empirical testing confirms or fails to confirm the relationships that would be predicted among concepts and, as such, provides more or less support for the construct validity of the instruments measuring those concepts. The establishment of construct validity is a complex process, often involving several studies and approaches. The hypothesis testing, factor analytical, convergent and divergent, and contrasted-groups approaches are discussed.

Hypothesis-Testing Approach

When the **hypothesis-testing approach** is used, the investigator uses the theory or concept underlying the measurement instrument's to validate the instrument. The investigator does this by developing hypotheses regarding the behavior of individuals with varying scores on the measure, gathering data to test the hypotheses, and making inferences on the basis of the findings, concerning whether the rationale underlying the instrument's construction is adequate to explain the findings.

For example, Resnick and Jensen (2000) used a hypothesis-testing approach to establish the construct validity of the Self-Efficacy for Exercise scale (SEE). The SEE is a revision of McAuley's (1990) self-efficacy barriers to exercise measure, a 13-item instrument that focuses self-efficacy expectations related to the ability to continue exercising in the face of barriers to exercise. This measure was initially developed for sedentary older adults in the community who participated in an outpatient exercise program including rowing, biking, and walking. Prior research demonstrated sufficient

evidence of reliability (alpha coefficient = 0.93) and validity, with efficacy expectations significantly correlated with actual participation in an exercise program (McAuley, 1992, 1993). The following two empirically supported hypotheses representing propositions related to measurement of exercise self-efficacy were used to assess the construct validity of the SEE:

1. Individuals with better health statuses are more likely to have stronger self-efficacy (Grembowski et al, 1989); and
2. Individuals with better mental health statuses are more likely to have stronger self-efficacy expectations (Bandura, 1997; Ruiz, 1992)

These two hypotheses were tested using the SEE and the 12-item Short Form Health Survey (SF-12), which is a valid and reliable measure of health status containing two scores—mental and physical health summary scores—that are health dimensions influencing exercise. As hypothesized, the SF-12 subscale scores, when controlled for age and gender, significantly predicted SEE scores (F = 38.9; p < .05; F = 24.3; p < 0.05). The SF-12 subscale scores for mental health accounted for 18% of the variance in SEE scores, and for an additional 4% of the variance in the SEE scores. When controlled for age and gender; SEE scores significantly predicted exercise activity (F = 78.8; p < 0.05), accounting for 30% of the variance in exercise activity. These findings provide support for the hypotheses and therefore preliminary support for the theoretical basis and conceptual accuracy of the SEE; individuals with better physical and mental health have stronger efficacy expectations about exercise activity. The homogeneous nature of the sample, however, suggests the need for further testing of the SEE with older adults from varied socioeconomic and cultural groups.

Convergent and Divergent Approaches

Two strategies for assessing construct validity include convergent and divergent approaches.

Convergent validity refers to a search for other measures of the construct. Sometimes two or more tools that theoretically measure the same construct are identified, and both are adminis-

TABLE **15-1**   Estimated LISREL Parameters of Construct Validity

	STANDARDIZED LOADINGS	ITEM/COMPOSITE RELIABILITY	2 × SE	VARIANCE EXTRACTED ESTIMATE
WARMTH AND REGARD				
		0.89*		0.48
#2	0.52	0.27	†	
#10	0.70	0.48	0.40	
#12	0.76	0.58	0.42	
#21	0.60	0.35	0.37	
#22	0.71	0.51	0.40	
#25	0.67	0.45	0.39	
#28	0.70	0.49	0.40	
#30	0.82	0.66	0.43	
#33	0.74	0.54	0.41	
INTRINSIC REWARDS OF GIVING				
		0.83*		0.49
#1	0.62	0.38	†	
#13	0.64	0.40	0.29	
#17	0.74	0.55	0.30	
#29	0.76	0.60	0.30	
#32	0.74	0.55	0.30	
LOVE AND AFFECTION				
		0.88*		0.64
#4	0.77	0.60	†	
#5	0.73	0.53	0.18	
#8	0.90	0.80	0.18	
#15	0.81	0.65	0.18	
BALANCE WITHIN FAMILY CAREGIVING				
		0.77*		0.47
#6	0.72	0.51	†	
#19	0.69	0.48	0.24	
#20	0.75	0.56	0.24	
#34	0.56	0.31	0.23	

From Carruth AK: Development and testing of the caregiver reciprocity scale, *Nurs Res* 45(2):92-97, 1996.
*Denotes composite reliabilities.
†Denotes value not estimated (parameter constrained at 1.0 in LISREL).

tered to the same subjects. A correlational analysis (i.e., test of relationship; see Chapters 16 and 17) is performed. If the measures are positively correlated, convergent validity is said to be supported. In the development of the Index of Professional Nursing Governance (IPNG), a tool to measure professional nursing governance of hospital-based nurses, Hess (1998) established convergent validity by correlating the IPNG with the Index of Centralization (IC), a nine-item tool that measures centralization as an organizational characteristic (e.g., allocation of decision making and hi-

erarchy of authority) that is similar but not identical to governance. The statistically significant but moderate correlation of 0.60 (n = 578, p = .005) between the IPNG and the IC supported the idea that the IPNG was measuring the distribution of nursing governance of hospitals. More recently, causal modeling has been used to establish convergent validity. In the development of the Caregiver Reciprocity Scale (CRS), Carruth (1996) established convergent validity using the causal modeling approach. As illustrated in Table 15-1, several indicators have been recommended to assess convergent validity: item loadings, composite reliability, average variance extracted by each construct, examining standard error, and t values. Table 15-1 presents data indicating significant findings between the CRS factor structure and the relevant causal modeling indicators, thereby offering support for the convergent validity of the items in each factor of the CRS.

Divergent validity uses measurement approaches that differentiate one construct from .others that may be similar. Sometimes researchers search for instruments that measure the opposite of the construct. If the divergent measure is negatively related to other measures, validity for the measure is strengthened. Hess (1998) assessed the divergent validity of the IPNG by using a one-tailed t test to compare professional governance between aggregated scores of nurses from hospitals with and without shared governance. The two groups were similar in demographic characteristics, but nurses from hospitals with shared governance reported significantly higher scores on the IPNG than those nurses from hospitals without shared governance (p = .0005, one-tailed), thereby supporting the divergent validity of the IPNG. More recently, the data from a factor analysis being conducted for other validity purposes can be used to determine divergent (sometimes called *discriminant*) validity. Carruth (1996) assessed the discriminant validity of the four factors (subscales) of the CRS by examining the correlations between each factor or subscale that appears in Table 15-1.

A specific method of assessing convergent and divergent validity is the **multitrait-multimethod approach.** Similar to the approach described, this method, proposed by Campbell and Fiske (1959), also involves examining the relationship between instruments that should measure the same construct and between those that should measure different constructs. A variety of measurement strategies, however, are used. For example, anxiety could be measured by the following:

- Administering the State-Trait Anxiety Inventory
- Recording blood pressure readings

- Asking the subject about anxious feelings
- Observing the subject's behavior

The results of one of these measures should then be correlated with the results of each of the others in a multitrait-multimethod matrix (Waltz, Strickland, and Lenz, 1991). In their classic study designed to develop, validate, and norm a measure of dimensions of interpersonal relationships (including social support, reciprocity, and conflict), Tilden, Nelson, and May (1990) used the multitrait-multimethod approach to validity assessment. The two traits of social support and conflict of the Interpersonal Relationship Inventory (IPRI) were each measured with two different methods—a subject self-report tool and an investigator-observation visual analog rating. Reciprocity was not included because of its high correlation with social support.

The use of multiple measures of a concept decreases systematic error. A variety of data-collection methods (e.g., self-report, observation, interview, and collection of physiological data) will also diminish the effect of systematic error.

Contrasted-Groups Approach

When the **contrasted-groups approach** (sometimes called the **known-groups approach**) to the development of construct validity is used, the researcher identifies two groups of individuals who are suspected to score extremely high or low in the characteristic being measured by the instrument. The instrument is administered to both the high- and low-scoring group, and the differences in scores are examined. If the instrument is sensitive to individual differences in the trait being measured, the mean performance of these two groups should differ significantly and evidence of construct validity would be supported. A t test or analysis of variance is used to statistically test the difference between the two groups. In the study by Bull, Luo, and Maruyama (2000) that sought to develop and assess the psychometric properties of the Care Continuity Instrument, a tool to measure continuity of posthospital care of elders, the contrasted-groups approach was used to compare continuity scores for elders in a telephone interview sample who were seen by the same physician postdischarge (continuity of provider) with those who were seen by different physicians. Elders who saw the same physician (n = 69) had significantly higher mean scores on continuity related to receiving information about care management (t = 2.64, p = .01) than elders who saw different physicians following discharge (n = 44). There was no statistically significant difference, however, between the two groups on continuity related to community services. The authors propose that the fact that the elders and their family caregivers indicated that they had received little information on services available might account for the lack of difference. These data suggest that there is some evidence of construct validity using the contrasted groups approach.

Factor Analytical Approach

A final approach to assessing construct validity is **factor analysis.** This is a procedure that gives the researcher information about the extent to which a set of items measures the same underlying construct or dimension of a construct. Factor analysis assesses the degree to which the individual items on a scale truly cluster together around one or more dimensions. Items designed to measure the same dimension should load on the same factor; those designed to measure differing dimensions should load on different factors (Anastasi, 1988; Nunnally and Bernstein, 1993). This analysis will also indicate whether the items in the instrument reflect a single construct or several constructs.

Swanson (1999) carried out a factor analysis during the establishment of construct validity of the Impact of Miscarriage Scale (IMS), an instrument developed to measure the impact of miscarriage on a woman's life. Phase III of IMS instrument development consisted of a principal components factor analysis with varimax rotation of the final 24 items. This analysis yielded four subscales (i.e., lost baby, personal significance, devastating event, and isolated) of five to seven items each, as indicated on Table 15-2. Findings from the factor analysis indicate that

the four-factor structure (subscale) of the IMS, presented in Table 15-2, accounts for 59.3% of the IMS's total variance, which is consistent with Swanson's (1993) phenomenologically derived middle-range caring theory, which provides the theoretical foundation of this study.

HELPFUL HINT When validity data about the measurement instruments used in a study are not included in a research article, you have no way of determining whether the intended concept is actually being captured by the measurement tool. Before you use the results in such a case, it is important to go back to the original source to check the instrument's validity.

The Critical Thinking Decision Path will help you assess the appropriateness of the type of validity and reliability selected for use in a particular research study.

RELIABILITY

Reliable people are those whose behavior can be relied on to be consistent and predictable. Likewise, the **reliability** of a research instrument is defined as the extent to which the instrument yields the same results on repeated measures. Reliability is then concerned with consistency, accuracy, precision, stability, equivalence, and homogeneity. Concurrent with the questions of validity or after they are answered, the researcher and the critiquer ask how reliable the instrument is. A reliable measure is one that can produce the same results if the behavior is measured again by the same scale. Reliability then refers to the proportion of accuracy to inaccuracy in measurement. In other words, if we use the same or comparable instruments on more than one occasion to measure a set of behaviors that ordinarily remains relatively constant, we would expect similar results if the tools are reliable. The three main attributes of a reliable scale are stability, homogeneity, and equivalence. The *stability* of an instrument refers to the instrument's ability to produce the same results with repeated testing. The *homogeneity* of an instrument means that all the items in a tool

TABLE **15-2** Psychometric Properties of the Impact of Miscarriage Scale Using Data Gathered at 1 Year

| ITEM NO. | H/L* | FACTOR LOADING SCORE | ITEM | SCALE SCORES | | | CRONBACH'S |
				n	MEAN	SD	
Impact of miscarriage: overall				198	59.8	15.4	0.93
Lost baby				196	17	4.87	0.86
21	H	0.87	Some women who miscarry feel they have lost a person, *but* some women who miscarry do not feel they have lost a person.				
19	H	0.85	Some women who miscarry feel there will always be a place in their heart for that baby, *but* some women who miscarry do not feel there will always be a place in their heart for that baby.				
18	H	0.70	Some women who miscarry do not feel they have lost a part of themselves, *but* some women who miscarry do feel they have lost a part of themselves.				
27	H	0.68	Some women would describe their miscarriage as just a loss of pregnancy *but* some women would not describe their miscarriage as just a loss of pregnancy.				
17	L	0.61	Miscarriage equals a loss of a part of my partner and me.				
24	H	0.59	Some women who have miscarried are irritated when their baby is called a fetus, *but* some women who have miscarried do not feel irritated when their baby is called a fetus.				
Personal significance				195	15.7	5.13	0.83
7	L	0.76	I have gotten through with dealing with my miscarriage.				
15	L	0.64	My miscarriage represents a major setback for me.				
8	L	0.63	I feel my body has betrayed me.				
6	L	0.59	My miscarriage destroyed my zest for life.				
13	L	0.58	When I think of my miscarriage, I still feel emotional pain.				
20	H	0.57	For some women miscarriage equals a lost chance to be a mother, *but* for some women miscarriage does not equal a lost chance to be a mother.				
3	L	0.52	After my miscarriage, I was feeling down for several days, but then I got over it.				

Item	Type	Loading	n	M		α
Devastating event			193	13.5	45	0.86
11	L	0.80	Miscarriage is like a nightmare.			
9	L	0.77	Miscarriage is like going from one extreme of happiness to the other, total unhappiness.			
1	L	0.73	My miscarriage was a horrendous devastating event.			
12	L	0.63	Miscarriage equals loss of hope.			
4	L	0.51	Miscarriage equals one big loss of control.			
Isolated			192	13.2	4.3	0.79
30	H	0.70	Some women who miscarry feel very isolated by their experience, *but* some women who miscarry are amazed at the number of people who shared in their loss.			
2	L	0.70	I felt very much alone in my loss.			
28	H	0.61	Some women feel guilt about their miscarriage, *but* some women do not feel guilt about their miscarriage.			
22	H	0.56	Some women who miscarry experience a loss of pride in themselves, *but* some women who miscarry do not experience a loss of pride in themselves.			
25	H	0.52	Some women dwell on the fact that their child will only exist in their memory, *but* some women do not dwell on the fact that their child will only exist in their memory.			
26	H	0.51	Some women who miscarry wonder "why did it happen to me," *but* some women who miscarry do not wonder "why did it happen to me."			

*H = Harter forced choice [really like me (1); sort of like me (2); but sort of like me (3); really like me (4)].
Likert [definitely true for me (1) to definitely not true for me(4)].

Determining the Appropriate Type of Validity and Reliability Selected for a Study

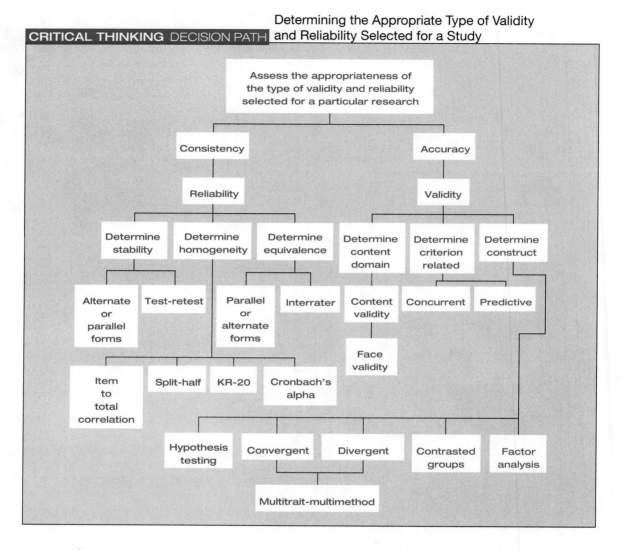

measure the same concept or characteristic. An instrument is said to exhibit *equivalence* if the tool produces the same results when equivalent or parallel instruments or procedures are used. Each of these attributes and the means to estimate them will be discussed. Before these are discussed, an understanding of how to interpret reliability is essential.

RELIABILITY COEFFICIENT INTERPRETATION

Because all of the attributes of reliability are concerned with the degree of consistency between scores that are obtained at two or more independent times of testing, they often are expressed in terms of a correlation coefficient. The reliability coefficient ranges from 0 to 1. The **reliability coefficient** expresses the relationship between the error variance, true variance, and the observed score. A zero correlation indicates that there is no relationship. When the error variance in a measurement instrument is low, the reliability coefficient will be closer to 1. The closer to 1 the coefficient is, the more reliable the tool. For example, a reliability coefficient of a tool is reported to be

BOX 15-2 Measures Used to Test Reliability

STABILITY
Test-retest reliability
Parallel or alternate form

HOMOGENEITY
Item-total correlation
Split-half reliability
Kuder-Richardson coefficient
Cronbach's alpha

EQUIVALENCE
Parallel or alternate form
Interrater reliability

0.89. This tells you that the error variance is small and the tool has little measurement error. On the other hand, if the reliability coefficient of a measure is reported to be 0.49, the error variance is high and the tool has a problem with measurement error. For a tool to be considered reliable, a level of 0.70 or higher is considered to be an acceptable level of reliability. The interpretation of the reliability coefficient, which is also called the alpha coefficient, depends on the proposed purpose of the measure. There are five major tests of reliability that can be used to calculate a reliability coefficient. The test(s) used depend(s) on the nature of the tool. They are known as **test-retest, parallel or alternate form, item-total correlation, split-half, Kuder-Richardson (KR-20), Cronbach's alpha,** and **interrater reliability.** These tests are discussed as they relate to the attributes of stability, equivalence, and homogeneity (Box 15-2). There is no best means to assess reliability in relationship to stability, homogeneity, and equivalence. The critiquer should be aware that the method of reliability that the researcher uses should be consistent with the investigator's aim.

STABILITY

An instrument is thought to be stable or to exhibit **stability** when the same results are obtained on repeated administration of the instrument. Researchers are concerned with an instrument's stability when they expect the instrument to measure a concept consistently over a period of time. Measurement over time is important when an instrument is used in a longitudinal study and therefore will be used on several occasions. Stability is also a consideration when a researcher is conducting an intervention study that is designed to effect a change in a specific variable. In this case, the instrument is administered once and then again later after the alteration or change intervention has been completed. The tests that are used to estimate stability are test-retest and parallel or alternate form.

Test-Retest Reliability

Test-retest reliability is the administration of the same instrument to the same subjects under similar conditions on two or more occasions. Scores from repeated testing are compared. This comparison is expressed by a correlation coefficient, usually a Pearson r (see Chapter 17). The interval between repeated administrations varies and depends on the concept or variable being measured. For example, if the variable that the test measures is related to the developmental stages in children, the interval between tests should be short. The amount of time over which the variable was measured should also be recorded in the report. An example of an instrument that was assessed for test-retest reliability is the Korean translation of the Exercise Self-Efficacy Scale (Shin, Jang, and Pender, 2001). The Exercise Self-Efficacy Scale was previously developed and tested for reliability and validity in other English speaking populations, and the translated version was assessed for use in a Korean population. The concept of test-retest is illustrated by the following: *"Test-retest reliability* measures were performed as a measure of instrument *stability* on a sample of 14 participants who were comparable to the study population. The *test-retest interval* was two weeks, and the *correlation coefficient* was .77" (Shin, Jang, and Pender, 2001). In this case, the interval was adequate 2 weeks between testing and the coefficient was above .70 (Nunnally and Bernstein, 1993).

Parallel or Alternate Form

Parallel or alternate form reliability is applicable and can be tested only if two comparable forms of the same instrument exist. It is like test-retest reliability in that the same individuals are tested within a specific interval, but it differs because a different form of the same test is given to the subjects on the second testing. Parallel forms or tests contain the same types of items that are based on the same domain or concept, but the wording of the items is different. The development of parallel forms is desired if the instrument is intended to measure a variable for which a researcher believes that "test-wiseness" will be a problem. For example, there are two alternate forms of the Partner Relationship Inventory (Hoskins, 1988) that may be used in a repeated-measures design. An item on one scale ("I am able to tell my partner how I feel") is consistent with the paired item on the second form ("My partner tries to understand my feelings"). Practically speaking, it is difficult to develop alternate forms of an instrument when one considers the many issues of reliability and validity of an instrument. If alternate forms of a test exist, they should be highly correlated if the measures are to be considered reliable.

HELPFUL HINT When a longitudinal design with multiple data-collection points is being conducted, look for evidence of test-retest or parallel form reliability.

INTERNAL CONSISTENCY/HOMOGENEITY

Another attribute of an instrument related to reliability is the **internal consistency** or **homogeneity** with which the items within the scale reflect or measure the same concept. This means that the items within the scale correlate or are complementary to each other. This also means that a scale is unidimensional. A unidimensional scale is one that measures one concept, such as exercise self-efficacy. A total score is then used in the analysis of data. The Self-Efficacy for Exercise Scale (Resnick and Jenkins, 2000) was tested for internal consistency, as well as for construct va-

BOX 15-3 Examples of Reported Cronbach's Alpha

Cronbach's coefficient alpha was calculated as a measure of internal consistency for the scale. A standardized alpha of .94 was obtained (Shin, Jang, and Pender, 2001).

"An alpha coefficient of .92 was sufficient evidence for the internal consistency of the Self-Efficacy for Exercise measure" (Resnick and Jenkins, 2000).

"Internal consistency reliability using Cronbach's coefficient alpha was computed for this sample. Results for the composite sample (.91–boys and .93–girls) as well as subsamples by grade and sex, are presented. . ." (Weber, 2000).

"Cronbach's alpha was .76 for the entire instrument" (Bull, Luo, and Maruyama, 2000).

lidity. The testing of the instrument revealed an alpha coefficient of .92. Because the alpha was above .70, it was sufficient evidence for supporting the internal consistency of the instrument. Homogeneity can be assessed by using one of four methods: item-total correlations, split-half reliability, Kuder-Richardson (KR-20) coefficient, or Cronbach's alpha (Box 15-3).

HELPFUL HINT When the characteristics of a study sample differ significantly from the sample in the original study, check to see if the researcher has reestablished the reliability of the instrument with the current sample.

Item to Total Correlations

Item to total correlations measure the relationship between each of the items and the total scale. When item to total correlations are calculated, a correlation for each item on the scale is generated (Table 15-3). Items that do not achieve a high correlation may be deleted from the instrument. Usually in a research study, all of the item to total correlations are not reported unless the study is a report of a methodological study. The lowest and highest correlations are typically reported. An example of an item to total correlation report is illustrated in the study by Jansen and Keller (1999) in which item to total correlations were computed

TABLE **15-3**   Examples of Item to Total Correlations from Computer-Generated Data

ITEM	ITEM TO TOTAL CORRELATION
1	0.5069
2	0.4355
3	0.4479
4	0.4369
5	0.4213
6	0.4216

for the 42-item Attentional Demand Survey, which measures the attentional demand of elders living in the community. The corrected item-scale correlations and alpha with item removed are reported. The individual items range from .44 to .65 and the subscales within the total scale range from .87 to .90, thus supporting the reliability of the scale (Nunnally and Bernstein, 1993).

Split-Half Reliability

Split-half reliability involves dividing a scale into two halves and making a comparison. The halves may be odd-numbered and even-numbered items or a simple division of the first from the second half, or items may be randomly selected into halves that will be analyzed opposite one another. The split-half provides a measure of consistency in terms of sampling the content. The two halves of the test or the contents in both halves are assumed to be comparable, and a reliability coefficient is calculated. If the scores for the two halves are approximately equal, the test may be considered reliable. A formula called the Spearman-Brown formula is one method used to calculate the reliability coefficient. In a study testing the Reynolds Adolescent Depression Scale, which is used to measure depression in clinical and community adolescents, the investigator computed a Spearman-Brown split-half reliability and found a reliability of .91 (Weber, 2000). The investigator also provided a rationale for the use of the test for this particular scale.

Kuder-Richardson (KR-20) Coefficient

The **Kuder-Richardson (KR-20) coefficient** is the estimate of homogeneity used for instruments that have a dichotomous response format. A dichotomous response format is one in which the question asks for a "yes/no" or "true/false" response. The technique yields a correlation that is based on the consistency of responses to all the items of a single form of a test that is administered one time. In a study investigating relationships among spirituality, perceived social support, death anxiety, and nurses' willingness to care for acquired immunodeficiency syndrome (AIDS) patients, Sherman (1996) uses the Templer Death Anxiety Scale (TDAS) (Templer, 1970), one of the most widely used measures of conscious death anxiety. Because the response format for the TDAS is binary ("true/false"), the KR-20 was used to determine the original internal consistency of the 15 items. A KR-20 reliability coefficient of 0.76 indicated a moderate level of internal consistency reliability. Because the original data were based on a sample of 31 college students and Sherman's study sample consisted of registered nurses, a pilot study was conducted and a reliability coefficient of 0.78 was calculated. When a KR-20 was calculated in the actual study, however, the reliability coefficient was computed at 0.63, certainly lower than was anticipated based on the results of the pilot study. In the discussion section of this article, Sherman (1996) comments on the low internal consistency reliability of the TDAS, suggesting that the "true/false" format that limits response possibilities may contribute to this phenomenon. She proposes that reformulation of the tool using a Likert scale format (see Chapter 11) may allow a researcher to better detect the real feelings of an individual, thereby increasing the reliability of the TDAS.

Cronbach's Alpha

The fourth and most commonly used test of internal consistency is **Cronbach's alpha.** Many tools used to measure psychosocial variables and attitudes have a Likert scale response format. A Likert scale format asks the subject to respond to

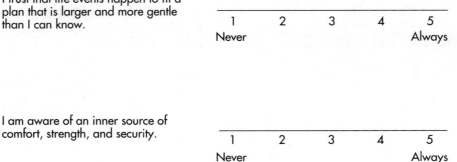

I trust that life events happen to fit a plan that is larger and more gentle than I can know.

| 1 | 2 | 3 | 4 | 5 |
| Never | | | | Always |

I am aware of an inner source of comfort, strength, and security.

| 1 | 2 | 3 | 4 | 5 |
| Never | | | | Always |

Figure 15-2   Examples of a Likert Scale. (Redrawn from Roberts KT, and Aspy CB: Development of the serenity scale, *J Nurs Measure* 1(2):145-164, 1993.)

a question on a scale of varying degrees of intensity between two extremes. The two extremes are anchored by responses ranging from "strongly agree" to "strongly disagree" or "most like me" to "least like me." The points between the two extremes may range from 1 to 5 or 1 to 7. Subjects are asked to circle the response closest to how they feel. Figure 15-2 provides examples of items from a tool that uses a Likert scale format. Cronbach's alpha simultaneously compares each item in the scale with the others. Examples of reported Cronbach's alpha are in Box 15-3.

HELPFUL HINT   If a research article provides information about the reliability of a measurement instrument but does not specify the type of reliability, it is probably safe to assume that internal consistency reliability was assessed using Cronbach's alpha.

EQUIVALENCE

Equivalence is either the consistency or agreement among observers using the same measurement tool or the consistency or agreement between alternate forms of a tool. An instrument is thought to demonstrate equivalence when two or more observers have a high percentage of agreement of an observed behavior or when alternate forms of a test yield a high correlation. There are two methods to test equivalence: interrater reliability and alternate or parallel form.

Interrater Reliability

Some measurement instruments are not self-administered questionnaires but are direct measurements of observed behavior. Instruments that depend on direct observation of a behavior that is to be systematically recorded must be tested for **interrater reliability.** To accomplish interrater reliability, two or more individuals should make an observation or one observer observe the behavior on several occasions. The observers should be trained or oriented to the definition and operationalization of the behavior to be observed. In the method of direct observation of behavior, the consistency or reliability of the observations between observers is extremely important. In the instance of interrater reliability, the reliability or consistency of the observer is tested rather than the reliability of the instrument. Interrater reliability is expressed as a percentage of agreement between scorers or as a correlation coefficient of the scores assigned to the observed behaviors.

In the study, "Patient Outcomes for the Chronically Critically Ill: Special Care Unit Versus Intensive Care Unit" (Rudy et al, 1995), the researchers carefully monitored interrater reliability because four out of six instruments used in the study depended on the accurate abstraction of data from patient records. Each member of the research team who participated in data collection was trained by the project director and had to achieve a 90% agreement on each measurement tool before independent data were collected. In addition, a detailed rulebook was kept so that reliability could be maintained. Interrater reliability was checked on a random selection of 10% of records and maintained at 90% agreement between coders. Whenever agreement dropped below 90%, differences in scoring were analyzed and resolved, usually through the construction of additional coding rules.

Another example of interrater reliability is given in the study conducted by Wikblad and Anderson (1995), who studied the differential effect on healing of three wound dressings in patients undergoing heart surgery. The first use of interrater reliability in this study consisted of five nurses from each of the units used in the study who were trained to examine the dressings. They rated the following parameters: (1) how well the incision could be seen through the dressing, (2) how much the dressing had loosened, (3) number of bandage changes and the reasons for those changes, (4) pain at removal of dressing on fifth day, and (5) difficulty in removing the dressing. They compared their results and discussed differing ratings. This procedure was repeated on five new patients until there was 100% agreement in the ratings. The second use of interrater reliability consisted of the evaluation of color photographs of the wound taken the fifth day after surgery. The actual evaluation was done by two independent raters, neither of whom was aware of the experimental conditions. The interrater reliability was calculated by use of the kappa coefficient. The kappa coefficient for ratings of wound healing was 0.81, and the agreement between the two raters was 91%. For ratings of redness, the agreement was 85% (with a kappa coefficient of 50.73).

Parallel or Alternate Form

Parallel or alternate form was described in the discussion of stability in this chapter. Use of parallel forms is then a measure of stability and equivalence. The procedures for assessing equivalence using parallel forms are the same.

CRITIQUING Reliability and Validity

Reliability and validity are two crucial aspects in the critical appraisal of a measurement instrument. Criteria for critiquing reliability and validity are presented in the Critiquing Criteria box. The reviewer evaluates an instrument's level of reliability and validity, as well as the manner in which these were established. In a research report, the reliability and validity for each measure should be presented. If these data have not been presented at all, the reviewer must seriously question the merit and use of the tool and the study's results.

CRITIQUING CRITERIA

1. Was an appropriate method used to test the reliability of the tool?
2. Is the reliability of the tool adequate?
3. Was an appropriate method(s) used to test the validity of the instrument?
4. Is the validity of the measurement tool adequate?
5. If the sample from the developmental stage of the tool was different from the current sample, were the reliability and validity recalculated to determine if the tool is still adequate?
6. Have the strengths and weaknesses of the reliability and validity of each instrument been presented?
7. Are strengths and weaknesses of the reliability and validity appropriately addressed in the Discussion, Limitations, or Recommendations sections of the report?

If a study does not use reliable and valid questionnaires, the results of a study can not be credible. It is the ethical responsibility of the critiquer to question the reliability and validity of instruments used in research studies and examine the findings in light of the quality of the instruments used and the data presented. The following discussion highlights key areas related to reliability and validity that should be evident to the critiquer in a research article.

Appropriate reliability tests should have been performed by the developer of the measurement tool and should then have been included by the current user in the research report. If the initial standardization sample and the current sample have different characteristics, the reader would expect the following: (1) that a pilot study for the present sample would have been conducted to determine if the reliability was maintained, or (2) that a reliability estimate was calculated on the current sample. For example, if the standardization sample for a tool that measures "satisfaction in an intimate heterosexual relationship" comprises undergraduate college students and if an investigator plans to use the tool with married couples, it would be advisable to establish the reliability of the tool with the latter group.

The investigator determines which type of reliability procedures are used in the study, depending on the nature of the measurement tool and how it will be used. For example, if the instrument is to be administered twice, the critiquer might determine that test-retest reliability should have been used to establish the stability of the tool. If an alternate form has been developed for use in a repeated-measures design, evidence of alternate form reliability should be presented to determine the equivalence of the parallel forms. If the degree of internal consistency among the items is relevant, an appropriate test of internal consistency should be presented. In some instances, more than one type of reliability will be presented, but the critiquer should determine whether all are appropriate. For example, the Kuder-Richardson formula implies that there is a single right or wrong answer, making it inappropriate to use with scales that provide a format of three or more possible responses. In such cases, another formula is applied, such as Cronbach's coefficient alpha formula. Another important consideration is the acceptable level of reliability, which varies according to the type of test. Coefficients of reliability of 0.70 or higher are desirable. The validity of an instrument is limited by its reliability; that is, less confidence can be placed in scores from tests with low reliability coefficients.

Satisfactory evidence of validity is probably the most difficult item for the reviewer to ascertain. It is this aspect of measurement that is most likely to fall short of meeting the required criteria. Validity studies are time-consuming, as well as complex, and sometimes researchers will settle for presenting minimal validity data. Therefore the critiquer should closely examine the item content of a tool when evaluating its strengths and weaknesses and try to find conclusive evidence of content validity. In the body of a research article, however, it is most unusual to have more than a few sample items available for review. Because this is the case, the critiquer should determine whether the appropriate assessment of content validity was used to meet the researcher's goal. Such procedures provide the critiquer with assurance that the tool is psychometrically sound and that the content of the items is consistent with the conceptual framework and construct definitions. Construct and criterion-related validity are some of the more precise statistical tests of whether the tool measures what it is supposed to measure. Ideally, an instrument should provide evidence of content validity, as well as criterion-related or construct validity, before a reviewer invests a high level of confidence in the tool.

The reader would also expect to see the strengths and weaknesses of instrument reliability and validity presented in the "Discussion," "Limitations," and/or "Recommendations" sections of a research article. In this context, the reliability and validity might be discussed in relation to other tools devised to measure the same variable. The relationship of the study's findings to the strengths and weaknesses in instrument reliability and validity are another important discussion point. Finally, recommendations for improving future studies in relation to instrument reliability and validity should be proposed. For example, in the "Instruments" and "Discussion" sections of a study investigating examining relationships among spirituality, perceived social support, death anxiety, and nurses' willingness to care for AIDS patients, Sherman (1996) appropriately reports the weaknesses in the reliability of the TDAS. She states that although the TDAS is often cited in the literature, the low internal consistency reliability of the scale (0.76) supports the recommendation that the instrument be pilot tested on the specific sample on which it will be administered. Because of the marginally acceptable reliability of the TDAS and because the study sample (i.e., registered nurses) differed from the original sample (i.e., college students) used for establishing reliability, a pilot study, yielding a marginally acceptable reliability coefficient of 0.78, was conducted using a sample of 30 nurses enrolled in a doctoral course. Sherman goes on, however, to comment that in the actual study, the TDAS's reliability coefficient of 0.63 was lower than anticipated, based on the results of the pilot study. Although Sherman appropriately addresses the low reliability of TDAS in relation to the psychometric properties of the tool and makes recommendations about revising the response format, she does not address this weakness in relation to the hypotheses and the findings of the study.

As you can see, the area of reliability and validity is complex. These aspects of research reports can be evaluated to varying degrees. The research consumer should not feel inhibited by the complexity of this topic but may use the guidelines presented in this chapter to systematically assess the reliability and validity aspects of a research study. Collegial dialogue is also an approach to evaluating the merits and shortcomings of an existing, as well as a newly developed, instrument that is reported in the nursing literature. Such an exchange promotes the understanding of methodologies and techniques of reliability and validity, stimulates the acquisition of a basic knowledge of psychometrics, and encourages the exploration of alternative methods of observation and use of reliable and valid tools in clinical practice.

Critical Thinking Challenges

Barbara Krainovich-Miller

➤ Discuss the three types of validity that must be established before a reviewer invests a high level of confidence in the tool. Include examples of each type of validity.
➤ What are the major tests of reliability? Is it necessary to establish more than one measure of reliability for each instrument used in a study? Which do you think is the most essential measure of reliability? Include examples in your answer.
➤ Is it possible to have a valid instrument that is not reliable? Is the reverse possible? Support your answer with instruments you might use in the clinical setting with your patients/clients.
➤ How do you think the concept of evidence-based practice has changed research utilization (RU) models? Do you think that the review of the literature is the same for developing a research proposal as it is for implementing the steps of RU or an evidence-based practice protocol? Support your position.

Key Points

- Reliability and validity are crucial aspects of conducting and critiquing research.
- Validity refers to whether an instrument measures what it is purported to measure, and it is a crucial aspect of evaluating a tool.
- Three types of validity are content validity, criterion-related validity, and construct validity.
- The choice of a validation method is important and is made by the researcher on the basis of the characteristics of the measurement device in question and its utilization.

- Reliability refers to the accuracy/inaccuracy ratio in a measurement device.
- The major tests of reliability are as follows: test-retest, parallel or alternate form, split-half, item to total correlation, Kuder-Richardson, Cronbach's alpha, and interrater reliability.
- The selection of a method for establishing reliability depends on the characteristics of the tool, the testing method that is used for collecting data from the standardization sample, and the kinds of data that are obtained.

REFERENCES

Anastasi A: *Psychological testing,* ed 6, New York, 1988, Macmillan.

Bakas T and Champion V: Development and psychometric testing of the Bakas Caregiving Outcomes Scale, *Nurs Res* 48(5):250-259, 1999.

Bandura A: *The self-efficacy: the exercise of control,* New York, 1997, WH Freedman.

Braden B and Bergstrom N: Predictive validity of the Braden Scale for pressure sore risk in a nursing home population, *Res Nurs Health* 17:459-470, 1994.

Bull MJ, Hansen HE, and Gross CR: A professional-patient partnership model of discharge planning with elders hospitalized with heart failure, *Appl Nurs Res* 13(1):19-28, 2000.

Bull MJ, Luo D, and Maruyama GM: Measuring continuity of elders' posthospital care, *J Nurs Measurement* 8(1):41-60, 2000.

Campbell D and Fiske D: Convergent and discriminant validation by the matrix, *Psychol Bull* 53:273-302, 1959.

Carruth AK: Development and testing of the caregiver reciprocity scale, *Nurs Res* 45(2):92-97, 1996.

Grembowski D et al: Self-efficacy and health behavior among older adults, *J Health Social Behav* 34:89-104, 1989.

Hess RG: Measuring nursing governance, *Nurs Res* 47(1):35-42, 1998.

Hoskins CN: *The partner relationship inventory,* Palo Alto, CA, 1988, Consulting Psychologists Press.

Hoskins CN, editor: *Developing research in nursing and health: quantitative and qualitative methods,* New York, 1998, Springer.

Jansen DA and Keller ML: An instrument to measure the attentional demands of community-dwelling elders, *J Nurs Measurement* 7:197-214, 1999.

Lyden CH et al: The Braden Scale for Pressure Ulcer Risk: evaluating the predictive validity in black and hispanic/latino elders, *Appl Nurs Res* 12(2):60-68, 1999.

McAuley E: Self-efficacy and the maintenance of exercise participation in older adults, *J Behavioral Med* 16(1):103-113, 1993.

McAuley E: The role of efficacy cognitions in the prediction of exercise in middle-aged adults, *J Behavioral Med* 15(1):65-88, 1992.

Nunnally JC and Bernstein IH: *Psychometric theory,* ed 3, New York, 1993, McGraw-Hill.

Resnick B and Jenkins LS: Testing the reliability and validity of the Self-Efficacy for Exercise Scale, *Nurs Res* 49:154-159, 2000.

Rudy EB et al: Patient outcomes for the chronically critically ill: special care unit versus intensive care unit, *Nurs Res* 44:324-331, 1995.

Ruiz B: Hip fracture recovery in older women: the role of self-efficacy and mood, Doctoral Dissertation, University of California, Los Angeles, 1992.

Sherman DW: Nurses' willingness to care for AIDS patients and spirituality, social support, and death anxiety, *Image* 28(3):205-213, 1996.

Shin YH, Jang HJ, and Pender N: Psychometric evaluation of the exercise self-efficacy scale among Korean adults with chronic illness, *Res Nurs Health* 24:68-77, 2001.

Stuppy DJ: The Faces Pain Scale: reliability and validity with mature adults, *Appl Nurs Res* 11(2):84-89, 1998.

Swanson KM: Effects of caring, measurement, and time on miscarriage impact and women's well-being, *Nurs Res* 48(6):288-298, 1999.

Swanson KM: Nursing as informed caring for the well being of others, *Image* 25(2):352-357, 1993.

Templer DI: The construction and validation of a death anxiety scale, *J Gen Psychol* 82:165-177, 1970.

Tilden VP, Nelson CA, and May BA: The IPR inventory: development and psychometric characteristics, *Nurs Res* 39(6):337-343, 1990.

U.S. Department of Health and Human Services (US DHHS): *Pressure ulcers in adults: prediction and prevention,* Rockville, Md., 1992, Public Health Service Agency for Health Care Policy and Research.

Waltz C, Strickland O, and Lenz E: *Measurement in nursing research,* ed 3, Philadelphia, 1991, FA Davis.

Weber S: Factor structure of the Reynolds adolescent depression scale in a sample of school-based adolescents, *J Nurs Measurement* 8:23-40, 2000.

Wikblad K and Anderson B: A comparison of three wound dressings in patients undergoing heart surgery, *Nurs Res* 44:312-316, 1995.

ADDITIONAL READINGS

Berk RA: Importance of expert judgment in content-related validity evidence, *West J Nurs Res* 12(5):659-671, 1990.

Elder JH: Videotaped behavioral observations: enhancing validity and reliability, *Appl Nurs Res* 12(4): 206-209, 1999.

Grubba CJ, Popovich B, and Jirovec MM: Reliability and validity of the Popovich scale in home health care assessments, *Appl Nurs Res* 3(4):161-163, 1990.

Laschinger HKS: Intraclass correlations as estimates of interrater reliability in nursing research, *West J Nurs Res* 14(2):246-251, 1992.

Meek PM et al: Psychometric testing of fatigue instruments for use with cancer patients, *Nurs Res* 49(4): 181-189, 2000.

Reineck C: Nursing research instruments: pathway to resources, *Appl Nurs Res* 4(1):34-45, 1991.

Shin YH and Colling KB: Cultural verification and application of the Profile of Mood States (POMS) with Korean elders, *West J Nurs Res* 22(1):68-83, 2000.

Thomas SD, Hathaway DK, and Arheart KL: Face validity, *West J Nurs Res* 14(1):109-112, 1992.

ANN BELLO

Descriptive Data Analysis

16

Key Terms

correlation
descriptive statistics
frequency distribution
interval measurement
kurtosis
levels of measurement
mean
measurement

measures of central tendency
measures of variability
median
modal percentage
modality
mode
nominal measurement
normal curve

ordinal measurement
percentile
range
ratio measurement
semiquartile range
 (semiinterquartile range)
standard deviation (SD)
Z score

Learning Outcomes

After reading this chapter, the student should be able to do the following:

- Define descriptive statistics.
- State the purposes of descriptive statistics.
- Identify the levels of measurement in a research study.
- Describe a frequency distribution.
- List measures of central tendency and their use.
- List measures of variability and their use.
- Critically analyze the descriptive statistics used in published research studies.

After carefully collecting data, the researcher is faced with the task of organizing the individual pieces of information so that the meaning is clear. It would be neither practical nor helpful to the reader to list individually each piece of data collected. The researcher must choose methods of organizing the raw data based both on the type of data collected and on the hypothesis or question that was tested.

Statistical procedures are used to give organization and meaning to data. Procedures that allow researchers to describe and summarize data are known as **descriptive statistics.** Procedures that allow researchers to estimate how reliably they can make predictions and generalize findings based on the data are known as inferential statistics (see Chapter 17). Descriptive statistical techniques reduce data to manageable proportions by summarizing them, and they also describe various characteristics of the data under study. Descriptive techniques include measures of central tendency, such as mode, median, and mean; measures of variability, such as modal percentage, range, and standard deviation (SD); and some correlation techniques, such as scatter plots. The research consumer does not need detailed knowledge of how to calculate these statistics but does need an understanding of their meaning, use, and limitations.

Measures of central tendency describe the average member of the sample, whereas **measures of variability** describe how much dispersion is in the sample. If a researcher reported that the average age of one nursing class was 22 years, with the youngest member 18 and the oldest 25, and that in another nursing class students had an average age of 22 years, but the youngest member was 17 and the oldest 45, the reader would form a very different picture of the two classes. In both cases the average member of the sample was the same, but in the second class there was much greater variation or dispersion in the age of the members of the class.

Descriptive statistics may be presented in several ways in a research report. The data may be reported in words in the text of the report or summarized in tables or graphs. Whatever the method of presentation, the report should give the reader a clear and orderly picture of the research results.

This chapter and the next are designed to provide an understanding of statistical procedures. This chapter focuses on the understanding and evaluation of descriptive statistical procedures, and the next chapter discusses inferential statistical procedures. To evaluate the appropriateness of the statistical procedures used in a study, the research consumer should have an understanding of the **levels of measurement** that are appropriate to each statistical technique.

LEVELS OF MEASUREMENT

Measurement is the assignment of numbers to objects or events according to rules. Every object that is assigned a specific number must be similar to every other object assigned that number. For example, male subjects may be assigned the number 1 and female subjects the number 2. The measurement level is determined by the nature of the object or event being measured. Levels of measurement in ascending order are nominal, ordinal, interval, and ratio. The **levels of measurement** are the determining factors of the type of statistics to be used in analyzing data.

The higher the level of measurement, the greater the flexibility the researcher has in choosing statistical procedures. Every attempt should be made to use the highest level of measurement possible so that the maximum amount of information will be obtained from the data as highlighted in Table 16-1. The Critical Thinking Decision Path illustrates the relationship between levels of measurement and appropriate choice of specific descriptive statistics.

NOMINAL MEASUREMENT

Nominal measurement is used to classify objects or events into categories. The categories are mutually exclusive; the object or event either has or does not have the characteristic. The numbers assigned to each category are nothing more than la-

TABLE **16-1** Level of Measurement Summary Table

MEASUREMENT	DESCRIPTION	MEASURES OF CENTRAL TENDENCY	MEASURES OF VARIABILITY
Nominal	Classification	Mode	Modal percentage, range, frequency distribution
Ordinal	Relative rankings	Mode, median	Range, percentile, semiquartile range, frequency distribution
Interval	Rank ordering with equal intervals	Mode, median, mean	Range, percentile, semiquartile range, standard deviation
Ratio	Rank ordering with equal intervals and absolute zero	Mode, median, mean	All

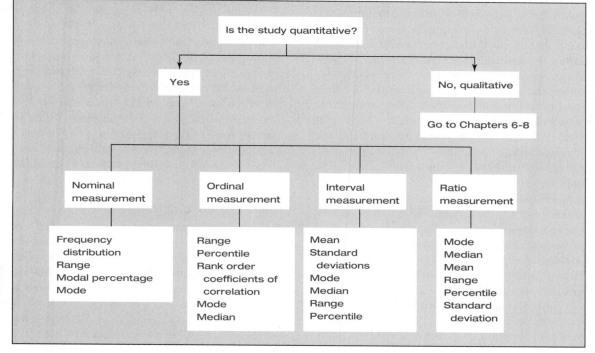

CRITICAL THINKING DECISION PATH Descriptive Statistics

bels; such numbers do not indicate more or less of a characteristic. Nominal level measurement can be used to categorize a sample on such information as gender, hair color, marital state, or religious affiliation. The Bull, Hansen, and Gross (2000) study of discharge planning for elders hospitalized with heart failure includes several examples of nominal level measurement, including marital status, race, caregiver relationship to patient, and sex (see Appendix A). The data may be presented in a table or in narrative form. Bull, Hansen, and Gross (2000) present the data in narrative form, whereas LoBiondo-Wood and associates (2000) present marital status in table form and race in narrative form (see Appendixes A and D). The nominal level of measurement allows the least amount of mathematical manipulation. Most commonly the frequency of each event is counted, as well as the percent of the total each category represents.

ORDINAL MEASUREMENT

Ordinal measurement is used to show relative rankings of objects or events. The numbers assigned to each category can be compared, and a member of a higher category can be said to have more of an attribute than one in a lower category. The intervals between numbers on the scale are not necessarily equal, and neither is zero an absolute zero. For example, ordinal measurement is used to formulate class rankings where one student can be ranked higher or lower than another. However, the difference in actual grade point average between students may differ widely. Another example is ranking individuals by their level of wellness and by their ability to carry out activities of daily living. Using the New York Heart Association classification of cardiac failure, individuals can be assigned to one of four classifications. Classification I represents little disease or interference with activities of daily living, while classification IV represents severe disease and little ability to carry out the activities of daily living independently but an individual in class IV cannot be said to be four times sicker than one in class I. A similar scale based on an individual's current health status is used to classify an individual's anesthesia risk.

Ordinal level data are limited in the amount of mathematical manipulation possible. In addition to what is possible with nominal data, medians, percentiles, and rank order coefficients of correlation can be calculated.

INTERVAL MEASUREMENT

Interval measurement shows rankings of events or objects on a scale with equal intervals between the numbers. The zero point remains arbitrary and not absolute. For example, interval measurements are used in measuring temperatures on the Fahrenheit scale. The distances between degrees are equal, but the zero point is arbitrary and does not represent the absence of temperature. Test scores also represent interval data. The differences between test scores represent equal intervals, but a zero does not represent the total absence of knowledge.

In many areas in the social sciences, including nursing, the classification of the level of measurement of intelligence, aptitude, and personality tests is controversial, with some regarding these measurements as ordinal and others as interval. The research consumer needs to be aware of this controversy and to look at each study individually in terms of how the data are analyzed (Knapp, 1990, 1993; Wang et al, 1999). Interval level data allow more manipulation of data, including the addition and subtraction of numbers and the calculation of means. This additional manipulation is why many argue for the higher classification level. The Family Inventory of Life Events and Changes and the Coping Health Inventory for Parents were used as interval measurements by LoBiondo-Wood and associates' (2000) study of family adaptation to a child evaluation for transplant surgery (see Appendix D).

RATIO MEASUREMENT

Ratio measurement shows rankings of events or objects on scales with equal intervals and absolute zeros. The number represents the actual amount of the property the object possesses. Ratio measurement is the highest level of measurement, but it is usually achieved only in the physical sciences. Examples of ratio level data are height, weight, pulse, and blood pressure. The Bull, Hansen, and Gross (2000) study used ratio measurement in reporting length of stay in the hospital (see Appendix A).

All mathematical procedures can be performed on data from ratio scales. Therefore the use of any statistical procedure is possible as long as it is appropriate to the design of the study (see Chapter 17).

TABLE **16-2**   Frequency Distribution

| INDIVIDUAL | | | GROUP | | |
SCORE	TALLY	FREQUENCY	SCORE	TALLY	FREQUENCY
90	I	1	>89	I	1
88	I	1			
86	I	1	80-89	ЖΤ ЖΤ ЖΤ	15
84	ЖΤ I	6			
82	II	2	70-79	ЖΤ ЖΤ ЖΤ	23
80	ЖΤ	5		ЖΤ III	
78	ЖΤ	5			
76	I	1	60-69	ЖΤ ЖΤ	10
74	ЖΤ II	7			
72	ЖΤ IIII	9	<59	II	2
70	I	1			
68	III	3			
66	II	2			
64	IIII	4			
62	I	1			
60		0			
58	I	1			
56		0			
54	I	1			
52		0			
50		0			
Total		51			51

Mean 73.1; standard deviation, +12.1; median, 74; mode, 72; range 36 (54-90).

HELPFUL HINT   The descriptive statistics calculated must be appropriate to both the purpose of the study and the level of measurement. Descriptive statistics assist in summarizing the data.

FREQUENCY DISTRIBUTION

One of the most basic ways of organizing data is in a frequency distribution. In a **frequency distribution** the number of times each event occurs is counted or the data are grouped and the fre-

quency of each group is reported. An instructor reporting the results of an examination could report the number of students receiving each grade or could group the grades and report the number in each group. Table 16-2 shows the results of an examination given to a class of 51 students. The results of the examination are reported in several ways. The columns on the left give the raw data tally and the frequency for each grade, whereas the columns on the right give the grouped-data tally and grouped frequencies. In their study of

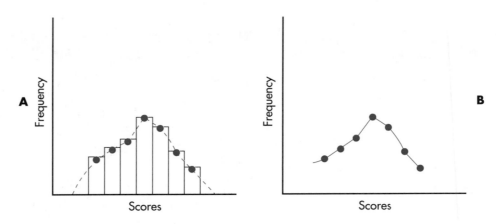

Figure 16-1   Frequency distributions. **A,** Histogram; **B,** frequency polygon.

discharge planning with elders, Bull, Hansen, and Gross (2000) group the elders by cohorts and report the results for each cohort rather than reporting the results for each patient (see Appendix A).

When data are grouped, it is necessary to define the size of the group or the interval width so that no score will fall into two groups and each group is mutually exclusive. The grouping of the data in Table 16-2 prevents overlap; each score falls into only one group. If the grouping had been 70 to 80 and 80 to 90, scores of 80 would have fallen into two categories. The grouping should allow for a precise presentation of the data without serious loss of information. Very large interval widths lead to loss of data information and may obscure patterns in the data. If the test scores in Table 16-2 had been grouped as 40 to 69 and 70 to 99, the pattern of the scores would have been obscured.

Information about frequency distributions may be presented in the form of a table, such as Table 16-2, or in graphic form. Figure 16-1 illustrates the most common graphic forms: the histogram and the frequency polygon. The two graphic methods are similar in that both plot scores or percentages of occurrence against frequency. The greater the number of points plotted, the smoother the resulting graph. The shape of the resulting graph allows for observations that

further describe the data. In their study of risk factors for cardiovascular disease in children with type 1 diabetes, Lipman and associates (2000) report the number of children in each body mass percentile and the number of children in each grouping of cholesterol level using histograms (Figure 16-2).

MEASURES OF CENTRAL TENDENCY

Measures of central tendency answer questions such as "What does the average nurse think?" and "What is the average temperature of patients on a unit?" They yield a single number that describes the middle of the group. They summarize the members of a sample. Therefore measures of central tendency are known as summary statistics and are sample specific. Because they are sample specific, they change with each sample. Table 16-3 shows how Mahon, Yarcheski, and Yarcheski (2000) in their study of positive and negative outcomes of anger in early adolescents list the means (M), standard deviations (SDs), and range for each of the study variables (see Appendix C). These scores represent the average of each variable, the amount of variation in the scores, and the range of the scores, respectively. For example, the state anger mean was 16.86 with

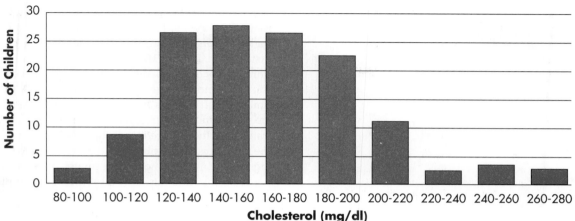

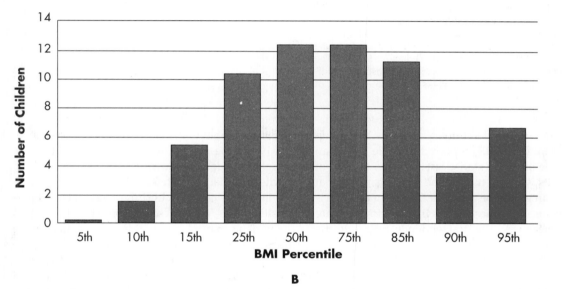

Figure 16-2   **A,** Total cholesterol levels in children with insulin-dependent diabetes mellitus (*n* = 140). **B,** Body mass index (BMI) of children with insulin-dependent diabetes mellitus (*n* = 67). (Reprinted from Lipman TH, et al: Risk factors for cardiovascular disease in children with type I diabetes, *Nurs Res* 49(3):164-165, 2000.

an SD (variation) of 9.56. This means that 68% of the adolescents scored between 7.3 and 26.42 on the measure of state anger.

Summary statistics also may be reported in narrative form as illustrated by the following excerpt from LoBiondo-Wood and associates' (2000)

study of family adaptation to a child's evaluation for transplant surgery (see Appendix D).

The subjects were 29 mothers, ranging in age from 19 to 44 years, whose children were being evaluated for a liver transplant. . . . All mothers were able to read and understand English. The sample comprised 17 Caucasian,

TABLE **16-3** Descriptive Statistics for Study Variables (*N* = 141)

VARIABLE	M	SD	RANGE
State anger*	16.86	9.56	10-40
Trait anger*	22.43	7.70	10-40
Change	8.53	2.85	1-16
Vigor	19.39	7.09	2-32
Symptom patterns	39.44	13.87	17-83
Well-being	138.81	29.80	47-193

*From Yarcheski A, Mahon NE, and Yarcheski TJ: An Empirical Test of alternative Theories of Anger in Adolescents, *Nurs Res* 23:17-24, 2000.

9 Afro-Americans, 1 American Indian, 1 Hispanic American, and 1 mother of unspecified ethnicity. Twenty (68.9%) of the mothers had attended or graduated from college. In the category of combined family income, 12 families (41.3%) earned below $20,000; 9 (31%) earned in the $20,001 to $30,000 range, and 5 earned above $30,001. The mean age of the children who were the transplant candidates was 3.3 years (SD, 4.3 years). Fifty-nine percent of the children were male.

The characteristics of a sample in a study are described in terms of summary statistics. The mean test score ($X = 73.1$) reported in Table 16-2 is an example of such a statistic. If a different group of students was given the same test, it is likely that the mean would be different. The term average is a nonspecific, general term. In statistics there are three measures of central tendency: the mode, the median, and the mean. Depending on the distribution, these measures may not all give the same answer to the question, "What is the average?" Each measure of central tendency has a specific use and is most appropriate to specific kinds of measurement and types of distributions.

HELPFUL HINT Careful review of the description of the sample will aid in deciding whether the study results are relevant to the population with whom the reader is working.

MODE

The **mode** is the most frequent score or result, and it can be obtained by inspection of the frequency distribution table or graph. A distribution can have more than one mode. The number of modes contained in a distribution is called the **modality** of the distribution. Figures 16-3, *A* and *D* and 16-4 show unimodal or one-peak distributions. Figure 16-3, *B*, shows a bimodal or two-peaked distribution. Multimodal distributions having two or more peaks are shown in Figure 16-3, *B* and *C*. Table 16-2 illustrates how the change in a few scores can change the modality of a distribution from unimodal to bimodal. The mode is most appropriately used with nominal data but can be used with all levels of measurement (see Table 16-1). The mode cannot be used for any subsequent calculations, and it is unstable; that is, the mode can fluctuate widely from sample to sample from the same population. A change in just one score in Table 16-2 would change the mode from 72.

MEDIAN

The **median** is the middle score or the score where 50% of the scores are above it and 50% of the scores are below it. The median is not sensitive to extremes in high and low scores. In the series of scores in Table 16-2, the twenty-sixth score will always be the median regardless of how high the highest or low the lowest score. It is best used when the data are skewed (see Normal Distribution in this chapter), and the researcher is interested in the "typical" score. For example, if age is a variable and there is a wide range with extreme scores that may affect the mean, it would be appropriate to also report the median. The median is easy to find either by inspection or calculation and can be used with ordinal or higher data as shown in Table 16-1. Bull, Hansen, and Gross (2000) report the median for preparedness of the elderly to manage their health care (see Appendix A).

MEAN

The **mean** is the arithmetical average of all the scores and is used with interval or ratio data (see Table 16-1). It is what is usually thought of when the term average is used in general conversation and is the most widely used measure of central tendency. Most tests of significance use the mean

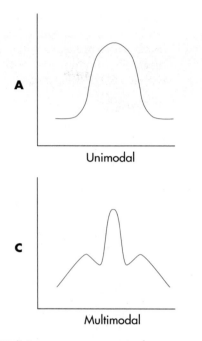

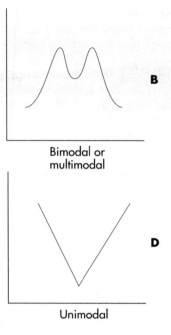

Figure 16-3   Symmetrical shapes.

(see Chapter 17). The mean is affected by every score but is more stable than the median or mode, and of the three measures of central tendency, it is the most constant or least affected by chance. The larger the sample size, the less affected the mean will be by a single extreme score. The mean is generally considered the single best point for summarizing data. In Table 16-2 the mean is the least affected by the change in the distribution from unimodal to bimodal. Bull, Hansen, and Gross (2000) report the means of demographic data and the means of all the variables except preparedness (see Appendix A).

When one compares the measures of central tendency, the mean is the most stable and the median the most typical of these statistics. If the distribution is symmetrical and unimodal, the mean, median, and mode will coincide. If the distribution is skewed, the mean will be pulled in the direction of the long tail of the distribution. With a skewed distribution, all three statistics should be reported. For example, national income in the

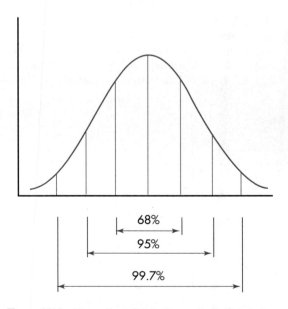

Figure 16-4   The normal distribution and associated standard deviations.

United States is skewed. The mean wage differs from the median wage, because the large salaries are so much greater than the low salaries.

> **HELPFUL HINT** Of the three measures of central tendency, the mean is the most stable, least affected by extremes, and most useful for other calculations. The mean can only be calculated with interval and ratio data.

NORMAL DISTRIBUTION

The concept of the normal distribution is a theoretical one, based on the observation that data from repeated measures of interval or ratio level data group themselves about a midpoint in a distribution in a manner that closely approximates the normal curve illustrated in Figure 16-4. In addition, if the means of a large number of samples of the same interval or ratio data are calculated and plotted on a graph, that curve also approximates the normal curve. This tendency of the means to approximate the normal curve is termed the sampling distribution of the means. The mean of the sampling distribution of the means is the mean of the population (see Chapter 17).

The **normal curve** is one that is symmetrical about the mean and is unimodal. The mean, median, and mode are equal. An additional characteristic of the normal curve is that a fixed per-centage of the scores falls within a given distance of the mean. As shown in Figure 16-4, about 68% of the scores or means will fall within 1 SD of the mean; 95% within 2 SD of the mean; and 99.7% within 3 SD of the mean.

SKEWNESS

Not all samples of data approximate the normal curve. Some samples are nonsymmetrical and have the peak off center. If one tail is longer than the other, the distribution is described in terms of skew. In a positive skew the bulk of the data are at the low end of the range and there is a longer tail pointing to the right or the positive end of the graph. Worldwide individual income has a positive skew, with most individuals in the low-to-moderate range and very few in the upper range. The mean in a positive skew is to the right of the median. In a negative skew, the bulk of the data are in the high range and the longer tail points to the left or the negative end of the graph. Age at death in the United States has a negative skew because most deaths occur at older ages. In a negative skew, the mean is to the left of the median. Figure 16-5 illustrates positive and negative skew. In each diagram the peak is off center and one tail is longer.

SYMMETRY

When the two halves of a distribution are folded over and they can be superimposed on each

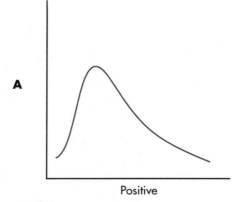
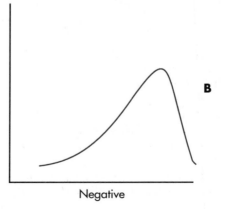

Positive

Negative

Figure 16-5 **A,** Positive skew; **B,** negative skew.

other, the distribution is said to be symmetrical. In other words, the two halves of the distribution are mirror images of each other. The overall shape of the distribution does not affect symmetry. Although the shapes in Figure 16-3 are different, they are all symmetrical; however, only Figure 16-3, *A* approximates the normal curve. Symmetry and modality are independent. Look at Figures 16-3, *A,* and 16-5, *A* and *B*. These are all unimodal, but Figure 16-5 *A* and *B* are skewed, whereas Figure 16-3, *A* is symmetrical.

KURTOSIS

Kurtosis is related to the peakness or flatness of a distribution. The peakness or flatness of a distribution is related to the spread of the data. The farther the data are spread out on a scale, the flatter the peak. The distribution that peaks sharply is called *leptokurtic,* whereas a broad, flat distribution is called *platykurtic.* Figure 16-6 illustrates kurtosis. Neither the leptokurtic nor the platykurtic distributions approximate the normal curve.

INTERPRETING MEASURES OF VARIABILITY

Variability or dispersion is concerned with the spread of data. Samples with the same mean could differ in both distribution (kurtosis) and skew.

Variability measures answer the questions "Is the sample homogeneous or heterogeneous?" and "Is the sample similar or different?" If a researcher measures oral temperatures in two samples, one sample drawn from a healthy population and one sample from a hospitalized population, it is possible that the two samples will have the same mean. However, it is likely that there will be a wider range of temperatures in the hospitalized sample than in the healthy sample. Measures of variability are used to describe these differences in the dispersion of data.

As with measures of central tendency, the various measures of variability are appropriate to specific kinds of measurement and types of distributions.

Modal percentage is used with nominal data and is the percentage of cases in the mode. A high modal percentage is indicative of decreased variability.

HELPFUL HINT Remember that descriptive statistics related to variability will enable you to evaluate the homogeneity or heterogeneity of a sample.

RANGE

The **range** is the simplest but most unstable measure of variability. Range is the difference between the highest and lowest scores. A change in either of

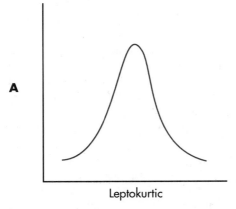

Leptokurtic

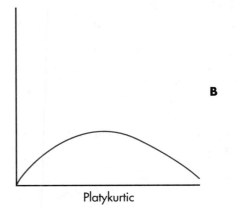

Platykurtic

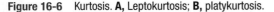

Figure 16-6 Kurtosis. **A,** Leptokurtosis; **B,** platykurtosis.

these two scores would change the range. The range should always be reported with other measures of variability. The range in Table 16-2 is 36, but this could easily change with an increase or decrease in the high score of 90 or the low score of 54. In Table 16-3 from the article by Mahon, Yarcheski, and Yarcheski (2000) the mean, SD, and range for all of the study variables are given (see Appendix C). This gives the reader the opportunity to see how much variability there is in the data.

SEMIQUARTILE RANGE

The **semiquartile range (semiinterquartile range)** indicates the range of the middle 50% of the scores. It is more stable than the range, because it is less likely to be changed by a single extreme score. It lies between the upper and lower quartiles, the upper quartile being the point below which 75% of the scores fall and the lower quartile being the point below which 25% of the scores fall. The middle 50% of the scores in Table 16-2 lies between 68 and 78, and the semiquartile range is 10.

PERCENTILE

A **percentile** represents the percentage of cases a given score exceeds. The median is the 50% percentile, and in Table 16-2 it is a score of 74. A score in the 90th percentile is exceeded by only 10% of the scores. The zero percentile and the 100th percentile are usually dropped.

STANDARD DEVIATION

The **standard deviation (SD)** is the most frequently used measure of variability, and it is based on the concept of the normal curve (see Figure 16-4). It is a measure of average deviation of the scores from the mean and as such should always be reported with the mean. The standard deviation takes all scores into account and can be used to interpret individual scores. Because the mean (X) and SD for the examination in Table 16-2 was $73.16 +/- 12.1$, a student should know that 68% of the grades were between 85.1 and 61. If the student received a grade of 88, he would know he did better than most of the class, whereas a grade of 58 would indicate he did not do as well as most of the

class. Table 16-3, from the study by Mahon, Yarcheski, and Yarcheski (2000) reports the mean, SD, and range of each study variable. As illustrated in this table, the mean score for the variable "trait anger" was 22.43, and the SD was 7.70. This means that 68% of the adolescents' trait anger scores would be expected to fall between 14.73 and 30.13. This table allows the reader to inspect the data and get a feel for the variation the data contain (see Appendix C).

The SD is used in the calculation of many inferential statistics (see Chapter 17). One limitation of the SD is that it is expressed in terms of the units used in the measurement and cannot be used to compare means that have different units. If researchers were interested in the relationship between height measured in inches and weight measured in pounds, it would be necessary for them to convert the height and weight measurements to standard units or Z scores. Bull, Hansen, and Gross (2000) calculated a composite score for outcome variables for each subject. The composite scores were then used to calculate the statistics (see Appendix A).

The **Z score** is used to compare measurements in standard units. Each of the scores is converted to a Z score, and then the Z scores are used to examine the relative distance of the scores from the mean. A Z score of 1.5 means that the observation is 1.5 SDs above the mean, whereas a score of -2 means that the observation is 2 SDs below the mean. By using Z scores, a researcher can compare results from scales that use different units, such as height and weight.

Many measures of variability exist. The modal frequency is the easiest to calculate, but the SD is the most useful. The SD and the semiquartile range always exist and are unique for each sample. The SD is the most stable statistic. Transformation of scores to Z scores allows comparison between scores that have different measurement units.

CORRELATION

Correlations are used to answer the question "To what extent are the variables related?" Correla-

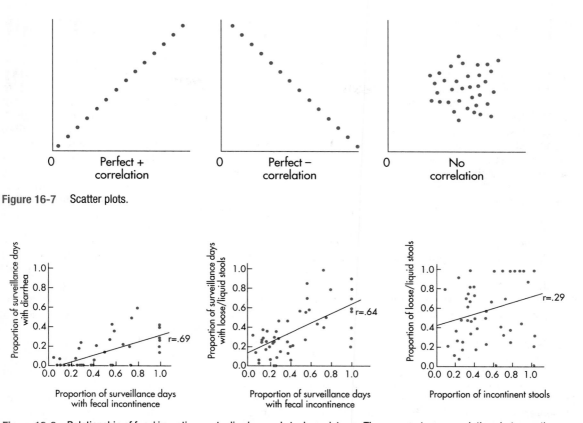

Figure 16-7 Scatter plots.

Figure 16-8 Relationship of fecal incontinence to diarrhea and stool consistency. There were strong correlations between the proportion of surveillance days with fecal incontinence and the proportion of surveillance days with diarrhea ($p < .001$), as well as between the proportion of surveillance days with fecal incontinence and the proportion of surveillance days with unformed and loose or liquid stools ($p < .001$). There was a significant relationship between the percentage of incontinent stools and the percentage of unformed and loose or liquid stools ($p = .04$). (From Bliss DZ, et al: Fecal incontinence in hospitalized patients who are acutely ill, *Nurs Res* 49(2):105, 2000.

tions are used most commonly with ordinal or higher level data. Most correlations are discussed in Chapter 15, but here we briefly mention scatter plots, which are visual representations of the strength and magnitude of the relationship between two variables. Figure 16-7 illustrates a perfect positive correlation, a perfect negative correlation, and no correlation. In most research, correlation results lie between these extremes. The strength of the correlation is demonstrated by how closely the data points approximate a straight line. In a *positive* correlation, the higher

the score on one variable, the higher the score on the other. Temperature and pulse are positively correlated; that is, a rise in temperature generally is associated with a rise in the pulse rate. In a *negative* correlation, the higher the score on one measure, the lower the score on the other measure. A decrease in blood volume is generally associated with a rise in the pulse rate. In the study of fecal incontinence by Bliss and associates (2000), the relationship of fecal incontinence to diarrhea and stool consistency was reported using scatter plots (Figure 16-8).

CRITIQUING Descriptive Statistics

Many students who have not had a course in statistics think they cannot critique descriptive statistics. However, students should be able to critically analyze the use of statistics even if they do not understand the derivation of the numbers presented. What is most important in critiquing this aspect of a research study is that the procedures for summarizing the data make sense in light of the purpose of the study (Critiquing Criteria box).

Before a decision can be made as to whether the statistics employed make sense, it is important to return to the beginning of the paper and determine the purpose of the study. Although all studies use descriptive statistics to summarize the data obtained, many studies go on to use identical statistics to test specific hypotheses (see Chapter 17). If a study is an exploratory one, it is possible that only descriptive statistics will be presented because their purpose is to describe the characteristics of a population.

Just as the hypotheses or question should flow from the problem and purpose of a study, so should the hypotheses or question suggest the type of analysis that will follow. The hypotheses should indicate the major variables that are expected to be presented in summary form. Each of the variables in the hypotheses should be followed in the results section with appropriate descriptive information.

After studying the hypotheses or question, the reader should proceed to the methods section. Using the operational definition provided, the level of measurement employed to measure each of the variables listed in the hypotheses or question need

to be identified. From this information it should be possible to determine the measures of central tendency and variability that should be employed to summarize the data. For example, you would not expect to see a mean used as a summary statistic for the nominal variable of gender. In all likelihood, gender would be reported as a frequency distribution. The means and SDs should be provided for measurements performed at the interval level. The sample size is another aspect of the methods section that is important when evaluating the researcher's use of descriptive statistics. The larger the sample, the less chance that one outlying score will affect the summary statistics.

Only after these aspects of the study have been examined should the results presented by the researcher be considered. Each important variable should have an appropriate measure of central tendency and variability presented. If tables or graphs are used, they should agree with the information presented in the text. The tables and the charts should be clearly and completely labeled. If the researcher presents grouped frequency data, the groups should be logical and mutually exclusive. The size of the interval in grouped data should not obscure the pattern of the data, nor should it create an artificial pattern. Each table and chart should be referred to in the text, but each should add to the text—not merely repeat it. Each table or graph should have an obvious connection to the study being reported. For example, one table may describe the sample and another may present data relevant to the hypotheses being studied. Table 16-3 illus-

CRITIQUING CRITERIA

1. Were appropriate descriptive statistics used?
2. What level of measurement is used to measure each of the major variables?
3. Is the sample size large enough to prevent one extreme score from affecting the summary statistics used?
4. What descriptive statistics are reported?
5. Were these descriptive statistics appropriate to the level of measurement for each variable?
6. Are there appropriate summary statistics for each major variable?
7. Is there enough information present to judge the results?
8. Are the results clearly and completely stated?
9. If tables and graphs are used, do they agree with the text and extend it, or do they merely repeat it?

trates a clearly presented table; each group is mutually exclusive, and the data in the table agree with the data in the text.

In reading a table such as Table 16-3 on page 338, the reader should first look at the heading. The title should give a valid indication of the information contained in the table. Next, the reader should review the column headings. Do these headings follow from the title? Is each heading clear and are any nonstandard abbreviations explained? Are the statistics contained in the table appropriate to the level of measurement used? In Table 16-3, the column heading follows from the title. Each study variable is listed along with its mean and SD as well as the range. Mean and SD are appropriate statistics because these data were regarded as interval data.

The results should be written so that they are understandable to the intended audience. The audience for nursing research is the average practicing nurse. Thus the descriptive information presented should be clear enough that the reader can determine the usefulness of the study in the individual practice situation.

Descriptive statistics cannot be critiqued apart from the study as a whole. Each part of the research paper must make sense in relation to the entire paper. Therefore each portion of the paper should be evaluated in relation to what has preceded it. As such, the evaluation of the descriptive statistics must precede the evaluation of the inferential statistics.

The following is a partial critique of the study by Bull, Hansen, and Gross (2000) that compared the professional-patient model of discharge planning with standard discharge planning; only one option is chosen at each step (see Appendix A):

Purpose of study: To examine differences in outcomes for elders hospitalized with heart failure and caregivers who participated in a professional-patient model of discharge planning compared with those who received the usual discharge planning.

Hypotheses: There are four hypotheses. They are all directional, research hypotheses.

Independent variable: For all four hypotheses, the independent variable is group participation; either professional-patient relationship partnership model of discharge planning (experimental group) or usual discharge planning (control group).

Dependent variable:

Hypothesis 1—Perceived health

Hypothesis 2—Satisfaction with discharge planning, perceptions of care continuity, preparedness, and difficulties managing care

Hypothesis 3—Caregivers' response to caregiving

Hypothesis 4—Resource use

Conceptual definition for hypothesis 4: Use of hospital services after discharge.

Operational definitions for hypothesis 4: Number of readmissions to the hospital and number of times the emergency room was used post-discharge.

Level of measurement: Nominal

Summary statistics:

Expected	Reported
Readmitted—percent each group	Percent readmitted—2 months and 2 weeks after discharge

Sample size: 180 elder/caregiver dyads

Conclusion: Reported statistics are appropriate for the problem, hypothesis, and level of measurement; sample size is large enough to prevent one score from having a large effect on the mean

---

Critical Thinking Challenges

Barbara Krainovich-Miller

➤ Discuss the ways a researcher might use the computer in analyzing data and presenting descriptive statistical results of a study.

➤ What is the relationship between the level of measurement a researcher uses and the choice of a statistical procedure?

➤ What type of visual representation can be used to demonstrate the use of correlations? Use examples from clinical practice to illustrate the difference between positive and negative correlations.

➤ A classmate from research class tells you that she thinks it is ridiculous for the instructor to ask the students to critique the descriptive statistics used in a study when none of the students have taken a statistics course. Would you agree or disagree with her claim? Defend your position.

Key Points

- Descriptive statistics are a means of describing and organizing data gathered in research.
- The four levels of measurement are nominal, ordinal, interval, and ratio. Each has appropriate descriptive techniques associated with it.
- Measures of central tendency describe the average member of a sample. The mode is the most frequent score, the median is the middle score, and the mean is the arithmetical average of the scores. The mean is the most stable and useful of the measures of central tendency, and with the standard deviation it forms the basis for many of the inferential statistics described in Chapter 17.
- The frequency distribution presents data in tabular or graphic form and allows for the calculation or observations of characteristics of the distribution of the data, including skewness, symmetry, modality, and kurtosis.
- In nonsymmetrical distributions, the degree and direction of the pull of the peak off center are described in terms of skew.
- In speaking of modality, the number of peaks is described as unimodal, bimodal, or multimodal.
- The relative spread of the data is described by kurtosis.
- Each characteristic of the frequency distribution is independent.
- Measures of variability reflect the spread of the data.
- The modal percentage is the percent of the cases in the mode.
- The ranges reflect differences between high and low scores.
- The standard deviation is the most stable and useful measure of variability. It is derived from the concept of the normal curve. In the normal curve, sample scores and the means of large numbers of samples group themselves around the midpoint in the distribution, with a fixed percentage of the scores falling within given distances of the mean. This tendency of means to approximate the normal curve is called the sampling distributions of the means. A Z score is the standard deviation converted to standard units.
- The scatter plot shows a measure of correlation.
- When critiquing published research reports, special emphasis should be given to the relationship of levels of measurement and appropriate descriptive techniques.

REFERENCES

Bliss DZ et al: Fecal incontinence in hospitalized patients who are acutely ill, *Nurs Res* 49(2): 101-108, 2000.

Bull MJ, Hansen HE, and Gross CR: A professional-patient partnership model of discharge planning with elders hospitalized with heart failure, *Appl Nurs Res* 13(1):19-28, 2000.

Knapp TR: Treating ordinal scales as interval scales: an attempt to resolve the controversy, *Nurs Res* 39(2): 121-123, 1990.

Knapp TR: Treating ordinal scales as ordinal scales, *Nurs Res* 42(3):184-186, 1993.

Lipman TH et al: Risk factors for cardiovascular disease in children with type 1 diabetes, *Nurs Res* 49(3):160-166, 2000.

LoBiondo-Wood G et al: Family adaptation to a child's transplant: pretransplant phase, *Prog Transplant* 10(2): 1-7, 2000.

Mahon NE, Yarcheski A, and Yarcheski TJ: Positive and negative outcomes of anger in early adolescents, *Res Nurs Health* 23:17-24, 2000.

Wang S et al: Bridging the gap between the pros and the cons in treating ordinal scales as interval scales from an analysis point of view, *Nurs Res* 48(4):226-229, 1999.

ADDITIONAL READINGS

Bluman AG: *Elementary statistics: a step by step approach,* ed 4, 2000, New York, McGraw-Hill Co.

Kerlinger FN and Lee HB: *Foundations of behavioral research,* ed 4, 1999, New York, Harcourt Brace Jovanovich.

Milton JS: *Statistical methods in the biological and health sciences,* ed 3, 1999, New York, McGraw-Hill Co.

Nunnally JC and Bernstein IH: *Psychometric theory,* ed 3, 1994, New York, McGraw-Hill Co.

SUSAN SULLIVAN-BOLYAI
MARGARET GREY

17

Inferential Data Analysis

Key Terms

analysis of covariance
(ANCOVA)
analysis of variance (ANOVA)
chi-square (X^2)
correlation
degrees of freedom
factor analysis
Fisher's exact probability test
inferential statistics
level of significance (alpha
level)
linear structural relationships
(LISREL)

multiple analysis of variance
(MANOVA)
multiple regression
nonparametric statistics
nonparametric tests of
significance
null hypothesis
parameter
parametric statistics
path analysis

Pearson correlation
coefficient (Pearson *r*;
Pearson product moment
correlation coefficient)
probability
sampling error
scientific hypothesis
standard error of the mean
t statistic
type I error
type II error

Learning Outcomes

After reading this chapter, the student should be able to do the following:

- Identify the purpose of inferential statistics.
- Distinguish between a parameter and a statistic.
- Explain the concept of probability as it applies to the analysis of sample data.
- Distinguish between type I and type II error and its effect on a study's outcome.
- Distinguish between parametric and nonparametric tests.
- List the commonly used statistical tests and their purposes.
- Critically analyze the statistics used in published research studies.

Inferential statistics are used to analyze the data collected in a research study. As a reader of research studies you need to understand the purpose and application of statistics. Although it may be useful also to understand how statistical procedures are conducted, such knowledge is not critical to understanding published research findings. The purpose of this chapter is to demonstrate how researchers use inferential statistics to make conclusions about larger groups (the population of interest) from sample data. Basic concepts and terminology are presented in the sections that follow so that the reader can begin to make sense of the statistics used in research papers. Those readers who desire a more advanced discussion should refer to the Additional Readings at the end of this chapter.

DESCRIPTIVE AND INFERENTIAL STATISTICS

Chapter 16 discussed descriptive statistics, which are the statistics used when the researcher needs to summarize the data. In this chapter our attention turns to the use of inferential statistics. Inferential statistics combine mathematical processes and logic that allow researchers to test hypotheses about a population using data obtained from probability samples. Statistical inference is generally used for two purposes—to estimate the probability that statistics found in the sample accurately reflect the population parameter and to test hypotheses about a population. In the first purpose, a **parameter** is a characteristic of a *population,* whereas a *statistic is* a characteristic of a *sample.* We use statistics to estimate population parameters. Suppose we randomly sample 100 people with chronic lung disease and use an interval level scale to study their knowledge of the disease. If the mean score for these subjects is 65, the mean represents the sample statistic. If we were able to study every subject with chronic lung disease, we also could calculate an average knowledge score and that score would be the parameter for the population. As you know, a researcher rarely is able to study an entire population, so inferential

statistics allow the researcher to make statements about the larger population from studying the sample.

The example given alludes to two important qualifications of how a study must be conducted so that inferential statistics may be used. First, it was stated that the sample was selected using probability methods (see Chapter 12). Because you are already familiar with the advantages of probability sampling, it should be clear that if we wish to make statements about a population from a sample, that sample must be representative. All procedures for inferential statistics are based on the assumption that the sample was drawn with a known probability. Second, it was stated that the scale had to reach the interval level of measurement. This is because the mathematical operations involved in doing inferential statistics require this level of measurement. The two Critical Thinking Decision Paths provide matrices that researchers use for statistical decision making.

HYPOTHESIS TESTING

The second and most commonly used purpose of inferential statistics is hypothesis testing. Statistical hypothesis testing allows researchers to make objective decisions about the outcome of their study. The use of statistical hypothesis testing allows researchers to answer such questions as "How much of this effect is a result of chance?" or "How strongly are these two variables associated with each other?"

The procedures used when making inferences are based on principles of negative inference. In other words, if a researcher studied the effect of a new educational program for patients with chronic lung disease, the researcher would actually have two hypotheses—the scientific hypothesis and the null hypothesis. The research or **scientific hypothesis** is that which the researcher believes will be the outcome of the study. In our example, the scientific hypothesis would be that the educational intervention would have a marked impact on the outcome in

CRITICAL THINKING DECISION PATH Inferential Statistics—Difference Questions

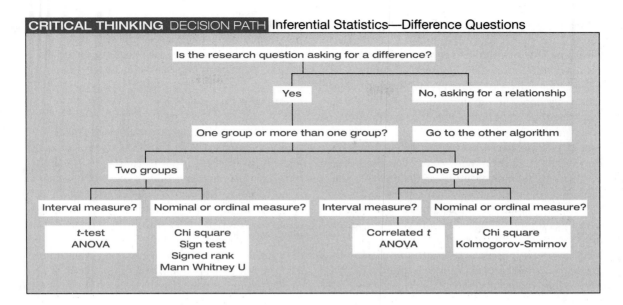

CRITICAL THINKING DECISION PATH Inferential Statistics—Relationship Questions

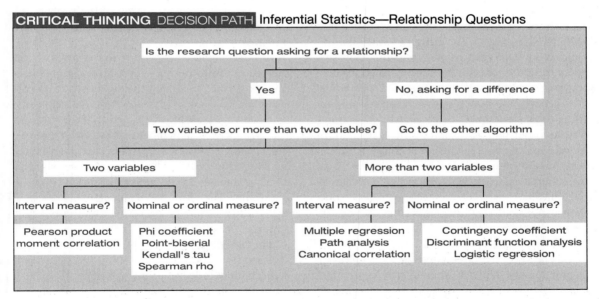

the experimental group beyond that in the control group. The **null hypothesis,** which is the hypothesis that actually can be tested by statistical methods, would state that there is no difference between the groups. Inferential statistics use the null hypothesis to test the validity of a scientific hypothesis in sample data. The null hypothesis states that there is no actual relationship between the variables and that any observed relationship or difference is merely a function of chance fluctuations in sampling.

The concept of the null hypothesis is often confusing. An example may help clarify this concept. The study by Bull, Hansen, and Gross (2000) (see

Appendix A) provides a good example. The authors were interested in determining whether elderly patients hospitalized for heart failure who received a discharge planning intervention would have better outcomes than those who received the usual discharge planning regimen. One of the four scientific hypotheses was that patients who received the intervention would have, at two weeks postdischarge, different perceived scores on client satisfaction with discharge planning, perceptions of care continuity, preparedness, and difficulties managing care than those who received the usual discharge planning regimen. This hypothesis was based on clinical knowledge and previous findings in the literature. On the basis of this hypothesis, the authors then determined whether the differences found on the various outcome variables differed significantly between the two groups. The researchers used the null hypothesis—that there were no differences between the groups of patients—to test this scientific hypothesis. The authors found that the patients in the intervention group reported significant differences (higher scores) in continuity and preparedness when compared to the traditional discharge planning group but no differences with satisfaction or difficulties managing care. In other words, although the investigators found that some of the differences in the scores between the groups with several of the variables (within that particular hypothesis) were large enough that they were unlikely to be caused by chance, not all of the variables predicted to be different in that particular hypothesis were so. Thus that null hypothesis could not be rejected.

All statistical hypothesis testing is a process of disproof or rejection. It is impossible to prove that a scientific hypothesis is true, but it is possible to demonstrate that the null hypothesis has a high probability of being incorrect. To reject the null hypothesis, then, is considered to show support for the scientific hypothesis and is the desired outcome of most studies reporting inferential statistics.

HELPFUL HINT Remember that most samples used in clinical research are samples of convenience, but most researchers use inferential statistics. Although such use violates one of the assumptions of such tests, the tests are robust enough so as to not seriously affect the results unless the data are skewed in unknown ways.

PROBABILITY

The researcher can never prove the scientific hypothesis but can show support for it by rejecting the null hypothesis, that is, by showing that the null hypothesis has a high probability of being incorrect. We have now introduced the theory underlying all of the procedures discussed in this chapter—probability theory. Probability is a concept that we talk about all the time, such as the chance of rain today, but we have a difficult time defining it. The **probability** of an event is the event's long-run relative frequency in repeated trials under similar conditions. In other words, the statistician does not think of the probability of obtaining a single result from a single study but rather of the chances of obtaining the same result from an idealized study that can be carried out many times under identical conditions. It is the notion of repeated trials that allows researchers to use probability to test hypotheses.

Statistical probability is based on the concept of **sampling error.** Remember that the use of inferential statistics is based on random sampling. However, even when samples are randomly selected, there is always the possibility of some errors in sampling. Therefore the characteristics of any given sample may be different from those of the entire population. Suppose a group of researchers has at their disposal a large group of patients with decubitus ulcers and they wish to study the average length of time for ulcers to heal with the usual nursing care. If the researchers studied the entire population, they might obtain an average healing time of 50 days, with a standard deviation (SD) of 10 days. Now suppose that the researchers did not have the money necessary to study all of the patients but wished instead to do several consecutive studies of these patients. For this study they first draw a sample of 25 patients, calculate the mean and SD, and replace the subjects in the pop-

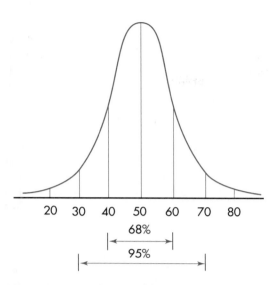

Figure 17-1   Sampling distribution of the means.

ulation before drawing the next sample. The researchers repeat this process many times so that they might end up with 50 different means. If the researchers then placed the means in a frequency distribution, it might appear as in Figure 17-1. This frequency distribution is a sampling distribution of the means. It illustrates that the researchers might find that one sample's mean might be 50.5, the next 47.5, the next 62.5, and so on. The tendency for statistics to fluctuate from one sample to another is known as sampling error.

Sampling distributions are theoretical. In practice, researchers do not routinely draw consecutive samples from the same population; usually they compute statistics and make inferences based on one sample. However, the knowledge of the properties of the sampling distribution—if these repeated samples are hypothetically obtained—permits the researcher to draw a conclusion based on one sample. This is possible because the sampling distribution of the means has certain known properties.

The sampling distribution of the means follows a normal curve, and the mean of the sampling distribution will be the mean of the population. As is discussed in the previous chapter,

the fact that the sampling distribution of the means is normal tells us several other important things. When scores are normally distributed, we know that 68% of the cases will fall between +1 SD and −1 SD or that the probability is 68 out of 100 that any one randomly drawn sample mean will lie within the range of values between ±1 SD. In the example given, if we drew only one sample, we would have a 68% chance of finding a sample mean that fell between 40 and 60. The SD of a theoretical distribution of sample means is called the **standard error of the mean.** The word error is used because the various means that make up the distribution contain some error in their estimates of the population mean. The error is considered to be standard because it implies the magnitude of the average error, just as a SD implies the average variation from one mean. The *smaller* the standard error, the *less* variable are the sample means and the *more accurate* are those means as estimates of the population value.

Although researchers rarely construct sampling distributions, standard error can be estimated because it bears a systematic relationship to the sample SD and the size of the sample. This tells us that increasing the size of the sample will increase the accuracy of our estimates of population parameters. It should make intuitive sense that to increase the size of a sample will decrease the likelihood that one outlying score will dramatically affect the sample mean (see Chapter 12). The other reason that the sampling distribution is so important is that there are sampling distributions for all statistics. Researchers consult these distributions when making determinations about rejecting the null hypothesis.

TYPE I AND TYPE II ERRORS

The researcher's decision to accept or reject the null hypothesis is based on a consideration of how probable it is that the observed differences are a result of chance alone. Because data on the entire population are not available, the researcher can never flatly assert that the null hypothesis is or is not true. Thus statistical inference is always based on incomplete information about a population, and it is possible for errors to occur when making this decision. There are two types of errors in statistical inference—type I and type II.

Let us return to the example of the study by Bull, Hansen, and Gross (2000) (see Appendix A) of elderly patients hospitalized with heart failure receiving a discharge planning intervention or traditional discharge planning. Remember that the null hypothesis of the study was that there would be no differences in outcomes between the two groups of patients. There were 40 patients in the intervention group and 70 in the traditional care group. The authors found no significant differences in patient satisfaction or difficulties in managing care, but differences in continuity and preparedness were significant. For simplification purposes, let us say that preparedness and continuity were the only two variables to be considered in the null hypothesis. If the differences found in preparedness and continuity were truly a function of chance (e.g., because this group of patients was unusual in some way) and if the number studied were too small, a type I error would occur. A **type I error** is the researchers' rejection of the null hypothesis when it is actually true. If on the other hand, the researchers had found that the groups did not differ but they had studied only a few patients, a type II error might occur. A **type II error** is the researchers' acceptance of a null hypothesis that is actually false. The relationship of the two types of errors is shown in Figure 17-2. When critiquing a study to see if there is a possibility of a type I error having occurred (rejecting the null hypothesis, when it is actually true), one should consider the reliability and validity of the instruments

used. For example, if the instruments did not accurately and precisely measure the intervention variables, one could conclude that the intervention made a difference when in reality it did not. It is critical to consider the reliability and validity of all the measurement instruments reported. In a practice discipline, type I errors usually are considered more serious because if a researcher declares that differences exist where none are present, the potential exists for patient care to be affected adversely. Type II errors (accepting the null hypothesis when it is false) may occur if the sample in the study is too small, thereby limiting the opportunity to measure a true difference between two groups. A larger sample size improves the ability to detect differences between two groups. If no significant difference is found between two groups with a large sample, it provides stronger evidence (than with a small sample) not to reject the null hypothesis.

HELPFUL HINT Decreasing the alpha level acceptable for a study increases the chance that a type II error will occur. Remember that when a researcher is doing many statistical tests, the probability of some of the tests being significant increases as the number of tests increases. Therefore, when a number of tests are being conducted, the researcher will often decrease the alpha level to 0.01.

LEVEL OF SIGNIFICANCE

The researcher does not know when an error in statistical decision making has occurred. It is possible to know only that the null hypothesis is indeed true or false if data from the total population are available. However, the researcher can control

	REALITY	
Conclusion of test of significance	Null hypothesis is true	Null hypothesis is not true
Not statistically significant	Correct conclusion	Type II error
Statistically significant	Type I error	Correct conclusion

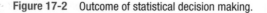

Figure 17-2 Outcome of statistical decision making.

the risk of making type I errors by setting the level of significance before the study begins (a priori). The importance of setting the level of significance before the study is conducted is explained in detail by Slakter, Wu, and Suzuki-Slakter (1991). The **level of significance (alpha level)** is the probability of making a type I error, the probability of rejecting a true null hypothesis. The minimum level of significance acceptable for nursing research is 0.05. If the researcher sets alpha, or the level of significance, at 0.05, the researcher is willing to accept the fact that if the study were done 100 times, the decision to reject the null hypothesis would be wrong 5 times out of those 100 trials. If as is sometimes done, the researcher wants to have a smaller risk of rejecting a true null hypothesis, the level of significance may be set at 0.01. In this case the researcher is willing to be wrong only once in 100 trials. The decision as to how strictly the alpha level should be set depends on how important it is to not make an error. For example, if the results of a study are to be used to determine whether a great deal of money should be spent in an area of nursing care, the researcher may decide that the accuracy of the results is so important that an alpha level of 0.01 is chosen. In most studies, however, alpha is set at 0.05.

Whatever level of significance is set, one either rejects or accepts the null hypothesis when comparing the statistical results to the preset alpha. For example in the Bull, Hansen, and Gross study (2000) (see Appendix A), the null hypothesis regarding client satisfaction, care continuity, preparedness, and difficulty managing care could not be rejected because not all of the variables listed in the hypothesis were significant at the 0.05 level or less. Client satisfaction and difficulty with managing care were not statistically different between the two groups.

Perhaps you are thinking that researchers should always use the lowest alpha level possible because it makes sense that researchers would like to keep the risk of both types of errors at a minimum. Unfortunately, decreasing the risk of making a type I error increases the risk of making a type II error. What this means is that the stricter the researcher is in preventing the rejection of a true null hypothesis, the more likely is the possibility that a false null hypothesis will be accepted. Therefore the researcher always has to accept more of a risk of one type of error when setting the alpha level.

Another method of determining level of significance and whether to accept or reject the null hypothesis is called the *critical values method*. In this method by calculating the estimates of population mean and SDs, a range of values is determined from which one can compare the sample mean findings and decide whether or not to reject the null hypothesis. Let us use the example of a study in which we want to know the importance of support groups for caregivers' of the elderly. We ask 100 caregivers to rate how important support groups are for them with an instrument that ranges from 0 (not important at all) to 100 (very important). If we use Figure 17-1 as the theoretical distribution for our study, we would see that 50 is the mean, 68% of the population would score between 40 and 60, and 95% would score between 30 and 70. Thus our null hypothesis would be that the mean scoring for the population of caregivers would be 50 and the alternative hypothesis would be greater or less than 50. After we do our measurement with our sample, we find that the sample mean score is 75. This mean is consistent with the alternative hypothesis, and we can be 95% sure that most of the time our sample mean would fall under this cutoff, thus giving us confidence in rejecting our null hypothesis. In other words, only 5 out of 100 times would we obtain this result by chance alone.

PRACTICAL VS. STATISTICAL SIGNIFICANCE

The reader should realize that there is a difference between statistical significance and practical significance. When a researcher tests a hypothesis and finds that it is statistically significant, this means that the finding is unlikely to have happened by chance. In other words, if the level of significance has been set at 0.05, the odds are 19 to 1 that the conclusion the researcher makes on the basis of the statistical test performed on sample data is correct. The researcher would reach the wrong conclusion only 5 times in 100.

Suppose a researcher is interested in the effect of loud rock music on the behavior of laboratory mice. The researcher could design an experiment to study this question and find that loud music makes the mice act strangely. A statistical test suggests that this finding is not the result of chance. However, such a finding may or may not have practical significance, even though the finding has statistical significance. Although some would argue that this study might have relevance to understanding the behavior of teenagers, some would argue also that the study has no practical value. Thus the findings of a study may have statistical significance, but they may have no practical value or significance. Although researchers should consider the practicality of a problem in the early stages of a research project (see Chapter 3), a distinction between the statistical and practical significance of the findings also should be made when discussing the results of a study. Some people believe that if findings are not statistically significant, they have no practical value. Consider the study by Rudy and associates (1995), who studied the outcomes in patients in two types of patient care systems. In this study some of the scientific hypotheses were also the null hypotheses, and the researchers indeed confirmed the null hypothesis that outcomes in the special care unit would not be worse than those of patients in traditional critical care units. These findings have practical importance because they reject common practice on the basis of scientific findings.

TESTS OF STATISTICAL SIGNIFICANCE

Tests of significance may be parametric or nonparametric. Most of the studies in nursing research literature use parametric tests that have the following three attributes:

1. They involve the estimation of at least one parameter.
2. They require measurement on at least an interval scale.

3. They involve certain assumptions about the variables being studied.

These assumptions usually include that the variable is normally distributed in the overall population. In contrast to parametric tests, **nonparametric tests of significance** are not based on the estimation of population parameters, so they involve less restrictive assumptions about the underlying distribution. Nonparametric tests usually are applied when the variables have been measured on a nominal or ordinal scale.

There has been some debate about the relative merits of the two types of statistical tests. The moderate position taken by most researchers and statisticians is that **nonparametric statistics** are best used when the data cannot be assumed to be at the interval level of measurement or when the sample is small and the normality of the underlying distribution cannot be inferred. If these assumptions can be made, however, most researchers prefer to use **parametric statistics** because they are more powerful and more flexible than nonparametric statistics.

Researchers use many different statistical tests of significance to test hypotheses. The procedure and the rationale for their use are similar from test to test. Once the researcher has chosen a significance level and collected the data, the data are used to compute the appropriate test statistic. For each test there is a related theoretical distribution that shows the probable and improbable values for that statistic. On the basis of the statistical result and the values in the distribution, the researcher either accepts or rejects the null hypothesis and then reports both the statistical result and its probability. Thus a researcher may perform a statistical test called a t test, obtain a value of 8.98, and report that it is statistically significant at the $p < .05$ level. This means that the researcher had 5 chances out of 100 to be wrong in concluding that this result could not have been obtained by chance. In addition, the likelihood of finding a statistic that is high enough to be statistically significant is increased as the sample size increases. This likelihood is indicated by the **degrees of freedom** that are often reported with the statistic and the probability value. Degrees of freedom is usually abbreviated as df.

TABLE **17-1**   Tests of Differences Between Means

LEVEL OF MEASUREMENT	ONE GROUP	TWO GROUPS		MORE THAN TWO GROUPS
		RELATED	INDEPENDENT	
NONPARAMETRIC				
Nominal	Chi-square	Chi-square Fisher exact probability	Chi-square	Chi-square
Ordinal	Kolmogorov-Smirnov	Sign test Wilcoxon matched pairs Signed rank	Chi-square Median test Mann-Whitney U	Chi-square
PARAMETRIC				
Interval or ratio	Correlated *t* ANOVA (repeated measures)	Correlated *t*	Independent *t* ANOVA	ANOVA ANCOVA MANOVA

TABLE **17-2**   Tests of Association

LEVEL OF MEASUREMENT	TWO VARIABLES	MORE THAN TWO VARIABLES
NONPARAMETRIC		
Nominal	Phi coefficient Point-biserial	Contingency coefficient
Ordinal	Kendall's tau Spearman rho	Discriminant function analysis
PARAMETRIC		
Interval or ratio	Pearson *r*	Multiple regression Path analysis Canonical correlation

Tables 17-1 and 17-2 show the most commonly used inferential statistics. The test used depends on the level of the measurement of the variables in question and the type of hypothesis being studied. Basically these statistics test two types of hypotheses—that there is a difference between groups (Table 17-1) or that there is a relationship between two or more variables (Table 17-2).

HELPFUL HINT   Just because a researcher has used nonparametric statistics does not mean that the study is not useful. The use of nonparametric statistics is appropriate when measurements are not made at the interval level or the variable under study is not normally distributed.

TESTS OF DIFFERENCE

Suppose a researcher has done an experimental study using an after-only design (see Chapter 10). What the researcher hopes to determine is that the two randomly assigned groups are different after the introduction of the experimental treatment. If the measurements taken are at the interval level, the researcher would use the *t* test to analyze the data. If the *t* statistic were found to be high enough as to be unlikely to have occurred by chance, the researcher would reject the null hypothesis and conclude that the two groups were indeed more different than would have been expected on the basis of chance alone. In other words, the researcher would conclude that the experimental treatment had the desired effect.

The study discussed earlier by Bull, Hansen, and Gross (2000) illustrates the use of the *t* statistic. The authors were studying the effects of the discharge planning intervention on hospitalized elders with heart failure. They used the *t* test to determine if at 2 weeks postdischarge there were differences in variables between the intervention and control groups. They found that the patients in the intervention group reported significantly higher scores in continuity and preparedness when compared to the traditional discharge planning group but no differences were found with satisfaction or difficulties managing care.

Parametric Tests

The *t statistic* is commonly used in nursing research. This statistic tests whether two group means are different. Thus this statistic is used when the researcher has two groups, and the question is whether the mean scores on some measure are more different than would be expected by chance. To use this test the variables must have been measured at the interval or ratio level, and the two groups must be independent. By independent we mean that nothing in one group helps determine who is in the other group. If the groups are related, as when samples are matched (see Chapter 12), and the researcher also wants to determine differences between the two groups, a paired or correlated *t* test would be used. Bull, Hansen, and Gross (2000) (see Appendix A) used this test to determine differences between the intervention and control groups.

The *t* statistic illustrates one of the major purposes of research in nursing—to demonstrate that there are differences between groups. Groups may be naturally occurring collections, such as age groups, or they may be experimentally created. The type of test used for any particular study depends primarily on whether the researcher is examining differences in one, two, or more groups and whether the data to be analyzed are nominal, ordinal, or interval (see Table 17-1).

Sometimes a researcher has more than two groups, or measurements are taken more than once, as in the Grey and associates (1999) study. Grey and associates wanted to know if a coping skills training (CST) intervention for adolescents with type 1 diabetes had an impact on their metabolic control, self-efficacy, coping abilities, depression, and quality of life over a 4-year period of time. Because some of the data are at the interval level, the researchers used **analysis of variance (ANOVA)**. Like the *t* statistic, it tests whether group means differ, but rather than testing each pair of means separately, ANOVA considers the variation among all groups. In other studies the researchers are interested in differences that occur before and after something occurs. This is the case in Grey and associates' (1999) study. They found that after 6 months the adolescents that received CST had better metabolic control, self-efficacy, less negative impact on their quality of life, and fewer worries about diabetes as compared to baseline and the control group. The appropriate statistic is the repeated measures analysis of variance, because this statistic takes into account the fact that multiple measures at several points in time affect the potential range of scores.

HELPFUL HINT A research report may not always contain the test that was done. The reader can find this information by looking at the tables. For example, a table with *t* statistics will contain a column for "t" values, and an ANOVA table will contain "F" values.

In other cases, particularly in experimental work, the researchers use *t* tests or ANOVA to determine whether random assignment to groups was effective in creating groups that are equivalent before introduction of the experimental treatment. In this case the researcher wants to show that there is no difference among the groups. In the Grey and associates (1999) study of the effects of CST on adolescents, the authors reported that the intervention and control groups were comparable at baseline except for the scores on the diabetes self-efficacy scale, which were lower in the intervention group. These results suggested that if differences were found between the two groups at follow-up, they were likely due to the intervention. Suppose, however, that these groups had differed on metabolic control at baseline. For the researchers to conclude that their intervention program was effective, they would need to control statistically for metabolic control. This is done by using the technique of **analysis of covariance (ANCOVA).** ANCOVA also measures differences among group means, and it uses a statistical technique to equate the groups under study on an important variable. Another expansion of the notion of analysis of variance is **multiple analysis of variance (MANOVA),** which also is used to determine differences in group means, but it is used when there is more than one dependent variable.

Nonparametric Tests

In the example from Grey and associates (1999), the researchers tested whether the subjects in the intervention and control group were similar by gender and treatment regimen. These two variables are not interval level data, so the researchers could not test this difference with any of the tests discussed thus far. When data are at the nominal level and the researcher wants to determine whether groups are different, the researcher uses another commonly used statistic, the **chi-square (X^2).** Chi-square is a nonparametric statistic used to determine whether the frequency in each category is different from what would be expected by chance. As with the t test and ANOVA, if the calculated chi-square is high enough, the researcher would conclude that the frequencies found would not be expected on the basis of chance alone, and the null hypothesis would be rejected. Although this test is quite robust and can be used in many different situations, it cannot be used to compare frequencies when samples are small and expected frequencies are less than 6 in each cell. In these instances the **Fisher's exact probability test** is used.

When the data are ranks, or are at the ordinal level, researchers have several other nonparametric tests at their disposal. These include the *Kol-mogorov-Smirnov test,* the *sign test,* the *Wilcoxon matched pairs test,* the *signed rank test for related groups,* the *median test,* and the *Mann-Whitney U test for independent groups.* Explanation of these tests is beyond the scope of this chapter; those readers who desire further information are referred to the Additional Readings at the end of the chapter.

A randomized clinical trial by Naylor and associates (1999) of the effects of a comprehensive discharge planning protocol and home follow-up implemented by a gerontological nurse specialist illustrates the use of several of these statistical tests. The researchers were interested in comparing the new method of discharge planning with usual discharge planning on readmissions, cost, depression, and patient satisfaction. Although the patients were randomly assigned to experimental and treatment groups, it was important to determine whether the random assignment procedure succeeded in creating equivalent groups. For data measured at the nominal level, such as gender and race, the chi-square statistic was used. For data measured at the interval level, such as age, the t test was used. Finally, to test the effect of the intervention, chi-square, t tests or Wilcoxon rank sum tests for number of readmissions, mean length of readmission stay, and ANOVA for measures of functional status, depression, and patient satisfaction were used, depending on the level of measurement.

TESTS OF RELATIONSHIPS

Researchers often are interested in exploring the *relationship* between two or more variables. Such studies use statistics that determine the **correlation,** or the degree of association, between two or more variables. Tests of the relationships between variables are sometimes considered to be descriptive statistics when they are used to describe the magnitude and direction of a relationship of two variables in a sample, and the researcher does not wish to make statements about the larger population. Such statistics also can be inferential when they are used to test hypotheses about the correlations that exist in the target population.

Null hypothesis tests of the relationships between variables assume that there is no relationship between the variables. Thus when a researcher rejects this type of null hypothesis, the conclusion is that the variables are in fact related. Suppose a researcher is interested in the relationship between the age of patients and the length of time it takes them to recover from surgery. As with other statistics discussed, the researcher would design a study to collect the appropriate data and then analyze the data using measures of association. In the example, age and length of time until recovery can be considered interval level measurements. The researcher would use a test called the **Pearson correlation coefficient, Pearson r,** or **Pearson product moment correlation coefficient.** Once the Pearson r is calculated, the researcher consults the distribution for this test to determine whether the value obtained is likely to have occurred by chance. Again the research reports both the value of the correlation and its probability of occurring by chance.

The interpretation of correlation coefficients often is difficult for students who are learning statistics. Correlation coefficients can range in value from −1.0 to +1.0 and also can be zero. A zero coefficient means that there is no relationship between the variables. *A perfect positive correlation* is indicated by a +1.0 coefficient, and a *perfect negative correlation* by a −1.0 coefficient. We can illustrate the meaning of these coefficients by using the example from the previous paragraph. If there were no relationship between the age of the patient and the time he or she required to recover from surgery, the researcher would find a correlation of zero. However, if the correlation were +1.0, this would mean that the older the patient, the longer it took him or her to recover. A negative coefficient would imply that the younger the patient, the longer it would take him or her to recover. Of course, relationships are rarely perfect. The magnitude of the relationship is indicated by how close the correlation comes to the absolute value of 1. Thus a correlation of −0.76 is just as strong as a correlation of +0.76, but the direction of the relationship is opposite. In addition, a correlation of

0.76 is stronger than a correlation of 0.32. When a researcher tests hypotheses about the relationships between two variables, the test considers whether the magnitude of the correlation is large enough not to have occurred by chance. This is the meaning of the probability value or the p value reported with correlation coefficients. As with other statistical tests of significance, the larger the sample, the greater the likelihood of finding a significant correlation. Therefore researchers also report the degrees of freedom associated with the test performed.

McCain and Cella (1995) conducted a cross-sectional study to examine the relationship among psychological distress, quality of life, uncertainty, coping patterns, stress, and CD4+ T-lymphocyte levels. The authors found that increased negative stress was correlated significantly with lower quality of life, with a correlation coefficient of 0.64, suggesting that as human immunodeficiency virus–positive (HIV+) patients experienced more negative stressors, they had lower quality of life. This reflects a moderately high correlation, and it indicates that approximately 41.94% (0.64 × 0.64) of the variability in quality of life is explained by negative stressful experiences.

Nominal and ordinal data also can be tested for relationships by nonparametric statistics. When two variables being tested have only two levels (e.g., male/female; yes/no), the phi coefficient can be used to express relationships. When the researcher is interested in the relationship between a nominal variable and an interval variable, the point-biserial correlation is used. Spearman rho is used to determine the degree of association between two sets of ranks, as is *Kendall's tau.* All of these correlation coefficients may range in value from −1.0 to +1.0. These tests are shown in Table 17-2.

Nursing problems are rarely so simple that they can be explained by only two variables. When researchers are interested in studying complex relationships among more than two variables, they use techniques other than those we have discussed thus far. When researchers are interested in understanding more about a problem than just the relationship between two variables, they often use a technique called **multiple regression,** which measures the relationship between one interval level dependent variable and several independent variables. Multiple regression is the expansion of correlation to include more than two variables, and it is used when the researcher wants to determine what variables contribute to the explanation of the dependent variable and to what degree. For example, a researcher may be interested in determining what factors help women decide to breastfeed their infants. A number of variables, such as the mother's age, previous experience with breastfeeding, number of other children, and knowledge of the advantages of breastfeeding, might be measured and then analyzed to see whether they, separately and together, predict the length of breastfeeding. Such a study would require the use of multiple regression. The results of a study such as this might help nurses know that a younger mother with only one other child might be more likely to benefit from a teaching program about breastfeeding than an older mother with several other children.

The reader of research reports often will see multiple regression techniques described as *forward solution, backward solution,* or *stepwise solution.* These are techniques used in multiple regression to find the smallest group of variables that will account for the greatest proportion of variance in the dependent variable. In the forward solution the independent variable with the highest correlation with the dependent variables is entered first, and the next variable is the one that will increase the explained variance the most. In the backward solution all variables are entered into the solution, and each variable is deleted to see whether the explained variance drops significantly. The stepwise solution is a combination of the two approaches. In general, all of the approaches give similar, although not identical, results (Bryk and Raudenbush, 1992).

Suppose the individual who was researching breastfeeding was interested in not just breastfeeding but also maternal satisfaction. *Canonical correlation* is used when there is more than one

dependent variable. If the data are nominal or ordinal, the contingency coefficient or discriminant function analyses are used. These last tests are beyond the scope of this text; further information can be found in the Additional Readings section.

Sachs and associates (1999) were interested in furthering the understanding of maternal depression and child abuse, and the factors influencing the potential for mothers in a rural setting to abuse their low-birth-weight infants. To do so, they needed to go beyond the analysis of relationships between two variables. Using multivariate regression including forward and backward analysis, the authors found that a high level of everyday stressors and lack of a support system were predictive of depressive symptoms in the mothers, and that these stressors had a direct effect on the potential for the mother to be abusive.

ADVANCED STATISTICS

Sometimes researchers are interested in even more complex problems. For example, Martinelli (1999) examined the effect of gender, self-efficacy, situational influences, and other health-promoting variables on the avoidance of passive smoke in young adults. On the basis of a proposed explanatory model for passive smoke avoidance, the author postulated that individual gender and general self-efficacy have direct and indirect effects on passive smoke avoidance. To test this mediating effect requires a type of advanced statistics called **path analysis.** In path analysis, the researcher hypothesizes the ways variables are related and in what order and then tests how strong those relationships or paths are. In this study, the author did find that performing health-promoting behaviors, having general and passive smoke avoidance self-efficacy, being female, and not living with a smoker had a direct effect on smoke avoidance.

This notion of testing specific relationships in a specific order can be extended further to test hypothesized variables that are made up of several measures. A technique called the analysis of **linear structural relationships (LISREL)** tests path models made up of variables that are not actually measured. For example, a researcher might study the concept of self-esteem and use three different measures to determine subjects' levels of self-esteem. The researcher would test how carefully these three measures actually measure self-esteem by testing a measurement model using LISREL. Because many of the variables of interest to nursing are not easily defined and measured and because we are ultimately interested in causal models, LISREL is becoming more commonly used in nursing studies; for examples, see Abel, Marion, and Seraphine (1998) and Estabrooks (1999). In both examples, the researchers were testing theories about complex problems and the LISREL technique allowed them the opportunity to study complex interactions among variables simultaneously.

Another advanced technique often used in nursing research is factor analysis. Factor analysis helps us understand concepts more fully and contributes to our ability to measure concepts reliably and validly (see Chapter 15). **Factor analysis** takes a large number of variables and groups them into a smaller number of factors. It is used to reduce a set of data so that it may be easily described and used. In addition, factor analysis is used for instrument development and theory development. In instrument development, factor analysis is used to group individual items on a scale into meaningful factors or subscales. Snyder-Halpern (1998), for example, was interested in determining health service organizations' readiness to be involved in clinical nursing research programs. She developed an Innovation Readiness Scale and pilot-tested the instrument for reliability and validity in two urban acute care settings. Factor analysis was used to determine whether the scale actually measured the concepts that they intended the instrument to measure.

Many other statistical techniques are available to nurse researchers. Consult any of the statistics sources listed in the Additional Readings section if further information is desired or if a test not discussed here is included in a study of interest to you.

CRITIQUING Inferential Statistical Results

Many students find that critiquing inferential statistics is difficult or even impossible if they have not taken a course in statistics. Although there is some merit to this feeling, there are aspects of the statistical analysis that may be critiqued without the benefit of years of statistics course work. Important questions to consider when critiquing the use of inferential statistics are listed in the Critiquing Criteria box.

CRITIQUING CRITERIA

1. Does the hypothesis indicate that the researcher is interested in testing for differences between groups or in testing for relationships?
2. What is the level of measurement chosen for the independent and dependent variables?
3. Does the level of measurement permit the use of parametric statistics?
4. Is the size of the sample large enough to permit the use of parametric statistics?
5. Has the researcher provided enough information to decide whether the appropriate statistics were used?
6. Are the statistics used appropriate to the problem, the hypothesis, the method, the sample, and the level of measurement?
7. Are the results for each of the hypotheses presented appropriately?
8. Do the tables and the text agree?
9. Are the results understandable?
10. Is a distinction made between practical significance and statistical significance? How?
11. What is the level of significance set for the study? Is it applied throughout the paper?

The first place to begin critiquing the statistical analysis of a research report is with the hypothesis. The hypothesis should indicate to you what type of statistics are used. If the hypothesis indicates that a relationship will be found, you should expect to find indices of correlation. If the study is experimental or quasiexperimental, the hypothesis would indicate that the author is looking for differences between the groups studied, and you would expect to find statistical tests of differences between means.

Then as you read the methods section of the paper, consider what level of measurement the author has used to measure the important variables. If the level of measurement is interval or ratio, the statistics most likely will be parametric statistics. On the other hand, if the variables are measured at the nominal or ordinal level, the statistics used should be nonparametric. Also consider the size of the sample, and remember that samples have to be large enough to permit the assumption of normality. If the sample is quite small, for example, 5 to 10 subjects, the researcher may have violated the assumptions necessary for inferential statistics to be used. Thus the important question is whether the researcher has provided enough justification to use the statistics presented.

Finally, consider the results as they are presented. There should be enough data presented for each hypothesis studied to determine whether the researcher actually examined each hypothesis. The tables should accurately reflect the procedure performed and be in harmony with the text. For example, the text should not indicate that a test reached statistical significance, while the tables indicate that the probability value of the test was above 0.05. If the researcher has used analyses that are not discussed in this text, you may want to refer to a statistics text to decide whether the analysis was appropriate to the hypothesis and the level of measurement.

There are two other aspects of the data analysis section that the reader should critique. The paper should not read as if it were a statistical textbook. The results of the study in the text of the paper should be clear enough to the average reader so that the reader can determine what was done and what the results were. In addition, the author should attempt to make a distinction between practical and statistical significance. Some results may be statistically significant, but their practical impor-

tance may be doubtful. If this is so, the author should note it. Alternatively, you may find yourself reading a research report that is elegantly presented, but you come away with a "so what?" feeling. Such a feeling may indicate that the practical significance of the study and its findings have not been adequately explained in the report.

Note that the critical analysis of a research paper's statistical analysis is not done in a vacuum. It is possible to judge the adequacy of the analysis only in relationship to the other important aspects of the paper: the problem, the hypotheses, the design, the data collection methods, and the sample. Without consideration of these aspects of the research process, the statistics themselves have very little meaning. Statistics can lie; thus it is most important that the researcher use the appropriate statistic for the problem. For example, a researcher may sometimes use a nonparametric statistic when it appears that a parametric statistic is appropriate. Because parametric statistics are more powerful than nonparametric, the result of the parametric analysis may not have been what the researcher expected. However, the nonparametric result might be in the expected direction, so the researcher reports only that result.

EXAMPLE OF THE USE AND CRITIQUE OF INFERENTIAL STATISTICS

Earlier in this chapter reference was made to the study by Bull, Hansen, and Gross (2000) (see Appendix A) comparing patient outcomes for those receiving a discharge planning intervention versus those receiving the usual discharge planning regimen. The statement of purpose implies that the authors were interested in looking at differences between groups. Therefore the reader should expect that the analysis will consist of statistical tests that examine differences between means, such as t tests or ANOVA.

Some of the demographic variables and predischarge measures of health were measured at the nominal level, so nonparametric statistics are used for these comparisons. Other major variables, such as preparedness, patient satisfaction, and difficulty with managing care were measured at the interval level, and differences between the two groups were determined using t tests. The hypotheses were tested using t tests or medians and ranks by Mann-Whitney U tests, depending on the level of measurement of the variable. These tests are appropriate to the problem because the researchers were interested in differences between the two groups. Results for each of the hypotheses are presented, and they suggest that there are differences in some of the outcomes between the two groups. Tables agree with the text, and the results are understandable to the reader. The discussion points out limitations to the study. Clear implications for practice are found, and they support the practical significance of the study. The statistical level of significance was set at 0.05 and is consistent throughout the paper. Therefore the researchers' statistics were appropriate to the study's purpose, method, sample, and levels of measurement.

Critical Thinking Challenges

Barbara Krainovich-Miller

➤ What assumption(s) is violated when a clinical research study uses a convenience sample and applies inferential statistics?
➤ What are the advantages and disadvantages of decreasing the alpha level for a study? What is the relationship between setting an alpha level and type I and type II errors?
➤ Discuss the parameters for using nonparametric statistics in a study and its impact on the usefulness of the findings.
➤ Discuss the way a reader of a research report can use the internet to determine if the appropriate inferential statistic was used.
➤ Is it ethical for a researcher to hire a statistician to perform the statistical analysis for his or her study?

KEY POINTS

- Inferential statistics are a tool to test hypotheses about populations from sample data.
- Because the sampling distribution of the means follows a normal curve, researchers are able to estimate the probability that a certain sample will have the same properties as the total population of interest. Sampling distributions provide the basis for all inferential statistics.
- Inferential statistics allow researchers to estimate population parameters and to test hypotheses. The use of these statistics allows researchers to make objective decisions about the outcome of the study. Such decisions are based on the rejection or acceptance of the null hypothesis, which states that there is no relationship between the variables.
- If the null hypothesis is accepted, this result indicates that the findings are likely to have occurred by chance. If the null hypothesis is rejected, the researcher accepts the scientific hypothesis that a relationship exists between the variables that is unlikely to have been found by chance.
- Statistical hypothesis testing is subject to two types of errors—type I and type II.
- Type I error occurs when the researcher rejects a null hypothesis that is actually true.

- Type II error occurs when the researcher accepts a null hypothesis that is actually false.
- The researcher controls the risk of making a type I error by setting the alpha level, or level of significance. Unfortunately, reducing the risk of a type I error by reducing the level of significance increases the risk of making a type II error.
- The results of statistical tests are reported to be significant or nonsignificant. Statistically significant results are those whose probability of occurring is less than 0.05 or 0.01, depending on the level of significance set by the researcher.
- Commonly used parametric and nonparametric statistical tests include those that test for differences between means, such as the t test and ANOVA, and those that test for differences in proportions, such as the chi-square test.
- Tests that examine data for the presence of relationships include the Pearson r, the sign test, the Wilcoxon matched pairs, signed rank test, and multiple regression.
- Advanced statistical procedures include path analysis, LISREL, and factor analysis.
- The most important aspect of critiquing statistical analyses is the relationship of the statistics employed to the problem, design, and method used in the study. Clues to the appropriate statis-

tical test to be used by the researcher should stem from the researcher's hypotheses. The reader also should determine if all of the hypotheses have been presented in the paper.

REFERENCES

Abel R, Marion LN, and Seraphine AE: The evaluation of motivation for sexual health among women, *West J Nurs Res* 20:166-179, 1998.

Bryk AS and Raudenbush SW: *Hierarchical linear models*, Newbury Park, CA, 1992, Sage.

Bull MJ, Hansen HE, and Gross CR: A professional-patient partnership model of discharge planning with elders hospitalized with heart failure, *Appl Nurs Res* 13:19-28, 2000.

Estabrooks CA: The conceptual structure of research utilization, *Res Nurs Health* 22:203-216, 1999.

Grey M et al: Coping skills training for youths with diabetes on intensive therapy, *Appl Nurs Res* 12:3-12, 1999.

Martinelli AM: Testing a model of avoiding environmental tobacco smoke in young adults, *Image J Nurs Sch* 31:237-242, 1999.

McCain NL and Cella DF: Correlates of stress in HIV disease, *West J Nurs Res* 17:141-155, 1995.

Naylor M et al: Comprehensive discharge planning and home follow-up of hospitalized elders, *JAMA* 281:613-620, 1999.

Rudy EB et al: Patient outcomes for the chronically critically ill: special care unit versus intensive care unit, *Nurs Res* 44:324-331, 1995.

Sachs B et al: Potential for abusive parenting by rural mothers with low-birth-weight children, *Image J Nurs Sch* 31:21-25, 1999

Slakter MJ, Wu YWB, and Suzuki-Slakter NS: *, **, and **[: statistical nonsense at the .00000 level, *Nurs Res* 40:248-249, 1991.

Snyder-Halpern R: Measuring organizational readiness for nursing research programs, *West J Nurs Res* 20:223-237, 1998.

ADDITIONAL READINGS

Blaloch HM: *Causal inferences in nonexperimental research*, New York, 1972, WW Norton.

Ferketich S and Muller M: Factor analysis revisited, *Nurs Res* 39:59-62, 1990.

Jacobson BS, Tulman L, and Lowery BJ: Three sides of the same coin: the analysis of paired data from dyads, *Nurs Res* 40:359-363, 1991.

Joreskog KG and Sorbom D: *Advances in factor analysis and structural equation models*, Cambridge, MA, 1979, Clark Abt.

Kerlinger FN and Pedhazur EJ: *Foundations of behavioral research*, ed 2, New York, 1986, Holt, Rinehart, and Winston.

Knapp TR: Treating ordinal scales as interval scales: an attempt to resolve the controversy, *Nurs Res* 39:121-125, 1990.

Knapp TR: Regression analysis: what to report, *Nurs Res* 43:187-189, 1994.

Lucke JF: Testing the homogeneity of correlated variances from a bivariate normal distribution, *Nurs Res* 43:314-315, 1994.

Nield M and Gocka I: To correlate or not to correlate: what is the question? *Nurs Res* 42:294-296, 1993.

Pedhazur EJ: *Multiple regression in behavioral research*, ed 2, New York, 1982, Holt, Rinehart, and Winston.

Schumacker RE and Lomax RG: *A beginner's guide to structural equation modeling*, New Jersey, 1996, Lawrence Erlbaum Associates, Inc.

Sidani S and Lynn MR: Examining amount and pattern of change: comparing repeated measures ANOVA and individual regression analysis, *Nurs Res* 42:283-286, 1993.

Stevens J: *Applied multivariete statistics for the social sciences*, New Jersey, 1996, Lawrence Erlbaum Associates, Inc.

GERI LOBIONDO-WOOD

Analysis of Findings

18

Key Terms

confidence interval
findings

generalizability
limitations

recommendations

Learning Outcomes

After reading this chapter, the student should be able to do the following:

- Discuss the difference between the *Results* section of a study and the *Discussion of the Results* section.
- Identify the format of the *Results* section.
- Determine if both statistically supported and statistically unsupported findings are discussed.
- Determine whether the results are objectively reported.
- Describe how tables and figures are used in a research report.
- List the criteria of a meaningful table.
- Identify the format and components of the *Discussion of the Results* section.
- Determine the purpose of the *Discussion* section.
- Discuss the importance of including generalizations and limitations of a study in the report.
- Determine the purpose of including recommendations in the study report.

The ultimate goals of nursing research are to develop nursing knowledge and evidence-based nursing practice, thereby supporting the scientific basis of nursing. From the viewpoint of the research consumer, the analysis of the results, interpretations, and generalizations that a researcher generates from a study becomes a highly important piece of the research project. After the analysis of the data the researcher puts the final pieces of the jigsaw puzzle together to view the total picture with a critical eye. This process is analogous to evaluation, the last step in the nursing process. The research consumer may view these last sections as an easier step for the investigator, but it is here that a most critical and creative process comes to the forefront. In the final sections of the report, after the statistical procedures have been applied, the researcher relates the statistical or numerical findings to the theoretical framework, literature, methods, hypotheses, and problem statements.

The final sections of published research reports are generally titled "Results" and "Discussion," but other topics, such as limitations of findings, implications for future research, and nursing practice, recommendations, and conclusions, may be separately addressed or subsumed within these sections. The presentation format of these areas is a function of the author's and the journal's stylistic considerations. The function of these final sections is to relate all aspects of the research process, as well as to discuss, interpret, and identify the limitations and generalizations relevant to the investigation, thereby furthering research-based practice. The process that both an investigator and the research consumer use to assess the results of a study is depicted in the Critical Thinking Decision Path. The goal of this chapter is to introduce the purpose and content of the final sections of a research investigation where data are presented, interpreted, discussed, and generalized. An understanding of what an investigator presents in these sections will help the research consumer to critically analyze an investigator's findings.

FINDINGS

The **findings** of a study are the results, conclusions, interpretations, recommendations, generalizations, and implications for future research and nursing practice, which are addressed by separating the presentation into two major areas. These two areas are the results and the discussion of the results. The "Results" section focuses on the results or statistical findings of a study, and the "Discussion of the Results" section focuses on the remaining topics. For both sections, the rule applies—as it does to all other sections of a report—that the content must be presented clearly, concisely, and logically.

RESULTS

The "Results" section of a research report is considered to be the data-bound section of the report and is where the researcher presents the quantitative data or numbers generated by the descriptive and inferential statistical tests. The results of the data analysis set the stage for the interpretations or "Discussion" section that follows the results. The "Results" section should then reflect the question and/or hypothesis tested. The information from each hypothesis or research question should be sequentially presented. The tests used to analyze the data should be identified. If the exact test that was used is not explicitly stated, then the values obtained should be noted. The researcher will do this by providing the numerical values of the statistics and stating the specific test value and probability level achieved (see Chapters 16 and 17). Examples of these can be found in Table 18-1. These numbers and their signs should not frighten the novice. These numbers are important, but there is much more to the research process than the numbers. They are one piece of the whole. Chapters 16 and 17 conceptually present the meanings of the numbers found in studies. Whether the consumer only superficially understands statistics or has an in-depth knowledge of statistics, it should be obvious that the results are clearly stated, and the presence or lack of statistically significant results should be noted. The "Additional Readings" list at the end

CRITICAL THINKING DECISION PATH Assessing Study Results

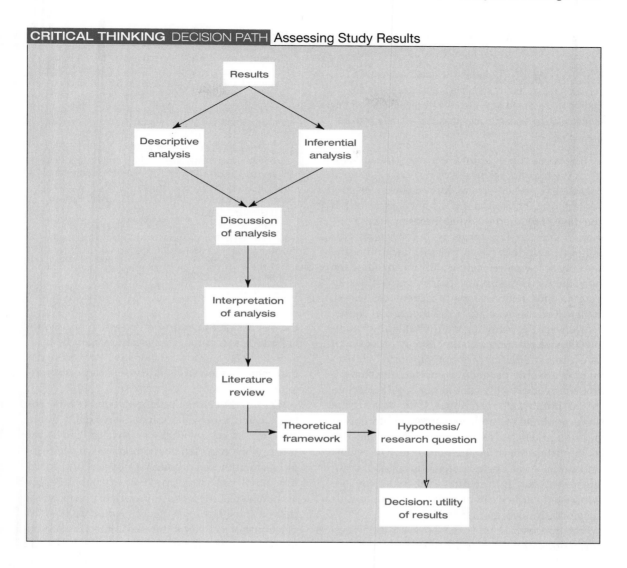

TABLE **18-1** Examples of Reported Statistical Results

STATISTICAL TEST	EXAMPLES OF REPORTED RESULTS
Mean	$m = 118.28$
Standard deviation	$SD = 62.5$
Pearson correlation	$r = 0.39, P < 0.01$
Analysis of variance	$F = 3.59, df = 2, 48, P < 0.05$
t test	$t = 2.65, P < 0.01$
Chi-square	$X^2 = 2.52, df = 1, P < 0.05$

of this chapter also provides further detail for those interested in the application of statistics.

HELPFUL HINT In the "Results" section of a research report, the descriptive statistics results are generally presented first, then the results of each of the hypotheses or research questions that were tested are presented.

The researcher is bound to present the data for all of the hypotheses posed or research questions asked (e.g., whether the hypotheses were accepted, rejected, supported, or not supported). If the data supported the hypotheses, it may be assumed that the hypotheses were *proven*, but this is not true. It does not necessarily mean that the hypotheses were proven; it only means that the hypotheses were supported and the results suggest that the relationships or differences tested, which were derived from the theoretical framework, were probably logical in that study's sample. Novice research consumers may think that if a researcher's results are not supported statistically or are only partially supported, the study is irrelevant or possibly should not have been published, but this also is not true. If the data are not supported, the research consumer should not expect the researcher to bury the work in a file. It is as important for a research consumer to review and understand unsupported studies as it is for the researcher. Information obtained from unsupported studies can often be as useful as data obtained from supported studies.

Unsupported studies can be used to suggest **limitations** of particular aspects of a study's design and procedures. Data from unsupported studies may suggest that current modes of practice, or current theory in an area may not be supported by research and therefore must be reexamined and researched further. Data helps generate new knowledge, as well as prevent knowledge stagnation. Generally, the results are interpreted in a separate section of the report. At times, the research critiquer may find that the "Results" section contains the results and the researcher's interpretations, which are generally found in the "Discussion" section. Integrating the results with

BOX 18-1 Example of Results Section

"Overall family stress as measured by the FILE and family adaptation (on the FAD) were positively and significantly related ($r = .58$, $p. < 01$)" (LoBiondo-Wood et al, 2000).

"For depression the predictor variables (resources and appraisal) accounted for 30% of the variance ($F = 8.45$, $p < .001$)" (Lee et al, 2001).

"Results of t-tests on the 2-week data indicated that caregivers in the intervention cohort reported higher scores on continuity of information about the elder's condition ($t = 2.28$, $p = .026$) and about services available ($t = 2.19$, $p = .03$)" (Bull, Hansen, and Gross, 2000).

"Abused women reported a higher previous incidence of STD than did nonabused women, primarily trichomonas (16.5% vs. 6.2%, $p < .001$) and chlamydia (24.2% vs. 16.35, $p < .02$)" (Dimmitt Champion et al, 2001).

the discussion in a report is the author's or journal editor's decision. Both sections may be integrated when a study contains several segments that may be viewed as fairly separate subproblems of a major overall problem.

The investigator should also demonstrate objectivity in the presentation of the results. A quote such as: "Women with lower physical and social functioning reported higher fatigue at all midpoints than those with higher physical and social function ($F = 3.8$ to 2.9, $p < 0.05$ to 0.001)" (Berger and Walker, 2001) is the appropriate means to express results. The investigators would be accused of lacking objectivity if they had stated the results in the following manner: "The results were not surprising as we found a significant relationship between lower physical and social functioning and higher fatigue, as we expected." Opinions or reactionary statements to the data in the "Results" section are therefore avoided. Box 18-1 provides examples of objectively stated results. The critiquer of a study should consider the following points when reading a "Results" section:

- The investigators responded objectively to the results in the discussion of the results.
- In the discussion of the results, the investigator interpreted the results, with a

TABLE **18-2** Sample Demographics (N = 29)

	MEAN AGE	RANGE
Mother	28.8	19-44
Father	30.5	21-45
Child	3.3	0.4-12.6
MARITAL STATUS	**N**	**%**
Single	4	13.8
Married	22	75.9
Divorced	3	10.3

careful reflection on all aspects of the study that preceded the results.

• The data presented are summarized. Much data is generated, but only the critical summary numbers for each test are presented. Examples of summarized data are the means and standard deviations of age, education, and income. Including all data is too cumbersome. The results can be viewed as a summation section.

• The condensation of data is done both in the written text and through the use of tables and figures. Tables and figures facilitate the presentation of large amounts of data.

• Results for the descriptive and inferential statistics for each hypothesis or research question are presented. No data should be omitted even if insignificant.

In their study, LoBiondo-Wood and associates (2000, see Appendix D) developed tables to present the results visually. Table 18-2 provides demographic descriptive results about the study's subjects. Table 18-3 provides the results of testing for a relationship between family variables of stress and coping and family adaptation. Tables allow researchers to provide a more visually thorough explanation and discussion of the results. If tables and figures are used, they must be concise. Although the text is the major mode of communicating the results, the tables and figures serve a supplementary but independent role. The role of tables and figures is to report results with some detail that the investigator does not enter

into the text. This does not mean that tables and figures should not be mentioned in the text. The amount of detail that the author uses in the text to describe the specific tabled data varies with the needs of the researcher. A good table is one that meets the following criteria:

• Supplements and economizes the text
• Has precise titles and headings
• Does not repeat the text

Another example of a table that meets these criteria can be found in the study by Bull, Hansen, and Gross (2000, see Appendix A). The research team wanted to report the comparisons of patient outcomes between the intervention and the control groups on a number of variables. Because of the number of variables, it is much easier for the reader to have a table that easily and clearly summarizes the results as this table does. To describe each one of these in the text of the article would not have economized space and would have been difficult to visualize. The table developed by the researchers (Table 18-4) allows the readers not only to visualize the variables quickly but also to assess the results.

HELPFUL HINT A well-written "Results" section is systematic, logical, concise, and drawn from all of the analyzed data. All that is written in the "Results" section should be geared to letting the data reflect the testing of the problems and hypotheses. The length of this section depends on the scope and breadth of the analysis.

DISCUSSION OF THE RESULTS

In the final section of the report, the investigator interprets and discusses the results of the study. In the discussion section, a skilled researcher makes the data come alive. The researcher gives the numbers in quantitative studies or the concepts in qualitative studies meaning and interpretation. The reviewer may ask where the investigator extracted the meaning that is applied in this section. If the researcher does the job properly, the reviewer will find a return to the beginning of the study. The researcher returns to the earlier points in the study where a problem statement was identified and independent and dependent variables were related

TABLE **18-3** Correlation among Family Variables and Family Adaptation

	FAD SUBSCALES AND GENERAL FUNCTIONING						
	AI	AR	BC	C	PS	R	GF
STRESS (FILE)							
Finance and business	.22	.06	.22	−.02	−.06	.37	.00
Marital strains	.62***	.62**	.07	.05**	.42**	.58**	.65***
Intrafamily strains	.06**	.73***	.17	.62**	.69***	.63***	.73***
Work-family transitions and strains	.05**	.48**	.27	.43**	.41*	.58**	.05**
Losses	.34	.43*	.23	.14	.29	.27	.36
Illness and family care strains	.36	.28	.03	.07	−.06	.28	.23
Pregnancy or childbearing strains	.19	.18	.04	.05	.14	.18	.07
Transition in and out	.54**	.20	−.03	.01	.06	.31	.25
Family legal violations	.47**	.01	−.13	.00	−.11	.23	.13
TOTAL	.68***	.60**	.18	.41*	.40*	.64***	.58**
COPING (CHIP)							
Family	−.53**	−.79***	−.32	−.53**	−.6**	−.22	−.68***
Medical	−.07	−.52**	−.24	−.38	−.56**	−.08	−.45**
Support	−.18	−.49*	−.24	−.48*	−.48*	−.15	−.47**
TOTAL	−.34	−.69***	−.31	−.54**	−.61**	−.19	−.62**

*$P < .05$; ** $P < .01$; *** $P < .001$

AI indicates affective involvement; *AR,* affective response; *BC,* behavior control; *C,* communications; *CHIP,* Coping Health Inventory for Parents; *FAD,* McMaster Family Assessment Device; *FILE.* Family Inventory of Life Events and Changes; *GF,* general functioning and total scale score; *PS,* problem solving; *R,* roles.

on the basis of a theoretical framework (Chapter 5) and literature review (Chapter 4). It is in this section that the researcher discusses the following:

- Both the supported and nonsupported data
- The limitations or weaknesses of a study in light of the design and the sample or data collection procedures
- How the theoretical framework was supported
- How the data may suggest additional or previously unrealized relationships

Even if the data are supported, the reviewer should not believe it to be the final word. It is important to remember that statistical significance is not the end point of a researcher's thinking and low *p* values may not be indicative of research breakthroughs. To the research critiquer, this means that statistical significance in a research study does not always mean that the results of a study are clinically significant. As the body of nursing research grows, so does the profession's ability to critically analyze beyond the test of significance and assess a research study's applicability to practice. Chapter 20 reviews methods used to analyze the usefulness of research findings. Within the nursing literature, discussion of clinical significance and evidence-based practice has also emerged (Goode, 2000; Ingersoll, 2000; Kovner, 1999; Rosswurm and Larabee, 1999; Titler et al, 1994).

As indicated throughout this text, many important pieces in the research puzzle must fit together for a study to be evaluated as a well-done project. Therefore researchers and reviewers should ac-

TABLE **18-4**   Scores for Elder Patients in Intervention and Control Groups 2 Weeks Postdischarge

MEASURES	INTERVENTION GROUPS, $n = 40$*	CONTROL GROUPS, $n = 71$	SIGNIFICANCE
SCALE AND SUBSCALE MEANS OR MEDIANS			
Continuity, information	27.51	23.50	.01
Continuity, services	9.40	6.40	.002
Preparedness (median)	58.54	43.53	.01
Difficulty	31.20	31.89	NS
Satisfaction CSQ	26.95	25.28	NS
General health (SF-36)	58.92	48.90	.04
Vitality (SF-38)	44.87	31.17	.004
Physical function (SF-36)	41.79	30.42	.03
Social function (SF-36)	66.16	61.25	NS
Mental health (SF-36)	77.64	75.27	NS
Role, physical (SF-36)	25.00	28.74	NS
Role, emotional (SF-36)	73.5	70.76	NS
Bodily pain (SF-36)	55.5	51.8	NS
COMPOSITE MEASURES			
Continuity (mean rank)	57.15	44.22	.027
Total health (mean rank)	55.87	37.95	.001

Note: Means are compared by *t*-tests, medians and ranks by Mann-Whitney *U* tests. Preparedness is the only median reported. *NS*, not significant.
*Sample size reflects those who received the complete intervention; in a few cases, patients were discharged before the intervention protocol was completed.

cept statistical significance with prudence. Statistically significant findings are not the sole means of establishing the study's merit. Remember that accepting statistical significances solely means that one is accepting that the sample mean is the same as the population mean, which may not be true (see Chapters 12 and 17). Another means to assess if the findings from one study can be generalized is to calculate a **confidence interval.** A confidence interval quantifies the uncertainty of a statistic or the probable value range within which a population parameter is expected to lie. The process used to calculate a confidence interval is beyond the scope of this text but references are provided for further explanation (Gardner and Altman, 1986,

1989; Wright, 1997). Other aspects, such as theory, sample, instrumentation, and methods, should also be considered.

When the results are not statistically supported, the researcher also returns to the theoretical framework and analyzes the earlier thinking process. Results of nonsupported hypotheses do not require the investigator to go on a fault-finding tour of each piece of the project. Such a course can become an overdone process. All research has weakness. This analysis is an attempt to identify the weaknesses and to suggest what the possible or actual problems were in the study. At times, the theoretical thinking is correct, but the researcher finds problems or limitations that could be attributed to the tools (see Chapters 14 and 15), the sampling methods (see Chapter 12), the design (see Chapters 9 to 11), or the analysis (see Chapters 16 and 17). Therefore when results are not supported, the investigator attempts to go on a fact-finding tour rather than a fault-finding one. The purpose of the discussion, then, is not to show humility or one's technical competence but rather to enable the reviewer to judge the validity of the interpretations drawn from the data and the general worth of the study. It is in the "Discussion" section of the report that the researcher ties together all the loose ends of the study and returns to the beginning to assess if the findings support, extend, or counter the theoretical framework of the study. It is from this point that reviewers of research can begin to think about clinical relevance, the need for replication, or the germination of an idea for further research study. Finally, the reviewer of a research project should find this section either in separate sections or subsumed within the "Discussion" section, and it should include generalizability and recommendations for future research, as well as a summary or a conclusion.

Generalizations **(generalizability)** are inferences that the data are representative of similar phenomena in a population beyond the study's sample. Reviewers of research are cautioned not to generalize beyond the population on which a study is based. Rarely, if ever, can one study be a recommendation for action. Beware of research studies that may overgeneralize. Generalizations that draw conclusions and make inferences within a particular situation and at a particular time are appropriate. An example of such a generalization is drawn from the study conducted by Lee and associates (2001) that was designed to study the relationship between empathy and caregiving appraisal and outcomes in informal caregivers of older adults. The researchers, when discussing the sample in light of the results, appropriately noted the following:

"Several limitations can be noted in this study. First, the results are drawn from a sample of primarily white caregivers with relatively high educational levels. Therefore, the results are only generalizable to those with similar backgrounds . . . Suggestions for future research would be to include subjects from varied ethnic backgrounds and to recruit subjects randomly from the community . . ."

This type of statement is important for reviewers of research. It helps to guide thinking in terms of a study's clinical relevance and also suggests areas for further research (see Chapter 20). One study does not provide all of the answers, nor should it. The final steps of evaluation are critical links to the refinement of practice and the generation of future research. Evaluation of research, like evaluation of the nursing process, is not the last link in the chain but a connection between findings that may serve to improve nursing theory and nursing practice.

HELPFUL HINT It has been said that a good study is one that raises more questions than it answers. So the research consumer should not view an investigator's review of limitations, generalizations, and implications of the findings for practice as lack of research skills.

The final area that the investigator integrates into the "Discussion" section is the recommendations. The **recommendations** are the investigator's suggestions for the study's application to practice, theory, and further research. This requires the investigator to reflect on the question "What contribution to nursing does this study make?" Box 18-2 provides examples of recommendations for future research and implications for nursing practice. This evaluation places the study into the realm of what is known and what needs to be known before being utilized. Nursing has grown tremendously over the last century through the efforts of many nursing researchers and scholars. This thought is critical and has been reaffirmed by many nurse researchers in the past decade, such as Donaldson (1998), Downs (1996), Hinshaw (2000), and Gortner (2000).

BOX 18-2 Examples of Research Recommendations and Practice Implications

RESEARCH RECOMMENDATIONS

"Based on data from this study and the long-term health care needs, further explorations of the short- and long-term impact of the child's transplant on the family are clearly needed to develop a picture of the child's and family's needs over time" (LoBiondo-Wood et al, 2000).

"Further directions for research are to determine whether the influences on fatigue supported in the trimmed models continue at later points in the treatment protocol and whether they are apparent in treatment for other cancer diagnoses" (Berger and Walker, 2001).

"Suggestions for future research would be to include subjects from varied ethnic backgrounds and to recruit subjects randomly from the community so that care-givers who do not have access to social services can be included. This sampling approach would increase the generalizability of the findings" (Lee et al, 2001).

PRACTICE IMPLICATIONS

"One consistent finding was noted when women with higher baseline role/physical function reported higher

fatigue at the first two cycle midpoints. Perhaps these women pushed themselves to continue to perform usual daily activities at pretreatment levels, leading to higher fatigue. Education on the use of energy conservation techniques may assist women of all lifestyles during chemotherapy" (Berger and Walker, 2001).

"The findings lead to the conclusion that interventions with the parents of this vulnerable group should focus not only on improving parenting quality, but also on promoting the physical and emotional health of mothers so as to reduce the frequency of caregiver changes. However, interventions need to be ethnically appropriate and include support, as well as education, for mothers" (Holditch-Davis et al, 2001).

"Nurse practitioners working with early adolescents who present with such symptoms need to consider anger as a possible precursor of the symptomatology. When assessments reveal this to be the case, early adolescents may be helped by teaching them to express their anger in ways that do not compromise their health, as suggested by Freeberg (1982)" (Mahon et al, 2000).

CRITIQUING the Results and Discussion

The results and the discussion of the results are the researcher's opportunity to examine the logic of the hypothesis(es) posed, the theoretical framework, the methods, and the analysis (see Critiquing Criteria). This final section requires as much logic, conciseness, and specificity as employed in the preceding steps of the research process. The consumer should be able to identify statements of the type of analysis that was used and whether the data statistically supported the hypothesis(es). These statements should be straightforward and not reflect bias (see Tables 18-3 and 18-4). Auxiliary data or serendipitous findings also may be presented. If such auxiliary findings are presented, they should be as dispassionately presented as were the hypothesis data. The statistical test used also should be noted. The numerical value of the obtained data also should be presented (see Tables 18-1, 18-3, and 18-4). The presentation of the tests, the numerical values found, and the statements of support or nonsupport should be clear, concise, and systematically reported. For illustrative purposes

that facilitate readability, the researchers should present extensive findings in tables.

The "Discussion" section should interpret the data, gaps, limitations, and conclusions of the study, as well as give recommendations for further research. Drawing these aspects into the study should give the consumer a sense of the relationship of the findings to the theoretical framework. Statements reflecting the underlying theory are necessary, whether or not the hypotheses were supported.

If the findings were not supported, the consumer should—as the researcher did—attempt to identify, without fault finding, possible methodological problems. Finally, a concise presentation of the study's generalizability and the implications of the findings for practice and research should be evident. The last presentation can help the research consumer begin to rethink clinical practice, provoke discussion in clinical settings (see Chapter 20), and find similar studies that may support or refute the phenomena being studied to more fully understand the problem.

CRITIQUING CRITERIA

1. Are the results of each of the hypotheses presented?
2. Is the information regarding the results concisely and sequentially presented?
3. Are the tests that were used to analyze the data presented?
4. Are the results presented objectively?
5. If tables or figures are used, do they meet the following standards?
   a. They supplement and economize the text.
   b. They have precise titles and headings.
   c. They are not repetitious of the text.
6. Are the results interpreted in light of the hypotheses and theoretical framework and all of the other steps that preceded the results?
7. If the data are supported, does the investigator provide a discussion of how the theoretical framework was supported?
8. If the data are not supported, does the investigator attempt to identify the study's weaknesses and strengths, as well as suggest possible solutions for the research area?
9. Does the researcher discuss the study's clinical relevance?
10. Are any generalizations made, and if so are they within the scope of the findings or beyond the findings?
11. Are any recommendations for future research stated or implied?

Critical Thinking Challenges   *Barbara Krainovich-Miller*

➤ Defend or refute the following statement: "All results should be reported and interpreted whether or not they support the hypothesis(es)."
➤ What type of knowledge does the researcher draw on to interpret the results of a study? Is the same type of knowledge used when the results of a study are not statistically significant?
➤ Do you agree or disagree with the statement that a good study is one that raises more questions than it answers? Support your view with examples.
➤ How is it possible for research consumers to critique the findings and recommendations of a reported study? How could you use the internet for critiquing the findings of a study?
➤ Now that nursing students and nurses have access to Cochrane reports of clinical problems (i.e., critiques of multiple studies available on a clinical topic) or critiques of individual studies of a clinical topic published in *Evidence-Based Nursing,* as well as published metaanalyses on clinical topics, why is it necessary for them to read and critique research studies on their own? Justify your response.

Key Points

- The analysis of the findings is the final step of a research investigation. It is in this section that the consumer will find the results printed in a straightforward manner.
- All results should be reported whether or not they support the hypothesis. Tables and figures may be used to illustrate and condense data for presentation.

- Once the results are reported, the researcher interprets the results. In this presentation, usually titled "Discussion," the consumer should be able to identify the key topics being discussed. The key topics, which include an interpretation of the results, are the limitations, generalizations, implications, and recommendations for future research.
- The researcher draws together the theoretical framework and makes interpretations based on

the findings and theory in the section on the interpretation of the results. Both statistically supported and unsupported results should be interpreted. If the results are not supported, the researcher should discuss the results reflecting on the theory, as well as possible problems with the methods, procedures, design, and analysis.

* The researcher should present the limitations or weaknesses of the study. This presentation is important because it affects the study's generalizability. The generalizations or inferences about similar findings in other samples also are presented in light of the findings.
* The research consumer should be alert for sweeping claims or overgeneralizations that a researcher may state. An overextension of the data can alert the consumer to possible researcher bias.
* The recommendations provide the consumer with suggestions regarding the study's application to practice, theory, and future research. These recommendations furnish the critiquer with a final perspective of the researcher on the utility of the investigation.

REFERENCES

Berger AN and Walker SN: An exploratory model of fatigue in women receiving adjuvant breast cancer chemotherapy, *Nurs Res* 50:42-52, 2001.

Bull MJ, Hansen HE, and Gross CR: A professional-patient partnership model of discharge planning with elders hospitalized with heart failure, *Appl Nurs Res* 13, 19-28, 2000.

Dimmitt Champion J et al: Minority women with sexually transmitted diseases: sexual abuse and risk for pelvic inflammatory disease, *Res Nurs Health* 24:38-43, 2001.

Donaldson S: Breakthroughs in nursing research, Invited presentation, Proceedings of the 25th Anniversary of the American Academy of Nursing, Acapulco, Mexico, 1998.

Downs FS: Research as a survival technique, *Nurs Res* 45:323, 1996.

Gardner MJ and Altman DG: Confidence intervals rather than p values: estimation rather than hypothesis testing, *Brit Med J Clin Res* 292:746-750, 1986.

Gardner MJ and Altman DG, editors: Statistics with confidence, London: *Brit Med J*, 1989.

Goode CJ: What constitutes the "evidence" in evidence-based practice, *Appl Nurs Res* 13(4):222-225, 2000.

Gortner S: Knowledge development in nursing: our historical roots and future opportunities, *Nurs Outlook* 48:60-67, 2000.

Hinshaw AS: Nursing knowledge for the 21st century: opportunities and challenges, *J Nurs Scholarship* 32(2):117-123, 2000.

Holditch-Davis D et al: Parental caregiving and developmental outcomes of infants of mothers with HIV, *Nurs Res* 50:5-14, 2001.

Ingersoll GL: Evidence-based nursing: what it is and what it isn't, *Nurs Outlook* 48:151, 2000.

Kovner CT: Making research-based practices changes based on . . ., *Appl Nurs Res* 12:167, 1999.

Lee HS, Brennan PF, and Daly BJ: Relationship of empathy to appraisal, depression, life satisfaction, and physical health in informal caregivers of older adults, *Res Nurs Health* 24:44-56, 2001.

LoBiondo-Wood G et al: The impact of transplantation on quality of life: a longitudinal perspective, *Progress in Transplantation* 10:81-87, 2000.

Mahon NE, Yarcheski A, and Yarcheski TJ: Positive and negative outcomes of anger in early adolescents, *Res Nurs Health* 23:17-24, 2000.

Rosswurm MA and Larabee JH: A model for change to evidence-based practice, *Image: J Nurs Scholar* 31:317-322, 1999.

Titler M et al: Infusing research into practice to promote quality care, *Nurs Res* 43:307-313, 1994.

Wright DB: *Understanding statistics: an introduction for the social sciences*, London, 1997, Sage Publications.

ADDITIONAL READINGS

Kirk RE: *Experimental design procedures for the behavioral sciences*, Pacific Grove, CA, 1995, Brooks/Cole.

Munro BH and Page EB: *Statistical methods for health care research*, ed 2, Philadelphia, 1993, JB Lippincott.

Myers JL and Well AD: *Research design and statistical analysis*, Hillsdale, NJ, 1995, Lawrence Erlbaum.

Pedhazer EJ: *Multiple regression in behavioral research*, ed 2, New York, 1986, Holt, Reinhardt, and Winston.

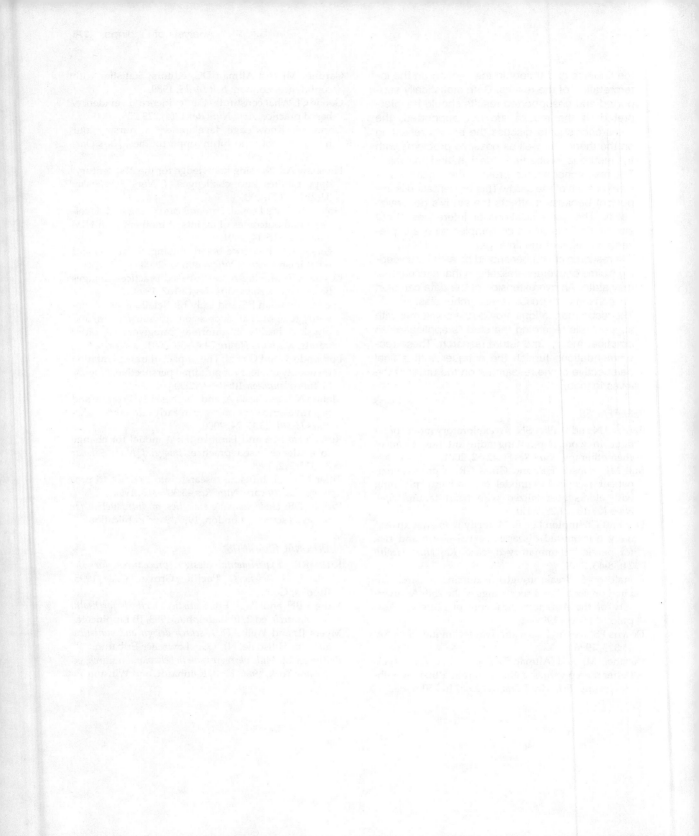

JUDITH A. HEERMANN
BETTY J. CRAFT

19

Evaluating Quantitative Research

Key Terms

replication   research base   scientific merit

Learning Outcomes

After reading this chapter, the student should be able to do the following:

- Identify the purpose of the critiquing process.
- Describe the criteria of each step of the critiquing process.
- Evaluate the strengths and weaknesses of a research report.
- Discuss the implications of the findings of a research report for nursing practice.
- Construct a critique of a research report.

Each component of a research study is examined to determine the merit of a research report. Criteria designed to assist the consumer in judging the relative value of a research report are found in previous chapters. An abbreviated set of questions summarizing the more detailed criteria, found at the end of each chapter, is used in this chapter as a framework for two sample research critiques (Table 19-1). These critiques are included to exemplify the process of evaluating reported research for potential application to practice, thus extending the **research base** for nursing. For clarification, readers are encouraged to refer to the earlier chapters for the detailed presentation of the critiquing criteria and explanations of the research process. The criteria and examples in this chapter apply to quantitative studies.

STYLISTIC CONSIDERATIONS

The evaluator should realize several important aspects related to the world of publishing before beginning to critique research studies. First, different journals have different publication goals and target specific professional markets. For example, *Nursing Research* is a journal that publishes articles on the conduct or results of research in nursing. Although *The Journal of Obstetric, Gynecologic, and Neonatal Nursing* also publishes research articles, it also includes articles related to the knowledge, experience, trends, and policies in obstetrical, gynecological, and neonatal nursing. The emphasis in the latter journal is broader in that it contains clinical and theoretical articles, as well as research articles. Consequently, the style and content of the manuscript vary according to the type of journal to which it is being submitted.

Second, the author of a research article prepares the manuscript using both personal judgment and specific guidelines. *Personal judgment* refers to the researcher's expertise that is developed in the course of designing, executing, and analyzing the study. As a result of this expertise, the researcher is in the position to judge which content is most important to communicate to the profession. The decision is a function of the following:

- The research design: experimental or nonexperimental
- The focus of the study: basic or clinical
- The audience to which the results will be most appropriately communicated

Guidelines are provided by each journal for preparing research manuscripts for publication. The following major headings are essential sections in the research report:

- Introduction
- Methodology
- Results
- Discussion

Depending on stylistic considerations related to authors' preferences and the publishing journal's requirements, specific content is included in each section of the research report. Stylistic variations (as factors influencing the presentation of the research study) are distinct from the focus of evaluating the reported research for **scientific merit.** Constructive evaluation is based on objective, unbiased, and impartial appraisal of the study's strengths and limitations. This is a step that precedes consideration of the relative worth of the findings for clinical application to nursing practice. Such judgments are the hallmark of promoting a sound evidence base for quality nursing practice.

TABLE **19-1**   Major Content Sections of a Research Report and Related Critiquing Guidelines

SECTION	QUESTIONS TO GUIDE EVALUATION
Problem statement and purpose (see Chapter 3)	1. What is the problem and/or purpose of the research study? 2. Does the problem or purpose statement express a relationship between two or more variables (e.g., between an independent and a dependent variable)? If so, what is/are the realtionship(s)? Are they testable? 3. Does the problem statement and/or purpose specify the nature of the population being studied? What is it? 4. What significance of the problem—if any—has the investigator identified?
Review of literature and theoretical framework (see Chapters 4 and 5)	1. What concepts are included in the review? Of particular importance, note those concepts that are the independent and dependent variables and how they are conceptually defined. 2. Does the literature review make the relationships among the variables explicit or place the variables within a theoretical/conceptual framework? What are the relationships? 3. What gaps or conflicts in knowledge of the problem are identified? How is the this study intended to fill those gaps or resolve those conflicts? 4. Are the references cited by the author mostly primary or secondary sources? Give an example of each. 5. What are the operational definitions of the independent and dependent variables? Do they reflect the conceptual definitions?
Hypothesis(es) or research question(s) (see Chapter 3)	1. What hypothesis(es) or research questions are stated in the study? Are they appropriately stated? 2. If research questions are stated, are they used in addition to hypotheses or to guide an exploratory study? 3. What are the independent and dependent variables in the statement of each hypothesis/research questions? 4. If hypotheses are stated, is the form of the statement statistical (null) or research? 5. What is the direction of the relationship in each hypothesis, if indicated? 6. Are the hypotheses testable?
Sample (see Chapter 12)	1. How was the sample selected? 2. What type of sampling method is used in the study? Is it appropriate to the design? 3. Does the sample reflect the population as identified in the problem or purpose statement? 4. Is the sample size appropriate? How is it substantiated? 5. To what population may the findings be generalized? What are the limitations in generalizability?
Research design (see Chapters 9 to 11)	1. What type of design is used in the study? 2. What is the rationale for the design classification? 3. Does the design seem to flow from the proposed research problem, theoretical framework, literature review, and hypothesis?
Internal validity (see Chapter 9)	1. Discuss each threat to the internal validity of the study. 2. Does the design have controls at an acceptable level for the threats to internal validity?
External validity (see Chapter 9)	1. What are the limits to generalizability in terms of external validity?

Continued

TABLE **19-1**   Major Content Sections of a Research Report and Related Critiquing Guidelines—cont'd

SECTION	QUESTIONS TO GUIDE EVALUATION
Research approach (see Chapters 13, 14, and 15)	
Methods (see Chapter 14)	1. What type(s) of data-collection methods(s) is/are used in the study? 2. Are the data-collection procedures similar for all subjects?
Legal-ethical issues (see Chapter 13)	1. How have the rights of subjects been protected? How? 2. What indications are given that informed consent of the subjects has been ensured?

Instruments (see Chapter 14)	1. Physiological measurement
	  a. Is a rationale given for why a particular instrument or method was selected? If so, what is it?
	  b. What provision is made for maintaining the accuracy of the instrument and its use, if any?
	2. Observational methods.
	  a. Who did the observing?
	  b. How were the observers trained to minimize bias?
	  c. Was there an observational guide?
	  d. Were the observers required to make inferences about what they saw?
	  e. Is there any reason to believe that the presence of the observers affected the behavior of the subjects?
	3. Interviews
	  a. Who were the interviewers? How were they trained to minimize bias?
	  b. Is there evidence of any interview bias? If so, what is it?
	4. Questionnaires
	  a. What is the type and/or format of the questionnaire(s) (e.g., Likert, open-ended)? Is(Are) it(they) consistent with the conceptual definition(s)?
	5. Available data and records
	  a. Are the records that were used appropriate to the problem being studied?
	  b. Are the data being used to describe the sample or for hypothesis testing?

Reliability and validity (see Chapter 15)	1. What type of reliability is reported for each instrument? 2. What level of reliability is reported? Is it acceptable? 3. What type of validity is reported for each instrument? 4. Does the validity of each instrument seem adequate? Why?

Continued

TABLE **19-1**   Major Content Sections of a Research Report and Related Critiquing Guidelines—cont'd

SECTION	QUESTIONS TO GUIDE EVALUATION

Analysis of data (see Chapters 16 and 17)	1. What level of measurement is used to measure each of the major variables?
	2. What descriptive or inferential statistics are reported?
	3. Were these descriptive or inferential statistics appropriate to the level of measurement for each variable?
	4. Are the inferential statistics used appropriate to the intent of the hypothesis(es)?
	5. Does the author report the level of significance set for the study? If so, what is it?
	6. If tables or figures are used, do they meet the following standards?
	   a. They supplement and economize the text.
	   b. They have precise titles and headings.
	   c. They do not repeat the text.

Conclusions, implications, and recommendations (see Chapter 18)	1. If hypothesis(es) testing was done, was/were the hypothesis(es) supported or not supported? 2. Are the results interpreted in the context of the problem/purpose, hypothesis, and theoretical framework/literature reviewed? 3. What does the investigator identify as possible limitations and/or problems in the study related to the design, methods, and sample? 4. What relevance for nursing practice does the investigator identify, if any? 5. What generalizations are made? 6. Are the generalizations within the scope of the findings or beyond the findings? 7. What recommendations for future research are stated or implied?
Application and utilization for nursing practice (see Chapter 20)	1. Does the study appear valid? That is, do its strengths outweigh its weaknesses? 2. Are there other studies with similar findings? 3. What risks/benefits are involved for patients if the research findings would be used in practice? 4. Is direct application of the research findings feasible in terms of time, effort, money, and legal/ethical risks? 5. How and under what circumstances are the findings applicable to nursing practice? 6. Should these results be applied to nursing practice? 7. Would it be possible to replicate this study in another clinical practice setting?

SAMPLE #1

The study, *Continuous Handrail Support, Oxygen Uptake, and Heart Rate in Women During Submaximal Step Treadmill Exercise* by Christman et al (2000), is critiqued. The article is presented in its entirety and is followed by the critique on p. 391.
(From *Research in Nursing & Health*, 23:35-42, 2000.)

CONTINUOUS HANDRAIL SUPPORT, OXYGEN UPTAKE, AND HEART RATE IN WOMEN DURING SUBMAXIMAL STEP TREADMILL EXERCISE

Sharon Klopfenstein Christman
Assistant Professor,
Department of Nursing,
Cedarville College,
Cedarville, OH

Anne Folta Fish
Associate Professor,
Barnes College of Nursing,
University of Missouri-St. Louis,
St. Louis, MO

Linda Bernhard
Associate Professor,
College of Nursing,
The Ohio State University,
Columbus, OH

David J. Frid
Assistant Professor,
College of Medicine and Public Health,
The Ohio State University,
Columbus, OH

Barbara A. Smith
Professor,
Marie L. O'Koren Endowed Chair of Nursing,
The University of Alabama at Birmingham,
Birmingham, AL

G. Lynn Mitchell
Biometrics Laboratory,
School of Public Health,
The Ohio State University,
Columbus, OH

Abstract: Past research suggests that continuous handrail support during exercise attenuates physiologic responses to exercise and reduces aerobic benefits; however, this phenomenon has not been systematically studied in women exercising on the step treadmill. The effects of three levels of handrail support (continuous light, continuous very light, or no handrail support) on oxygen uptake and heart rate during step treadmill exercise were examined in 15 healthy women. Measures were obtained during 6 bouts of exercise, 3 bouts at 25 steps/min followed by 3 bouts at 33 steps/min. At both step rates, mean oxygen uptake was significantly reduced during continuous light and continuous very light handrail support as compared with no handrail support, and mean heart rate was significantly reduced during continuous light versus no handrail support. At 25 steps/min only, mean heart rate was significantly re- duced during continuous very light versus no handrail support. Findings indicate that women who use even continuous light or continuous very light handrail support attenuate physiologic responses during step tread- mill exercise, thereby reducing aerobic requirements and gaining suboptimal benefits from exercise.

Keywords: handrail support; oxygen uptake; heart rate; step treadmill; stepping

Health care professionals at wellness centers and women's health clinics emphasize the beneficial effects of aerobic exercise in preventing cardiovascular disease in women (U.S. Department of Health and Human Services, 1996; Fletcher, 1997; Healy, 1995; Leon, 1997; Writing Group of the 1996 AAN Expert Panel on Women's Health,

1997). The use of several modes of exercise, including stepping, is recommended to provide variety in exercise routines. A stepping modality gaining increased popularity is the step treadmill, a fixed-height vertical treadmill with a revolving staircase that provides an aerobic workout and simulates actual stair climbing of 8-in. steps. The step treadmill has adjustable step rates (25–138 steps/min) and two side handrails (Christman, Fish, Frid, Smith, & Bryant, 1998).

Although the manufacturer's recommendations for the proper use of the step treadmill include a statement that handrails may be used intermittently for balance only, exercisers in health club settings often are observed using continuous handrail support (heavy, light, or very light) during exercise (Peterson & Bryant, 1995). Moreover, in our laboratory, 8 of 10 women interviewed stated that, given a choice, they would prefer to use continuous light or continuous very light handrail support while exercising on the step treadmill. There is a paucity of literature on which to base clinical guidelines or research protocols about the use of handrail support, with only one study conducted in a sample of young women exercising on the treadmill, not the step treadmill (von Duvillard & Pivirotto, 1991). Therefore, the extent to which continuous handrail support, even light or very light support, affects women's physiologic responses to step treadmill exercise is not known. The aim of this study was to determine, in women, the effects of three levels of handrail support (continuous light, continuous very light, or no handrail support) on oxygen uptake and heart rate during submaximal step treadmill exercise.

This study extends the work of von Duvillard and Pivirotto (1991) who studied continuous handrail support in young women during treadmill exercise, as well as the work of Howley, Colacino, and Swensen (1992) who studied continuous handrail support in a small group of men during stepper exercise. The stepper and the step treadmill differ in that the stepper has two pedals, not a revolving staircase, and the stepper requires repetitive vertical stepping-down leg motion

without the horizontal work of stepping forward as is the case of the step treadmill. The current study is the first in which the effect of continuous handrail support on physiologic responses to submaximal exercise in middle-aged women exercising on the step treadmill is examined, and in which light and very light handrail support is contrasted to the no handrail support condition in the same group of women.

In the absence of handrail support, physiologic responses to submaximal exercise are highly reproducible and have been well-described in healthy adults (Brooks, Fahey, & White, 1996). Oxygen uptake and heart rate rise predictably in a parallel fashion in response to increases in exercise intensity, for example, increases in step rate (American College of Sports Medicine [ACSM], 1995). In addition, at a constant step rate, the within-subject variability of measures of oxygen uptake and heart rate is minimal (Bruce, Kusumi, & Hosmer, 1973). In contrast to no handrail support, attenuation of oxygen uptake and heart rate during continuous handrail support has been reported in studies using the treadmill or stepper, and may occur due to alterations in the body's normal biomechanics during submaximal exercise. In other words, the pressure of the hands or fingers on the handrails and the unloading of work from the legs and feet may attenuate physiologic responses of the body during submaximal exercise (Peterson & Bryant, 1995). According to Brooks et al., work is defined as the product of a force (mass × acceleration) acting through a distance. Unloading of work from the legs and feet may reduce three important components of force: weight of the body, muscle force, and friction force of the feet against the exercise surface (ACSM, 1998). Therefore, if an exerciser supports the weight of the arms or hands continuously on the handrails, the work of the legs is reduced, the aerobic requirement of exercising muscle is reduced, and the physiologic responses to exercise are attenuated (McConnell, Foster, Conlin, & Thompson, 1991). Theoretically, unloading of work from the legs and feet also would lead to reduced fatigue in the exercising muscles. In

Table 1.   Summary of Literature on Percent Reduction in Oxygen Uptake and Heart Rate Responses to Submaximal Exercise During Continuous Handrail Support

Physiologic Variables	Continuous Handrail Support Conditions			
	Heavy Versus Light	Heavy Versus No	Light Versus No	Very Light Versus No
Oxygen uptake (FHRS/treadmill)		9-30%[5]	16-18%[2,3]	19%[4]
Heart rate (FHRS/treadmill)			8-10%[2,3]	ns[4]
Oxygen uptake (SHRS/treadmill)			ns[5]	
Heart rate (SHRS/treadmill)			ns[5]	
Oxygen uptake (SHRS/stepper)	11%[1]	12%[1]	ns[1]	
Heart rate (SHRS/stepper)	5%[1]	5%[1]	ns[1]	

Note. Results taken from studies by [1]Howley et al., 1992; [2]McConnell et al., 1991; [3]Ragg et al., 1980; [4]von Duvillard & Pivirotto, 1991; and [5]Zeimetz et al., 1985. FHRS = front handrail support; SHRS = side handrail support; ns = no statistically significant reduction.

support of this thesis, researchers found that subjects could indeed exercise longer when using continuous handrail support than when using no handrail support (Gardner, Skinner, & Smith, 1991; von Duvillard & Pivirotto, 1991).

A summary of literature regarding oxygen uptake and heart rate responses to submaximal exercise during continuous handrail support is presented in Table 1. For comparison purposes, findings are presented as percent reduction in either oxygen uptake or heart rate. Continuous heavy handrail support refers to supporting weight on the arms on the handrails. Continuous light handrail support refers to placing the hands on the handrails, whereas continuous very light handrail support refers to placing the fingers barely in contact with the handrails (Butts, Dodge, & McAlpine, 1993; Holland, Hoffmann, Vincent, Mayers, & Caston, 1990; Howley et al., 1992; Luketic, Hunter, & Feinstein, 1993). The review includes research using continuous front or side handrail support on the treadmill and continuous side handrail support conditions on the stepper. Although front handrail support requires a pulling motion and side handrail support requires a pushing motion, these maneuvers are thought to yield the same result (i.e., unloading of work from the legs and feet). Across studies, percent reductions in oxygen uptake were consistently greater than percent reductions in heart rate, although authors did not comment on this trend.

In contrast to no handrail support, continuous handrail support attenuated oxygen uptake and heart rate in young men (mean age = 24 years) and in a combined group of middle-aged men and women (mean age = 46 years), during submaximal exercise on the treadmill (McConnell et al., 1991; Zeimetz, McNeill, Hall, & Moss, 1985). Using a spring-loaded mechanism to quantify continuous front handrail support on the treadmill, a strong negative correlation ($r = -0.98$) was reported between increasing levels of resistance (handrail support) and oxygen uptake (Zeimetz et al., 1985). Even continuous very light handrail support attenuated oxygen uptake in a sample of 45 young women (ages 18–25 years) during submaximal exercise on the treadmill (von Duvillard & Pivirotto, 1991). During submaximal stepper exercise, continuous heavy handrail support was found to attenuate both oxygen uptake and heart rate in contrast to no handrail support in 5 healthy young men (ages 20–33 years) (Howley et al., 1992).

The literature supports the phenomenon of attenuated physiologic responses to submaximal exercise during continuous handrail support conditions. In no studies were mean increases in oxygen uptake or heart rate found during continuous handrail support versus no handrail support. The greatest deviations from normal oxygen uptake during submaximal exercise accompanied the heaviest continuous handrail support condition (Zeimetz et al., 1985). Finally, reductions in oxygen uptake or heart rate were widespread; observed in studies using various exercise modes (treadmill or stepper) and using various subgroups (men, women, or combined groups of men and women) (Howley et al., 1992; Ragg, Murray, Karbonit, & Jump, 1980; von Duvillard & Pivirotto, 1991).

Before handrail support recommendations can be made for women exercising on the step treadmill, research must be conducted. Therefore, the research question for the current study was: Does continuous light or continuous very light handrail support reduce oxygen uptake and/or heart rate compared with no handrail support in women during submaximal step treadmill exercise?

METHOD

A within-subject quasi-experimental design with the order of conditions (continuous light, continuous very light, and no handrail support) randomly assigned was used. The study was specifically designed with at least 10 min of seated rest between exercise bouts so that there would be a low likelihood of carryover effect.

Sample

Seventeen healthy women volunteered to participate in the study. Two of the women were excluded because of inability to tolerate step treadmill exercise at 25 steps/min, an indication of profoundly low physical fitness (ACSM, 1995). The sample consisted of 15 healthy women. Subjects were nonsmokers, had no history or evidence of cardiac or respiratory disease, and were taking no medication with cardiovascular effects. About half of the women had exercised on a step treadmill in the past. The mean age was 45.3 years ($SD = 7.4$), mean body mass index was 28 ($SD = 4.3$), mean resting systolic blood pressure was 126 mmHg ($SD = 12.7$), mean resting diastolic blood pressure was 82 mmHg ($SD = 7.4$), and mean resting heart rate was 72 beats/min ($SD = 9.6$). None of the women had dysrhythmias or untoward cardiac events during the study protocol.

Posthoc power analysis revealed a power of greater than 95% to detect differences in oxygen uptake among the three handrail support conditions at both 25 and 33 steps/min with a sample size of 15 (Hintze, 1996). Similar results were found for heart rate at both 25 and 33 steps/min. All power analyses were performed with $\alpha = .05$.

Measures

Oxygen uptake was measured during bouts of submaximal exercise on a Gauntlet step treadmill (StairMaster Sports/Medical Products, Kirkland, Washington). Oxygen uptake is defined as the amount of oxygen used by the body to perform physical work; measurements of oxygen uptake reflect the aerobic requirement (aerobic demand) of exercising muscles (ACSM, 1995). Submaximal was defined as oxygen uptake during exercise not exceeding 75% of maximal oxygen uptake, calculated with a commonly used percent maximal heart rate equation (ACSM, 1995). Mixed expiratory gases were sampled for analysis using a metabolic cart (SensorMedics MMC Horizon System, Anaheim, California), a rubber mouthpiece, and a nonrebreather valve (Hans Rudolph 2700 Series, Kansas City, Missouri). Oxygen uptake was recorded as the average of oxygen uptake during the last 30 s of each bout. The test-retest reliability for maximal oxygen uptake during step treadmill exercise was $r = .83$ (Holland et al., 1990). Values for submaximal oxygen uptake were not found in the literature. Concurrent validity has been established for oxygen uptake on the step treadmill and treadmill (Holland et al.).

A continuous electrocardiogram was performed during submaximal exercise bouts using a 10 lead ECG system (SensorMedics ECG Horizon System, Anaheim, California) in order to be able to view leads other than Lead II in the event of dysrhythmias or ST-segment change. Heart rate was recorded and averaged the last 30 s of each exercise bout. The test-retest reliability for heart rate during step treadmill exercise was .99 (Holland et al., 1990). Concurrent validity has been established for heart rate on the step treadmill and treadmill (Holland et al, 1990).

Procedures

The study was approved by the Human Subjects Institutional Review Board and all subjects provided written informed consent after an explanation of the study was provided. Two resting blood pressures were taken manually 2 min apart in the same quiet room after 5 min of seated rest, and then averaged (National Institutes of Health, 1997). A Random Zero sphygmomanometer was used (Hawksley, MKII, New York). Women were oriented to correct techniques for mounting and dismounting the step treadmill and were oriented to using the handrail support conditions. The protocol for the handrail support conditions was adopted from the literature (Butts et al., 1993; Holland et al., 1990; Howley et al., 1992) and is presented in Table 2. A plumb bob and line were used to assure that women were standing with erect posture on the step treadmill, not leaning forward, and also were at the same point or height on the stairs when stair climbing. The handrails were marked with tape to ensure that women's hands were placed in the correct positions for each handrail condition. A heavy handrail support condition was not tested in the current study, as this condition is difficult to standardize, and women could perform a Valsalva maneuver when supporting their weight, thereby altering heart rate (Folta, Metzger, & Therrien, 1989).

Women attended two additional sessions to practice using the step treadmill and to correctly demonstrate the three handrail support conditions. After women were able to demonstrate the handrail support conditions properly, one 2-hr afternoon session was scheduled for data collection. Women were instructed not to eat for 3 hr prior to the appointment and not to exercise strenuously 24 hr before the appointment (ACSM, 1995).

The order of handrail support conditions was randomly assigned. A standard set of warm-up exercises was performed for 3 min. The metabolic cart was calibrated using known gases. Ten electrodes were applied to the anterior chest and the headgear and mouthpiece were positioned for oxygen uptake measurement. Baseline resting oxygen uptake and heart rate were measured si-

Table 2. Protocol for Handrail Support Conditions

Continuous light handrail support condition
  Arms flexed at the elbows with the palms resting on, and the fingers loosely wrapped around, the rubberized portion of the handrail
  Weight not supported, elbows not locked, and the Valsalva maneuver not performed
Continuous very light handrail support condition
  Arms flexed at the elbows with the tips of the thumb and the first two fingers resting on the top of the rubberized portion of the handrail
  Fourth finger and fifth finger flexed under the palm
No handrail support condition
  Arms rested at sides and arms hanging straight down or slightly flexed at the elbows
  Hands and arms not touching the handrail, except rarely to catch balance

Note: Handrail support conditions adapted from Butts et al., 1993; Holland et al., 1990; and Howley et al., 1992.

multaneously after 3 min of seated rest. Women were asked to step onto the step treadmill without pulling on the handrails. Women began stepping at 25 steps/min using the first assigned handrail support condition. All exercise bouts and rest periods were timed with a stopwatch. During exercise women were assessed by one nurse who continuously monitored the handrail support condition and by another nurse who monitored the oxygen uptake and heart rate response.

Because a "steady state" of exercise is achieved by about 4.5 min in an untrained individual (McArdle, Katch, & Katch, 1986), oxygen uptake and heart rate for each condition were recorded simultaneously at 5.5 min and at 6 min of exercise and averaged for that condition. To control for the fact that, with repeated testing, women might anticipate the end of each exercise period at 6 min and thereby have altered physiologic responses, the timer on the console was hidden from view and the protocol was continued until 6.5 min to assure accurate 6 min measurements. After 6.5 min of exercise, the step rate was slowed, and the woman stepped off the step treadmill and rested quietly in a chair for 10 min between conditions. Baseline measures of oxygen uptake and heart rate were obtained simultaneously before each exercise bout. Oxygen uptake and heart rate were recorded simultaneously and averaged according to the protocol for the second and then the third predetermined handrail support condition.

After 15 min of rest and recalibration of the metabolic cart, women were asked to repeat the exercise protocol using the same order of handrail support conditions while stepping at 33 steps/min. Potential hazards were minimal because women were familiar with using the step treadmill and the monitoring equipment.

Twenty-five and 33 steps/min were chosen because these step rates are typically used by sedentary women who begin an exercise program. Women stepped at a rate of 25 steps/min then at 33 steps/min, because women typically progress from 25 to 33 steps/min as they increase the amount of exercise they can perform over time in their exercise programs.

Data Analysis

Descriptive statistics were used to analyze sociodemographic data, variability of oxygen uptake during steady-state exercise, and percent reduction in oxygen uptake and heart rate. Paired *t* tests were used to determine, within the no handrail support condition, differences in oxygen uptake and heart rate between the two step rates. Oxygen uptake and heart rate values were analyzed separately at each step rate using repeated measures analysis of variance to construct a pooled within-subject variance based on the dependence of the observations. This pooled variance was used to compare mean response at each level of handrail support and Tukey post hoc comparisons were calculated. Repeated measures analysis was conducted separately at each step rate because investigators were studying responses at two different step rates and not between step rates. A *p* value of $< .05$ was considered statistically significant.

RESULTS

All women completed all handrail support conditions. In all cases, oxygen uptake and heart rate returned to baseline during rest periods. By 4.5 min into each exercise period, women reached steady state, in other words, between 4.5 and 6 min, variability in oxygen uptake was minimal (.4%), reflecting constant workloads. Although women were told that they could reach for the handrail if they felt that they were falling, no attempt was made to grab the handrails during the last 1.5 min of any handrail condition. Thus, the practice sessions, which each of the women underwent to learn correct handrail support conditions, were effective.

In the no handrail support condition, mean oxygen uptake and mean heart rate were greater in response to step treadmill submaximal exercise at 33 steps/min compared with 25 steps/min ($p < .05$) (Table 3). This finding demonstrated that the 33 steps/min rate provided a significantly higher submaximal exercise intensity than the 25 steps/min rate (74 and 65% of maximal oxygen uptake, respectively, in these physically untrained women).

At 25 steps/min, there was a significant reduction (7–8%) in mean oxygen uptake during both continuous light and continuous very light handrail support as compared with no handrail support ($p < .05$) (Table 3). At 33 steps/min, mean oxygen uptake was significantly reduced by 6% during continuous light versus no handrail support and by 4% during continuous very light versus no handrail support.

At 25 steps/min, mean heart rate was significantly reduced by 4.5% during continuous light versus no handrail support and by 1.2% during continuous very light versus no handrail support (Table 3). At 33 steps/min, mean heart rate was significantly reduced by 4.8% during continuous light versus no handrail support. In contrast, at 33 steps/min mean heart rate was not significantly reduced during continuous very light versus no handrail support (2.5%).

DISCUSSION

Findings from previous studies indicate that continuous handrail support attenuates oxygen uptake and heart rate during submaximal exercise

Table 3. Physiologic Responses to Submaximal Step Treadmill Exercise During Handrail Support Conditions

	Handrail Support Conditions					
	Continuous Light ($N = 15$)		Continuous Very Light ($N = 15$)		No ($N = 15$)	
Variables	M	SEM	M	SEM	M	SEM
Oxygen uptake (ml/kg/min) at 25 steps/min	13.9[a]	0.2	14.0[a]	0.2	15.1	0.2
Oxygen uptake (ml/kg/min) at 33 steps/min	15.8[a]	0.2	16.2[a]	0.1	16.8	0.1
Heart rate (beats/min) at 25 steps/min	108[a]	2.3	111[a]	2.4	113	2.3
Heart rate (beats/min) at 33 steps/min	123[a]	2.6	126	3.2	129	3.3

[a]Significantly less than no handrail support, $p < .05$.

on the treadmill or stepper. The current study has added important dimensions to the handrail support literature by confirming that continuous handrail support, even light or very light handrail support, attenuates oxygen uptake, and in most cases heart rate, in middle-aged women performing submaximal exercise on the step treadmill. Specifically, decreases in oxygen uptake found in the current study are consistent with previous research (McConnell et al., 1991; Ragg et al., 1980; Zeimetz et al., 1985). Reductions in heart rate found in the current study were similar in direction but less pronounced than those found by other researchers (McConnell et al., 1991; Ragg et al., 1980). However, the lack of significant reductions in heart rate during very light handrail support at 33 steps/min in the current study is similar to other findings reported in women (von Duvillard & Pivirotto, 1991).

Findings of the current study were not consistent with the findings of Howley et al. (1992) who found that oxygen uptake and heart rate were not significantly decreased during continuous light versus no handrail support in healthy males on the stepper. Although Howley et al. concluded that light handrail support did not compromise effectiveness of stepper exercise for men, the results of the current study do not support that conclusion for women using the step treadmill. The discrepancy in findings between the two studies may be due to differences in gender, physical fitness of subjects, or in the type of stepping machine employed.

In agreement with published studies, percent reduction in oxygen uptake was consistently more pronounced than percent reduction in heart rate (McConnell et al., 1991, Ragg et al., 1980). In agreement with a trend in the literature (Zeimetz et al., 1985), greater changes in percent reduction in oxygen uptake and heart rate tended to occur with the more extreme continuous handrail support condition; in this case continuous light handrail support. Also consistent with the literature for women (von Duvillard & Pivirotto, 1991), even the least extreme handrail support condition, continuous very light handrail support, resulted in a significant decrease in oxygen uptake.

The phenomenon of attenuated physiologic responses to submaximal exercise during continuous handrail support is important. For example, in research and clinical practice settings, clinicians may use protocols with cardiac patients that allow for handrail support during exercise. However, once the exercise test or supervised portion of the exercise program is completed, the patient may begin to exercise in a gym where they become more comfortable with the equipment and stop using the handrails. Once the patient decides to stop holding the handrails, the aerobic requirement of the activity increases (i.e. greater exercise intensity), and they may be at risk for arrhythmias, angina, or other cardiac events.

In community settings, healthy adults typically look at the lighted console on the step treadmill for feedback about the step rate and number of calories burned, which is based on predictive equations. In the no handrail support condition, this information on both step rate and calories burned is accurate. However, during a continuous handrail support condition, the step rate on the console is accurate but the readout for calories burned over-estimates the actual aerobic requirement of the exercise. This discrepancy results in a perception of burning more calories than are actually burned. At a time when busy women are encouraged to get the most out of an exercise program, exercising in a way that reduces exercise benefits is counterproductive (Bailey, 1994).

One approach to control for the effect of handrail support in any setting is to ask women to practice the no handrail support condition and use intermittent contact with the handrails to catch their balance only. Women who have experience using exercise equipment usually can exercise without handrail support after one practice session. For those who do not regularly use exercise equipment, practicing three times may be necessary to exercise comfortably without continuous handrail support. Gardner et al. (1991) were successful in using the no handrail support condition during treadmill exercise in a combined group of men and women who had a mean age of 71 years and also had peripheral vascular disease. However, if handrail support must be used, the degree of support should be consistently maintained and documented.

Recently, manufacturers have begun producing some stepping machines without the side handrails. A much smaller and higher handrail in front of the exerciser by the console has replaced the side handrails. In this way, for purposes of safety, women can still touch the handrail for balance but cannot conveniently hold on to or lean on the new style of handrail (Peterson & Bryant, 1995).

Although the homogeneity of this group of women limits the generalizability of the results, the findings do provide support for discussing directions for future research, and present direction for developing handrail support protocols. First, when studies include combined groups of men and women, analysis by gender must be conducted (McConnell et al., 1991). Second, further study will be needed to determine the effects of continuous handrail support on physiologic responses in women from ethnically diverse cultures, in women exercising at higher step rates than those used in the current study, and in highly fit women such as competitive athletes or firefighters (O'Connell, Thomas, Cady, & Karwasky, 1986). Finally, handrail support requires improved quantification, perhaps using biomechanical techniques, to determine the degree of lower extremity unloading that occurs with handrail support. This information would be helpful when prescribing stepping exercise, for example, as a treatment for osteoporosis in midlife or older women. Weight-bearing exercise is known to slow or prevent the development of osteoporosis (U.S. Department of Health and Human Services, 1996), and determining the amount of lower extremity unloading that occurs with continuous handrail support would help practitioners develop handrail support protocols specific to desired outcomes.

REFERENCES

American College of Sports Medicine. (1995). ACSM's guidelines for exercise testing and prescription (5th ed.). Baltimore: Williams & Wilkins.

American College of Sports Medicine. (1998). ACSM's resource manual for guidelines for exercise testing and prescription. Baltimore: Lippincott, Williams & Wilkins.

Bailey, C. (1994). Smart exercise. Boston: Houghton Mifflin.

Brooks, G.A., Fahey, T.D., & White, T.P. (1996). Exercise physiology: Human bioenergetics and its applications (2nd ed.). Mountain View, California: Mayfield.

Bruce, R.A., Kusumi, I., & Hosmer, D. (1973). Maximal oxygen intake and normographic assessment of functional aerobic impairment in cardiovascular disease. American Heart Journal, 85, 506-560.

Butts, N.K., Dodge, C., & McAlpine, M. (1993). Effect of stepping rate on energy costs during StairMaster exercise. Medicine and Science in Sports and Exercise, 25, 378-382.

Christman, S.K., Fish, A.F., Frid, D.J., Smith, B.A., & Bryant, C.X. (1998). Stepping as an exercise modality for improving fitness and function. Applied Nursing Research, 11, 49-54.

Fletcher, G.F. (1997). How to implement physical activity in primary and secondary prevention: A statement for healthcare professionals from the task force on risk reduction, American Heart Association. Circulation, 96, 355-357.

Folta, A., Metzger, B.L., & Therrien, B. (1989). Preexisting physical activity level and cardiovascular responses across the Valsalva maneuver. Nursing Research, 38, 139-143.

Gardner, A.W., Skinner, J.S., & Smith, L.K. (1991). Effects of handrail support on claudication and hemodynamic responses to single-stage and progressive treadmill protocols in peripheral vascular occlusive disease. American Journal of Cardiology, 68, 99-105.

Healy, B. (1995). A new prescription for women's health. New York: Viking Penguin.

Hintze, J.L. (1996). PASS 6.0 user's guide: Power analysis and sample size for windows. Kaysville, Utah: NCSS.

Holland, G.J., Hoffmann, J.J., Vincent, W., Mayers, M., & Caston, A. (1990). Treadmill vs step treadmill ergometry. The Physician and Sportsmedicine, 18(1), 79-85.

Howley, E.T., Colacino, D.L., & Swensen, T.C. (1992). Factors affecting the oxygen cost of stepping on an electronic stepping ergometer. Medicine and Science in Sports and Exercise, 24, 1055-1058.

Leon, A.S. (Ed.). (1997). National Institutes of Health: Physical activity and cardiovascular health. Champaign, IL: Human Kinetics.

Luketic, R., Hunter, G.R., & Feinstein, C. (1993). Comparison of StairMaster and treadmill heart rates and oxygen uptakes. Journal of Strength and Conditioning Research, 7, 34-38.

McConnell, T.R., Foster, C., Conlin, N.C., & Thompson, N.N. (1991). Prediction of functional capacity during treadmill testing: Effect of handrail support. Journal of Cardiopulmonary Rehabilitation, 11, 255-260.

McArdle, W.D., Katch, F.I., & Katch, V.L. (1986). Exercise physiology: Energy, nutrition, and human performance. Philadelphia: Lea & Febiger.

National Institutes of Health. (1997). The sixth report of the Joint National Committee on Prevention, Detection, Evaluation, and Treatment of High Blood Pressure (NIH Publication No. 98-4080). Washington, DC: U.S. Department of Health and Human Services.

O'Connell, E.R., Thomas, P.C., Cady, L.D., & Karwasky, R.J. (1986). Energy costs of simulated stair climbing as a job-related task in fire fighting. Journal of Occupational Medicine, 28, 282-284.

Peterson, J.A., & Bryant, C.X. (1995). The StairMaster fitness handbook. Champaign, IL: Sagamore.

Ragg, K.E., Murray, T.F., Karbonit, L.M., & Jump, D.A. (1980). Errors in predicting functional capacity from a treadmill exercise stress test. American Heart Journal, 100, 581-583.

U.S. Department of Health and Human Services. (1996). Physical activity and health: A report of the Surgeon General. Atlanta, GA: U.S. Department of Health and Human Services, Centers for Disease Control and Prevention, National Center for Chronic Disease Prevention and Health Promotion.

von Duvillard, S.P., & Pivirotto, J.M. (1991). The effect of front handrail and nonhandrail support on treadmill exercise in healthy women. Journal of Cardiopulmonary Rehabilitation, 11, 164-168.

Writing Group of the 1996 AAN Expert Panel on Women's Health (1997). Women's health and women's health care: Recommendations of the 1996 AAN expert panel on women's health. Nursing Outlook, 45(1), 7-15.

Zeimetz, G.A., McNeil, J.F., Hall, J.R., & Moss, R.F. (1985). Quantifiable changes in oxygen uptake, heart rate, and time to target heart rate when hand support is allowed during treadmill exercise. Journal of Cardiopulmonary Rehabilitation, 5, 525-530.

INTRODUCTION TO CRITIQUE #1

The article, *Continuous Handrail Support, Oxygen Uptake, and Heart Rate in Women During Submaximal Step Treadmill Exercise,* is examined in terms of its quality and the potential usefulness of the findings for application to nursing practice.

PROBLEM AND PURPOSE

The authors state that the aim or purpose of this study "was to determine, in women, the effects of three levels of handrail support (continuous light, continuous very light, or no handrail support) on oxygen uptake and heart rate during submaximal step treadmill exercise" (Christman et al, 2000). The independent variable is the three levels of support that affect the dependent variables oxygen uptake and heart rate. The purpose specifies a population of women, is appropriately stated, and provides direction for statistical analyses. The significance of the problem is establishing evidence-based recommendations for handrail support to maximize aerobic benefits of step treadmill use in preventing cardiovascular disease in women.

REVIEW OF LITERATURE AND DEFINITIONS

Christman et al (2000) develop a framework for this study based on Brooks, Fayey, and White's definition of work and the effect of support in reducing force. Thus "if an exerciser supports the weight of the arms or hands continuously on the handrails, the work of the legs is reduced, the aerobic requirement of exercising muscle is reduced, and the physiologic responses to exercise are attenuated" (Christman et al, 2000).

The concepts include handrail support, the physiologic responses of heart rate and oxygen uptake, and submaximal exercise. Levels of continuous handrail support are defined as follows: "heavy" is supporting weight on one's arms on the handrails, "light" is placing hands on the handrails, and "very light" is barely placing fingers in contact with the handrails. "Oxygen uptake is defined as the amount of oxygen used by the body to perform physical work. . . Submaximal was defined as oxygen uptake during exercise not exceeding 75% of maximal oxygen uptake."

Gaps justifying the research include the lack of information on the effect of handrail support on women's physiologic responses to step treadmill exercise. Prior studies were limited to young women using a treadmill and a small group of men using a stepper. The present study examined the effect of light, very light, and no handrail support in a population of middle-aged women who used a step treadmill for submaximal exercise.

The references used appear to be balanced between primary and secondary sources. The reference to von Duvillard and Pivirotto (cited by Christman et al, 2000) is an example of a primary source because it is identified as a study of handrail support affecting oxygen uptake and heart rate. The reference selected to illustrate the use of a secondary source is the Fletcher publication. This is a task force report on risk reduction through implementing physical activity in primary and secondary prevention (cited by Christman et al, 2000).

The independent variable of continuous handrail support condition was operationalized by adoption of a protocol reported in the literature. "Continuous light handrail support" was defined as flexion of arms at elbows, palms resting on and fingers loosely wrapped around the rubberized portion of the handrail; "very light handrail support" was defined as flexion of arms at elbows and tips of thumb and first two fingers only resting on top of rubberized portion of the handrail with the fourth and fifth fingers flexed under the palm; "no handrail support" specified arms resting at sides and hanging straight down or slightly flexed at elbows with no touching of handrail except rarely for balance.

The dependent variables were the oxygen uptake and heart rate. "Oxygen uptake was recorded as the average of oxygen uptake during the last 30 of each bout" (Christman et al, 2000). Heart rate was recorded via continuous electrocardiogram and averaged over the last 30 seconds of each exercise bout. The operational definitions reflect the conceptualization of the respective independent and dependent variables.

HYPOTHESES AND/OR RESEARCH QUESTIONS

A research question—rather than a hypothesis—is used to guide this quasi-experimental study. The question is as follows: "Does continuous light or continuous very light handrail support reduce oxygen uptake and/or heart rate compared with no handrail support in women during submaximal step treadmill exercise?" (Christman et al, 2000). The question is appropriately stated to include both the independent and dependent variables, as well as to provide a predicted direction.

SAMPLE

The convenience sample consisted of 17 healthy women who volunteered to participate in this study, two of whom were excluded because of low physical fitness. The sampling method is acceptable for the quasi-experimental research design, but the use of a nonprobability sample limits generalizability to the sample itself. The sample selected for inclusion in the research project matches the population proposed in the purpose statement, which specifies women. The mean age of 45.3 years is consistent with the intent to fill the gap in studying physiologic responses in middle aged women. The range of ages, however, although not reported, would appear to be 30 to 60 years given the standard deviation of 7.4. Christman and associates (2000) report that a post hoc power analysis for a sample of 15 revealed a power of greater than 95% to detect differences in oxygen uptake and heart rate at both 25 and 33 steps per minute, which supports adequacy of sample size.

RESEARCH DESIGN

The three criteria, as follows, for a quasi-experiment are met in the design of this study: (1) The patients who signed informed consent were randomly assigned to the order of handrail conditions; (2) The research subject served as her own control; and (3) Manipulation of the independent variable was met by varying handrail support from light to very light to none. The choice of a quasi-experimental design flows from the purpose and its accompanying framework of comparing the effects of three levels of handrail support on the physiologic responses of oxygen uptake and heart rate. The design allows for answering the research question, which asks if there are differences in oxygen uptake and/or heart rate using continuous light or very light handrail support compared with no handrail support in women during submaximal step treadmill exercise.

Internal Validity

Examination of threats to internal validity reveals no indication of difficulty associated with the history or maturation of this adult population of women during this one-time intervention study. Selection bias is controlled by exclusion of smokers, those who had a history or evidence of cardiac or respiratory disease or who were taking medication with cardiovascular effects, and by randomly assigning subjects to experimental conditions. Two of the volunteers were excluded because of intolerance to step treadmill exercise at 25 steps/minute, the lowest exercise rate used in the study. Mortality is probably not a threat, because the subjects served as their own control and the 15 remaining subjects completed the study protocol. Potential threats due to instrumentation and testing appear controlled through use of a standardized procedure to ensure consistency in observation and measurement of variables. The threats identified seem minimal.

External Validity

Generalizability of findings is limited by the use of a nonprobability sampling technique. The findings may be generalized only to the sample.

RESEARCH APPROACH
Methods

Data-collection methods include physiologic measures of the dependent variables (i.e., oxygen uptake and heart rate) that are specified and appear consistent and systematic throughout the study. Sample descriptions included demographic data, body mass index (BMI), and blood pressure. Blood pressure and BMI are physiologic measures. Consistency of blood pressure measurement is described, but information on BMI is not included. Demographics were likely obtained by interview or questionnaire, though this is not stated.

Legal-Ethical Issues

The study was approved by the Human Subjects Institutional Review Board. Written informed consent was obtained after the study was explained.

Instruments

The only rationale provided for instrument use was the selection of a 10-lead ECG system that allowed view of leads other than lead II in the event of dysrhythmias or ST-segment changes. Information on maintenance of instrument accuracy was provided only for the measurement of oxygen uptake. Oxygen uptake was measured based on samples of mixed expiratory gases through use of a metabolic cart which was calibrated using known gases before each 25 steps per minute exercise period, and again before the 33 steps per minute exercises. Demographic data were likely obtained by either interview or questionnaire. Body mass index was reported for the sample although data collection and calculation were not specified. The potential for bias does exist, although there is no discussion of evidence for such bias in the research report.

Reliability and Validity

Test-retest reliabilities for both maximal oxygen uptake and heart rate during step treadmill exercise are reported with acceptable levels of .83 and .99 respectively. Concurrent validity has been established for both oxygen uptake and heart rate on the step treadmill and treadmill as reported by Holland and associates (as cited in Christman et al, 2000). No judgment about the adequacy of validity can be made without further information.

ANALYSIS OF DATA

Oxygen uptake is measured as milliliters per kilogram per minute, and heart rate is measured as the number of beats per minute, both of which are ratio level measurements. Descriptive statistics reported are means, standard error of means, and percent reduction in oxygen uptake and heart rate. Inferential tests used include repeated measures analysis of variance at each step rate and Tukey post hoc comparisons. Paired *t* tests were used within the no handrail support condition to compare means between the step rates. The inferential and descriptive statistics used are appropriate for the ratio level of measurement. The inferential statistics used are appropriate to answer the research question posed in this study. The level of significance set for the study is specified as 0.05.

Three tables are used to present additional information. The tables are precisely titled and headed. Table 1 summarizes the information from literature reviewed; Table 2 delineates the protocol for handrail support conditions; and Table 3 supplements the content on data analyses presented in the narrative. Unnecessary repetition is avoided.

CONCLUSIONS, IMPLICATIONS, AND RECOMMENDATIONS

The authors answer their research question affirmatively for a significant reduction of oxygen uptake in continuous light or continuous very light handrail support conditions compared with no handrail support. The heart rate was significantly reduced in all conditions except for the 33 steps per minute condition where the mean heart rate was not significantly reduced during continuous very light vs. no handrail support.

The authors appropriately interpret the findings in relation to the study's aim—that is, determining the effects of handrail support on oxygen uptake rate and heart rate in women during submaximal step treadmill exercise. Christman and associates (2000) integrate the results of their study with that of earlier researchers noting both consistencies and inconsistencies. A methodological limitation acknowledged by the authors is the inadequacy of quantification of the degree of handrail support. The authors also discussed the homogeneity of the sample, which limited generalizability related to gender, ethnic diversity, and fitness level in women.

Christman and associates (2000) identify the relevance for nursing practice when they discuss the need to develop exercise protocols that incorporate empirical data on the attenuation of oxygen uptake and heart rate during submaximal exercise using handrail support on the step treadmill. A generalization made is "that continuous handrail support, even light or very light handrail support, attentuates oxygen uptake, and in most cases heart rate, in middle-aged women performing submaximal exercise on the step treadmill." This generalization appears within the scope of the findings assuming agreement that a mean age of 45.3 years is representative of middle-age. The authors' suggestions for further research are as follows: (1) to conduct analysis by gender in studies including both men and women; (2) to expand the sample population to include ethnically diverse women, women exercising at higher step rates, and highly fit women; and (3) to improve quantification of handrail support, perhaps using biomechanical techniques to determine the degree of lower extremity unloading.

APPLICATION TO NURSING PRACTICE

Validity of the study is supported by the strengths that are evident in the design and conduct of the research, outweighing its weaknesses. The results confirm previous research that indicated the attenuation of oxygen uptake in continuous handrail support. The inconsistencies noted are thought to be due to differences in gender, physical fitness, or type of stepping machine used. Christman and associates (2000) identify a potential risk related to failure to prepare patients who go from supervised exercise practice using handrail support to unsupervised exercise without continued use of handrail support. Exercise intensity increases without handrail support and could increase the risk for arrhythmias, angina, and other cardiac events. The potential for benefit from use of the research findings accrues from accurate estimates of energy expenditure with variations in handrail support conditions.

Direct application of the research findings is feasible in protocols for women using step treadmill exercisers assuming adequate replication. The time, effort, and cost of incorporating information on the use of continuous handrail support would be minimal. Nurses in teaching situations related to exercise programs could apply the results in their practice. The protocol and measures are clearly defined and would allow for replication of the research.

SAMPLE #2

The study "Depression: A Comparison Study Between Blind and Sighted Adolescents" by Sonia G. Koenes, RN, MSN and Judith F. Karshmer, PhD, RN, CNS, published in *Issues in Mental Health Nursing* (2000) is critiqued. The article is presented first and followed by the critique on p. 402. From *Issues in Mental Health Nursing* 21:269-279, 2000.)

DEPRESSION: A COMPARISON STUDY BETWEEN BLIND AND SIGHTED ADOLESCENTS

Sonia G. Koenes, RN, MSN

Judith F. Karshmer, PhD, RN, CNS
Department of Nursing,
New Mexico State University,
Las Cruces, NM

An exploratory study was conducted to identify whether the incidence of depression was greater among blind adolescents than among a sighted comparison group. A convenience sample of 22 adolescents, legally blind since birth, and 29 sighted adolescents participated in the study. The adolescents in both samples were between the ages of 12 and 18. The Beck Depression Inventory (BDI) was used to measure depression. The findings indicated that the incidence of depression among the blind adolescents was significantly higher than the incidence of depression among the sighted adolescents ($t = 2.937, df = 50, p < .005$). Mean BDI score was 7.103 for the sighted group and 13.652 for the blind group. There were no significant relationships between demographic variables and depression. This study serves as a pilot for more extensive research that can expand the empirical base for understanding depression and its relationship to visual impairment among adolescents.

Visually impaired adolescents have a unique set of challenges that can have a major impact on their overall mental health and emotional well being. Perhaps most significant is the relationship between the tasks of adolescence and the demands of blindness which could contribute to the incidence of depression among this population. Depression is the most common mental disorder in the United States affecting between 15–25% of the adult population (Zung, Broadhead, & Roth, 1993). Recently it has become apparent that depression is also a major behavioral health problem among adolescents (Brage, 1995). Twenty percent of adolescents in the United States experience significant and persistent mental disorders (Kools, 1998). Symptoms that were traditionally viewed as manifestations of a normal maturational process among teenagers and usually ignored must be considered as potentially diagnostic of clinically significant depression (Peterson et al., 1993). Convincing evidence suggests that school-aged children and adolescents suffer from depressive disorders and these conditions disrupt healthy functioning in a variety of areas (Birmaher et al., 1996a; Birmaher et al., 1996b; Garrison et al., 1997; Kovacs, 1996).

In addition to having to meet the developmental demands of adolescence, the blind teen encounters a host of other challenges. Although it seems reasonable to assume that having a visual impairment might pose a significant threat to healthy psychosocial development of the adolescent, there have been a limited number of studies exploring these relationships. It is difficult to determine how frequently symptoms of depression in the blind adolescent go unrecognized. The intersection of the two worlds—adolescence and blindness—provides an important area of research. If visually impaired adolescents are particularly prone to experience depression, it is important for mental health nurses to actively assess for signs and symptoms in order to initiate early intervention and treatment.

LITERATURE REVIEW
Depression in Adolescents

In the past, the early warning signs of depression were often overlooked during adolescence—chalked up to "growing pains" (Substance Abuse and Mental Health Services Administration, SAMHSA, 1998). However, the study of depression among adolescents has grown to become a major focus of research within psychology, psychiatry, and related mental health fields (Brage, 1995; Lahey et al., 1996; Mufson & Fairbanks, 1996; Reynolds, 1994). Factors associated with the onset, duration, and recurrence of depression at an early age have been considered in multiple studies. A number of categories of variables have been found to contribute including psychopathology, demographic, familial, psychosocial, genetic, and environmental factors (Birmaher et al., 1996a; Jensen et al., 1993).

In spite of these findings, available evidence suggests that depression in adolescence is often overlooked, ignored, or viewed as symptomatic of other problems. The parents of adolescents report significantly fewer depressive symptoms among their teenage children than those that are self-reported (Reynolds, 1994). Mood swings, withdrawal, changes in eating, sleeping, difficulty concentrating, reduced engagement in reinforcing activities, fatigue, and irritability are often judged as part of normal adolescent behavior, rather than symptoms of depression (Birmaher et al., 1996b). Such findings indicate that even when adolescents are symptomatic, their depression goes undetected and untreated. Reynolds (1994) suggests several reasons for this oversight. Adolescents tend to internalize much of their depressive symptomology. The norm exists that adolescence is supposed to be a period of turmoil and emotional instability. Many teens are hesitant to call attention to their feelings and avoid seeking relationships with adults in which they might have to explain themselves.

Epidemiological studies suggest that a substantial number of adolescents suffer from depression. Approximately 4 out of 100 teenagers get seriously depressed each year (DEPRESSION Awareness, Recognition, and Treatment, D/ART, 1998). The depression potentiates a number of harmful behaviors, including impairment in school performance and in relationships with others, an increased risk of suicidal behaviors and homicidal ideation, tobacco use, and abuse of alcohol and other drugs (Birmaher et al., 1996b; Golombek, Hebert, Tamplin, Secher, & Pearson, 1997). A recent SAMHSA (1998) study reported that adolescents with psychosocial problems are more likely to use cigarettes, engage in binge drinking and are much more likely to use marijuana than those with little or no indication of problems.

Jensen and his colleagues (1993) found that there has been a substantial increase in the prevalence of depression in recent years and that the age of onset is younger. For some, the earlier onset of depression is a precursor to serious mental health problems and psychosocial dysfunction in adulthood (Reynolds, 1994). A study done by Pine, Cohen, Gurley, Brook, and Ma (1998) found that experiencing a depressive disorder during adolescence confers a strong risk for a recurrent episode during early adulthood. The younger age of onset also seems to be related to the manner in which depression is expressed. The social and cognitive level of an individual directly influences the depressive symptomology and pervasive behavioral characteristics (Weiss et al., 1992). Earlier experiences with depression can disrupt cognitive and social development. Depression that is experienced at a young age can have long-term negative effects because of the significant disruption that takes place in learning, academic performance, and social adaptation (Kovacs & Goldston, 1991). The duration of a depressive experience in children and adolescents is also significant. A number of studies have suggested that the longer an episode of major depression persists, the greater the risk for adverse effects on subsequent normal social and cognitive development (Golombek et al., 1997).

Recognition of depression as a significant psychological disturbance in adolescents has led to investigations of youngsters at risk for educational, physical, and mental health problems (Reynolds, 1994). It seems obvious that the complexities associated with maturation, the demands of education, tension in peer and family relationships, and issues of self-esteem place a high level of stress on teens and suggest that adolescents are at increased risk for depression (Birmaher et al., 1996b). Although research has explored how specific factors including gender, ethnicity, and sexual orientation correlate with the risk for depression, there have been relatively few studies focusing on the unique variables inherent in adolescence (Peterson et al., 1993).

Depression Among Individuals with Disabilities

The literature suggests that there is a link between the psychological experience of depression and physical conditions. A number of studies have demonstrated that depression affects physical disease, and physical disease likewise affects depression (Jensen et al., 1993). Additionally, physical disability and poor physical health has been identified among potential risk factors for depression (Reinherz et al., 1989). However, there have been few studies exploring the relationships between adolescence, physical disability, and depression. And there are even fewer that focus on blindness, adolescence, and depression. MacCuspie (1992) found that children with a visual impairment were more likely than sighted children to experience social isolation. On the other hand, Huurre and Aro (1998) compared a group of 54 adolescents with visual impairments to a control group of 385 normally sighted adolescents. Self-reports indicated that the adolescents with a visual impairment did not differ

from the control group in the frequency of depression, distress symptoms, or in their relationships with parents and siblings. However, they did have greater feelings of loneliness and more difficulty in making friends. These somewhat inconsistent findings underscore the need for continued research that explores the nature of the interaction of visual impairment, adolescence, and depression.

MacCuspie (1992) found that people who are visually impaired are socially isolated. This isolation among blind adolescents became more apparent as an increasing number were integrated into mainstream schools (Hoben & Lindstrom, 1980). A person without sight has extensive perceptual, behavioral, cognitive, and emotional challenges (Dodds et al., 1994). Those who are visually impaired are already at risk for problems related to social learning and adaptation (Kovacs & Goldston, 1991). For adolescents such adjustments are layered with the demands inherent in an exacting developmental phase. Understanding how a visual impairment contributes to the adolescence experience and to the incidence of depression among adolescents provides important baseline information for planning primary prevention and early intervention strategies.

PURPOSE

The purpose of this pilot study was to explore whether the incidence of depression is greater among adolescents who are legally blind than among adolescents who are sighted. Relationships of demographic variables to depression were also examined.

METHODOLOGY
Sample

A convenience sample of 22 adolescents who had been legally blind since birth and were currently enrolled in a residential school for the blind, and 29 sighted adolescents participated in the study. The blind adolescents met the state standard for legal blindness (State of New Mexico, 1993). All participants were between 12 and 18 years old and had no mental retardation. Approval was secured from school administrators and parents or guardians, who had to provide written consent for subject participation. Actual student involvement was entirely voluntary. They were invited to participate in a study designed to "explore stress and its impact in adolescence." The researcher explained to the students that they had the right to withdraw from the study at any time and that participation was not linked to any academic evaluation or school expectations, and that there were no negative consequences for refusing.

Measures

Two instruments were used in the study. The Beck Depression Inventory (Beck, 1967) was used to measure depression. A short demographic survey, developed by the researcher, was used to collect information on subjects' age, gender, ethnicity, family composition, academic standing, participation in extracurricular activities, health problems, and use of prescription medications. The BDI is a 21-item instrument, designed to include the symptoms integral to the depressive constellation and provides a mechanism to grade their intensity. A total BDI score represents a combination of identified symptoms and their perceived intensity and ranges from 0 to 36—the higher the score, the more significant the depression. The BDI has been used extensively and its validity and reliability are well documented (Beck, 1967). Interrater consistency for the instrument has been established at $r = .86$, $p \leq .001$ (Beck, 1967). Stability has been documented by robust consistency between scores on the instrument and external clinical ratings.

Originally designed for use with adults, the BDI has been evaluated for use with adolescents (Bennett et al., 1997). The scores of 328 adolescents referred to a depression clinic were factor analyzed to test the discriminant validity of each factor. Their results indicate the BDI is a valid screening tool for adolescent depression, regardless of the presence of comorbid conditions. The BDI was further by evaluated by Olsson and von Knorring (1997). Students aged 16–17 years in the first year of high school completed the instrument

(n = 2270). Cronbach's reliability coefficient alpha was 0.89, and there were strong correlations between individual item scores and total scores. A diagnostic interview that focused on depression experiences during the previous year of high school was conducted with all of the students with scores of 16 or higher (n = 199) and with the same number of participants in the control group with low scores. The diagnosis of depression was confirmed in 73% of high scorers. Thus, the BDI has psychometric properties that make it an appropriate tool of the present study. In addition, the manner in which it is administered makes it extremely well suited to the sample under consideration. The BDI is designed for use by a trained interviewer who reads each statement in each category aloud and then asks the subject to select the statement that seems to best fit his or her current experiences. As a result, both sighted and nonsighted subjects have a similar testing experience and the administration process does not introduce any additional testing bias. Because of this common approach, the findings from this study may be compared to the findings of other studies using the BDI. The demographic survey was administered in the same fashion; the researcher read each question and range of answers aloud. The subject was then asked to choose the answer that best fit his or her situation.

RESULTS

The blind group consisted of 12 males (55%) and 10 (45%) females. The age range was 12–18 and the mean age was 15 years. The sighted group had 13 (45%) males and 16 females (55%) with an age range of 14–18 and mean of 16 years. Both groups had a diverse ethnic distribution (see Table 1), and had similarly variable academic standing, involvement in extracurricular activities, family composition, and use of prescription medication.

The findings indicated that the incidence of depression among blind adolescents was significantly higher than the incidence of depression among the sighted adolescents ($t = 2.937$, $df = 50$, $p < .005$). Mean BDI score was 7.103 for the

Table 1.   Distribution of Demographic Variables for Visually Impaired and Sighted Subjects

	Visually impaired		Sighted	
	N	%	N	%
Males	12	55%	13	45%
Females	10	45%	16	55%
Hispanic	6	27%	11	37%
Native Am	7	32%	3	10%
Anglo	5	23%	14	48%
African Am	1	4%	1	3%
Other/NA	3	14%	0	0%
Age range	12-18		14-18	
Average age	15 years		16 years	

sighted group and 13.652 for the visually impaired group. Schwab, Bialow, Martin, and Holzer (1967) established 10 as the cut-off point between "depressed" and "nondepressed." Subjects who score above 10 are more likely to have symptoms of clinical depression.

Correlation coefficients were computed to analyze the relationships between depression and key demographic variables including gender, ethnicity, use of prescription medications, family composition, academic standing, and involvement in extracurricular activities. Nonsignificant relations were found among these variables and depression. Even gender, a variable that has been tied to an increased risk for depression, was not a discriminating variable. Roberts, Roberts, and Chen (1997) found that among an ethnically diverse sample of adolescents, females had higher prevalence of depression than males. Brage (1995) has also documented that depression occurs more often in female adolescents than male adolescents. In the recent study however, even though the mean BDI score was higher for females (11.231) than for males (8.769), the difference was not statistically significant ($t = 1.037$, $df = 50$, $p < .305$).

Limitations

There are a number of limitations to the generalizability of the findings. The sample size was relatively small. Although checklist and rating scales are widely used in child psychiatry because they offer the practitioner a cost-effective method of obtaining extensive clinical information in a relatively short period of time, they have their limitations. A significant limitation of the current study is that the BDI was administered only once to the subjects. Although this is accepted practice (Beck, 1967; Bennett et al., 1997; Olsson & von Knorring, 1997), the one-shot assessment of an adolescent's feelings cannot be evidence of a condition over time. The fact that the inventory was administered verbally introduced a potential bias of social desirability. Perhaps of greatest concern to the generalizability of the findings was the potentially confounding variable that all of the blind subjects were enrolled in a residential school for the visually impaired and lived away from home during the week, returning to their families on the weekend. In the future, this study must be replicated with a sample including sighted subjects who attend a residential school and visually impaired subjects who live at home.

DISCUSSION

The results of this exploratory study suggest that the incidence of depression among blind adolescents is greater than among sighted adolescents. Although this may not be surprising, it has important ramifications for those working with the visually impaired. In accord with the current philosophy to mainstream those with visual impairments, the ironic consequence may be that the blind adolescent's behavior that would be indicative of depression is now viewed as normal.

The nurse or teacher working with visually impaired teens may be directed to look for similarities across groups and conclude that sullen, withdrawn, even asocial behavior is a consequence of typical adolescent defiance.

However, the findings of this study suggest that blind adolescents are even more likely to be depressed than sighted teens. Therefore, the negative consequences of missing key signs and symptoms are particularly profound. Academic difficulties, social isolation, increased stress, and altered self-esteem are but a few of the immediate concerns of adolescents experiencing depression. The subtleties of depression become more apparent and certainly more costly as long-term effects lead to substance abuse, suicide or homicide involvement, and other psychiatric problems. Emotional and social dysfunctions become an ever greater problem when depression is left untreated.

Directions for Future Research

This study establishes a base for future inquiry. An extension of the study is essential to explore whether the finding of an increased incidence of depression among blind adolescents extends to other physically challenged populations. Of particular interest is whether other chronic conditions such as hearing impairments and deafness, musculoskeletal problems, and even diabetes and asthma contribute to a level of risk for depression to the already vulnerable adolescent population. A study conducted by Leung and his colleagues (1997) found that for adolescents with chronic illness, it is the perception of illness severity that is an important indicator of psychosocial well-being. Perhaps it is those blind adolescents who have not resolved the angst created by blindness that are more likely to experience depression than those who have achieved some level of acceptance. Research involving in-depth interviews of these adolescents about their lived experience of blindness would be very useful.

SUMMARY

There is a growing body of knowledge that documents the nature and extent of depression among adolescents. However, there appears to be a paucity of empirical studies that explores the interaction of physical challenges among adolescents in relation to depression. Nurses must take an active role to focus the attention of health care professionals on such populations at "double-risk." The cost of undetected and untreated depression to both the individual and society is enormous. Early recognition of the signs and symptoms of depression is key in order to ameliorate the negative biological, social, and emotional consequences of the disease.

The nurse is in the ideal situation to educate teachers and parents about the prevalence of unrecognized depression in adolescents. He or she spans educational and medical systems. Viewed as a valued expert, the nurse can help families and schools differentiate between the behaviors that are normal manifestations of teen years and those that are indicative of depression. The visually impaired adolescent's actions and behavior must be viewed from within the context that he or she is part of a vulnerable population. Troubleshooting at-risk behavior facilitates early detection and timely intervention and can be the most significant contribution of the nurse to the mental health of this population.

REFERENCES

Beck, A. T. (1967). *Depression causes and treatment.* Philadelphia: University of Pennsylvania Press.

Bennett, D., Ambrosini, P., Bianchi, M., Barnett, D., Metz, C., & Rabinovich, H. (1997). Relationship of Beck Depression Inventory factors to depression among adolescents. *Journal of Affective Disorders, 45*(3), 127-134.

Birmaher, B., Ryan, N., Williamson, D., Brent, D., Kaufman, J., Dahl, R., Perel, J., & Nelson, B. (1996a). Childhood and adolescent depression: A review of the past 10 years: Part I. *Journal of the American Academy of Child and Adolescent Psychiatry, 35*(11), 1427-1439.

Birmaher, B., Ryan, N., Williamson, D., Brent, D., Kaufman, J., Dahl, R., Perel, J., & Nelson, B. (1996b). Childhood and adolescent depression: A review of the past 10 years: Part II. *Journal of the American Academy of Child and Adolescent Psychiatry, 35*(12), 1575-1583.

Brage, D. G. (1995). Adolescent depression: A review of the literature. *Archives of Psychiatric Nursing, 9*(1), 45-55.

DEPRESSION Awareness, Recognition, and Treatment (D/ART). (1998). Let's talk about . . . DEPRESSION. DEPRESSION Awareness, Recognition, and Treatment Homepage. [On-line]. Available FTP: Hostname: http://www.nimh.nih.gov/dart/index.html.

Dodds, A., Ferguson, E., Ng, L., Flannigan, G., Hawes, G., & Yates, L. (1994). The concept of adjustment: A structural model. *Journal of Visual Impairment and Blindness, 88*(6), 4487-4497.

Garrison, C. Z., Waller, J. L., Cuffe, S. P., Mc Keown, R. E., Addy, C. L., & Jackson, K. L. (1997). Incidence of major depressive disorder and dysthymia in young adolescents. *Journal of the American Academy of Child and Adolescent Psychiatry, 36*(4), 458-465.

Golombek, I. M., Hebert, J., Tamplin, A., Secher, S. M., & Pearson, J. (1997). Short-term outcome of major depression: II. Life events, family dysfunction, and friendship difficulties as predictors of persistent disorder. *Journal of the American Academy of Child Adolescent Psychiatry, 36*(4), 474-480.

Hoben, M., & Lindstrom, V. (1980). Evidence of isolation in the mainstream. *Journal of Visual Impairment and Blindness, 74,* 289-292.

Huurre, T., & Aro, H. (1998). Psychosocial development among adolescents with visual impairment. *European Child and Adolescent Psychiatry, 7*(2), 73-78.

Jensen, P. S., Koretz, D., Locke, B. Z., Schneider, S., Radke-Yarrow, M., Richters, J. E., & Rumsey, J. M. (1993). Child and adolescent psychopathology research: Problems and prospects for the 1990s. *Journal of Abnormal Child Psychology, 21*(5), 551-580.

Kools, S. (1998). Prevention of mental health problems in adolescence. *Annual Review of Nursing Research, 16,* 83-116.

Kovacs, M. (1996). Presentation and course of major depressive disorder during childhood and later years of the life span. *Journal of the American Academy of Child and Adolescent Psychiatry, 35*(6), 705-715.

Kovacs, M., & Goldston, D. (1991). Cognitive and social cognitive development of depressed children and adolescents. *Journal of the American Academy of Child and Adolescent Psychiatry, 30*(3), 388-392.

Lahey, B. B., Flagg, E. W., Bird. H. R., Schwab-Stone, M. E., Canino, G., Dulcan, M. K., Leaf, P. J., Davies, M., Brogan, D., Bourdon, K., Horwitz, S. M., Rubio-Stipec, M., Freeman, D. H., Lichtman, J. H. Shaffer, D., Goodman, S. H., Narrow, W. E., Weissman, M. M., Kandel, D. B., Jensen, P. S., Richters, J. E., & Regier, D. A. (1996). The NIMH methods for the epidemiology of child and adolescent mental disorders (MECA) study: Background and methodology. *Journal of the American Academy of Child and Adolescent Psychiatry, 35*(7), 855-864.

Leung, S., Steinbeck, K., Morris, S., Kohn, M., Towns, S., & Bennett, D. (1997). Chronic illness perception in adolescence: Implications for the doctor-patient relationship. *Journal of Paediatric Child Health, 33*(2) 107-112.

MacCuspie, P. A. (1992). The social acceptance and interactions of visually impaired children in integrated settings. In S. Sacks, L. Kekelis, & R. J. Gaylord Ross (Eds.) *The development of social skills by blind and visually impaired students* (pp. 83-102). New York: American Foundation for the Blind.

Mufson, L., & Fairbanks, J. (1996). Interpersonal psychotherapy for depressed adolescents: A one year-naturalistic follow-up study. *Journal of the American Academy of Child and Adolescent Psychiatry, 35*(9) 1145-1155.

Olsson, G., & von Knorring, A. (1997). Beck's Depression Inventory as a screening instrument for adolescent depression in Sweden: Gender differences. *Acta Psychiatric Scandinavica, 95*(4), 277-282.

Peterson, A. C., Compas, B. E., Brooks-Gunn, K., Stemmler, M., Ey, S., & Grant, K. E. (1993). Depression in adolescence. *American Psychologist, 48*(2) 155-168.

Pine, D., Cohen, P., Gurley, D., Brook, J., & Ma. Y. (1998). The risk for early-adulthood anxiety and depressive disorders in adolescents with anxiety and depressive disorders. *Archives of General Psychiatry, 55*(1), 56-64.

Reinherz, H., Stewart-Berghauer, G., Pakiz, B., Frost, A., Moeykens, B., & Holmes, W. (1989). The relationship of early risk and current mediators to depressive symptomatology in adolescence. *Journal of the American Academy of Child and Adolescent Psychiatry, 28*, 942-947.

Reynolds, W. M. (1994). Depression in adolescents: Contemporary issues and perspectives. *Advances in Clinical Child Psychology, 16*, 261-316.

Roberts, R., Roberts, C., & Chen, Y. (1997). Ethnocultural differences in prevalence of adolescent depression. *American Journal Community Psychology, 25*(1), 95-110.

Substance Abuse and Mental Health Services Administration (SAMHSA). (1998). *National Household Survey on Drug Abuse.* Washington, DC: SAMHSA Press Office.

Schwab, J. J., Bialow, M., Martin, P. C., & Holzer, C. (1967). A comparison of two rating scales for depression. *Journal of Clinical Psychology, 23*, 94-96.

State of New Mexico. (1993). *Technical assistance/best practices manual.* Santa Fe, NM: Author.

Weiss, B., Weisz, J. R., Politano, M., Carey, M., Nelson, W. M., & Finch, A. J. (1992). Relations among self-reported depressive symptoms in clinic-referred children versus adolescents. *Journal of Abnormal Psychology, 101*(3), 391-397.

Zung, W., Broadhead, E., & Roth, E. (1993). Prevalence of depression symptoms in primary care. *The Journal of Family Practice, 37*(4), 337-344.

INTRODUCTION TO CRITIQUE #2

This critique examines the research reported by Koenes and Karshmer (2000) that compared the occurrence of depression in blind and sighted adolescents. The purpose of this critique is to determine the quality of the research on the basis of the information provided in the report, as well as its potential usefulness for nursing practice.

PROBLEM AND PURPOSE

The identified purpose is "to explore whether the incidence of depression is greater among adolescents who are legally blind than among adolescents who are sighted" and to examine the "relationships of demographic variables to depression." The statement suggests comparing two groups to test the relationships among the identified variables in a population of legally blind and sighted adolescents. The authors appropriately identify the significance of the problem of depression in adolescence and document the additional risks for depression in adolescents who are visually impaired. Furthermore, sources providing evidence of the increasing prevalence and younger age of onset of depression in adolescents are reported.

REVIEW OF LITERATURE AND DEFINITIONS

The concepts included in the literature review provide a framework for the relationship of adolescence, depression, and disabilities (i.e., blindness). Blindness is conceptually defined as "without sight"; depression is evidenced in adolescents by "mood swings, withdrawal, changes in eating, sleeping, difficulty concentrating, reduced engagement in reinforcing activities, fatigue and irritability" (Koenes and Karshmer, 2000). The relationship of these variables is based on the developmental demands of adolescence combined with the challenge of visual impairment. In addition, presence of symptoms of the psychiatric diagnosis of depression has been linked to physical conditions. Increased social isolation and loneliness in visually impaired adolescents have been demonstrated empirically and may offer insight into the mechanism of increased risk for depression.

The authors identify a gap in the literature as the limited study of threats to healthy psychosocial development in adolescents who are blind. Most sources cited by these authors are primary. The reference by Mufson and Fairbanks reports results of a 1-year naturalistic follow-up study which constitutes a primary source (cited in Koenes and Karshmer, 2000). The article by Brage is a review of literature on adolescent depression (cited in Koenes and Karshmer, 2000) and provides an example of a secondary source.

Measurement or operationalization of the variables is accomplished as follows: the Beck Depression Inventory (BDI) is used to measure depression, and adolescents are individuals between the ages of 12 and 18 years. The state standard for legal blindness is referred to, but details of the operational definition are not provided. Demographic variables are operationalized as age, gender, ethnicity, family composition, academic standing, participation in extracurricular activities, health problems, and use of prescription medications. The operational definitions are congruent with conceptual definitions.

HYPOTHESES AND/OR RESEARCH QUESTIONS

No research questions or research hypotheses are stated. The inferred hypothesis is: "The incidence of depression is greater among adolescents who are legally blind than among adolescents who are sighted" (Koenes and Karshmer, 2000). This hypothesis is stated in the form of a purpose "to explore" and is used to guide the study. The independent variable is sighted or legally blind, and the dependent variable is depression. The research hypothesis predicts the direction of greater incidence of depression in blind adolescents and is testable.

SAMPLE

The convenience sample of 22 adolescents was selected from students enrolled in a residential school for the blind. The setting for the convenience sample of 29 sighted adolescents is not reported. The sample reflects the population of sighted and legally blind adolescents designated in the purpose and is appropriate to an exploratory design. This is a nonprobability convenience sample, necessitating caution in generalizing beyond the sample. No justification is provided for the sample size, which is small, but the authors do identify a relatively small sample size as a limitation of the study. The size, however, may be considered adequate for a pilot study.

RESEARCH DESIGN

Koenes and Karshmer (2000) use a nonexperimental design—specifically, an exploratory design. Exploratory designs are nonexperimental because there is no manipulation of an independent variable. This type of design permits comparing the incidence of depression in adolescents who are sighted and those who are legally blind. The design is consistent with the purpose of exploring how the occurrence of depression relates to visual acuity and allows testing the relationships proposed in the literature review and the inferred research hypothesis.

Internal Validity

Although the threats to internal validity are most clearly applicable to experimental research designs, attention to the relationships among the identified variables and rival interpretations that might potentially compromise the study is necessary for nonexperimental designs, as well. Possible threats of history, maturation, and mortality are not identified for this study. Testing is not a problem because measures are taken only once. Potential bias associated with instrumentation exists due to differences in verbal administration of the BDI. Interviewer training is not discussed. Selection bias is noted as the major threat to internal validity because of the use of a small convenience sample. The lack of random selection negates control for such variables as differences in subjects' life experiences. Overall, few threats to internal validity are identified that would inordinately decrease confidence in the results.

External Validity

Generalizability is limited to the sample because of the effect of sample selection.

RESEARCH APPROACH

Methods

Koenes and Karshmer (2000) used structured interviews as indicated in the statements that "the researcher read each question and range of answers aloud. The subject was then asked to choose the answer that best fit his or her situation." No further details about the data-collection procedure are provided.

Legal-Ethical Issues

The rights of the subjects appear to have been well-protected. "Approval was secured from school administrators and parents or guardians, who had to provide written consent for subject participation" (Koenes and Karshmer, 2000). In addition, student involvement was voluntary, and students were informed of their right to withdraw from the study at any time. Assurance was provided that participation in the study was not a school requirement and academic evaluation would not be affected by not participating.

Instruments

Two questionnaires are used as interview guides—the items were read to the subjects and their responses recorded. The investigator is reported as collecting data with no description of training before conducting the interviews. It is not known whether data were collected by one or more of the researchers. No evidence is provided to indicate any interviewer bias. It is not known whether any inflections in the voice or clarification of items occurred that might have influenced responses. The authors identify the possibility of bias due to social desirability of responses when the questions are asked by interview rather than read by the respondent.

The BDI is a 21-item instrument that includes depressive symptoms and a means to grade their intensity with possible scores ranging from 0 to 36: "the higher the score the more significant the depression" (Koenes and Karshmer, 2000). The format of the demographic questionnaire is not described but includes items on "age, gender, ethnicity, family composition, academic standing, participation in extracurricular activities, health problems and use of prescription medications."

Reliability and Validity

Koenes and Karshmer (2000) report a Cronbach's reliability coefficient alpha of .89 for the BDI and support of internal consistency of the BDI based on strong item-total correlations from the work of Olsson and von Knorring with 16- and 17-year-old students. The report of interrater consistency for the BDI established at $r = .86$, $p \leq .001$ seemed unclear as discussed in Koenes and Karsher. Review of the source cited (Beck, 1967) provided clarification. Internal consistency determined through split-half reliability yielded a reliability coefficient of .86. Item-total analysis provided correlations between each item and the total scale score that were significant at the .001 level. Beck (1967) describes an indirect method of measuring stability using variations of interrater reliability and test-retest. A high degree of consistency was found among interviewers' ratings of clinical depression compared with the scores obtained on the depression inventory on two different occasions.

Criterion-related validity is reported based on diagnostic interviews with 199 students who scored 16 or higher and 199 students who scored low as a control group. Depression was confirmed in 73% of high scorers. Discriminate validity provided support to the use of the BDI with adolescents who also had other psychiatric diagnoses. These reports are indicative of acceptable levels of reliability and validity.

ANALYSIS OF DATA

The BDI constitutes an interval level of measure. The only demographic variables with identifiable levels of measure are gender and ethnicity, which are nominal. Information was not provided about measures of use of prescription medications, family composition, academic standing, and involvement in extracurricular activities. Descriptive statistics reported are frequencies and percents of gender and ethnicity of samples; range and means of age; and means of BDI for each group— sighted and visually impaired. Inferential statistics were *t* tests looking at differences in means of BDI, which is appropriate for level of measure and purpose. The appropriateness of the use of correlations analyzing the relationships of depression and the demographic variables cannot be determined without further information on the measurement of other demographic variables and the type of correlation used. Level of significance set for the study is not reported.

One table was used to summarize information on gender, ethnicity, and age for visually impaired and sighted groups. This table has precise titles and headings with little repetition of the text.

CONCLUSIONS, IMPLICATIONS, AND RECOMMENDATIONS

The purpose of the "study was to explore whether the incidence of depression is greater among adolescents who are legally blind than among adolescents who are sighted" (Koenes and Karshmer, 2000). The hypothesis implied within the purpose was supported by finding higher levels of depression among the legally blind. The results are discussed in terms of the framework, which supports the expectation that adolescent development combined with a physical impairment (i.e., blindness) would increase the incidence of depression. The inconsistency of the failure to find significant differences in depression by gender in this study was contrasted with literature reviewed.

Koenes and Karshmer noted a number of limitations in their study. The generalizability of findings was discussed in terms of the small sample and the selection of a sample of blind adolescents that was limited to students enrolled in a residential school who were away from home during the week. The administration of the BDI was once viewed as a limitation based on failure to obtain evidence of a condition over time, and the administration by interview was viewed as introducing the potential bias of social desirability.

The relevance for nursing practice from this study is the need for those working with the visually impaired to be aware of the increased likelihood of depression in blind adolescents, as well as to be aware of the emotional and social dysfunctional problems that may be further exaggerated when depression is untreated. The generalization is kept within the scope of the findings by the authors' use of the qualifying phrase that "the results of this exploratory study suggest," and by discussion of specific limitations to the generalizability.

Koenes and Karshmer (2000) state that "this study must be replicated with a sample including sighted subjects who attend a residential school and visually impaired subjects who live at home." Qualitative research has been recommended that focuses on the lived experience of adolescents who are blind. Another avenue of research is also suggested to determine if there is an increased incidence of depression with other physically challenged populations of adolescents.

APPLICATION TO NURSING PRACTICE

The study has merit, given the stage of the research program. The strengths include identification of a problem for which Koenes and Karshmer (2000) establish significance not only for the individual but also for society, particularly when depression is overlooked and untreated. The BDI has established reliability and validity. The weaknesses of this study are the limitations acknowledged by the investigators. The major limitations of a small sample size and limited representativeness of the sample are acknowledged and serve to direct the need for future research. While results are congruent with studies relating visual impairment and social isolation, results are inconsistent with a cited study that did not find differences in depression in groups of sighted and visually impaired adolescents.

Minimal risks are apparent in nurses assessing for depression in adolescents. Benefits of identifying and referring for treatment of depression in adolescents are likely to outweigh the cost of the effects of untreated depression. Individual administration of the BDI would require time, effort, and money. Although direct application is not appropriate given the exploratory nature of the research, conceptual or cognitive application of the results from this pilot exploratory study to clinical practice are legitimate from the perspective of Stetler's (1994) model of research utilization. Replication of the study is feasible and necessary using a larger sample of visually impaired and sighted adolescents drawn from other settings (i.e., living at home or residential living arrangements).

Critical Thinking Challenges

Barbara Krainovich-Miller

➢ Discuss the ways stylistic considerations of a journal impact on the researcher's ability to present research findings of a quantitative study.
➢ Are critiques of quantitative studies by consumers of research, either in the role of student or practicing nurse, valid? What level quantitative study is best for consumers of research to critique? What assumptions did you use to make this determination?
➢ What is essential for the consumer of research to use when critiquing a quantitative research study? Discuss the ways you might use internet resources now or in the future when critiquing studies.

REFERENCES

Beck AT: *Depression: causes and treatment*, Philadelphia, 1967, University of Pennsylvania Press.

Christman SF et al: Continuous handrail support, oxygen uptake, and heart rate in women during submaximal step treadmill exercise, *Res Nurs Health* 23:35-42, 2000.

Koenes SG and Karshmer JF: Depression: a comparison study between blind and sighted adolescents, *Iss Ment Health Nurs* 21:269-279, 2000.

Stetler CM: Refinement of the Stetler/Marram model for application of research findings to practice, *Nurs Outlook* 42:15-25, 1994.

ADDITIONAL READINGS

American Psychological Association: *Publication manual of the American Psychological Association,* ed 4, Washington, DC, 1994, The Association.

Funk SG, Tornquist EM, and Champagne MT: A model for improving the dissemination of nursing research, *West J Nurs Res* 11:361-367, 1989.

Larson E: Using the CURN project to teach research utilization in a baccalaureate program, *West J Nurs Res* 11:593-599, 1989.

Nolan MT et al: A review of approaches to integrating research and practice, *Appl Nurs Res* 7:199-207, 1994.

Titler MG and Goode CJ, editors: Research utilization, *Nurs Clin North Am* 30(3), 1995.

FOUR

APPLICATION OF RESEARCH: EVIDENCE-BASED PRACTICE

RESEARCH VIGNETTE
Merle H. Mishel

CHAPTER **20**
Use of Research in Practice

Research Vignette

Use of Middle-Range Theory in Nursing Research

Introducing concepts into nursing begins with identifying the concept in patient care and then working to define and measure the concept. In that way, my work on the concept of uncertainty in illness began when I spoke with patients about their understanding and comprehension about what was happening to them during their illness. It was apparent that many patients did not understand their illness or treatment plan and had many unknowns about the outcome. I decided that the experience of uncertainty needed more attention in nursing. However, it was during my doctoral study that I defined the concept and developed an instrument to measure uncertainty.

My work has blended research, theory, and instrumentation. My early work focused on developing and testing a measure of uncertainty in illness. It was clear from early qualitative work that uncertainty had several dimensions that reflected the focus of uncertainty over the course of an illness. The Uncertainty in Illness Scale was developed from interviews with hospitalized patients. Description of the process of scale development and early findings were published in *Nursing Research* in 1981. Since that time, other versions of the scale have been developed, and the scale has been translated into eight languages and is used throughout the world.

Development of a measure to study uncertainty enabled me to conduct a series of studies with cancer patents, patients with lupus, caregivers of Alzheimer's patients, patients with rheumatoid arthritis, and patients with multiple sclerosis to study uncertainty. The benefit of having a measure of uncertainty is that it allowed me to conduct studies in which the findings were used to further refine the conceptualization of uncertainty and to test early propositions about how the concept functions. These studies were used to form some initial theory about uncertainty to explain how the concept functioned, what it was related to, and why it was important. Using a retroductive approach, findings from these early studies generated new questions that were further tested. Drawing on this early work and that of other investigators using the uncertainty scale, along with theories from psychology and information processing, the Uncertainty in Illness Theory was developed. After publication of the theory in 1988, I continued to test the theory and to revise it as findings accumulated across studies. Tests of the theory on women with cancer supported that uncertainty was increased when symptoms changed and fluctuated over time, and uncertainty was decreased by support systems and by good communication with health care providers. As other researchers used the uncertainty in illness scales, more information about the concept emerged. It became clear that uncertainty was usually an aversive experience and related to anxiety, depression, and reduced optimism. The effects of uncertainty on emotional status were found in many studies with different populations. All of these studies supported the uncertainty theory.

The findings about uncertainty were mainly limited to those with acute illness. From some of my qualitative work exploring uncertainty in chronic illness and from the work of other investigators, it became apparent that uncertainty functioned differently in acute versus chronic illness. In chronic illnesses, where the course of the illness fluctuates over time, uncertainty is a constant companion. Findings from qualitative work seemed to show that enduring uncertainty leads to a change in one's orientation toward the world and a change in value systems. Instead of expecting predictable events, some people with chronic illness begin to expect uncertainty as a major theme in their life. Based on these findings, I developed another theory of uncertainty in illness that applied to those with chronic illness. The publication in 1990 referred to a reconceptualization of the uncertainty theory. This theory did not replace the original uncertainty theory that applies to those with an acute illness. Instead, the new theory was to be applied to those with the enduring uncertainty found in chronic illness.

As the research on uncertainty accumulated as a result of my studies and the work of other researchers in nursing and other disciplines, the need to develop some methods to help people handle the uncertainty in acute illness became apparent. I developed the Uncertainty Management Intervention, which is a theory-based strategy. By being theory-based, it is drawn from the original theory of uncertainty in illness. The components of the intervention follow the original model in the theory. The principles of the intervention are based on the theory.

There have been five funded studies, funded by the National Institute for Nursing Research and the National Cancer Institute, testing the intervention across age groups, ethnic groups, different gender, and different cancers. The intervention is telephone delivered with a weekly call to the patient for 8 to 10 weeks. The telephone interview is the intervention and it follows a defined protocol. It begins with an assessment of the patient's problems or concerns guided by the antecedents of uncertainty portion of the theory. The assessment is designed to tap into the concerns of the

specific target populations and is defined by the protocol. After identifying a problem, the intervener classifies it with the patient's information according to the nature of the uncertainty. The third phase is determining the degree of threat the patient is experiencing about the uncertainty. This follows the appraisal section of the Uncertainty in Illness Theory. The intervention is then delivered based on the assessment, and it is structured to either provide information, resources, or management and communication skills.

The intervention has been tested with both older and younger white, black, and Mexican-American women treated for breast cancer. Two studies have focused on testing the intervention with white and black men with either localized or recurrent and advanced prostate cancer. Although the outcomes differ in some ways across the studies, the Uncertainty Management Intervention helps cancer patients problem solve, reevaluate their situation as manageable, gain cancer knowledge, improve patient-provider communication, and improve management of treatment side effects.

The research career I have described contains the components of conceptualization, measurement, theory development, descriptive qualitative and quantitative studies, and development and testing of a theory-based intervention. The plans now are to continue publishing the findings from the intervention studies and to disseminate the intervention into clinical practice.

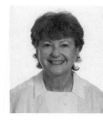

Merle H. Mishel PhD, RN, FAAN
Kenan Professor of Nursing,
School of Nursing,
University of North Carolina at
 Chapel Hill,
Chapel Hill, NC

MARITA G. TITLER*

Use of Research in Practice

20

Key Terms

conduct of research
diffusion
dissemination
evidence-based guidelines

evidence-based practice
integrative research review
knowledge-focused triggers
problem-focused triggers

research-based practice
research-based protocols
research utilization

Learning Outcomes

After reading this chapter, the student should be able to do the following:

- Differentiate among conduct of nursing research, research utilization, and evidence-based practice.
- Cite examples of evidence-based practices (EBPs) that have improved quality of care and contained costs.
- Identify examples of evidence-based practice models.
- List key steps when undertaking evidence-based practice.
- Identify three barriers to evidence-based practice and strategies to address each.
- Use research findings and other forms of evidence to improve the quality of care.

*The author would like to acknowledge Kim Jordan for her superb assistance in preparing this manuscript for publication.

The conduct of research is of little value unless findings are used in practice to improve patient care. Contributions of nursing to improve patient outcomes can be optimized by the use of evidence-based practice (EBP) guidelines and research-based nursing treatments. Several studies have demonstrated that use of research-based interventions is more likely to result in better outcomes than ritual-based nursing care (Heater, Becker, and Olson, 1988; Titler et al, 1992). Incorporation of research findings and other forms of evidence into practice, however, is a difficult and challenging process. Experts note that, in many ways, EBP presents more challenges to overcome than does the conduct of research (Prevost, 1994; Stetler et al, 1998a). Influencing behavior of multiple caregivers to let go of ritual-based practices is not an easy task (Titler, 1997). The benefits of EBP for nurses and patients, however, make the challenges worthwhile. This chapter presents an overview of EBP and research utilization and the relationship to conduct and dissemination of research, describes the steps of EBP, and sets forth future directions for EBP including a Center of EBP and Translational Research.

OVERVIEW OF EVIDENCE-BASED PRACTICE AND RESEARCH UTILIZATION

Research utilization began with Florence Nightingale who used data to change practices that contributed to high mortality rates in hospitals and communities (Nightingale, 1858,1859,1863a, 1863b). In the early 1900s, however, few nurses built on the solid foundation of research utilization exemplified by Nightingale. Separation of conduct and use of research is rooted in the 1930s and 1940s, a period in nursing when there were few educationally qualified nurse researchers, most nursing research was done by nonnurses, and hospitals were used as the primary setting for nursing education. During the mid-1900s, nurses were being prepared as researchers in fields other than nursing and most research focused on nurses rather than patients (Titler, 1993). Today more nurses are being prepared

as researchers in nursing, and the scientific body of nursing knowledge is growing. It is now every nurse's responsibility to facilitate the use of that knowledge in practice.

In the 1970s, 1980s, and early 1990s, as nursing science became available to guide practice, research utilization was advanced by demonstration projects and programs such as the Conduct and Utilization of Research in Nursing (CURN) project (Horsley et al, 1983), the Western Interstate Commission for Higher Education in Nursing (WICHEN) regional program on nursing research development (Kreuger, 1978; Kreuger, Nelson, and Wolanin, 1978; Lindeman and Krueger, 1977), the Nursing Child Assessment Satellite Training project (NCAST) (King, Barnard, and Hoehn, 1981), the Moving New Knowledge into Practice Project (Cronenwett, 1995; Funk, Tornquist, and Champagne, 1989), and the Orange County Research Utilization in Nursing Project (Rutledge and Donaldson, 1995). From these works (Table 20-1), **research utilization** became known as a process of using research findings to improve patient care. It encompasses dissemination of scientific knowledge; critique of studies; synthesis of research findings; determining applicability of findings for practice; developing a **research-based practice** standard or guideline; implementing the standard; and evaluating the practice change with respect to staff, patients, and cost/resource utilization (Stetler et al, 1995; Titler et al, 1994a). In comparison to research utilization, the **conduct of research** is the analysis of data collected from a homogenous group of subjects who meet study inclusion and exclusion criteria for the purpose of answering specific research questions or testing specified hypotheses. Research design, methods, and statistical analyses are guided by the state of the science in the area of investigation. Traditionally, conduct of research has included **dissemination** of findings via research reports in journals and at scientific conferences. Research utilization begins when nurses are exposed to this new knowledge. The relationships among conduct, dissemination, and utilization of research are illustrated in Figure 20-1.

Parallel to nursing's work in research utilization, physicians have focused on evidence-based

TABLE **20-1** Demonstration Project and Studies in Research Utilization

PROJECT	DESCRIPTION	RESULTS
WICHEN Regional Program on Nursing Research Development (Kreuger, 1978; Kreuger et al, 1978; Lindeman and Kreuger, 1977).	• This project used the linker model and series of workshops for pairs of clinical nurses and researchers from academia to learn methods of planned change and research utilization. • Participants were challenged to implement changes in patient care based on research. • Finding studies that addressed the identified clinical problems was a challenge.	• Linker model published reports of projects (Axford and Cutchen, 1977; Dracup and Breu, 1978) • Education of clinicians and educators
• Conduct and Utilization of Research in Nursing (CURN). • Directed by the Michigan Nurses Association.	• This project focused on the development of research-based protocols for practice. • Implementation occurred in acute care hospitals.	• Ten research-based clinical protocols • Guide that describes, from an organizational perspective, how to advance nursing practice via research utilization • Increased use of research findings in experimental sites
• Nursing Child Assessment Satellite Training (NCAST) project (King et al, 1981).	• NCAST was a three-phase, 10-year project. • Phase I focused on testing use of a communication satellite for disseminating research results focused on health assessment techniques for children. • Phase II focused on adding videotaped parent-child interactions and written materials. • Phase III focused on teaching public health nurses use of research-based health assessment practices in follow-up care of preterm infants and their families.	• Improved health assessment practices • Improved follow-up care of preterm infants • Research-based health assessment practice guide for infants and children
• Moving New Knowledge into Practice (Funk et al, 1989, 1991a, 1991b, 1995a, 1995b).	• This project involved a series of five national conferences each with a specific theme (e.g., chronic illness) that brought together nurse scientists and clinicians. • The foci of conferences were to examine the state of the science, share the latest research findings, and discuss implications for practice.	• Five conference monograph texts • Barriers to research utilization scale • Description of barriers to using research in practice
• Orange County Research Utilization in Nursing Project (Rutledge and Donaldson, 1995).	• This project created a regional network of 20 hospitals and home health nursing service organizations (NSOs) and 6 schools of nursing. • Its purpose was to provide research utilization networking and continuing education to RNs employed by participating NSOs, and to promote a strategic commitment of NSOs to research-based practice.	• Completion of at least one RU project by each NSO • Use of AHCPR guidelines • Use of a more scientific approach with clinical data
• Retrieval and application of research in nursing.	• Stanford University Hospital provides hospital-based computer terminals linked to the internet for access to national databases and retrieval of key studies applicable to practice.	• Staff use of computers to access scientific information for practice

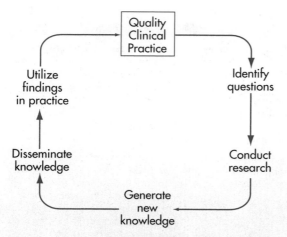

Figure 20-1   The model of the relationship among conduct, dissemination, and use of research. (Redrawn from Weiler K, Buckwalter K, and Titler M: Debate: is nursing research used in practice? In McCloskey J and Grace H, editors: *Current issues in nursing,* ed 4, St Louis, 1994 Mosby.)

medicine (EBM) to promote synthesis and use of research findings from randomized clinical trials (Long and Harrison, 1996; Mion, 1998; Rochon, Dikinson, and Gordon, 1997). EBM has been defined by some experts as the synthesis and use of scientific findings from randomized clinical trials only (Dickersin and Manheimer, 1998; Estabrooks, 1998; Geyman, 1998; Long and Harrison, 1996; Mion, 1998), while others define EBM more broadly to include use of empirical evidence from other scientific methods (e.g., descriptive studies) and use of information from case reports and expert opinion (Cook, 1998; Sackett et al, 1996). Sackett and colleagues (2000) define EBM as "the integration of best research evidence with clinical expertise and patient values."

The term *evidence-based practice* in nursing has become widely adopted in recent years by the nursing profession (Estabrooks, 1998). The terms *research utilization* and *evidence-based practice* are sometimes used interchangeably (Titler et al, 1999a). Although these two terms are related, they are not "one and the same" (Titler et al, 1999a). Adopting the definition of EBP as the conscience and judicious use of the current "best" evidence in

the care of patients and delivery of health care services, research utilization is a subset of EBP that focuses on the application of research findings. **Evidence-based practice** is a broader term that not only encompasses research utilization but also includes use of case reports and expert opinion in deciding the practices to be used in health care. When enough research evidence is available, it is recommended that the evidence base for practice be based on the research. In some cases, a sufficient research base may not be available, and the health care provider may need to supplement research findings with other types of evidence such as expert opinion and case reports when developing an EBP guideline. As more research is done in a specific area, the research evidence can be used to update and refine the guideline.

USE OF EVIDENCE IN PRACTICE

Cronenwett (1995) describes two forms of using research evidence in practice: conceptual and decision driven. Conceptual driven forms of using evidence in practice influence the thinking of the health care provider, not necessarily action. Exposure to new scientific knowledge occurs, but the new knowledge may not be used to change or guide practice. An integrative review of the literature, formulation of a new theory, or generating new hypotheses may be the result. Use of knowledge in this way is referred to as knowledge creep or cognitive application. It is often used by individuals who read and incorporate research into their critical thinking (Weiss, 1980). Decision-driven forms of using evidence in practice encompass application of scientific knowledge as part of a new practice, policy, procedure, or intervention. In this type of application of research findings, a critical decision is reached to change or endorse current practice based on review and critique of studies applicable to that practice. Examples of decision-driven models of using research in practice are the Iowa Model of Research Based Practice to Promote Quality Care (Titler et al, 1994b), the Stetler model (Stetler, 1994), and the Conduct and Utilization of Research in Nursing (CURN) project.

EBP can be undertaken from an individual and/or organizational perspective. Specifically, a nurse can read and synthesize research, seek expert opinions of others, read case reports in the literature, and then use the information in his or her practice. In contrast, an organization (e.g., hospital) or health care system (e.g., University of Iowa Health Care) can make an organizational commitment to incorporate research into their agency, resulting in practice policies and procedures that are evidence-based (Goode and Titler, 1996).

MODELS OF EVIDENCE-BASED PRACTICE

Several models of EBP have been explicated recently (Goode and Piedalue, 1999; Rosswurm and Larrabee, 1999; Soukup, 2000; Titler et al, in press), and most are extensions of earlier research utilization models (Barnsteiner, Ford, and Howe, 1995; Goode et al, 1987; Stetler, 1994; Titler et al, 1994b). Although a thorough discussion of these models is beyond the scope of this chapter, three models are presented here as examples.

The Iowa Model of Evidence-Based Practice is an organizational, collaborative model developed by the University of Iowa Hospitals and Clinics and the University of Iowa College of Nursing. The model incorporates conduct of research, use of research evidence, and use of other types of nonresearch evidence (Figure 20-2) (Titler et al, in press). The Iowa Model of Evidence-Based Practice is a revision of the original research utilization model, the Iowa Model of Research-Based Practice to Promote Quality of Care (Titler et al, 1994b). Revisions of the original model were based on feedback from over 100 users of the model nationwide and a review of the literature on EBP. Authors of the revised Iowa model adopted the definition of EBP as the conscientious and judicious use of current best evidence to guide health care decisions (Sackett et al, 1996). Levels of evidence range from randomized clinical trials to case reports and expert opinion. In this model, knowledge- and problem-focused "trigger(s)" lead staff members to question current nursing practice and whether patient care can be improved through the use of research findings. If through the process of literature review and critique of studies, it is found that there is not a sufficient number of scientifically sound studies to use as a base for practice, consideration is given to conducting a study. Nurses in practice collaborate with scientists in nursing and other disciplines to conduct clinical research that addresses practice problems encountered in the care of patients. Findings from such studies are then combined with findings from existing scientific knowledge to develop and implement these practices. If there is insufficient research to guide practice, and conducting a study is not feasible, other types of evidence (e.g., case reports, expert opinion, scientific principles, theory) are used and/or combined with available research evidence to guide practice. Priority is given to projects in which a high proportion of practice is guided by research evidence. Practice guidelines usually reflect research and nonresearch evidence and therefore are called EBP guidelines.

An EBP guideline is developed from the available evidence. The recommended practices, based on the relevant evidence, are compared to current practice, and a decision is made about the necessity for a practice change. If a practice change is warranted, changes are implemented using a process of planned change. The practice is first implemented with a small group of patients, and an evaluation is carried out. The EBP is then refined based on evaluation data, and the change is implemented with additional patient populations for which it is appropriate. Patient/family, staff, and fiscal outcomes are monitored. Organizational and administrative support facilitates the success of using this model.

The Evidence-Based Practice Model from the Center for Advanced Nursing Practice was developed and used by the Bryan LGH Medical Center in Lincoln, Nebraska (Soukup, 2000). It is a dynamic model that includes four interactive phases: evidence-triggered, evidence-supported, evidence-observed, and evidence-based phases. The model is inclusive of all forms of evidence that support practice, including clinician perspectives and external benchmarking.

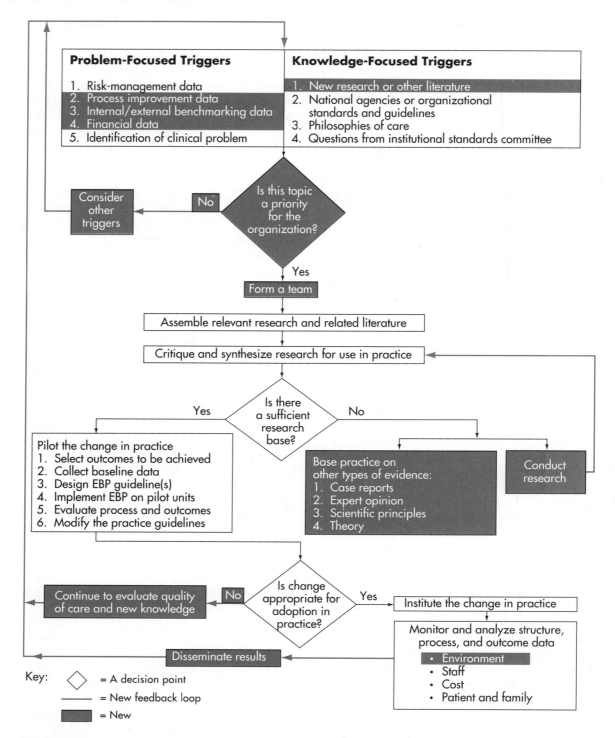

Figure 20-2 The Iowa model of evidence-based practice to promote quality care. (Redrawn from Titler M et al: *Evidence-Based Practice and the Iowa Model of Research-Based Practice to Promote Quality Care* [in press].)

In the evidence-triggered phase, practice and knowledge triggers provide the basis for areas of practice that might benefit from EBP. Practice triggers, similar to the problem-focused triggers of the Iowa model, are clinical questions, practice patterns, or organizational data that suggest opportunities for improvement. Knowledge triggers refer to emergent knowledge related to developments in clinical practice, advances in technology, and program development. The outcome of the evidence-triggered phase is a clear description of the practice area in question and the trigger data used to arrive at this area of practice. For example, if pain management for a specific patient population is the area of focus for the EBP, performance data on pain management practices and the American Pain Society principles (APS, 1999a) for use of analgesics may be among the trigger sources used to identify this area. The evidence-supported phase focuses on review of existing evidence for best practice. Multiple sources are used and include research, authoritative literature, national clinical standards and guidelines, and best practices reported by experts. During the evidence-observed phase of the model, the proposed practice or comprehensive program initiative is designed and implemented. Appropriate methods and measurements are used and may include piloting the change in practice, and/or performing a clinical study, a point prevalence study, product evaluation, or cost/benefit analysis. The evidence-based phase encompasses a critical analysis to determine if the EBP is being used. This phase addresses the critical question, "Has best practice been achieved and based on what evidence?" (Soukup, 2000). The model serves as a catalyst for promoting the scholarship of practice and empowers clinicians to optimize patient outcomes across the continuum of care.

A model for change to EBP was developed and tested by Rosswurm and Larrabee (1999) at the West Virginia University School of Nursing in collaboration with nurses from the Charleston Area Medical Center. The model is derived from theoretical and research literature related to EBP,

research utilization, and change theory. The model guides practitioners through the process of EBP, beginning with assessment of the need for the change and ending with integration of an evidence-based protocol in practice (Figure 20-3). Step 1 of the process is assessing the need for change by examining data from internal agency sources such as customer satisfaction surveys, utilization, risk surveillance, quality improvement monitors, and staff performance. Internal data are then compared with external benchmarking data to determine if there is an opportunity to improve practice and to clearly identify the problem. Step 2 of the model is further defining the problem using a standardized nursing classification system and then linking the problem with standard classifications of interventions and outcomes. For example, a problem of acute confusion in the elderly may be linked with the nursing treatment of Delirium Management from the Nursing Interventions Classification, and with nursing outcomes of Cognitive Orientation and Safety from the Nursing Outcomes Classification. Linking the problem with interventions and outcomes provides some focus for Step 3—synthesis of the best evidence. The problem, potential interventions, and outcomes become the major variables for reviewing the research literature. Practitioners evaluate the strength and weaknesses of the studies, gaps in the science, and conflicts in the available knowledge. The purpose of the synthesis of the studies is to determine whether the strength of the evidence supports a change in practice. Step 4 is designing a change in practice. This step uses the synthesis of the best evidence to describe the sequence of care activities, usually in the form of a protocol, procedure, or standard. Other components of Step 4 are identification of resources needed to change practice, planning the implementation process, and defining outcomes that will be used to measure the effect of the change in practice. Step 5 is implementing and evaluating a change in practice using a pilot study. The decision to adapt, adopt, or reject the change in practice is based on the outcome indicator data, feedback from staff, cost data, and

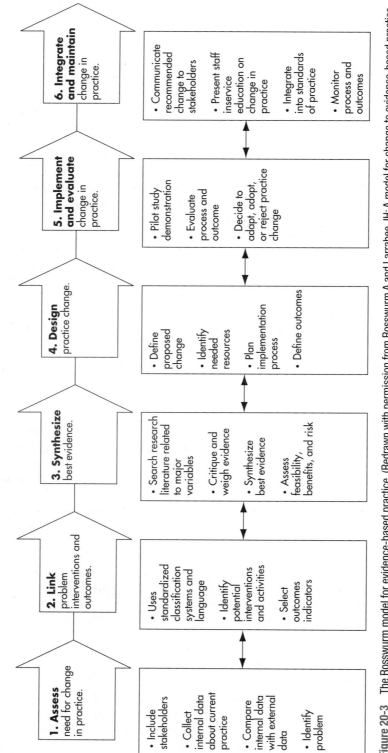

Figure 20-3 The Rosswurm model for evidence-based practice. (Redrawn with permission from Rosswurm A and Larrabee JH: A model for change to evidence-based practice. *Image: J Nurs Schol* 31(4):317-322).

recommendations from key stakeholders. Step 6 is to integrate and maintain the change in practice, depending on the results of the pilot study. This model may be applicable for various health care settings (Rosswurm and Larrabee, 1999).

STEPS OF EVIDENCE-BASED PRACTICE

The Iowa Model of Evidence-Based Practice (see Figure 20-2) serves as the organizing framework for discussing the steps of EBP. A group approach is most helpful in fostering a specific EBP with one person in the group providing the leadership for the project.

SELECTION OF A TOPIC

The first step in carrying out an EBP project is to select a topic. Ideas for EBP come from several sources categorized as problem- and knowledge-focused triggers. **Problem-focused triggers** are those identified by staff through quality improvement, risk surveillance, benchmarking data, financial data, or recurrent clinical problems. An example of a problem-focused trigger is increased incidence of deep venous thrombosis and pulmonary emboli in trauma and neurosurgical patients (Blondin and Titler, 1996; Stenger, 1994). **Knowledge-focused triggers** are ideas generated when staff read research, listen to scientific papers at research conferences, or encounter EBP guidelines published by federal agencies or specialty organizations. Examples initiated from knowledge-focused triggers include pain management, prevention of skin breakdown, assessing placement of nasogastric and nasointestinal tubes, and use of saline to maintain patency of arterial lines. Sometimes topics arise from a combination of problem- and knowledge-focused triggers such as the length of bed rest time after femoral artery catheterization. In selecting a topic, it is essential that nurses consider how the topic fits with organization, department, and unit priorities in order to garner support from leaders within the organization and the necessary resources to successfully complete the project.

BOX 20-1   Selection Criteria for an Evidence-Based Practice Project

1. The priority of this topic for nursing and for the organization
2. The magnitude of the problem (small, medium, large)
3. Applicability to several or few clinical areas
4. Likelihood of the change to improve quality of care, decrease length of stay, contain costs, or improve patient satisfaction
5. Potential "landmines" associated with the topic and capability to diffuse them
6. Availability of baseline quality improvement or risk data that will be helpful during evaluation
7. Multidisciplinary nature of the topic and ability to create collaborative relationships to effect the needed changes
8. Interest and commitment of staff to the potential topic

Individuals should work collectively to achieve consensus in topic selection. Working in groups to review performance improvement data, brainstorm about ideas, and achieve consensus about the final selection is helpful. For example, a unit staff meeting may be used to discuss ideas for EBP, quality improvement committees may identify three to four practice areas in need of attention based on quality improvement data (e.g., urinary tract infections in elderly, restraint reduction, preventing constipation in the elderly), an EBP task force may be appointed to select and address a clinical practice issue (e.g., pain management), or a Delphi survey technique may be used to prioritize areas for EBP. Criteria to consider when selecting a topic are outlined in Box 20-1. Figure 20-4 shows a helpful chart for selecting a topic.

HELPFUL HINT   No matter what method is used to select an EBP topic, it is critical that the staff members who will implement the potential practice changes are involved in selecting the topic and view it as contributing significantly to the quality of care (Cole and Gawlinski, 1995).

Topic ideas	Priority for:		Magnitude of the problem (small = 1; large = 5)	Applicability (narrow =1; broad = 5)	Likelihood to:		
	Nursing (1= low; 5 = high)	Organization (1= low; 5 = high)			Improve quality of care (1= low; 5 = high)	Decrease length of stay/contain costs (1= low; 5 = high)	Improve satisfaction (1= low; 5 = high)
Chest physiotherapy							
Diarrhea in tube-fed patients							
Clogged small-bore feeding tubes							
Treatment of pressure ulcers							

Figure 20-4   Tool to use in selecting a topic for evidence-based practice.

FORMING A TEAM

A team is responsible for development, implementation, and evaluation of the EBP. The team or group may be an existing committee such as the quality improvement committee, the practice council, or the research committee. A task force approach also may be used, in which a group is appointed to address a specific practice issue and use research findings or other evidence to resolve the issue or improve practice. The composition of the team is directed by the topic selected and should include interested stakeholders in the delivery of care. For example, a team working on EB pain management should be interdisciplinary and include pharmacists, nurses, physicians, and psychologists. In contrast, a team working on the EBP of bathing might include a nurse expert in skin care, assistive nursing personnel, and staff nurses.

LITERATURE RETRIEVAL

Once a topic is selected, relevant research and related literature need to be retrieved and should include clinical studies, metaanalyses, integrative literature reviews, and existing EBP guidelines. As more evidence is available to guide practice, professional organizations and federal agencies are developing and making available EBP guidelines (Lang, 1999). It is important that these guidelines are accessed as part of the literature retrieval process. The Agency for Healthcare Research and Quality (AHRQ), formerly the Agency for Health Care Policy and Research, funds 12 Evidence-Based Practice Centers (Box 20-2) that develop evidence reports in selected clinical topics. AHRQ also sponsors a National Guideline Clearinghouse where abstracts of EBP guidelines are set forth on a web site (http://www.guideline.gov). Other professional organizations that have EBP guidelines available are the American Pain Society (http://www.ampainsoc.org); Oncology Nursing Society (http://www.ons.org); the American Association of Critical Care Nurses (http://www.aacn.org); the Association for Women's Health, Obstetrics, and Neonatal Nursing (http://www.

Agency for Healthcare Research and Quality Evidence-Based 20-2 Practice Centers*

1. Blue Cross and Blue Shield Association, Technical Evaluation Center (TEC), Chicago, Illinois
2. Duke University, Durham, NC
3. ECRI, Plymouth Meeting, PA
4. Johns Hopkins University, Baltimore, MD
5. McMaster University, Hamilton, Ontario, Canada
6. MetaWorks, Inc., Boston, MA
7. New England Medical Center, Boston, MA
8. Oregon Health Sciences University, Portland, OR
9. Research Triangle Institute and University of North Carolina at Chapel Hill, NC
10. Southern California Evidence-based Practice Center—RAND, Santa Monica, CA
11. University of California, San Francisco and Stanford University, Stanford, CA
12. University of Texas Health Science Center, San Antonio, TX

*http://www.ahrq.gov

awhonn.org); the Gerontological Nursing Interventions Research Center (http://www.nursing.uiowa.edu/gnirc); and the American Thoracic Society (http://www.thoracic.org).

In addition to using traditional methods of finding published literature (e.g., card catalogs, health indexes), other sources of information include bibliographies of integrative reviews, abstracts published as part of conference proceedings, master's theses and doctoral dissertations, direct written or verbal communication with scientists who are investigating a particular topic but have not yet published the results, and others who may have completed an EB project on the same topic. A number of health care indexes, such as MEDLINE, and the Cumulative Index to Nursing and Allied Health Literature (CINAHL), have electronic databases available to assist with the search process. Current best evidence from specific studies of clinical problems can be found in an increasing number of electronic databases such as the Cochrane Library (http://update.cochrane.co.uk; www.updateusa.com), the Centers for Health Evidence (www.

cche.net), and Best Evidence (www.acponline.com) (Sackett et al, 2000). Another electronic database, Evidence-based Medicine Reviews (EBMR) from Ovid Technologies (http://www.ovid.com) combines several electronic databases including the Cochrane Database of Systematic Reviews, Best Evidence, Evidence-Based Mental Health, Evidence-Based Nursing, Cancerlit, Healthstar, Aidsline, Bioethicsline and MEDLINE, plus links to over 200 full text journals. EBMR links these databases to one another; if a study on a topic of interest is found on MEDLINE and also has been included in a systematic review in the Cochrane Library, then the review also can be readily and easily accessed (Sackett et al, 2000). The On-Line Journal of Knowledge Synthesis for Nursing is also helpful, because each article provides a synthesis of the research and an annotated bibliography for selected references. The Best Practices Network (http://www.best4health.org) disseminates practices from several nursing organizations (see Chapter 4).

In using these sources, it is important to identify key search terms and to use the expertise of health science librarians in locating publications relevant to the project. Further information regarding location of publications is in Chapter 4.

Once the literature is located, it is helpful to classify the articles as clinical (nonresearch), integrative research reviews, theory articles, research articles, and EBP guidelines. Before reading and critiquing the research, it is useful to read theoretical and clinical articles to have a broad view of the nature of the topic and related concepts, and to then review existing EBP guidelines. It is helpful to read articles in the following order:

1. Integrative review articles to understand the state of the science
2. Clinical articles to understand the state of the practice
3. Theory articles to understand the various theoretical perspectives and concepts that may be encountered in critiquing studies
4. EBP guidelines and evidence reports
5. Research articles including metaanalyses

SCHEMAS FOR GRADING THE EVIDENCE

There is no consensus among professional organizations or across health care disciplines in methods used for denoting the type of evidence for a specific practice or the grading schemas to denote the quality of evidence (Brown, 1999; Lohr and Carey, 1999). For example, The Joint ACCP/AACVPR Pulmonary Rehabilitation Guidelines Panel (1997) used an A, B, C rating scale to reflect the quality of the studies, including study designs and the consistency of the results of the scientific evidence: A = scientific evidence provided by well-conducted, controlled trials (randomized and nonrandomized) with statistically significant results that consistently support the recommendation; B = scientific evidence provided by observational studies or by controlled trials with less consistent results; and C = expert opinion because available scientific evidence did not present consistent results or because controlled trials were lacking. In contrast, the AHCPR guideline on cancer pain (1994) used a Roman numeral system to denote the type of evidence (e.g., I = metaanalysis of multiple, well-designed controlled studies, to V = case reports and clinical examples) and a letter grading system to denote the strength and consistency of the evidence (e.g., A = evidence of type I or consistent findings from multiple studies of types II, III, or IV, to D = little or no evidence or type V evidence only). A summary of various rating systems is found in Table 20-2. Findings from qualitative research are noticeably missing in many of these rating systems.

Prior to critiquing research articles, reading relevant literature, and reviewing EBP guidelines, it is imperative that an organization or group responsible for the review agree on the method used for noting the type of research and grading the evidence set forth in practice recommendations (Stetler et al, 1998b). It is also important to decide how the method will be reflected in the guideline. For example, the pulmonary rehabilitation guidelines set forth the practice recommendation and evidence grade, followed by a narrative summary of the research evidence, with reference citations, to support the recommendation: "A program of exercise training of the muscles of ambulation is recommended as a part of pulmonary rehabilitation for patients with COPD. Strength of evidence = A" (ACCP/AACVPR, 1997). In a recently developed guideline for acute pain management in the elderly (Herr et al, 2000), the practice recommendation is followed by the reference citations in APA format and the evidence grade.

CRITIQUE OF EVIDENCE-BASED PRACTICE GUIDELINES

As the number of EBP guidelines proliferate, it becomes increasingly important that nurses critique these guidelines with regard to the methods used for formulating them and consider how they might be used in their institution (Brown, 1999; Cluzeau and Littlejohns, 1999; Cluzeau et al, 1997; Liddle, Williamson, and Irwig, 1996). Critical areas that should be assessed when critiquing EBP guidelines include (1) data of publication or release, (2) authors of the guideline, (3) endorsement of the guideline, (4) a clear purpose of what the guideline covers and patient groups for which it was designed, (5) types of evidence (research, nonresearch) used in formulating the guideline, (6) types of research included in formulating the guideline (e.g., "we considered only randomized and other prospective controlled trials in determining efficacy of therapeutic interventions . . .") (7) a description of the methods used in grading the evidence, (8) search terms and retrieval methods used to acquire research and nonresearch evidence used in the guideline, (9) well-referenced statements regarding practice, (10) comprehensive reference list, (11) review of the guideline by experts, and (12) whether the guideline has been used or tested in practice, and if so, with what types of patients and in what types of settings. **Evidence-based guidelines** that are formulated using rigorous methods provide a useful starting point for nurses to understand the evidence base of certain practices. However, more research may be available since the publication of the guideline and refinements may be needed. Although information in well-developed, national, EB guidelines is a helpful reference, it is usually necessary to localize the guideline using institution-specific EB policies, procedures, or standards before application within a specific setting.

CRITIQUE OF RESEARCH

Critiques of research articles are undertaken next. Integrative review articles such as "Drawing Coagulation Studies from Arterial Lines" (Laxson and Titler, 1994) and "Nasogastric and Nasointestinal Feeding Tube Placement" (Rakel et al, 1994) provide a good foundation for critique of research published subsequent to the integrative review article. The original research, cited in the integrative review, may warrant a critique with a forward look toward application of findings in practice (Pettit and Kraus, 1995).

Critique of each study should use the same methodology, and the critique process should be a shared responsibility. It is helpful, however, to have one individual provide leadership for the project and design strategies for completing critiques. A group approach to critiques is recommended because it distributes the workload, helps those responsible for implementing the changes to understand the scientific base for the change in practice, arms nurses with citations and research-based sound bites to use in effecting practice changes with peers and other disciplines, and provides novices an environment to learn critique and application of research findings. Methods to make the critique process fun and interesting include the following:

- Using a journal club to discuss critiques done by each member of the group
- Pairing a novice and expert to do critiques
- Eliciting assistance from students who may be interested in the topic and want experience doing critiques
- Assigning the critique process to graduate students interested in the topic
- Making a class project of critique and synthesis of research for a given topic

- Several resources available to assist with the critique process include the following:
  Reading Research: A User-Friendly Guide for Nurses and Other Health Professionals (Davies and Logan, 1993)
  Knowledge for Health Care Practice. A Guide to Using Research Evidence (Brown, 1999)
  Evidence-Based Medicine and accompanying compact disc (Sackett et al, 2000)

> **HELPFUL HINT** Keep critique processes simple, and encourage participation by staff members who are providing direct patient care.

SYNTHESIS OF RESEARCH FINDINGS

Once studies are critiqued, a decision is made regarding use of each study in the synthesis of research findings for application in clinical practice. Factors that should be considered for inclusion of studies in the synthesis of findings are overall scientific merit of the study; type (e.g., age, gender, pathology) of subjects enrolled in the study and the similarity to the patient population to which the findings will be applied; and relevance of the study to the topic of question. For example, if the practice area is prevention of deep venous thrombosis in postoperative patients, a descriptive study using a heterogeneous population of medical patients is not appropriate for inclusion in the synthesis of findings.

To synthesize the findings from research critiques, it is helpful to use a summary table (see also summary tables in Chapters 18 and 19), in which critical information from studies can be documented. Essential information to include in such summaries is the following:

- Study purpose
- Research questions/hypotheses
- The variables studied
- A description of the study sample and setting
- The type of research design
- The methods used to measure each variable
- Detailed description of the independent variable/intervention tested
- The study findings

TABLE **20-2** Summary of Evidence-Based Practice Rating Systems

MANAGEMENT OF CANCER PAIN (AHCPR, 1994) AND GUIDELINE FOR THE MANAGEMENT OF ACUTE AND CHRONIC PAIN IN SICKLE-CELL DISEASE (APS, 1999b)	AHCPR PANEL FOR THE PREDICTION AND PREVENTION OF PRESSURE ULCERS IN ADULTS (1992b)	ACCP/AACVPR PULMONARY REHABILITATION GUIDELINE PANEL (1997)	AMERICAN ASSOCIATION OF CRITICAL-CARE NURSES (1998)
TYPE OF EVIDENCE	**STRENGTH OF EVIDENCE**	**STRENGTH OF EVIDENCE**	**STRENGTH OF EVIDENCE**
I. Metaanalysis of multiple well-designed controlled studies	A. Good research-based evidence supports the recommendation	A. Scientific evidence provided by well-designed, well-conducted, controlled trials (randomized and nonrandomized) with statistically significant results that consistently support the guideline recommendation	I. Manufacturer's recommendations only
II. At least one well-designed experimental study	B. Fair research-based evidence supports the recommendation		II. Theory-based, no research data to support recommendations; recommendations from expert consensus group may exist
III. Well-designed, quasiexperimental studies, such as nonrandomized controlled, single-group prepost, cohort, time series, or matched-case controlled studies	C. The recommendation is based on expert opinion and panel consensus	B. Scientific evidence provided by observational studies or by controlled trials with less consistent results to support the guideline recommendation	III. Laboratory data only, no clinical data to support recommendations
IV. Well-designed nonexperimental studies such as comparative and correlational descriptive and case studies		C. Expert opinion that supports the guideline recommendation because the available scientific evidence did not present consistent results or because controlled trials were lacking	IV. Limited clinical studies to support recommendations
V. Case reports and clinical examples			V. Clinical studies in more than one or two different patient populations and situations to support recommendations
STRENGTH AND CONSISTENCY OF EVIDENCE			VI. Clinical studies in a variety of patient populations and situations to support recommendations
A. Evidence of type I or consistent findings from multiple studies of types II, III, or IV			
B. Evidence of types II, III, or IV, and findings are generally consistent			
C. Evidence of types II, III, or IV, but findings are inconsistent			
D. Little or no evidence, or there is type V evidence only			

TABLE **20-2** Summary of Evidence-Based Practice Rating Systems—cont'd

GERONTOLOGICAL NURSING INTERVENTIONS RESEARCH CENTER, RESEARCH DISSEMINATION CORE (1999)	STETLER ET AL (1998a; STETLER ET AL 1998b)	ROSSWURM AND LARRABEE (1999)	U.S. PREVENTATIVE SERVICES TASK FORCE (1996)
STRENGTH AND CONSISTENCY OF GRADING THE EVIDENCE	**STRENGTH OF EVIDENCE**	**QUALITY OF EVIDENCE**	**QUALITY OF EVIDENCE**
A. Evidence from well-designed metaanalysis.	I. Metaanalysis of multiple controlled studies	I. a. Metaanalysis of randomized controlled trials	I. Evidence obtained from at least one properly randomized controlled trial
B. Evidence from well-designed controlled trials, both randomized and nonrandomized, with results that consistently support a specific action (e.g., assessment), intervention, or treatment	II. Individual experimental study	b. One randomized controlled trial	II-1. Evidence obtained from well-designed controlled trials without randomization
	III. Quasiexperimental study such as nonrandomized controlled single group prepost test, time series, or matched case-controlled studies	II. a. One well-designed controlled study without randomization	II-2. Evidence obtained from well-designed cohort or case-control analytic studies preferably from more than one center or research group
C. Evidence from observational studies (e.g., correlational descriptive studies) or controlled trials with inconsistent results	IV. Nonexperimental study, such as correlational descriptive research and qualitative or case studies	b. One other type of well-designed quasiexperimental study	II-3. Evidence obtained from multiple time series with or without the intervention. Dramatic results in uncontrolled experiments (such as the results of the introduction of penicillin treatment in the 1940s) also could be regarded as this type of evidence.
D. Evidence from expert opinion or multiple case reports	V. Case report or systematically obtained, verifiable quality, or program evaluation data	III. Comparative, correlational, and other descriptive studies	III. Opinions of respected authorities, based on clinical experience; descriptive studies and case reports; or reports of expert committees
	VI. Opinions of respected authorities; or the opinions of an expert committee, including their interpretation of nonresearch-based information	IV. Evidence from expert committee reports and expert opinions	

Citation	Purpose and research questions	Research design	Sample	Independent variables and measures	Dependent variables and measures	Statistical tests	Results	Impli-cations	General strengths	General weaknesses	Summary statements for practice

Figure 20-5   Example of a summary table for research critiques.

An example of a summary form is illustrated in Figure 20-5.

HELPFUL HINT Use of a summary form helps identify commonalities across several studies with regard to study findings and the types of patients to which study findings can be applied.

SETTING FORTH EVIDENCE-BASED PRACTICE RECOMMENDATIONS

Based on the critique of EBP guidelines and synthesis of research, recommendations for practice are set forth. The type and strength of evidence used to support the practice needs to be clearly delineated. The following are examples of practice recommendation statements:
- Avoid massage over bony prominences (strength of evidence = B) (AHCPR, 1992b).
- Any individual assessed to be at risk for developing pressure ulcers should be placed when lying in bed on a pressure-reducing device such as foam, alternating air, gel, or water mattresses (strength of evidence = B) (AHCPR, 1992b).

DECISION TO CHANGE PRACTICE

After studies are critiqued and synthesized and EBPs are set forth, the next step is to decide if findings are appropriate for use in practice. Criteria to consider in making these decisions include the following:
- Relevance of research findings for practice
- Consistency in findings across studies
- A significant number of studies with sample characteristics similar to those to which the findings will be used
- Consistency among evidence from research and other nonresearch evidence
- Feasibility for use in practice
- The risk/benefit ratio (risk of harm; potential benefit for the patient)

It is recommended that practice changes be based on several studies with similar findings.

Synthesis of study findings and other evidence may result in supporting current practice, making minor practice modifications, undertaking major practice changes, or developing a new area of practice. For example, a project on gauze versus transparent dressings did not result in a practice change because the studies reviewed substantiated current practice (Pettit and Kraus, 1995). In comparison, a pediatric intravenous (IV) infiltration guideline was developed from a combination of research findings and expert consultation because few studies used pediatric subjects, sample sizes were small, and research results were inconclusive (Montgomery and Budreau, 1996). This project resulted in a new EBP for treatment of IV infiltrations, resulting in a significant reduction in tissue damage.

DEVELOPMENT OF EVIDENCE-BASED PRACTICE

The next step is to put in writing the evidence base of the practice (Haber et al, 1994) using the grading schema that has been agreed upon. When results of the critique and synthesis of evidence support current practice or suggest a change in practice, a written EBP protocol is warranted. A written EBP protocol (e.g., standard; policy; procedure) is necessary so that individuals know (1) that the practices are based on evidence and (2) the type of evidence (e.g., randomized clinical trial, expert opinion) used in developing the protocol. Several different formats can be used to document EBP changes. The format chosen is influenced by what and how the document will be used. Written EBPs should be part of the organizational policy and procedure manual and should include detailed references to the parts of the policy and procedure that are based upon research and non-research evidence.

Clinicians (e.g., nurses, physicians, pharmacists) who adopt EBPs are influenced by the perceived participation they have had in developing and reviewing the protocol (Baker and Feder, 1997; Bauchner and Simpson, 1998; Bero et al, 1998; Shortell et al, 1995; Soumerai et al, 1998; Titler, 1995). It is imperative that once the EBP protocol is written, key stakeholders have an opportunity to review it and provide feedback to the individual(s) responsible for writing it. Use of focus groups is a useful way to provide discussion about the EBP protocol and to identify key areas that may be potentially troublesome during the implementation phase. Key questions that can be used in the focus groups are in Box 20-3.

> **HELPFUL HINT** Use a consistent approach to writing EBP standards and referencing the research and related literature.

BOX 20-3 Key Questions for Focus Groups

1. What is needed by (nurses, physicians) to use the protocol with patients in units (specify unit)?
2. In your opinion, how will this protocol improve patient care in your unit/practice?
3. What modifications would you suggest in the evidence-based protocol before using it in your practice?
4. What content in the protocol is unclear or needs revision?
5. What would you change about the format of the protocol?
6. What part of this protocol/practice change do you view most challenging?
7. Do you have any other suggestions?

IMPLEMENTING THE PRACTICE CHANGE

If a practice change is warranted, the next steps are to make the EB changes in practice. Rogers' seminal work on diffusion of innovations (Rogers, 1995) is extremely useful in facilitating adoption of EBPs. Rogers' model was developed from review of over 4000 studies on innovation adoption and has undergone empirical testing by various disciplines (Camiletti and Huffman, 1998; Carroll et al, 1997; Funk et al, 1995a; Schnelle et al, 1998). According to this model, **diffusion** of an innovation (e.g., an EBP) is influenced by the nature of the innovation and the manner in which it is communicated (communication process) to members (health care providers) of a social system (e.g., acute care hospital, nursing unit) (Rogers, 1995). Strategies for promoting adoption of EBPs must address these four areas within a context of participative, planned change.

Nature of the innovation, in this case the characteristics of the EBP, influence health care providers' use of practices in delivery of patient care. Traditional barriers to use of research evidence to guide practice include (1) conflicting research results, (2) research reports that are difficult for staff to understand, (3) relevant studies not being compiled in one place, and (4) isolation from colleagues knowledgeable about research (Atkins et al, 1998; Carroll et al, 1997; Funk et al, 1995b; Mion, 1998; Wells and Baggs, 1994). Development of EBP guidelines has improved access to research evidence but changing standards, policies, or procedures to be evidence-based does not guarantee that they will be adopted in practice. Developing a positive attitude and a commitment among clinicians to be involved is an important first step. This goes beyond making new knowledge available to staff. It encompasses attitudinal changes in which staff are encouraged to think critically about their current practice and to question if perhaps there is a more scientific approach to a certain aspect of care. Involvement of staff in selecting the EBP topic and helping to determine methods by which research will be reviewed, critiqued, and translated into practice is particularly effective.

EBP standards or guidelines may be lengthy in order to include essential research citations and practice recommendation grades. A number of studies have demonstrated that clinical systems, computer decision support systems, and prompts that support the EBP, such as decision-making algorithms or equianalgesic charts, have a significant positive effect on improving adherence to EBPs (Chambers et al, 1989; Cohen et al, 1982; Hunt et al, 1998; Oxman et al, 1995; Titler et al, 1999a). Computer-based decision support systems can automate physician and nurse reminders and detail the evidence base of practice recommendation in settings that have automated medical records (Schneider and Eisenberg, 1998; Soumerai and Avorn, 1990). Other settings may rely on written practice prompts or quick reference guides. To move evidence from the "book to the bedside," information from EB guidelines, policies, procedures, or standards must be integrated into daily patient care processes, and information must be readily available and observable for practitioners. Those responsible for implementing the EBP standard need to consider use of practice prompts, decision support systems, and quick reference guides as part of the implementation process. An example of a quick reference guide is shown in Table 20-3.

Methods of communicating the EBP standard to those delivering care affects adoption of the practice (Carroll et al, 1997; Funk et al, 1995b;

Rogers, 1995; Wells and Baggs, 1994). Education of staff, use of opinion leaders, change champions, core groups, and consultation by experts in the content area (e.g., advanced practice nurse) are essential components of the implementation process. Interactive and didactic education used in combination with other practice-reinforcing strategies have a more positive effect in changing behavior than educational sessions alone (Bero et al, 1998; Bookbinder et al, 1996; Oxman et al, 1995; Schneider and Eisenberg, 1998).

It is important that staff know the scientific basis for the changes in practice, and improvements in quality of care anticipated by the change. Disseminating this information to staff needs to be done creatively using various educational strategies. A staff in-service may not be the most effective method nor reach the majority of the staff. Although it is unrealistic for all staff to have participated in the critique process or to have read all studies used to develop the EBP, it is important that they know the myths and realities of the practice. Education of staff also must include ensuring that they are competent in the skills necessary to carry out the new practice. For example, if using pH to check placement of nasogastric and nasointestinal tubes is to be used rather than auscultation, staff knowledge and skill to obtain aspirate from small-bore feeding tubes is essential (Rakel et al, 1994).

One method of communicating information to staff is through use of colorful posters that identify myths and realities or describe the essence of the change in practice (Titler et al, 1994a). Visibly identifying those who have learned the information and are using the EBP (e.g., buttons, ribbons, pins) stimulates interest in others who may not have internalized the change. As a result, the "new" learner may begin asking questions about the practice and be more open to learning the EBP. Other educational strategies such as train-the-trainer programs, computer-assisted instruction, and competency testing are helpful in education of staff.

Several studies have demonstrated that opinion leaders are effective in changing behaviors of health care practitioners (Bero et al, 1998; Oxman

TABLE **20-3**   Using Nonpharmacological Treatment for Managing Acute Pain in the Elderly

GENERAL PRINCIPLES:

- Offer nonpharmacological strategies to complement, not replace, pharmacological treatments.
- Selection of nonpharmacological interventions should be based on the older adult's cognitive and functional abilities and on his/her level of pain.
- Encourage use of constructive pain-coping strategies that have been successful in managing prior episodes of pain.
- Promote patient choice in the selection of nonpharmacological treatments.

NONPHARMACOLOGICAL INTERVENTIONS FOR MILD, MODERATE, AND SEVERE PAIN		
MILD PAIN (0-3)	MODERATE PAIN (4-6)	SEVERE PAIN (7-10)
Breathing	Breathing	Breathing
Distraction	Distraction	Environmental modification
Environmental modification	Environmental modification	Heat/cold application
Heat/cold application	Heat/cold application	Positioning/repositioning
Music	Music	
Positioning/repositioning	Positioning/repositioning	
Relaxation and imagery	Relaxation and imagery	
Spiritual practices	Spiritual practices	
Superficial massage	Superficial massage	
	TENS[1]	

NONPHARMACOLOGICAL TREATMENTS FOR ACUTE PAIN MANAGEMENT IN THE ELDERLY	
TREATMENT	BRIEF DESCRIPTION OF TREATMENT
Breathing	Slow, deep breathing can benefit patients who are tense and in pain. • The patient should be instructed to take a deep breath and let it out slowly. • Rhythmic breathing can be combined with peaceful imagery.
Distraction	Can include a variety of actions: • Talking with others • Watching TV • Reading • Singing • Humor
Environmental Modification	Can include a variety of interventions: • Decreasing noise • Providing planned blocks of time for undisturbed rest • Decreasing lights
Cold/Heat Application	Application of cold or heat might require a physician order. Be cautious to prevent skin injury in the elderly. • Cold or heat can be applied to the site of pain or to a site proximal, distal or contralateral to the pain. • Cold or heat usually is applied for 20-30 minutes; the minimal effective time is 5-10 minutes. • Cold can be applied via waterproof bags, terry cloth dipped in ice water, gel packs or homemade cold packs (e.g., frozen peas). • Cold is preferred to heat in the presence of acute trauma, but patients may be reluctant to use it. • Cold usually works better than heat because it relieves pain faster, it relieves more pain, and pain relief lasts longer after cold is removed. • Heat can be applied via hot packs, immersion in water, or retention of body heat using plastic wrap.

[1]Although TENS is effective for both mild and moderate pain, the cost of the treatment decreases its appropriateness for mild pain.

Continued

TABLE **20-3** Using Nonpharmacological Treatment for Managing Acute Pain in the Elderly—cont'd

NONPHARMACOLOGICAL TREATMENTS FOR ACUTE PAIN MANAGEMENT IN THE ELDERLY—cont'd	
TREATMENT—cont'd	BRIEF DESCRIPTION OF TREATMENT—cont'd
Music	Music is related to release of endorphins in the brain and provides distraction. • Can be used to decrease pain intensity and to enhance sleep. • When used therapeutically, music provides psychological support. • Patient preference regarding music should be respected.
Positioning/ Repositioning	Involves maintaining anatomically correct position in a manner that enhances comfort and minimizes pain or further injury. • When patients are on their backs, elevating the legs with pillows has been related to decreased reports of pain in older adults with hip fractures. • When patients are side-lying, placing a pillow between the legs prevents adduction of the hips and improves comfort.
Relaxation and Imagery	*Patient instructions for jaw relaxation technique:* 1. Let your lower jaw drop slightly, as though you were starting a small yawn. 2. Keep your tongue quiet and resting in the bottom of your mouth. 3. Let your lips get soft. 4. Breathe slowly and rhythmically with a three-rhythm pattern of inhale, exhale, rest. 5. Allow yourself to stop forming words; do not even think words. *Guided imagery* • Imagery can be used to ease anxiety, promote relaxation, and decrease pain. • Guided imagery tapes are an excellent alternative for one-to-one instruction.
Spiritual Practices	May include the following activities: • Prayer • Meditation • Visit time with clergy
Superficial Massage	Decreases pain mainly by relaxing muscles. • Most common sites are the back and shoulders. • Hands and feet also may be massaged. • Vibration can have a soothing effect similar to massage and can provide numbing of an area that is stimulated for extended periods.
TENS (Transcutaneous Electrical Nerve Stimulation)	TENS may relieve pain by stimulating endorphin levels, by activating a complex neural inhibitory system, or by stimulating large diameter sensory neurons. • TENS must be prescribed by a physician. • The success rate of TENS varies and is strongly dependent upon the skill of the person administering it. • Almost any pain that is reasonably well-localized may respond to TENS.

et al, 1995; Soumerai et al, 1998). Opinion leaders are from the local health care setting and are viewed as an important and respected source of influence amongst their peer group. The key characteristic of an opinion leader is that he or she is trusted to evaluate new information in the context of group norms. To do this, an opinion leader must be considered by associates as technically competent and a full and dedicated mem-

ber of the local group (Oxman et al, 1995; Soumerai et al, 1998). Opinion leaders influence behavior of their peer group by role modeling the new practice, peer influence, and altering group norms (Goodpastor and Montoya, 1996). If the EBP change that is being implemented is interdisciplinary in nature (e.g., pain management), it is recommended that an opinion leader be selected for each discipline (nursing, medicine, pharmacy). Role expectations of an opinion leader are in Box 20-4.

Use of change champions is another useful strategy for implementing EBP changes (Backer, 1987,1995; Rogers, 1995; Shively et al, 1997; Titler and Mentes, 1999b; Titler et al, 1994a). Change champions are practitioners within a group who continually promote adoption of the changes. The change champion believes in an idea; will not take "no" for an answer; is undaunted by insults and rebuffs; and above all, persists (Greer, 1988). The following characteristics describe successful change champions:

1. Expert clinicians
2. Viewed as informal leaders by their peers
3. Have positive working relationship with other nurses and health professionals
4. Are passionate about the topic of the practice change
5. Are committed to providing quality patient care

Change champions circulate information, encourage peers to align their practice with the evidence, convene committees, and orient new personnel to the idea. For potential research-based changes in practice to reach the bedside, it is imperative that one or two "change champions" be identified for each patient care unit or service where the change is being made (Scott and Rantz, 1994). Staff nurses are some of the best change champions for EBP.

Using a "core group" in conjunction with change champions is another helpful strategy for implementing the practice change (Barnason et al, 1998; Schmidt et al, 1996; Titler et al, 1994a). A core group is a select group of practitioners with the mutual goal of disseminating information regarding a practice change and facilitating the change in practice by other staff in their unit or peer group. Success of the core group approach requires that core group members work well with the change champion and represent various shifts, days of the week, and tenure in the practice setting. Core group members become knowledgeable about the scientific basis for the practice, assist with disseminating the EB information to other staff, and reinforce the practice change on a daily basis. The

BOX 20-4   Role Expectations of an Opinion Leader*

1. Be/become an expert in the evidence-based practice.
2. Provide organizational/unit leadership for adopting the evidence-based practice.
3. Implement various strategies to educate peers about the evidence-based practice.
4. Work with peers, other disciplines, and leadership staff to incorporate key information about the evidence-based practice into organizational/unit standards, policies, procedures, and documentation systems.
5. Promote initial and ongoing use of the evidence-based practice by peers.

*From AHRQ funded study on acute pain management in the elderly (Titler PI; 5 RO1 HS10482).

change champion educates the core group members and assists them in changing their practices. Each member of the core group, in turn, takes the responsibility for effecting the change in two to three of their peers. Core group members provide positive feedback to their assigned staff who are changing their practices and encourage those reluctant to change to try the new practice. Core group members also are able to assist the change champion in identifying the best way to teach staff about the practice change and to proactively solve issues that arise (Titler et al, 1994a). Using a core group approach in conjunction with a change champion results in a critical mass of practitioners promoting adoption of the EBP.

Outreach and consultation by an expert in the practice has been shown to promote positive changes in practice behaviors of nurses and physicians (Hendryx et al, 1998). Advanced practice nurses (APNs) can provide one-on-one consultation to staff regarding use of the EBP with specific patients, assist staff in troubleshooting issues in application of the practice, and provide feedback on provider performance regarding use of the EBPs. Studies have demonstrated that use of APNs as facilitators of change promote adherence to the EBP (Bauchner and Simpson, 1998; Hendryx et al, 1998).

Members of a social system influence how quickly and widely EBPs are adopted. Staff nurses and other health care providers within an organization may become barriers to using research in practice if they perceive that the aspect of care is not important, do not understand the reasons for the practice change, do not perceive that they have the authority to make practice changes, or feel powerless in effecting change in their clinical setting (Funk et al, 1995b). Audit and feedback of performance data, performance gap assessment, and trying the EBP changes are strategies that promote adoption of EBPs (Berwick and Coltin, 1986; Eisenberg, 1986; Lomas et al, 1991; Rogers, 1995; Titler et al, 1994b).

Performance gap assessment is baseline evaluation of the practices that are being changed and providing this information to health care providers when initiating implementation. Specific practice indicators selected for performance gap assessment are related to the practices that are the focus of change such as documentation of pain intensity for acute pain management.

Monitoring of critical performance indicators and feedback to staff (audit and feedback) is an important strategy to use throughout the implementation process in order for staff to be aware of improvements in practices and patient outcomes. Audit and feedback should be done at regular intervals throughout the implementation process (e.g., every 2 to 4 weeks).

Users of an innovation usually try it for a period of time before adopting it in their practice (Meyer and Goes, 1988; Rogers, 1995). When "trying an EBP" (piloting the change) is incorporated as part of the implementation process, users have an opportunity to use it for a period of time, provide feedback to those in charge of implementation, and modify the practice if necessary. Piloting the EBP as part of implementation has a positive influence on the extent of adoption of the new practice (Rogers, 1995; Shively et al, 1997; Titler et al, 1994b).

The social system in which an EBP is implemented has a high degree of influence on adoption of the practice (Rogers, 1995). Leadership support, at both the upper and middle levels, is essential for adoption of EBPs (Backer, 1995; Katz, 1999; Maxwell, 1995; Shortell et al, 1995; Stetler et al, 1998a; Stetler et al, 1998b). Such support is expressed verbally but must also include provision of financial support to purchase educational materials and time for staff to participate in committee meetings and fulfill assigned responsibilities.

The role of the nurse manager is critical in making EBP changes a reality for staff at the bedside. Nurse managers must expect that staff will participate in EBP activities, role model the change in their practice, and provide written and verbal support for the practice change. When selecting a potential topic, it is important that the nurse manager values the idea and supports the potential changes.

APNs are critical to helping staff retrieve and critique the studies and other evidence on the selected topic. Although staff nurses are often willing to participate, the APN provides significant leadership in the process by facilitating synthesis of the research and other evidence, critically analyzing what practices should be changed, assisting staff to communicate these changes to their peers, and role modeling the changes in his or her practice.

As part of the work of implementing the change, it is important that the social system—unit, service line, and clinic—ensure that policies, procedures, standards, clinical pathways, and documentation systems support the use of the EBPs. Documentation forms or clinical information systems may need revision to support changes in practice; use of documentation systems that fail to readily support the new practice thwarts change. For example, if staff members are expected to reassess and document pain intensity within 30 minutes following administration of an analgesic agent, then documentation forms must reflect this practice standard. It is the role of upper and middle level leadership to ensure that organizational documents and systems are flexible and supportive of the EBPs.

In summary, making an EB change in practice involves a planned change process incorporating:
- Unfreezing old behaviors or attitudes
- Adopting new behaviors or practices
- Refreezing or integrating the change into the work role of the unit or practice setting

BOX **20-5**   Steps of Evaluation for Evidence-Based Projects

1. Identify process and outcome variables of interest.
Example: Process variable—Patients >65 years of age will have a Braden scale completed upon admission
Outcome variable—Presence/absence of nosocomial pressure ulcer; if present—stage I, II, III, IV
2. Determine methods and frequency of data collection.
Example: Process variable—Chart audit of all patients >65 years old, 1 day a month
Outcome variable—Patient assessment of all patients >65 years old, 1 day a month
3. Determine baseline and follow-up sample sizes.

4. Design data-collection forms.
Example: Process chart audit abstraction form
Outcome variable—pressure ulcer assessment form
5. Establish content validity of data-collection forms.
6. Train data collectors.
7. Assess interrater reliability of data collectors.
8. Collect data at specified intervals.
9. Provide "on-sight" feedback to staff regarding the progress in achieving the practice change.
10. Assist feedback of analyzed data to staff.
11. Use data to assist staff in modifying or integrating the evidence-based practice change.

Implementing the change will take several weeks to months, depending on the nature of the practice change. It is important that those leading the project are aware of change as a process and continue to encourage and teach peers about the change in practice. The new practice must be continually reinforced and sustained or the practice change will be intermittent and soon fade, allowing more traditional methods of care to return.

EVALUATION

Evaluation provides an opportunity to collect and analyze data with regard to use of a new EBP and then to modify the practice as necessary. It is important that the EB change is evaluated, both on the pilot area and when the practice is changed in additional patient care areas. The importance of the evaluation cannot be overemphasized; it provides information for performance gap assessment, audit and feedback, and provides information necessary to determine if the EBP should be retained, modified, or eliminated.

A desired outcome achieved in a more controlled environment, when a researcher is implementing a study protocol to a homogeneous group of patients (conduct of research), may not result in the same outcome when the practice is implemented in the natural clinical setting, by several caregivers, to a more heterogeneous patient population. Steps of the evaluation process are summarized in Box 20-5.

Evaluation should include both process and outcome measures (Goode, 1995; Lepper and Titler, 1999; Rosswurm and Larrabee, 1999). The process component focuses on how the EBP change is being implemented. It is important to know if staff are using the practice in care delivery and if they are implementing the practice as noted in the written EBP standard. Evaluation of the process also should note (1) barriers that staff encounter in carrying out the practice (e.g., lack of information, skills, or necessary equipment), (2) differences in opinions among health care providers, and (3) difficulty in carrying out the steps of the practice as originally designed (e.g., shutting off tube feedings 1 hour before aspirating contents for checking placement of nasointestinal tubes). Process data can be collected from staff and/or patient self-reports, medical record audits, or observation of clinical practice. Examples of process and outcome questions are shown in Table 20-4.

Outcome data are an equally important part of evaluation. The purpose of outcome evaluation is to assess whether the patient, staff, and/or fiscal outcomes expected are achieved. Therefore it is important that baseline data be used for a pre/post comparison. The outcome variables measured should be those that are projected to change as a result of changing practice (Goode, 1995; Rosswurm and Larrabee, 1999; Soukup, 2000). For example, research demonstrates that less restricted family

TABLE **20-4** Examples of Evaluation Measures

EXAMPLE PROCESS QUESTIONS					
NURSES' SELF-RATING	SD	D	NA/D	A	SA
1. I feel well prepared to use the Braden Scale with older patients.	1	2	3	4	5
2. Malnutrition increases patient risk for pressure ulcer development.	1	2	3	4	5
EXAMPLE OUTCOME QUESTION					
PATIENT					
1. On a scale of 0 (no pain) to 10 (worst possible pain), how much pain have you experienced over the past 24 hours? _____ (pain intensity)					

SD, Strongly disagree; *D*, disagree; *NA/D*, neither agree nor disagree; *A*, agree; *SA*, strongly agree.

visiting practices in critical care units result in improved satisfaction with care. Thus patient and family member satisfaction should be an outcome measure that is evaluated as part of changing visiting practices in adult critical care units. Outcome measures should be measured before the change in practice is implemented, after implementation, and every 6 to 12 months thereafter. Findings must be provided to clinicians to reinforce the impact of the change in practice and to ensure that they are incorporated into quality improvement programs. For example, an organizational task force to institute EBPs for pain management included members from the Department of Nursing Quality Improvement Committee. Data collection focused on adequacy of pain control and patient satisfaction with pain management. Representatives from divisional quality improvement committees were responsible for collecting data from at least 20 patients per unit or clinical area. Results of the quality improvement monitor were distributed to each nursing unit, and staff were encouraged to use this information in identifying ways to improve pain management practices (Schmidt, Alpen, and Rakel, 1996).

When collecting process and outcome data for evaluation of EBP change, it is important that the data-collection tools are user-friendly, short, concise, easy to complete, and have content validity. Focus must be on collecting the most essential data. Those responsible for collecting evaluative data must be trained on the methods of data collection and be assessed for interrater reliability (see Chapter 14). It is our experience that those in-

dividuals who have participated in implementing the protocol can be very helpful in evaluation by collecting data, providing timely feedback to staff, and assisting staff to overcome barriers encountered when implementing the changes in practice.

One question that often arises is how much data are needed to evaluate this change. The preferred number of patients *(N)* is somewhat dependent on the size of the patient population affected by the practice change. For example, if the practice change is for families of critically ill adult patients and the organization has 1000 adult critical care patients annually, then 50 to 100 satisfaction responses preimplementation, and 25 to 50 responses postimplementation, at 3 and 6 months should be adequate to look for trends in satisfaction and possible areas that need to be addressed in continuing this practice (e.g., more bedside chairs in patient rooms). The rule of thumb is to keep the evaluation simple, because data often are collected by busy clinicians who may lose interest if the data collection, analysis, and feedback are too long and tedious.

The evaluation process should include planned feedback to staff who are making the change. The feedback needs to include verbal and/or written appreciation for the work and visual demonstration of progress in implementation and improvement in patient outcomes. The key to effective evaluation is to ensure that the EB change in practice is warranted (e.g., will improve quality of care) and that the intervention does not bring harm to patients (Goode, 1995;

BOX

Use of Saline to Flush Peripheral Intravenous Devices: Cost and Quality

20-6

- Use of saline flush is an effective method for maintaining patency, decreasing incidence of phlebitis, and increasing duration of peripheral IV catheter placement.
- By using saline flush rather than heparin for peripheral IV catheters, risks related to heparin use are reduced.
- Use of saline flush saves $20,000 to $40,000 per hospital per year.
- Patients report that saline does not burn as much as heparin flush.
- Use of saline flush for peripheral intermittent infusion devices improves quality of care and contains cost (Goode et al, 1991, 1993).

Lepper and Titler, 1999). For example, when instituting a research-based protocol for using saline flush rather than heparin flush for peripheral intravenous locks (Box 20-6), it was important to inform staff that the use of saline did not result in increased loss of patency, saved the organization $38,000 annually, and resulted in fewer complaints of pain and burning while flushing the lock (Goode et al, 1991, 1993).

HELPFUL HINT Include patient outcome measures (e.g., pressure ulcer prevalence) and cost (e.g., cost savings, cost avoidance) in evaluation.

CREATING A CULTURE OF EVIDENCE-BASED PRACTICE

Creating a culture of EBP in health care agencies requires an organizational commitment and commitment of nurses employed in the setting. This is an interactive process because the expectations of the organization are a reflection of the individuals employed in the setting (Stonestreet and Lamb-Havard, 1994; Van Mullem et al, 1999).

For EBP to be a reality in health care, organizations must make a commitment to provide an infrastructure to support it (Horsley, Crane, and Bingle, 1978; Stetler et al, 1998a). Three essential ingredients of this infrastructure are (1) access to

information, (2) access to individuals who have skills necessary for EBP, and (3) verbal and written commitment to EBP, particularly the use of research evidence, as part of the organization's operations in provision of patient care. EBPs improve patient outcomes, contain costs, and assist in meeting requirements of the Joint Commission on Accreditation of Healthcare Organizations (JCAHO) (Anders et al, 1997; Cook, 1998; Titler et al, 1994b; Titler et al, 1999a).

INFORMATION

Access to information includes computer access to research publications, evidence papers, EB guidelines, and quality data for evaluating practice. Use of research list servers and computerized literature databases are two examples of increasing access by nurses to research information. Journals that emphasize reporting research in a manner that facilitates use in practice are available. These include *Applied Nursing Research, Clinical Nursing Research,* and specialty journals such as the *American Journal of Critical Care.* Research columns also are printed in many clinical journals and provide a starting point for EBP. The *Annual Review of Nursing Research* publishes **integrative research reviews** that are helpful in understanding the state of the science in an area and the components of the science that may be ready for practice. A growing number of journals summarize the best evidence, using explicit criteria for scientific merit (Sackett et al, 2000). They provide structured abstracts of the best studies, and expert commentaries regarding the context of the studies and clinical applicability of the findings. These journals include: *Evidence-Based Medicine; Evidence-Based Mental Health; Evidence-Based Nursing; Evidence-Based Health Care Policy and Practice;* and *Evidence-Based Cardiovascular Medicine.*

We need to make better use of the electronic superhighway to access and share research-based information and to minimize current duplicative efforts of critiquing and synthesizing research (Crane, 1995; Cronenwett, 1995). It is essential that staff be taught how to access electronic sources such as the AHRQ National

Guideline Clearinghouse (http://www.guideline.gov) as part of their professional education and development (see Chapter 4).

HUMAN RESOURCES

Access to people with expertise in critique and synthesis of research and translating research findings into practice is also important. Such experts can be employed within the organization, shared with a nearby collegiate setting, or contracted on an as-needed basis. Nurses with master's degrees often have the skill set to lead projects and can seek consultation from doctorally prepared researchers employed outside the organization, when necessary. Masters-prepared nurses are not, however, substitutes for doctorally prepared researchers. Nurse executives should not expect the same type of outcomes as can be achieved with employment of a doctorally prepared clinical nurse researcher who has more extensive research knowledge and skill and who can serve as a consultant to address practice-based research issues (Kirchhoff and Titler, 1994).

ORGANIZATIONAL CLIMATE

An organizational climate conducive to EBP must state, in the mission, philosophy, goals, and organizational performance standards, the value of using research evidence and data-based decision making. The type of research activities that nurse executives can integrate into the practice setting are influenced by the implicit and explicit value statements found in these documents. Nurse executives (NEs) set the climate for nursing practice, and if they are not supportive of EBP, particularly application of research evidence, EBP is not likely to occur. Thus NEs have a responsibility to influence the nature of the organizational documents to encompass value statements regarding research (Kirchhoff and Titler, 1994).

Incorporation of behaviors about EBP in job descriptions and performance appraisals is an important strategy for facilitating use of research findings in practice. Examples of such behaviors include identifying potential topics for EBP projects, participating in the critique of research, and serving on the EBP committees or work groups.

BOX 20-7 Options for Integrating Research into a Nursing Department

Listed in order from limited enactment to fuller enactment:
1. Research committees
   a. Ad hoc
   b. Standing
2. Consultation
   a. Contractual agreements
   b. Pooled resources of practice agencies to hire consultative services of a nurse scientist
3. Use of existing personnel
   a. Advanced practice nurses
   b. Nurse managers
   c. Education specialist
4. Collaboration
   a. Doctorally prepared advanced practice nurses
   b. Consortium arrangements
   c. Joint appointment
5. Doctorally prepared research scientist
   a. Part-time
   b. Full-time
6. Research department
   a. Budgeted staff positions
   b. Supply budget
   c. Travel budget

Modified from Kirchhoff K and Titler MG: Responsibilities of nurse executives for research in practice. In Spitzer-Layman R, editor: *Nursing management desk reference*, Philadelphia, 1994, WB Saunders.

Such behaviors must be used in performance appraisals of staff.

NEs communicate the value of research by legitimizing research activities. This includes instituting recognition programs for participating in research, encouraging staff to participate in research courses, providing verbal and written feedback to staff who conduct studies or participate in EBP projects, encouraging staff to attend regional and national meetings to present research and EBP projects, and nominating staff for regional and national research awards.

An important responsibility of nurse executives is exploring options for integration of research into practice. Practice-based research can be enacted at various levels using different strategies as outlined in Box 20-7 (Kirchhoff and Titler, 1994).

Individuals within the organization can influence the organizational climate by reading professional journals, questioning tradition-based practices, serving as change champions, and disseminating research-based information to their peers (Van Mullem et al, 1999). For example, a nurse reads a study on accuracy of coagulation profiles drawn from heparinized arterial lines (Laxson and Titler, 1994). She approaches the nurse manager and medical director about this issue, and questions if perhaps this is an area of practice where improvements might occur. Having received the preliminary support of the nurse manager and medical director, she proceeds to discuss this issue with her co-workers and seeks additional studies that have been done on this topic. Finding several studies, she seeks the consultation of an APN to assist with the critique and synthesis of the research findings. The nurse continues to provide leadership in making the practice change and serves as the change champion in her unit. This nurse, by her individual interest in research and commitment to research-based practice, will have a ripple effect on the organization and use of research to improve the quality of care.

Criteria for evaluating the success of integrating EBPs into an organization's culture include a combination of traditional scientific criteria, effect on the organizational climate, and improvements in providing cost-effective quality care (Van Mullem et al, 1999). These criteria are summarized in Box 20-8. EBPs such as use of saline to flush peripheral IV devices in adults and appropriate use of sequential compression devices for prevention of deep vein thrombosis (DVT) have resulted in improved quality of care while containing costs (Stenger, 1994).

FUTURE DIRECTIONS

Use of research across health care systems for improving quality of care is essential. **"What we really want to get at is *not* how many reports have been done, but how many people's lives are being bettered by what has been accomplished. In other words, is it (the science) being used, is it being followed, is it actually being given to pa-**

> **BOX 20-8   Outcomes of Integrating Evidence-Based Practice into Organizational Culture**
>
> **SCIENTIFIC CRITERIA**
>
> 1. The number of evidence-based practice projects
> 2. The number of evidence-based practice publications
> 3. The number of grants submitted and funded in which staff are investigators
>
> **ORGANIZATIONAL CLIMATE CRITERIA**
>
> 1. Number of evidence-based practice protocols used by staff
> 2. Number of staff participating in research and evidence-based practice activities
> 3. Climate of inquiry whereby staff question their practice
> 4. Increased number of professional nurses recruited and retained
> 5. Return of nurses to school for baccalaureate or higher degrees
> 6. National reputation, consultations, and visits to the organization
>
> **COST AND QUALITY OF CARE**
>
> 1. Decreased length of stay
> 2. Cost avoidance
> 3. Cost savings
> 4. Improved quality of care (e.g., decreased nosocomial urinary tract infections, improved pain management, decrease in nosocomial pressure ulcer development, increased satisfaction of families of critically ill patients)

tients? What effect is it having on people?" (Congressman John Porter, 1998, former Chairman of the House Appropriations Subcommittee on Labor, Health and Human Services, and Education). This quotation demonstrates the importance of translating into practice the science of health care. As the profession continues to understand the science of nursing and synthesize this science for application in practice, it will become increasingly necessary that we test and understand how to best promote the use of this science in daily practice. Twenty-seven studies have been funded by AHRQ on translating research into practice (Table 20-5), and as the results of these studies are disseminated, we will know

TABLE **20-5** Translating Research into Practice Studies Funded by the Agency for Healthcare Research and Quality

TITLE OF STUDY	NAME OF INSTITUTION	PRINCIPAL INVESTIGATOR(S)	PROJECT PERIOD
1. An Internet Intervention to Increase Chlamydia Screening	University of Alabama	Allison, Jeroan J.	9/30/00-9/29/03
2. Point of Care Delivery of Research Evidence	University of Missouri–Columbia	Balas, E. A.	9/01/00-8/31/03
3. Improving Quality with Outpatient Decision Support	Brigham and Women's Hospital	Bates, David W.	9/30/00-8/31/03
4. Improving Utilization of Ischemic Stroke Research	Minneapolis Medical Res Inst	Borbas, Catherine	9/30/00-8/31/03
5. Improving Diabetes Care Collaboratively in the Community	University of Chicago	Chin, Marshall H.	9/30/99-9/29/02
6. MCO Use of a Pediatric Asthma Management Program	University of Connecticut	Cloutier, Michelle M.	9/11/00-8/31/03
7. Pediatric EBM—Getting Evidence Used at the Point of Care	University of Washington	Davis, Robert L.	9/01/00-8/31/03
8. Evidence-Based 'Reminders' in Home Health Care	VNSNY	Feldman, Penny H.	9/30/99-3/30/02
9. Better Pediatric Outcomes Through Chronic Care	University of Connecticut	Fifield, Judith	9/30/00-9/29/03
10. Diabetes Education Multimedia for Vulnerable Populations	University of Illinois at Chicago	Gerber, Ben S.	9/01/00-8/31/03
11. Reducing Adverse Drug Events in the Nursing Home	University of Massachusetts Medical Center	Gurwitz, Jerry H.	7/01/00-6/30/03
12. Translating Research: Patient Decision Support/Coaching	Michigan State University	Holmes-Rovner, Margaret M.	9/30/00-11/30/03
13. Evidence-Based Surfactant Therapy for Preterm Infants	University of Vermont	Horbar, Jeffrey D.	9/30/99-9/29/02
14. Implementing Adolescent Preventive Guidelines	University of California–San Francisco	Irwin, Charles E.	9/30/00-8/31/03

Continued

more about the specific strategies that are most helpful in promoting EBP.

For organizations to take full advantage of EBP projects undertaken at various sites throughout the country, a National Center for Evidence-Based Practice and Translational Research is needed. Such a center would encompass a computerized database of EBP protocols that includes the relevant policy and procedure, the population to which it applies, the quality improvement indicators and data-collection forms used in evaluation, a list of references, suggested strategies for change, the type of institutions where the protocol has been implemented, contact people at each agency, and the protocol content expert. This information should be available on-line through electronic communications such as a dedicated list serve, the Virtual Hospital System, or some other form of electronic media. Such a center could facilitate networking among health care professionals working on similar EB projects and provide lists of consultants and edu-

TABLE **20-5** Translating Research into Practice Studies Funded by the Agency for Healthcare Research and Quality—cont'd

TITLE OF STUDY	NAME OF INSTITUTION	PRINCIPAL INVESTIGATOR(S)	PROJECT PERIOD
15. Improving Pain Management in Nursing Homes	University of Colorado Health Center	Jones, Katherine R.	9/27/00-8/31/03
16. Improving the Evidence for Unstable Angina Guidelines	University of Wisconsin	Katz, David A.	9/01/00-8/31/02
17. Translating Prevention Research into Practice	Meharry Medical College	Levine, Robert A.	9/30/00-9/29/03
18. Optimizing Antibiotic Use in Long-Term Care	McMaster University	Loeb, Mark B.	9/30/00-8/31/02
19. Smoking Control in MCH Clinics: Dissemination Strategies	University of Illinois at Chicago	Manfredi, Clara	9/01/00-8/31/03
20. Interventions to Improve Pain Outcomes	Mount Sinai School of Medicine	Morrison, R. Sean	7/01/00-6/30/03
21. Primary and Secondary Prevention of CHD and Stroke	Medical University of South Carolina	Ornstein, Steven M.	9/30/00-8/31/03
22. Do Urine Tests Increase Chlamydia Screening in Teens	University of California–San Francisco	Shafer, Mary-Ann	9/30/99-9/29/02
23. Practice Profiling to Increase Tobacco Cessation	Main Medical Assessment Foundation	Swartz, Susan H.	9/30/99-9/29/02
24. Translating Chlamydia Screening Guidelines into Practice	Center for Health Studies	Thompson, Robert S.	9/30/00-6/30/03
25. Evidence Based Practice: From Book to Bedside	University of Iowa	Titler, Marita	9/30/99-9/29/02
26. Developing an Asthma Management Model for Head Start CHI	Arkansas Children's Hosp Res Inst	Vargas, Perla A.	9/26/00-8/31/03
27. A Model for Use of the UI Guideline in US Nursing Homes	University of Rochester	Watson, Nancy M.	9/1/00-8/31/03

cational materials that may be helpful to those beginning to use research findings in their practice (Titler, 1997). This center also would provide data regarding the interventions/strategies that have been tested to translate research into practice and provide a "tool kit" of these interventions for use by all types of health care agencies. For example, the tool kit on use of opinion leaders to translate research into practice might include a definition of opinion leader, characteristics of opinion leaders, how to select an opinion leader, the function of the opinion leader, in what types of settings and projects opinion leaders have been used effectively, and methods to evaluate the effect of using opinion leaders in promoting adoption of a certain EBP. Lastly, such a center also would provide consultation and conduct translational research, that is, research on interventions for translating research into practice.

Education of nurses must include knowledge and skills in the use of research evidence in practice. Nurses are increasingly being held

| **Critical Thinking Challenges** | *Barbara Krainovich-Miller* |

➤ Do you agree or disagree with the following statement: "Much of nursing's research 'sits on shelves in libraries.' " Support your position with examples.

➤ There are several classic research utilization (RU) demonstration projects. Discuss the similarities and differences among these classic RU projects. Include in your discussion the Agency for Healthcare Research and Quality guidelines for various clinical problems. Include what technology you might use to assist you in your answer.

➤ Discuss the role of technology in implementing the steps of RU. Include in your discussion how computer electronic databases might help you; support your position with examples.

---

accountable for practices based on scientific evidence. Thus, we must communicate and integrate into our profession the expectation that it is the professional responsibility of every nurse to read and use research in their practice and to communicate with nurse scientists the many and varied clinical problems for which we do not yet have a scientific base.

Key Points

• The term research utilization and evidence-based practice are sometimes used interchangeably. These terms though related are not one and the same. *Research utilization* is the process of using research findings to improve practice. *Evidence-based practice (EBP)* is a broad term that not only encompasses research utilization but also includes use of case reports and expert opinion in deciding best practice.

• There are two forms of research evidence used: conceptual and decision driven.

• There are several models of evidence-based practice. A key feature of all models is the judicious review and synthesis of research regarding a nursing practice in order to develop evidenced based practice.

• The steps of EBP using the Iowa Model of Evidence-Based Practice are: selection of a topic, forming a team, literature retrieval, schemas for grading the evidence, critique of EBP guidelines, critique of research articles, synthesis of research findings, developing EBP, and implementing the change.

• Adoption of EBP standards requires education and dissemination to staff, and use of change strategies such as opinion leaders, change champions, use of a core group, and use of consultants.

• Overall EBP change involves: unfreezing old behaviors or attitudes, adopting new behaviors or practices, refreezing or integrating the change into the work role or practice setting.

• It is important to evaluate the change. Evaluation provides information for performance gap assessment, audit, and feedback and provides information necessary to determine if the practice should be retained.

• Evaluation includes both process and outcome measures.

• It is important for organizations to create a culture of EBP. To create this culture requires an interactive process. To provide this culture organizations need to provide access to information, access to individuals who have skills necessary for EBP and a written and verbal commitment to EB practice in the organization's operations.

REFERENCES

ACCP/AACVPR: Special report: pulmonary rehabilitation, joint ACCP/AACVPR evidence-based guidelines, *Chest* 112(5):1363-1396, 1997.

Agency for Health Care Policy and Research (AHCPR): Acute pain management: operative or medical procedures and trauma. Clinical practice guideline number 1, Rockville, Maryland, 1992a, U.S. Department of Health and Human Services, Public Health Services, Agency for Health Care Policy and Research, AHCPR Pub. No. 92-0032.

Agency for Health Care Policy and Research (AHCPR): Pressure ulcers in adults: prediction and prevention. Clinical practice guideline, number 3, Rockville, Maryland, 1992b, U.S. Department of Health and Human Services, Public Health Services, Agency for Health Care Policy and Research, AHCPR publication no. 92-0047.

Agency for Health Care Policy and Research (AHCPR): Management of cancer pain. Clinical practice guideline number 9, Rockville, Maryland, 1994, U.S. Department of Health and Human Services, Public Health Service, Agency for Health Care Policy and Research, AHCPR Publication No. 94-0592.

American Association of Critical Care Nurses (ACCN): *Protocols for practice: creating a healing environment*, Aliso Viejo, Calif, 1998, ACCN.

American Pain Society (APS): *Principles of analgesic use in the treatment of acute pain and cancer pain*, ed 4, Glenville, Ill, 1999a, APS.

American Pain Society (APS): *Guidelines for the management of acute and chronic pain in sickle cell disease*, Glenview, Ill, 1999b, APS.

Anders RL et al: Development of a scientifically valid coordinated care path, *J Nurs Admin* 27(5):45-52, 1997.

Atkins DM, Kamerow DM, and Eisenberg JMM: Evidence-based medicine at the Agency for Health Care Policy and Research, *ACP Journal Club* Mar-April, 128:A1214, 1998.

Axford R and Cutchen L: Using nursing research to improve preoperative care, *J Nurse Admin* 7(10):16-20, 1977.

Backer TE: Research utilization and managing innovation in rehabilitation organizations, *J Rehabil* 54:18-22, 1987.

Backer TE: Integrating behavioral and systems strategies to change clinical practice, *Joint Commission Journal on Quality Improvement* 21(7):351-353, 1995.

Baker R and Feder G: Clinical guidelines: Where next?, *Int J Qual Health Care* 9(6):399-404, 1997.

Barnason S et al: Utilizing an outcomes approach to improve pain management by nurses: A pilot study, *Clinical Nurse Specialist* 12(1):28-36, 1998.

Barnsteiner JH, Ford N, and Howe C: Research utilization in a metropolitan children's hospital, *Nurs Clin North Am* 30(3):447-455, 1995.

Bauchner H and Simpson L: Specific issues related to developing, disseminating, and implementing pediatric practice guidelines for physicians, patients, families, and other stakeholders, Health Services Research 33(4):1161-1177, 1998.

Bero LA al: Closing the gap between research and practice: An overview of systematic reviews of interventions to promote the implementation of research findings, *Br Med J* 317:465-468, 1998.

Berwick DM and Coltin KL: Feedback reduces test use in a health maintenance organization, *JAMA* 255:1450-1454, 1986.

Blondin MM and Titler MG: Deep vein thrombosis and pulmonary embolism prevention: What roles do nurses play? *Medsurg Nurs* 5(3):205-208, 1996.

Bookbinder M et al: Implementing national standards for cancer pain management: Program model and evaluation, *J Pain Symptom Manag* 12(6):334-347, 1996.

Brown SJ: *Knowledge for health care practice: A guide to using research evidence*, Philadelphia, 1999, WB Saunders Company.

Camiletti YA and Huffman MC: Research utilization: Evaluation of initiatives in a public health nursing division, *Can J Nurs Admin* 11(2):59-77, 1998.

Carroll DL et al: Barriers and facilitators to the utilization of nursing research, *Clinical Nurse Specialist* 11(5):207-12, 1997.

Chambers CV et al: Microcomputer-generated reminders: Improving the compliance of primary care physicians with mammography screening guidelines, *J Fam Pract* 29:273-80, 1989.

Cluzeau FA and Littlejohns P: Appraising clinical practice guidelines in England and Wales: The development of a methodologic framework and its application to policy, *J Qual Imp* 25(10):514-521, 1999.

Cluzeau F et al: *Appraisal instrument or clinical guidelines, version 1 user guide*, London, 1997, St. George's Hospital Medical School.

Cohen DI et al: Improving physician compliance with preventive medicine guidelines, *Med Care* 20:1040-1045, 1982.

Cole KM and Gawlinski A: Animal-assisted therapy in the intensive care unit, *Nurs Clin North Am* 30(3):529-537, 1995.

Cook D: Evidence-based critical care medicine: A potential tool for change, *New Horizons* 6(1):20-25, 1998.

Crane J: The future of research utilization, *Nurs Clin North Am* 30(3):565-577, 1995.

Cronenwett LR: Effective methods for disseminating research findings to nurses in practice, *Nurs Clin North Am* 30(3):429-438, 1995.

Davies B and Logan J: *Reading research: a user-friendly guide for nurses and other health professionals*, Ottawa, Ontario, Canada, 1993, Canadian Nurses Association.

Dickersin K and Manheimer E: The Cochrane Collaboration: evaluation of health care and services using systematic reviews of the results of randomized controlled trials, *Clin Obstet Gynecol* 41(2):315-31, 1998.

Dracup KA and Breu CS: Using nursing research findings to meet the needs of grieving spouses, *Nurs Res* 27(4):212-216, 1978.

Eisenberg JM: *Other approaches to changing physicians' practice: doctors' decisions and the cost of medical care: The reasons for doctors' practice patterns and ways to change them,* Ann Arbor, MI, 1986, Health Administration Press Perspectives.

Estabrooks CA: Will evidence-based nursing practice make practice perfect?, *Can J Nurs Res* 30(1): 15-36, 1998.

Funk SG, Tornquist EM, and Champagne MT: A model for improving the dissemination of nursing research, *West J Nurs Res* 11:361-367, 1989.

Funk SG, Tornquist EM, and Champagne MT: Barriers and facilitators of research utilization: An integrative Review, *Nurs Clin North Am* 30:395-408, 1995b.

Funk SG et al: Administrators' views on barriers to research utilization, *Appl Nurs Res* 8(1):44-49, 1995a.

Gerontological Nursing Interventions Research Center (GNIRC): *Guidelines for writing evidence-based practice protocols,* Iowa City, Iowa, 1999, University of Iowa Gerontological Nursing Interventions Research Center, Research Dissemination Core.

Geyman JP: Evidence-based medicine in primary care: an overview. *J Am Board Fam Pract* 11(1):46-56, 1998.

Goode CJ: Evaluation of research-based nursing interventions, *Nurs Clin North Am* 30(3), 1995.

Goode CJ and Piedalue F: Evidence-based clinical practice, *JONA* 29(6):15-21, 1999.

Goode CJ and Titler MG: Moving research-based practice throughout the health care system, *Medsurg Nurs* 5(5):380-383, 1996.

Goode CJ et al: Use of research based knowledge in clinical practice, *J Nurs Admin* 17(12):11-18, 1987.

Goode CJ et al: A meta-analysis of effects of heparin flush and saline flush: quality and cost implications, *Nurs Res* 40(6):324-330, 1991.

Goode CJ et al: Improving practice through research: the case of heparin vs. saline for peripheral intermittent infusion devices, *Medsurg Nurs* 2(2):23-27, 1993.

Goodpastor WA and Montoya ID: Motivating physician behavior change: Social influence versus financial contingencies, *Int J Health Care Quality Assurance* 9(6):4-9, 1996.

Greer AL: The state of the art versus the state of the science, *Intl J Technol Assessment in Health Care* 4:5-26, 1988.

Haber J et al: Shaping nursing practice through research-based protocols, *J NY State Nurs Assoc* 25(3):3-8, 1994.

Heater BS, Becker AM, and Olson RK: Nursing interventions and patient outcomes: a meta-analysis of studies, *Nurs Res* 37(5):303-307, 1988.

Hendryx MS et al: Outreach education to improve quality of rural ICU care: results of a randomized trial, *Am J Respir Crit Care Med* 158(2):418-423, 1998.

Herr K et al: Evidence-based guideline: acute pain management in the elderly In Lisa Grant, editor: *From book to bedside: acute pain management in the elderly,* 1 R01, HS10482-01, Iowa City, Iowa, 2000, The University of Iowa.

Horsley J, Crane J, and Bingle JD: Research utilization as an organizational process, *J Nurs Admin* 8(7):4-6, 1978.

Horsley J et al: *Using research to improve nursing practice: A guide,* Philadelphia, 1983, WB Saunders.

Hunt DL et al: Effects of computer-based clinical decision support systems on physician performance and patient outcomes: A systematic review, *JAMA* 280(15): 1339-1346, 1998.

Katz DA: Barriers between guidelines and improved patient care: An analysis of AHCPR's unstable angina clinical practice guideline, *HSR* 34(1):337-389, 1999.

King D, Barnard KE, and Hoehn R: Disseminating the results of nursing research, *Nurs Outlook* 29:164-169, 1981.

Kirchhoff K and Titler MG: Responsibilities of nurse executives for research in practice. In Spitzer-Layman R (ed): *Nursing management desk reference,* Philadelphia, 1994, WB Saunders.

Kreuger JC: Utilization of nursing research: The planning process, *J Nurs Admin* 8:6-9, 1978.

Kreuger JC, Nelson AH, and Wolanin MO: *Nursing research: development, collaboration, and utilization,* Germantown, Md, 1978, Aspen.

Lang NM: Discipline-based approaches to evidence-based practice: a view from nursing, *J Qual Imp* 25(10):539-544, 1999.

Laxson CJ and Titler MG: Drawing coagulation studies from arterial lines: an integrative literature review, *Am J Crit Care* 3(1):16-22, 1994.

Lepper HS and Titler MG: Program evaluation. In Mateo MA and Kirchhoff KT, editors: *Using and conducting nursing research in the clinical setting,* ed , Philadelphia, 1999, WB Saunders.

Liddle J, Williamson M, and Irwig L: *Improving health care and outcomes: method for evaluating research guideline evidence,* Sydney, 1996, NSW Health Department, State Health Publication No. (CEB) 96-204.

Lindeman CA and Kreuger JC: Increasing the quality, quantity, and use of nursing research, *Nurs Outlook* 25(7):450-454, 1977.

Lohr KN and Carey TS: Assessing "best evidence": Issues in grading the quality of studies for systematic reviews, *J Qual Imp* 25(9):470-479, 1999.

Lomas J et al: Opinion leaders vs. audit and feedback to implement practice guidelines: Delivery after previous cesarean section, *JAMA* 265:2202-2207, 1991.

Long A and Harrison S: Evidence-based decision making, *Health Services Journal* 106(5486, Health Manage Guide):1-12, 1996.

Maxwell LE: Innovation Adoption: introducing IV patient controlled analgesia to the nursing workplace, *Can J Nurs Admin* 8(4):59-75, 1995.

Meyer AD and Goes JB: Organizational assimilation of innovations: a multilevel contextual analysis, *Academy of Management Journal* 31:897-923, 1988.

Mion LC: Evidence-based health care practice, *J Gerontol Nurs* 24(12):5-6, 1998.

Montgomery LA and Budreau GK: Implementing a clinical practice guideline to improve pediatric intravenous infiltration outcomes, *AACN Clin Iss* 7(3):411-424, 1996.

Nightingale F: *Notes on matters affecting the health, efficiency, and hospital administration of the British Army*, London, 1858, Harrison and Sons.

Nightingale F: *A contribution to the sanitary history of the British Army during the late war with Russia*, London, 1859, John W. Parker and Sons.

Nightingale F: *Notes on hospitals*, London, 1863a, Longman, Green, Roberts, and Green.

Nightingale F: *Observation on the evidence contained in the statistical reports submitted by her to the Royal Commission on the Sanitary State of the Army in India*, London, 1863b, Edward Stanford.

Oxman AD et al: No magic bullets: A systematic review of 102 trials of interventions to improve professional practice, *Can Med Assoc J* 153(10):1423-1431, 1995.

Pettit DM and Kraus V: The use of gauze versus transparent dressing for peripheral intravenous catheter sites, *Nurs Clin North Am* 30(3):495-506, 1995.

Prevost SS: Research-based practice in critical care, *AACN Clin Iss Crit Care Nurs* 5(2):101, 1994.

Rakel BA et al: Nasogastric and nasointestinal feeding tube placement: An integrative review of research, *AACN Clin Iss Crit Care Nurs* 5(2):194-206, 1994.

Rochon PA, Dikinson E, and Gordon M: The Cochrane Field in health care of older people: Geriatric medicine's role in the collaboration, *JAGS* 45(2):241-243, 1997.

Rogers E: *Diffusion of innovations*, New York, 1995, The Free Press.

Rosswurm MA and Larrabee JH: A model for change to evidence-based practice, *Image: J Nurs Schol* 31(4):317-322, 1999.

Rutledge DN and Donaldson NE: Building organizational capacity to engage in research utilization, *J Nurs Admin* 25(10):12-16, 1995.

Sackett D et al: Evidence based medicine: What it is and what it isn't, *Br Med J* 312:71-72, 1996.

Sackett DL et al: *Evidence-based medicine: how to practice and teach EBM*, London, 2000, Churchill Livingstones.

Schmidt KL, Alpen MA, and Rakel BA: Implementation of the Agency for Health Care Policy and Research pain guidelines, *AACN Clin Iss Crit Care* 7(3):425-435, 1996.

Schneider EC and Eisenberg JM: Strategies and methods for aligning current and best medical practices: The role of information technologies, *West J Med* 168(5):311-318, 1998.

Schnelle JF et al: Developing rehabilitative behavioral interventions for long-term care: Technology transfer, acceptance, and maintenance issues, *J Am Geriatrics Soc* 46(6):771-777, 1998.

Scott J and Rantz M: Change champions at the grassroots level: Practice innovation using team process, *Nurs Admin Q* 18(3):7-17, 1994.

Shively M et al: Testing a community level research utilization intervention, *Appl Nurs Res* 10(3):121-127, 1997.

Shortell SM et al: Assessing the impact of continuous quality improvement/total quality management: Concept versus implementation, *Health Services Research* 30:377-401, 1995.

Soukup SM: The center for advanced nursing practice evidence-based practice model, *Nurs Clin North Am* 35(2):301-309, 2000.

Soumerai S and Avorn J: Principles of educational outreach ('academic detailing') to improve clinical decision making, *JAMA* 263(4):549-556, 1990.

Soumerai SB et al: Effect of local medical opinion leaders on quality of care for acute myocardial infarction: A randomized controlled trial, *JAMA* 279(17): 1358-1363, 1998.

Stenger K: Putting research to good use, *Am J Nurs* 94(Suppl):30-38, 1994.

Stetler CB: Refinement of the Stetler/Marram model for application of research findings to practice, *Nurs Outlook* 42:15-25, 1994.

Stetler CB et al: Enhancing research utilization by clinical nurse specialists, *Nurs Clin North Am* 30(3):457-473, 1995.

Stetler CB et al: Evidence-based practice and the role of nursing leadership, *JONA* 28(7/8):45-53, 1998a.

Stetler CB et al: Utilization-focused integrative reviews in a nursing service, *Appl Nurs Res* 11(4):195-206, 1998b.

Stonestreet JS and Lamb-Havard J: Organizational strategies to promote research-based practice, *AACN Clin Iss Crit Care* 5(2):133-146, 1994.

Titler MG: Critical analysis of research utilization (RU): an historical perspective, *Am J Crit Care* 2(3):264, 1993.

Titler MG: Changing visiting practices in critical care units, *MedSurg Nurs* 4(1):65-68, 1995.

Titler MG: Research utilization: necessity or luxury? In McCloskey JC and Grace H, editors: *Current issues in nursing*, ed 5, St Louis, 1997, Mosby.

Titler MG and Mentes JC: Research utilization in gerontological nursing practice, *J Gerontol Nurs* 25(6):6-9, 1999b.

Titler MG et al: Nursing research in times of economic cutbacks: implications for nurse administrators, *Series Nurs Admin* 4:167-182, 1992.

Titler MG et al: Research utilization in critical care: an exemplar, *AACN Clin Iss Crit Care* 5(2):124-132, 1994a.

Titler MG et al: Infusing research into practice to promote quality care, *Nurs Res* 43(5):307-313, 1994b.

Titler MG et al: From book to bedside: putting evidence to use in the care of the elderly, *J Qual Imp* 25(10):545-556, 1999a.

Titler MG et al: The Iowa model of evidence-based practice to promote quality care, *Crit Care Clin North Am*, (in press).

US Preventive Services Task Force: *Guide to clinical preventive services*, ed 2, Washington, DC, 1996, US Department of Health and Human Services.

Van Mullem C et al: Strategic planning for research use in nursing practice, *JONA* 29(12):38-45, 1999.

Weiss CH: Knowledge creep and decision accretion, *Knowledge Creation Diffusion Utilization* 1:381-404, 1980.

Wells N and Baggs JG: A survey of practicing nurses' research interests and activities, *Cinical Nurse Specialist* 8:145-151, 1994.

Appendix A

From *Applied Nursing Research* 13(1):19-28, 2000.

A PROFESSIONAL-PATIENT PARTNERSHIP MODEL OF DISCHARGE PLANNING WITH ELDERS HOSPITALIZED WITH HEART FAILURE

Margaret J. Bull, PhD, RN, FAAN
School of Nursing,
University of Maryland,
Baltimore, MD

Helen E. Hansen, PhD, RN
School of Nursing,
University of Minnesota,
Minneapolis, MN

Cynthia R. Gross, PhD
School of Nursing,
College of Pharmacy,
University of Minnesota,
Minneapolis, MN

Despite efforts to improve the discharge planning process and subsequent outcomes, existing mechanisms fail to accurately identify elders' needs for follow-up care. Studies report rehospitalization rates ranging from 12 to 50%. The two aims of this study were to (1) examine the difference in outcomes for elders hospitalized with heart failure and caregivers who participated in a professional-patient partnership model of discharge planning compared to those who received the usual discharge planning and (2) examine differences in costs associated with hospital readmission and use of the emergency room following hospital discharge. A before-and-after nonequivalent control group design was used for this study. Data were collected from the control and the intervention cohorts before discharge and at 2 weeks and 2 months postdischarge. One hundred and fifty-eight patient-caregiver dyads completed both the predischarge and 2-weeks postdischarge interviews; 140 also completed a 2-month follow up. The average age of elders was 73.7 years; the average age of the caregivers was 58.5 years. The findings indicated that elders in the intervention cohort felt more prepared to manage care, reported more continuity of information about care management and services, felt they were in better health, and when readmitted spent fewer days in the hospital than the control cohort. Caregivers in the intervention cohort also reported receiving more information about care management and having a more positive reaction to caregiving 2 weeks postdischarge than the control cohort. (Copyright © 2000 by W.B. Saunders Company.)

More than 2 million Americans have heart failure and 400,000 new cases are diagnosed each year. Heart failure is the most common medical diagnosis in hospitalized elders and the incidence increases with advancing age (Guerra-Garcia, Taffeta, & Protas, 1997). In 1992 more than $5.6 billion was spent on hospital care for Medicare patients admitted for heart failure. An estimated $230 million was spent on medications (USDHHS, 1994). Efforts to curtail costs have resulted in shortened lengths of hospital stays. With shortened lengths of stay, health professionals have less time in which to identify elders' needs for follow-up care and less time to arrange aftercare (National Center for Health Statistics,

1997). Identifying these needs and arranging appropriate follow-up care are critical to helping elders maintain independent living and preventing costly hospital readmissions.

Discharge planning, a process of identifying patient needs for follow-up care and arranging for that care, might be expected to address this problem. Despite efforts to improve the discharge-planning process and subsequent outcomes, existing mechanisms fail to accurately identify elders' needs for follow-up care; and studies report rehospitalization rates ranging from 12 to 50% (Bull, Maruyama, & Luo, 1995; Happ, Naylor, & Roe-Prio, 1997; Lockery, Dunkle, Kart, & Coulton, 1993). One study also showed that elders who were more independent in activities of daily living were more likely to be readmitted to the hospital than elders who were functionally impaired but receiving home health services (Bull, 1994a). This suggests that there may be difficulty with accurately identifying needs and planning for follow-up care.

The aims of this study were as follows:

1. examine differences in outcomes for elders and caregivers who participated in a professional-patient partnership model of discharge planning compared to those who received the usual discharge planning, and

2. examine differences in costs associated with hospital readmission and use of the emergency room following hospital discharge.

It was hypothesized that at 2 weeks postdischarge:

1. Scores on perceived health will be different for clients in the intervention and control cohorts.

2. Client satisfaction with discharge planning, perceptions of care continuity, preparedness and difficulties managing care will differ for the intervention and control cohorts.

3. Caregivers' response to caregiving will be different for the experimental and control cohorts.

4. Resource use will be different for the control and intervention cohorts.

The same hypotheses were posited for 2 months postdischarge. The professional-patient partnership model is an intervention designed to facilitate identification of elders' needs for follow-up care and to provide a mechanism for identifying those who require more in-depth assessments. It provides nursing staff with a means of getting to know the patient quickly, provides a structure for elder patient and caregivers participation in planning, and promotes interaction between health professionals and patients.

BACKGROUND

The conceptual framework for this study (see Figure 1) is based on an evaluation approach that incorporates structure, process, and outcome (Donabedian, 1966). As indicated in Figure 1, the intervention occurs within the hospital's organizational context and is likely to be influenced by both patient and caregiver characteristics. Previous research suggests that three structural factors influence the extent to which elder patients participate in discharge planning: their health status, health locus of control, and the hospital environment. Elder patients who were more functionally impaired were less likely to participate in discharge planning decisions (Lockery, Dunkle, Kart, & Coulton, 1993). In such situations health professionals often relied on caregivers in planning posthospital care. Patients' participation in discharge planning also was positively correlated with locus of control—i.e., the belief that what they do influences their health (Lockery, Dunkle, Kart, & Coulton, 1993). Perceived lack of control over discharge decisions was associated with posthospital psychological distress for elders who scored high on the locus of control scale (Coulton, Dunkle, Haug, Chow, & Vielhaber, 1989); these patients also were more likely to take control of their health, seek health information, be knowledgeable about their diseases, and maintain their physical well-being (Wallston, Wallston, Devellis, & Peabody, 1978). Previous studies have not examined factors that influence

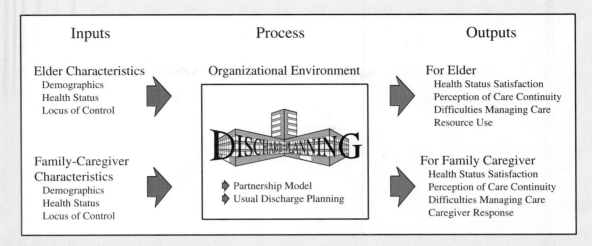

Figure 1.   Conceptual framework of the study.

caregiver participation in planning for discharge; however, caregivers' health status, locus of control, and demographics might influence their participation.

The discharge-planning process for elder patients is fragile and vulnerable to breakdown. The effects of breakdown frequently manifest themselves in the unmet needs and problems elders and their caregivers experience following discharge and readmission. Poor communication among hospital staff, physicians, elders, their caregivers, and community agencies has been identified as the root of discontinuity and difficulties elders and caregivers encounter postdischarge (Bull & Kane, 1996; Jewell, 1993). In fact 80% of elders reported unmet information needs 1 week following hospital discharge (Mistriaen, Duijnhouwer, Wijkel, deBont, & Veeger, 1997). Interventions aimed at improving communication might lead to better outcomes.

In previous studies, the outcomes most often examined in relation to the discharge-planning process were readmission, costs of care, and length of hospital stay. Early referral to social service resulted in shorter lengths of hospital stay for some patients (Evans, Hendricks, Lawrence-Umlauf, & Bishop, 1989; Schrager, Halmon, Myers, Nichols & Rosenblum, 1978). Hospital discharge-planning programs increased lengths of stay for patients with congestive heart failure and emphysema but decreased length of stay for patients admitted with hip fractures and strokes (Cable & Mayers, 1983). Use of geriatric consultation services also have resulted in fewer readmissions within 1 month of discharge (Campion, Jette, & Berkman, 1983). Use of advanced practice nurses as case managers in planning for discharge has been linked with positive outcomes (Brooten et al., 1996). For the most part, case management tends to target elder patients who are frail and severely impaired in their functional ability. Although there is lack of agreement on who needs case management, and it is generally agreed that not all patients require it, all patients do need to have their needs for follow-up care assessed.

Although some previous studies emphasize outcomes in terms of resource consumption, others emphasize outcomes important to the elder patients such as the continuity of information, the ability to function in their environment, having access to services to assist them with managing their care, and satisfaction with the plan of care (Bull, 1994a; Proctor, Morrow-Howell, Albaz, & Weir, 1992). Similar outcomes seem appropriate for caregivers who assist elders in managing their

Table 1. Design of Study and Dyads Enrolled

Elder/Caregiver Cohorts	Preintervention Period Data Collection Times			Intervention Period Data Collection Times		
	Predischarge, n	2 Weeks Postdischarge, n	2 Months Postdischarge, n	Predischarge, n	2 Weeks Postdischarge, n	2 Months Postdischarge, n
Control						
Hospital 1	29	22	22			
Hospital 1[a]				54	46	39
Hospital 2	42	40	39			
Intervention						
Hospital 2				55	45[b]	40

[a]This cohort was dropped from the analysis since the implementation of a critical pathway during this time period changed the discharge planning protocol at this site.
[b]Ten of the 55 dyads were discharged before they could complete all elements of the protocol and were not included in the analysis of 2-week and 2-month outcomes.

care following discharge. Addressing the needs of caregivers is a vital component in meeting elder's needs and maintaining their independent living arrangements (Bull, Maruyama, & Luo, 1995).

METHODS
Design

A before-and-after nonequivalent control group design was used for this study. Two hospitals were matched in terms of size, type, and discharge-planning practices used in cardiac units; Hospital 1 served as a control site and Hospital 2 implemented the intervention. Data were collected on four elder/caregiver cohorts—control cohorts from each hospital prior to the intervention, the intervention cohort, and a cohort of elder patients at the control hospital at the same time as the intervention cohort. Unfortunately, Hospital 1 (the site of one of the control cohorts) implemented a congestive heart failure critical pathway during the final months of data collection; as a result, data from cohort four was not included in the analysis for this article. Table 1 summarizes the design and the number of dyads in each cohort.

Setting

Cardiac units from two large community hospitals (between 400 and 500 bed facilities) located in a midwest metropolitan area with a population of 2 million served as sites for the study. The

principal investigator randomly selected one institution for implementation of the partnership model (Hospital 2) and the other for the control group (Hospital 1).

Sample

The sample consisted of 180 elder/caregiver dyads. The criteria for sample selection were (a) elder patient hospitalized with heart failure, (b) participants able to speak and understand English, (c) patient at least 55 years of age, (d) patient able to identify a family member or friend who would help her or him with aftercare following hospitalization, and (e) patient achieved a score indicating cognitive competence on a mental status questionnaire (Kahn, Goldfarb, Pollack & Peck, 1960). One hundred and fifty-eight dyads completed both the predischarge and 2-week postdischarge interviews; 140 also completed a 2-month follow up. Sample mortality was attributed to the elder's death, readmission to the hospital, inability to participate because of illness or being too confused to participate, and relocation out-of-state with a change in caregiver.

The average age of the elders was 73.7 years ($SD = 8.8$; range 55 to 94) and education level ranged from seventh grade through graduate school with a mean of 12 years ($SD = 2.5$). The majority of patients (94.4%) were White. Caregivers ranged in age from 20 to 86 years with a mean of 58.5 years ($SD = 14.9$) and their mean level of education was 12.9 years ($SD = 2.2$). The majority of caregivers were White (93.6%) and female (73%). Half of the caregivers were spouses of the elder patient, 28.6% were daughters, 9.8% were sons, 7.1% were siblings or grandchildren, and 4.5% were friends. The patients had been hospitalized for either a primary (67.2%) or secondary (32.8%) diagnosis of congestive heart failure.

Intervention

Nurses and social workers at the hospital implementing the intervention received an orientation to the partnership model and assistance with its implementation. The intervention had the following components:

1. An educational program for nurses and social workers included information on discharge-planning assessment, patient and caregiver participation, and use of the patient and caregiver self-administered Discharge Planning Questionnaire (DPQ) to identify needs for follow-up care (Bull, 1994b).
2. Elders and caregivers were asked to complete the DPQ approximately 1 to 2 days after the elder was admitted to the participating medical unit.
3. Elders and caregivers viewed a videotape on preparing to leave the hospital and were given structured questions related to managing posthospital care to discuss with their doctor, nurse, or social worker.
4. Elders were given a form to list medication information and a brochure on how to access community services.

The extent to which patients and health care professionals made use of the intervention was monitored by asking nurses to complete a form for each patient and by asking elders and caregivers whether plans for discharge were discussed with them, when they were discussed, and by whom.

Procedures

The approval of the universities' and hospitals' institutional review boards were obtained. A member of the research team checked with the charge nurse daily to identify potential participants and obtained permission to introduce the study to elders who met the study criteria. Potential participants were contacted 1 to 2 days following admission to the medical unit and the study was explained. If the elder agreed to participate, the family member or friend who assisted with managing their care also was contacted and invited to participate in the study. Only data from consenting dyads were included in this analysis.

Data were collected on the elder's and caregiver's health status through in-person interviews approximately 1 day before discharge. Telephone interviews were conducted 2 weeks and 2 months postdischarge. Interviews with the elder required 20 to 25 minutes before discharge and 30 to 35 minutes at 2 weeks and at 2 months following hospitalization. Interviews with the caregiver or friend required 20 minutes prior to discharge and 40 to 50 minutes at 2 weeks and at 2 months postdischarge.

Instruments

Description of the instruments used to collect data, psychometric properties, and time points for data collection appear in Table 2. Demographic information was collected for elders and their caregivers at the interview prior to discharge. Demographics included age, race, education level, income, and type of health insurance. In addition, information was gathered on elders' length of hospital stay and length of time since they had been diagnosed with congestive heart failure.

Data Analysis

Independent group comparisons for single variables were made using t-tests, Mann-Whitney U or X^2 tests, depending on the level of measurement of the independent variables of interest. Relationships among scales were examined using the Pearson Product Moment correlation statistic. Statistical significance was determined using the traditional .05 cutoff for two-tailed p values. To

Table 2. Instruments, Time Points, and Psychometrics

Instrument	Time Point	Description	Alpha Coefficients	Alpha Coefficients for This Study
Short Form-36 (SF-36)[a]	Predischarge Two weeks postdischarge Two months postdischarge	36 items, eight health concepts: a) physical functioning, b) general health, c) role functioning, d) bodily pain, e) mental health, f) social functioning, and g) vitality. Scores are 0 to 100. Higher score indicates better health. It requires approximately 15 minutes to complete.	.77 to .90	.76 to .91 elders .79 to .93 caregivers
Symptom Questionnaire[b]	Predischarge Two weeks postdischarge Two months postdischarge	Psychological distress subscales of anxiety, depression, anger-hostility, and somatic symptoms. 23 items per subscale.	.86 to .92	.90 caregivers .91 elders
Health Locus of Control[c]	Predischarge	Global scale oriented to health: 6 items	.77	.78 caregivers .84 elders
Client Satisfaction Questionnaire (CSQ)[d]	Two weeks postdischarge	Measure of general satisfaction with health services: 8 items. Higher scores indicate greater satisfaction. Modified to specifically address discharge planning.	.84 to .95	.84 elders .89 caregivers
Care continuity[a]	Two weeks postdischarge Two months postdischarge	12 items measure perceptions of care continuity. Higher scores indicate greater continuity.	.75 to .84	.80 to .84
Difficulties managing care	Two weeks postdischarge Two months postdischarge	Number and type of difficulties experienced in managing care: 13 items. Higher scores indicate more difficulty.	.85 to .88	.88 elder .89 caregiver
Preparedness	Two weeks postdischarge	Overall rating in response to one question about how prepared they felt to manage care post-discharge on a scale from 0 to 10.	NA	NA
Resource use	Two weeks postdischarge Two months postdischarge	Readmission to the hospital and use of the emergency room postdischarge. Medicare allowance was used as a standard.	NA	NA
Caregiver response[f]	Two weeks postdischarge Two months postdischarge	21 items measure family reaction to caregiving. Four subscales are negative reaction (NA), role responsibility (RR), impact on finances (F), and impact on schedule (S).	NA .84 to .89 RR .80 to .84 F .80 to .84 S .81 to .87	NA .90 RR .81 F .75 S .88

[a]Ware & Sherbourne, 1992, McHorney, Ware, Rogers, Rucksack, & Lu, 1992.
[b]Kellner 1987.
[c]Wallston, Wallston, Devellis, & Peabody, 1978.
[d]Pascoe & Attkisson, 1983.
[e]Bull, Luo, & Maruyama, 1997.
[f]Given, Stommel, Collins, King, & Given, 1990.

control Type 1 errors and provide a summary comparison of between-group differences, multivariate comparisons between intervention and control groups were made using the nonparametric method of O'Brien (1984), which involves ranking all subjects on each outcome variable, one at a time, and then summing the ranks across variables within a domain of interest. The sum is then divided by the number of variables within a domain to obtain a composite score for each subject. Composite scores were compared for the intervention and control cohorts using a Mann-Whitney U test. This method has greater power and requires fewer assumptions than alternative approaches such as Bonferroni adjustment or Hotelling's t-test. Based on the final sample size at 2 weeks, this study had approximately 80% power for two-tailed tests to detect moderate differences between intervention and control groups (effect size of $>.6$) and moderate to large effects between caregiver groups (effect size of $>.7$).

RESULTS

There were no statistically significant differences in demographics, length of hospital stay, or predischarge measures of health for the three cohorts of elders. Because the control elder cohorts from both hospitals were not significantly different on summary health status measures and health locus of control predischarge or at 2 weeks or 2 months postdischarge, the control cohorts were combined for this analysis. Control caregiver cohorts from the two hospitals differed significantly on measures of health, difficulties managing care, and care continuity scores postdischarge; however, caregivers in the control and intervention cohorts from Hospital 2, which implemented the partnership model, were not significantly different on demographics or predischarge measures of health. Consequently each control cohort of caregivers was compared separately with the intervention cohort.

At 2 weeks postdischarge, 9.5% of the sample had been readmitted to the hospital and 8.1% had visited the emergency room. At 2 months postdischarge, approximately 20% had been readmitted

to the hospital and 18% had visited the emergency room. Approximately 50% of the elders and 60% of the caregivers acknowledged difficulty evaluating and managing symptoms and recognizing complications of illness at 2 weeks and at 2 months following hospitalization. Health locus of control was positively related to elders' perception of care continuity 2 weeks postdischarge ($r = .35$, $p = .001$) and inversely related to length of hospital stay ($r = -.29$, $p = .007$). Elders with higher scores on locus of control had shorter lengths of stay; however, the relationship between locus of control and caregiver participation in discharge planning was not significant.

Aim 1

Outcomes for elder patients were examined initially by comparing control and intervention cohorts on each of 20 subscales including health, satisfaction, preparedness, continuity, difficulty managing care, anxiety, depression, and resource use. Based on measures at 2 weeks, the results indicated that elders in the intervention cohort reported significantly higher mean scores than the control cohort on preparedness ($t = 4.30$, $p = .04$), continuity in receipt of information about the elder's condition ($t = 2.80$, $p = .006$), continuity in services ($t = 3.15$, $p = .002$), measure of general health perception ($t = 2.0$, $p = .04$), and vitality ($t = 2.99$, $p = .004$). Elders in the intervention group felt more prepared to manage their care, reported receiving more explanation about their condition and medications, more information about community services, and feeling in better health 2 weeks postdischarge than the control cohort. Although the intervention cohort reported higher mean scores on satisfaction than the control cohort, the difference was not statistically significant ($t = -1.35$, $p = .18$). The group means appear in Table 3. At 2 months postdischarge, elders in the intervention cohort also reported significantly higher scores (better continuity) than the control cohort on continuity of care ($t = 3.31$, $p = .002$ for continuity of information; $t = 5.20$, $p = .001$ for continuity of services). Elder outcomes also were examined by calculating

Table 3. Scores for Elder Patients in Intervention and Control Groups Two Weeks Postdischarge

Measures	Intervention Groups, $n = 40^a$	Control Groups, $n = 71$	Significance
Scale and subscale means or medians			
Continuity, information	27.51	23.50	.01
Continuity, services	9.40	6.40	.002
Preparedness (median)	58.54	43.53	.01
Difficulty	31.20	31.89	NS
Satisfaction CSQ	26.95	25.28	NS
General health (SF-36)	58.92	48.90	.04
Vitality (SF-36)	44.87	31.17	.004
Physical function (SF-36)	41.79	30.42	.03
Social function (SF-36)	66.16	61.25	NS
Mental health (SF-36)	77.64	75.27	NS
Role, physical (SF-36)	25.00	29.74	NS
Role, emotional (SF-36)	73.50	70.76	NS
Bodily pain (SF-36)	55.50	51.80	NS
Composite measures			
Continuity (mean rank)	57.15	44.22	.027
Total health (mean rank)	55.87	37.95	.001

Note. Means are compared by *t*-tests, medians and ranks by Mann-Whitney *U* tests. Preparedness is the only median reported. *NS*, not significant.
[a]Sample size reflects those who received the complete intervention; in a few cases patients were discharged before the intervention protocol was completed.

composite scale scores and forming six measures: (1) total health, (2) care continuity, (3) difficulties managing care, (4) resource use, (5) satisfaction, and (6) preparedness (Fairclough, 1997; O'Brien, 1984). The scales of the SF-36 plus the anxiety and depression scales were transformed to ranks and summed to form a total health score. The continuity subscales were transformed and combined in the same way. Results of comparing control cohorts with the intervention cohort 2 weeks postdischarge using the Mann-Whitney statistic indicated that elders in the intervention group reported significantly higher scores on continuity of care, preparedness, and total health than the control groups (see composite scores in Table 3). Although elders in the intervention group reported higher mean scores on satisfaction at 2 weeks and total health at 2 months postdischarge than the controls, the differences were not statistically significant at the .05 level. There were no statistically significant differences in the elders' scores on difficulties in managing care at 2 weeks or 2 months postdischarge.

Outcomes for caregivers also were examined in two phases: first comparing control and intervention cohorts on each scale using *t*-tests and then forming composite scores. Results of *t*-tests on the 2-week data indicated that caregivers in the intervention cohort reported higher scores on continuity of information about the elder's condition ($t = 2.28, p = .026$) and about services available ($t = 2.19, p = .03$). They also reported higher scores on general health perceptions ($t = 1.96, p = .05$), vitality ($t = 2.62, p = .01$), and on mental health ($t = 2.04, p = .046$) than the control cohort. Caregivers in the intervention cohort reported significantly less negative reaction to caregiving 2 weeks postdischarge than the control cohort ($t = -2.49, p = .015$). Although the intervention group reported higher scores on satisfaction, the differences were not statistically significant ($t = -1.80, p = .076$). Caregivers in the intervention group also reported significantly higher scores on care continuity scales at 2 months postdischarge, indicating that they received more explanation about the elder's medications, condition, and in-

Table 4.   Scores for Caregivers in Intervention and Control Groups

Measures	Intervention Group, $n = 40$	Control Groups		Significance*	
		Hospital 2, $n = 42$	Hospital 1, $n = 29$	Intervention vs. Control Hospital 1	Intervention vs. Control Hospital 2
Scale and subscale means 2 weeks postdischarge					
Continuity, information	26.45	22.07	24.59	.026	NS
Continuity, services	8.42	6.10	8.36	.03	NS
Mental health (SF-36)	80.00	69.68	81.09	.046	NS
General health (SF-36)	77.31	68.57	75.81	.05	NS
Vitality (SF-36)	63.12	48.38	63.63	.01	NS
Scale and subscale means 2 months postdischarge					
Continuity, information	28.52	21.65	21.06	.001	.005
Continuity, services	9.63	6.32	8.18	.005	NS
Difficulty	32.00	36.59	25.87	NS	.01
Composite measures (mean ranks)					
Total health, 2 weeks	39.62	29.66	19.38	.04	.004
Total health, 2 months	33.48	24.93	13.63	.05	.001
Continuity, 2 weeks	39.62	32.82	21.75	NS	.018
Continuity, 2 months	36.95	26.41	15.56	.05	.009

Note. Means are compared by *t*-tests, medians and ranks by Mann-Whitney *U* tests. Table includes only measures that were statistically significant across the three groups. *NS*, not significant.

formation about community services. The mean and median scores for each cohort appear in Table 4; composite scores indicated that caregivers in the intervention cohort reported significantly better health and higher scores on continuity of care than the control cohort at 2 weeks and 2 months postdischarge.

Aim 2

Although there were no statistically significant differences between intervention and control cohorts on readmission to the hospital and use of the emergency room at 2 weeks postdischarge, the intervention group was readmitted less often (6.7% for the control group versus 4% for the intervention group). At 2 months postdischarge 3.2% of the elders who received the complete intervention had been readmitted compared to 17% of the controls. At 2 weeks postdischarge, percentages of elders who visited the emergency room show that there were fewer elders from the intervention cohort (6.9%) than from the controls (8.3%). However, none of the elders had more than one visit to the emergency room at the

2-week time period. At 2 months postdischarge, use of the emergency room was slightly higher for the intervention cohort (8.8%) than the controls (8.3%). Translating resource use to costs using a standard charge of $800 for a 1-day uncomplicated hospital stay, $238 for an emergency room visit, and subtracting the cost of the intervention, the average cost savings per person in the partnership model was approximately $4,300.

DISCUSSION

With shortened lengths of hospital stay and time constraints on health professionals, it often becomes easier to make discharge plans for patients rather than with them. Nurses can play a key role in shaping the extent to which patients and caregivers are involved in planning for discharge. The findings from this study suggest that the professional-patient partnership model can facilitate elder and caregiver participation in planning. The partnership model promoted elder and caregiver participation in identifying their postdischarge needs, their preferences, and encouraging them to seek answers to questions about the elder's condition and care management before they left the hospital. The partnership model participants felt more prepared to manage their care and received more information about care management than the control group. Nurses in practice might incorporate elements of this model in helping patients plan for discharge. For instance, they might encourage patients and caregivers to express their perspectives on postdischarge needs and preferences, encourage them to ask questions about care management before discharge, and refer them to resources for getting questions answered or concerns addressed following discharge.

In spite of better perceived continuity of care, more than half the elders and caregivers in both the intervention and control cohorts reported difficulty evaluating and managing symptoms following hospitalization. Some of the elders who reported no difficulty evaluating symptoms reported having adverse symptoms such as "fluid build up" (edema) but did not seem to associate the symptom with their dietary intake or their medical condition. For instance, elders who had been eating foods high in salt did not realize that sodium contributes to fluid retention or that fluid retention is a symptom of heart failure. This suggests that nurses need to teach patients and caregivers not only about the symptoms and what to do to promote comfort or relief, but also about the process of recognizing symptoms. Because some elders were successful in evaluating symptoms, knowing information about the process they used to evaluate symptoms might help to refine discharge planning interventions.

When readmitted, elders in the partnership model spent fewer days in the hospital than the control group. Perhaps these cohorts were more likely to continue to ask questions about their condition, diet, and medications and consequently received information that helped them manage their care at home.

Caregivers in the intervention cohort may have derived short-term benefits that facilitated their caregiving role. Receiving information about the elder's condition, medication, and diet might have reduced frustrations of caregiving during the first 2 weeks at home and contributed to their positive response to caregiving. It is possible that the reduced frustration might also have impacted the caregivers' mental health and vitality.

Nurse administrators might want to evaluate the feasibility of the partnership model for their facility or consider a system-wide discharge-planning mechanism that incorporates the importance of considering patient preferences and the critical role of caregivers in discharge planning. Implementation of the partnership model's discharge-planning protocol required approximately 20 to 25 minutes of personnel time per elder/caregiver dyad. This included showing the video, having the elder and caregiver complete the DPQ, orienting them to the medication form and structured question guide, and providing information about community services. Although these tasks were conducted by a member of the research team in order to track the time involved and completeness of the intervention components, the dimensions could be incorporated in clinical practice. To do so, however, it would be vital for nurse managers to include documentation and monitoring systems that emphasize the staff nurses role in discharge planning. It is also essential to provide staff with an orientation to discharge planning and the importance of patient and caregiver participation and develop a mechanism for monitoring adverse effects of the discharge planning intervention. Although the intervention cohort in this study did not score worse on any outcome measure than the controls, thereby suggesting the intervention was not harmful, use of the partnership approach with some cultural groups might tear at the fabric of their culture or have an adverse effect such as increasing anxiety or the caregiver's burden. Thoughtful reflection on the cultural practices of populations served by an acute care hospital is a critical element in evaluating the feasibility of using an intervention such as the partnership model.

Nurse educators might want to evaluate the extent to which content on discharge planning and continuity of care is emphasized in the curriculum. What sort of tools do students learn to use to identify and evaluate elders' needs for follow-up care? How well do the students' assessment of the elder's need match the elder's and caregiver's perception of their need? To what extent are patient's preferences for care considered in discharge planning? Although partnering with clients in planning for care is inherent in Standards of Gerontological Nursing, the beginning student or novice practitioner might benefit from a structured guide to help them implement the standards.

Even though the potential cost saving from this approach might be attractive, it is important to consider the limitations of this study. The sample was predominantly White and had, on average, a high-school education. Although participation in planning might have been culturally acceptable for this group, the idea of asking questions of health care professionals might not be considered acceptable in other cultures. Further testing of the tenets of the partnership model with other cultures and with persons hospitalized for other conditions is necessary to delineate the context in which the model works.

Further research is needed to evaluate the long-term benefits of the partnership model. Explicating the process of symptom recognition might provide information for refining the intervention that could have long-term implications for reducing hospital readmissions for elders who have heart failure.

Acknowledgment

This project was funded by the Retirement Research Foundation of Chicago.

References

Berkman, B., Dumas, S., Gastfriend, J., Poplawski, J., & Southworth, M. (1987). Predicting hospital readmission of elderly patients. *Health and Social Work, 12*, 221-228.

Brooten, D., Naylor, M., Brown, L., York, R., Hollingsworth, A., Cohen, S., Roncoli, M. & Jacobsen, B. (1996). Profile of postdischarge rehospitalization and acute care visits for seven patient groups. *Journal of Public Health Nursing, 13*(2), 128-134.

Bull, M.J. (1994a). Use of formal community services by elders and their family caregivers two weeks following hospital discharge. *Journal of Advanced Nursing, 19*, 503-508.

Bull, M.J. (1994b). Patients' and professionals' perceptions of quality in discharge planning. *Journal of Nursing Care Quality, 8*(2), 47-61.

Bull, M.J. (1994c). A discharge planning questionnaire for clinical practice. *Applied Nursing Research, 7*(4), 193-207.

Bull, M.J., Maruyama, G., & Luo, D. (1995). Testing a model for posthospital transition of family caregivers. *Nursing Research, 44*(3), 131-138.

Bull, M.J., Luo, D., & Maruyama, G. (1997). Developing an instrument to measure continuity of care for elders. Paper presented at Sigma Theta Tau Biennial Convention, Indianapolis, IN. December 3, 1997.

Bull, M.J., & Kane, R.L. (1996). Gaps in discharge planning. *Journal of Applied Gerontology, 15*(4), 506-520.

Cable, E., & Mayers, L. (1983). Discharge planning effect on length of hospital stay. *Archives of Physical Medical Rehabilitation, 64*, 57-60.

Campion, E., Jette, A., & Berkman, B. (1983). An interdisciplinary geriatric consultation service: A controlled trial. *Journal of the American Geriatrics Society, 31*, 792-796.

Coulton, C., Dunkle, R., Haug, M., Chow, J., & Vielhaber, D. (1989). Locus of control and decision making for posthospital care. *The Gerontologist, 29*, 627-632.

Donabedian, A. (1966). Evaluating the quality of medical care. *Milbank Memorial Fund Quarterly, 44*, 194-196.

Evans, R., Hendricks, R., Lawrence-Umlauf, K., & Bishop, D. (1989). Timing of social work interventions and medical patients' length of hospital stay. *Health and Social Work, 14*(4), 277-282.

Evans, R., & Hendricks, R. (1993). Evaluating hospital discharge planning: A randomized clinical trial. *Medical Care, 31*(4), 358-370.

Fairclough, D. (1997). Summary of measures and statistics for comparison of quality of life in a clinical trial of cancer therapy. *Statistics in Medicine, 16,* 1197-1209.

Given, B., Stommel, M., Collins, C., King, S., & Given, C. (1990). Responses of elderly spouse caregivers. *Research in Nursing and Health, 13,* 7785.

Guerra-Garcia, M., Taffeta, G., & Protas, E. (1997). Considerations related to disability and exercise in elderly women with congestive heart failure. *Journal of Cardiovascular Nursing, 11*(4), 60-74.

Happ, M., Naylor, M., & Roe-Prior, P. (1997). Factors contributing to rehospitalization of elderly patients with heart failure. *Journal of Cardiovascular Nursing, 11*(4), 75-84.

Jewell, S.E. (1993). Discovery of the discharge process: A study of patient discharge from a care unit for elderly people. *Journal of Advanced Nursing, 18,* 1288-1296.

Kahn, R.L., Goldfarb, M., Pollack, M., & Peck, A. (1960). Brief objective measures for the determination of mental status in the aged. *Advanced Journal of Psychiatry, 117,* 326-328.

Kellner, R. (1987). A symptom questionnaire. *Journal of Clinical Psychiatry, 48*(7), 268-274.

Lockery, S., Dunkle, R., Kart, C., & Coulton, C. (1993). Factors contributing to the early rehospitalization of elderly people. *Health & Social Work, 19*(3), 182-191.

Mahoney, C., Ware, J., Rogers, W., Rucksack, A., & Lu, J. (1992). The validity and relative precision of Mos short-and long-form health status scales and Dartmouth coop charts. *Medical Care, 30*(5), MS253-265.

Mistriaen, P., Duijnhouwer, E., Wijkel, D., deBont, M., Veeger, A. (1997). The problems of elderly people at home one week after discharge from the acute care setting. *Journal of Advanced Nursing, 25,* 1233-1240.

National Center for Health Statistics. (1994). *Prevention Profile, Health United States 1993.* Public Health Services, Hyattsville, Maryland.

O'Brien, P. (1984). Procedures for comparing samples with multiple endpoints. *Biometrics 40,* 1079-1087.

Pascoe, G., & Attkisson, C. (1983). The evaluation ranking scale: A new methodology for assessing satisfaction. *Evaluation and Program Planning, 6,* 335-347.

Proctor, E., Morrow-Howell, N., Albaz, R., & Weir, C. (1992). Patient and family satisfaction with discharge plans. *Medical Care, 30*(3), 262-274.

Schrager, J., Halmon, M., Myers, D., Nichols, R., & Rosenblum, L. (1978). Impediments to the course and effectiveness of discharge planning. *Social Work and Health Care, 4*(1), 65-79.

U.S. Department of Health and Human Services. Public Health Service. (1994) *Heart Failure: Evaluation and Care of Patients With Left-Ventricular Systolic Dysfunction.* Rockville, MD: Agency for Health Care Policy Research.

Wallston, K., Wallston, B., Devellis, R., & Peabody. (1978). Development of the multidimensional health locus of control (MHLC) scales. *Health Education Monographs, 6*(2), 160-170.

Ware, J., & Sherbourne, D. (1992). The Mos 36-item short-form health survey (SF36). *Medical Care, 30,* 473-483.

Appendix B

From *Oncology Nursing Forum* 27(3): 473-480, 2000.

Bone Marrow Transplantation: The Battle for Hope in the Face of Fear

Marlene Zichi Cohen, PhD, RN
John S. Dunn, Sr., Distinguished Professor in Oncology Nursing,
University of Texas Health Science Center,
School of Nursing;
Coordinator of Applied Nursing Research,
M.D. Anderson Cancer Center,
University of Texas,
Houston, TX

Cathaleen Dawson Ley, RN, MN
Doctoral student,
University of Maryland,
School of Nursing,
Baltimore, MD

Purpose/Objectives: To describe patients' experience of having an autologous bone marrow transplantation (BMT).

Design: Hermeneutic phenomenologic, descriptive, and interpretive.

Setting: Outpatient treatment area of a comprehensive cancer center in the Southwest.

Sample: 20 adult survivors of autologous BMT, 15 women and 5 men, with a mean age of 46 years.

Methods: Content analysis of verbatim transcriptions of open-ended interviews using hermeneutic phenomenology, which combines descriptive and interpretive phenomenology.

Conclusions: These patients illustrate that fear, a predominant reality when undergoing autologous BMT, is balanced with hope for survival. The overarching fear, fear of death, often was related to the unknown, including cancer recurrence. The fear of the unknown also came from being unprepared physically and emotionally. Losses were intertwined with these fears and included loss of both control and trust in one's body. Patients discussed fear of leaving the hospital and not having someone "constantly looking at you to make sure that the cancer isn't back." These fears and losses changed patients' view of life and led to a need for help in bringing closure to the experience.

Implications for Nursing Practice: Specific nursing actions to help allay fear include providing information about both feelings and procedures, giving opportunities to discuss fears and losses, arranging meetings with others who have had a BMT or suggesting an appropriate support group, and including family in all interventions, as appropriate. Reducing fears with these interventions helped patients maintain hope. By understanding the relationship between hope and fear, nurses caring for people having BMT can use specific strategies to decrease fear, hence increasing hope in patients. Nursing education can emphasize the need to adequately prepare patients. Further research is indicated to explore the effectiveness of interventions to prepare patients for BMT and the interplay between hope and fear.

Key Points . . .

- Maintaining hope for patients with cancer is a nursing challenge.
- Fear, specifically of the unknown and death, is a usual and appropriate reaction to the prospect of undergoing bone marrow transplant (BMT).
- No amount of pre-BMT preparation is sufficient to help patients understand what to expect;

however, creative efforts should be employed to give patients some idea of what is to come.

- The extent to which fears can be allayed will help determine the ability of the individual to maintain hope.

> *Faith—is the pierless bridge*
> *Supporting what We see*
> *Unto the Scene that We do not.*
> —Emily Dickinson

Bone marrow transplantation (BMT) rapidly is becoming a standard treatment for a variety of malignant and hematologic diseases. In 1995, 29,000 BMTs were performed worldwide, as compared to only 10 years earlier when less than 4,000 were performed (International Bone Marrow Transplant Registry, 1996). The number of autologous BMTs has increased annually and currently surpasses the number of allogeneic BMTs performed (International Bone Marrow Transplant Registry). The need to focus research efforts on the long-term psychological and social factors involved in autologous BMT has become more evident.

A number of studies in the past 15 years have examined the impact of BMT on patients' quality of life, physical and psychological status, and psychosocial adjustment. Several comprehensive reviews have been published (Andrykowski, 1994; Hjermstad & Kaasa, 1995; Whedon & Ferrell, 1994).

In addition, several studies were designed to understand the perspective of BMT recipients. Shuster, Steeves, Onega, and Richardson (1996) used hermeneutic inquiry to describe the meaning of BMT for hospitalized patients. The patients' struggle with their disease and with the BMT process was seen as a fight between body (nature) and mind (culture). The body was perceived as a source of the problem as well as the cure. In addition, patients perceived the body as an entity that could heal itself and the mind as an entity that could produce an attitude that would not interfere with the body's healing process.

Steeves (1992) also used a hermeneutic approach to explore the process of "meaning making" and life interpretation with a group of BMT recipients. Two major themes were identified: negotiating a new social position and struggling to understand the experience. Feelings of loss of control were expressed as well as a willingness to relinquish power to physicians in the belief that physicians would tell patients what they needed to know. The medical center was viewed as a "safe haven"; consequently, patients feared leaving the protective environment of the inpatient setting upon discharge.

Although these studies have provided useful information about aspects of patients' perspectives of the BMT process, only one informant in these previous interpretive studies had an autologous BMT; all others had allogeneic transplants. Another difference is that treatments and survival statistics continue to change considerably. Further research is needed to explore the lived experience of patients who have undergone autologous BMT and to address the question of how nurses can provide the most effective care to these patients. Phenomenologic philosophy guided this investigation of the experience of patients undergoing autologous BMT to better understand the effect of this treatment on their lives and how nursing care can best meet their needs.

METHODS

Hermeneutic phenomenologic research, which combines features of descriptive and interpretive phenomenology, guided this study (Cohen, Kahn, & Steeves [in press]; van Manen, 1994). Phenomenologic inquiry was used to explore patient experiences with the autologous BMT process by people who had undergone this procedure at a comprehensive cancer center. This in-depth exploration of patients' perspectives of having an autologous BMT provides useful insights into their perspectives. A number of themes emerged from these data; however, this article will focus on themes related to fears and hope. Other themes have been reported elsewhere (Cohen, Headley, & Sherwood [in press]; Tarzian, Iwata, & Cohen, 1999).

Sample

All patients who had undergone and survived an autologous BMT on a relatively new and small hospital unit were asked to participate. The five patients who were unwilling to participate all said they did not have time for the interviews.

Procedure

Interviews were conducted in a private room at the hospital after participants signed informed consents. Measures were taken to protect anonymity, such as altering identifying information. In this article, pseudonyms have replaced references to proper names.

An opening question guided patient interviews: "What was it like to have a bone marrow transplant?" Patients described their experience of having an autologous BMT. The interview questions were as open as possible to ensure that the content discussed was determined by the person being interviewed rather than the interviewer. Reflections of what the informant said were used to encourage the person to continue. Commonly used probes were "Please say more about that"; "What did that mean to you?"; "How did you feel about that?"; and "How was that helpful (or not helpful)?" Cohen conducted the interviews and also worked with graduate students to train and supervise them throughout the process to ensure interviews were equivalent.

Data Analysis and Interpretation

Texts were analyzed following the hermeneutic phenomenologic approach based on the Utrecht School of phenomenology (van Manen, 1994). The researchers immersed themselves in the data, listened to the tapes, and read the verbatim transcripts several times. Transcripts were examined line-by-line, and tentative theme names were penciled in the margins. The narrative passages then were grouped or clustered under the tentative theme names. This procedure was followed for each participant. The passages and themes were compared with passages and themes of all other informants, across themes, and with other passages in the same theme.

To reduce bias and increase data accuracy and trustworthiness in the findings, the interviewers were not members of the autologous BMT staff. Patients were assured that what they said would not be reported to the staff in a way that identified either the patient or staff members. In addition, themes were cross-validated with other researchers, and an agreement of identified themes was achieved.

FINDINGS

Subjects

Twenty patients were interviewed, 15 women and 5 men, with a mean age of 46 years. The mean number of months post-autologous BMT was 16 (range = 2-49.5 months). The patients were well educated, with at least a high school education, and approximately half were professionals. Patients were primarily Caucasian but included two African Americans, two Asian Americans, one Latina, and one Greek. Nine had breast cancer, six had lymphoma, two had leukemia, two had myeloma, and one had Hodgkin's disease.

Fear of Death and Hope for Survival

The prevailing theme of the participants in this study was the experience of being fearful. Surprisingly, little literature on BMT addresses the topic of fear in patients in general and fear in patients undergoing autologous BMT specifically. Monika, a 50-year-old woman, poignantly discussed her fear of having an autologous BMT.

I was very sick, but something inside me kept thinking, well I have to do that bone marrow, and I was terrified. I was very scared. I'm a chicken. I'm such a coward to begin with. I'm very chicken. I was more scared than anything. And I think I was scared I wasn't going to make it through. . . . I wanted to run away. Bone marrow transplant, just the word itself . . . I've had a few things in my life that were pretty bad, but this had to have been one of the worst things I've had to face. And you're still facing it. You still do. I know they've done absolutely everything they can do and so far so good. I come in for my checkups and it's okay. I do a lot of praying, a lot of praying. But I was afraid.

This statement embodies the overriding fear of dying that study participants identified. All of the participants, regardless of age, gender, ethnicity, or length of time since autologous BMT, articulated a fear of death. Participants vividly recalled and discussed their fears of dying from the procedure.

If the fear of dying was so strong, why did these individuals choose to undergo an autologous BMT? The hope alluded to in Monika's statement ("so far so good . . .") may begin to answer that question. Ned, a 55-year-old man, summarized his rationale for having the autologous BMT by reasoning that selecting an autologous BMT was not a choice but, instead, the "last best chance of survival." In their quest for survival, patients had unsuccessfully pursued all other treatment options. With no other treatment options remaining, an autologous BMT was the final treatment option that offered hope for recovery. Amanda, a 62-year-old woman whose lymphoma had recurred, expressed her feelings.

So in my mind there was never any question but that I would have it. I just thought, it's the only way to stay alive . . . made me realize that I probably wouldn't live long if I didn't have a bone marrow transplant. So I approached it. It interrupted my life, but, on the other hand, I would have probably died had I didn't have a bone marrow transplant.

Despite their fears about dying, the participants believed the probability of dying without the autologous BMT seemed certain. Eileen, a 47-year-old mother of three young children, expressed the realization that undergoing an autologous BMT was the only choice remaining if she hoped to live to raise her children.

You're weighing the unknown with the known and, yet, you don't know the time frame of the unknown. But, what I had to tell myself was, okay, you've got a 15% (chance of survival), but then you got an 85% chance of coming out dead. It's like, would you get on an airplane if they said there's a 15% chance it will not crash? Could you think that there's an 85% chance that it wouldn't (work)? No, you wouldn't choose to make that . . . I was not in that position. . . . I know that if I didn't do it, if I didn't take that 15% chance, I would crash eventually.

Fear of the Unknown: Uncharted Physical, Mental, and Emotional Territory

The threat to survival was magnified by the fear of not knowing what to expect either during the autologous BMT procedure or recovery. Partici-

pants frequently expressed the feeling of not being prepared physically or emotionally for what laid ahead. Ana, a 44-year-old woman, was quite unprepared for the intensity of the autologous BMT, despite previously undergoing both a radical mastectomy and chemotherapy.

That was a big surprise to me that the emotional feelings about the whole experience would be so strong, would last so long. Maybe they're lasting a long time because they never really got released anywhere. . . . You let it out a little tiny bit at a time. I didn't realize that the chemotherapy would be so difficult as it was physically and mentally and emotionally. It was very, very difficult.

Ana, like other participants, expressed anger toward the nursing staff for not being honest about the intensity of pain that was experienced during the procedure. Use of euphemisms such as "pressure" and "discomfort" to describe pain failed to adequately prepare the participants. Instead, "sugarcoating" the experience only seemed to amplify the fear.

The transplant—I didn't expect it to be as scary as it was. Because when it was being described to me, some of the symptoms that were described to me were with using words like discomfort, and that doesn't begin to describe it. That's like going to the dentist and he says 'You're going to feel a little pressure,' and then he sticks the drill right where the nerve is. That is not pressure. That is pain. I think that surprised me because some of the words that were used were "discomfort" and 'you won't have an appetite' when, in fact, it isn't 'you won't have an appetite,' it's 'you will be throwing up constantly.' It isn't "discomfort," it's "pain."

In addition to not being prepared for the intensity of pain experienced during the procedure, participants expressed distress at not knowing how long they would suffer with pain post-treatment. Monika recalled the fear she experienced because she did not know that the pain would last so long following treatment.

You don't know what to expect. Stem cells? What the heck is that? (Having a catheter inserted for stem cell administration) was painful for me. This was painful for me. The only thing I wished they had told me was that the pain was going to last longer than what it was, 'cause I kept saying 'five days, it should be gone.' It was two weeks! That went on for a long time. But after that, it was fine. And going through that was fine, but you know you're working all the way up to this big major thing. . . . It's overwhelming.

When not given adequate advance preparation, even relatively minor procedures became fraught with fear and apprehension about what to expect. Monika described how she became tormented with fear during a urinary catheterization procedure because of a lack of information about what to expect.

What are they going to do? Then to think they put the catheter in you. And I thought, 'Oh my God, one more thing.' You know, you're not even halfway over. I made it bigger than what it was . . . I thought it was just going to be terrible.

This fear of the unknown was related not only to a perception of being unprepared but also to the commonly accepted belief that each patient's experience was unique. Many patients expressed the idea that each autologous BMT experience is unique because everyone is different and, therefore, many believed it was impossible to fully prepare beforehand. Maintaining this belief was analogous to groping through the dark on an uncharted course with the image of unfathomable pain and suffering lurking ahead. Odessa, a 37-year-old woman who had undergone a mastectomy and chemotherapy within 15 months prior to having the autologous BMT, articulated this fear.

The chemo itself wasn't worrisome. I was scared about the BMT because I didn't know what that would be like. Chemo I had gone through, and I just figured it would be worse, but it was a known quantity. To me, the things that were the most scary were the ones that I hadn't gone through and I had no idea what it would be like.

Paradoxically, although too little preparation or the wrong type of information left patients feeling unprepared and terrified of the prospects that laid ahead, too much information was considered equally intimidating. The consent-for-treatment form was described as a particularly "disturbing piece of paper" because it contained details of every "remotely possible adverse reaction." Participants expressed being "scared" and "terrified" after reading the document. Eileen cogently asserted her feelings.

Terrified—I mean, I think that's just a normal part of it. I mean, yes, I was terrified. I mean, just looking at that consent form is enough to make you turn and run.

An especially grievous experience for the participants was the recollection of being handed the consent form shortly before the procedure and being expected not to be frightened, as was 46-year-old Connie's experience.

And then when I went in for the transplant, I get this paper, five-page letter like this, and they're like, 'read it over.' I read it over. After I read it I said, 'I'm not having it. No way.' And they're like 'you have one hour, because we're starting the general.' And I said, 'I'm not signing it.' I mean, they give you the worst possible thing that could happen to you, and I said that's not fair because no one told me this a month ago before I came prepared. So that, to me, was scary.

However, even when given information to prepare for the procedure and the recovery, the participants expressed the belief that no amount of education could have fully prepared them for the intensity of the experience of undergoing an autologous BMT. Despite having previous invasive and painful procedures that may have been equally life threatening, the participants approached the autologous BMT with more apprehension than previous procedures. Connie explained.

I didn't know really what to expect. I think that when you go through a treatment, although it is explained, I think you really don't know what you're getting yourself into until you're in the midst of it. You really don't know what the feeling is going to be like. You might know the semantics of this is going to happen, your counts are going to go low, they are going to take you to the brink of death, and they're going to give you four days of chemotherapy. Well, even though I had chemotherapy with the five different treatments I had, I had no way of knowing the severity of it and how I would feel for so many days. I think you have to go through it to really be able to know.

Loss of Control

This sense of not knowing what to expect because of inadequate or inappropriate preparation contributed significantly to a feeling of loss of control over one's life. Participants, therefore, believed that a measure of control could have been regained if they had been adequately prepared in advance. Ana discussed the need to preserve personal control through knowledge.

I think the worst thing that happens, and maybe that's just by my standards, is you lose control over your life or your lifestyle or your quality of life. You lose control. And the more you know the less control you will lose. If you know everything there is to know about how to prepare for an earthquake, and you prepare for it appropriately and you are very, very knowledgeable, then when and if it happens, I'd like to think you won't be in as bad of shape. You won't lose as much control. But if you're totally oblivious to it, you've never even heard of an earthquake, and you're in the middle of an earthquake, you're just going to go stark-raving mad. You're going to go bananas, you're going to have no control whatsoever. I think that's the same kind of thing with any medical procedure, including a bone marrow transplant.

Loss of control of bodily functioning was a particularly devastating experience for some of the participants. Feelings of vulnerability, personal exposure, and shame were described when recounting the memory of no longer having control. Monika revealed feelings of vulnerability and embarrassment about vomiting during treatment.

I used to be afraid I would get sick during the treatment, and I'd be so embarrassed if I ever had to start throwing up. I don't know if it bothers anyone else but it does me. And then you're in this room with all these people and then you think 'Oh my God, I can't let anything like that happen.' I mean it's bad enough you're in there. You have no hair. You have no eyelashes. You have no eyebrows. You have this ridiculous thing on your head cause you don't want to walk around bald and then you have to worry about 'am I going to vomit here in front of everybody?' Well, it happened once. And I just was in tears. I felt terrible, and they weren't fast enough to close those curtains, and people were around me.

Witnessing the dramatic physical changes in their bodies post-autologous BMT brought forth a wide range of painful emotions in patients, ranging from bewilderment to shock. Cindy, a 28-year-old woman diagnosed with leukemia, recalled the horror she experienced post-treatment.

I got to the point where I couldn't hardly talk. I couldn't move my hands. I couldn't dress myself. The skin when it turned—it was like laying out in the sun for four days bare naked. You just got this major sunburn everywhere. Everywhere . . . under your arms, everywhere. You turn beet red and it all fell off. My fingerprints fell off. Every-

thing fell off. I still don't have any hair. Then all my hair fell out, eyelashes, everything.

In addition to loss of control from physical changes, some spoke of the emotional loss of control resulting from the loss of dignity they experienced while going through treatment. Ana felt that having an autologous BMT was so difficult that she would not put herself through it again.

I wouldn't go through it again because of the discomfort, and I wouldn't go through it again because of the emotional . . . I couldn't live through the emotional difficulty of it. I couldn't go through that again. I don't think I could come through it a second time. I don't think I could be a trooper for that long, that hard, again. I wouldn't put my family through that. I guess my feeling is if it didn't work, I would rather just deal with the consequences. There were so many times during the bone marrow transplant that I just wanted to give up because I felt like just give me some dignity. There was such lack of dignity that you suffer through. You lose control of your bowels. You lose control of everything. Physically you lose control of everything. You have nothing that you can control. You can't control your emotions. You can't control whether you're awake or semiconscious. You can't control your bodily functions and it's just . . . I couldn't go through it again. I wouldn't.

All the participants, however, did not hold this view. Others, such as Eileen, felt that despite the hardship she had endured, the BMT had saved her life, and she felt grateful for this.

I think I am a better person for it in that I do appreciate maybe more. I appreciate life more. I'm not the least bit vindictive or 'Woe is me, oh why did this have to happen to me?' Anything like that. I'm just grateful that I'm here. And I realize that if it hadn't been for this, I wouldn't be here.

Fear of Discharge/Fear of Recurrence

Being discharged was a time of great ambivalence. Participants described being torn between longing to return to the "outside world" again and fearing leaving the hospital setting. Within the hospital, a perceived sense of security existed as they were under the constant watchful eyes of the staff members if their cancer should reemerge. Once discharged from this protected environment, a sense of vulnerability and lingering fear replaced this security.

After the bone marrow transplant and the radiation, it's like, for a while you feel like Dr. Jekyll and Mr. Hyde because a part of you says 'I'm so glad to be finished with it, and if I never see that place again it will be too soon' type of thing. So part of you feels that way. And then another part of you feels that you have an umbilical cord to this place and you're terrified not to be here, because as long as you're here, somebody constantly is looking at you to make sure that the cancer isn't back. And so you're terrified, I suppose, like a kid whose parents tell him he has to move out of the house. You're terrified that "how do I know it isn't growing back right this very second." Nobody is looking at it.

Once discharged, a persistent concern occurred about the length of time it took to recover and feel "normal again." Steve, a 62-year-old man with multiple myeloma, was three months post-autologous BMT and expressed concern for the pace of his recovery.

The only thing that you're not sure of after you go through it and you get home . . . I think I should be getting well faster but everybody tells me (that after) what you've been through you shouldn't. I think that's the thing, you've just got to be patient. . . . I'm not gaining weight. I know I'm feeling better and I'm looking better, but you want to know if you're doing what everybody else does. Are you advancing as fast? And of course, is it working?

This heightened awareness of symptoms fueled the anguish and fear of the return of cancer. Lorraine, a 54-year-old woman with an aggressive form of lymphoma, revealed her feelings.

Going home was traumatic. It was traumatic. It was wonderful to be home, but (I) feel very frail and fragile. I think you have a lot of time to think of all the terrible things that could be going on inside your body as you lay there at home. All of a sudden you go from people checking on you every half hour to going through a 24-hour day with a lot of time on your hands.

Participants described living with the dread that their cancer would return. Slight aches and pains and occasional lack of appetite that might be ignored by people who had not had cancer became threatening. A year following her autologous BMT, Eileen still became alarmed by changes she experienced in her appetite.

It was very strange because I had never had trouble with appetite. In fact, I was always the opposite, you know. How could I not eat? And so that kind of alarmed me, because, being that I always wanted to eat more than I should, you know, suddenly not wanting food was worrisome to me.

Living with the dread of the cancer recurring did not appear to abate with time. Instead, the experience of having an autologous BMT and living with uncertainty was described as a life-altering experience. Lorraine revealed, "It was momentous, because it made everything seem more mortal. Made me feel more mortal having a bone marrow transplant." The participants' perceptions of their personal security and continued existence became profoundly and irrevocably altered. They experienced an elevated awareness of both life's finiteness and the fragility of human life. For Eileen, living daily with an unceasing awareness of her own mortality was experienced as a loss.

It's like a loss because there's always like an emptiness because something has been lost. Whether it's just time, a breast, or whatever, there's always that element of a little bit of fear . . . which, really, any of us should have. You know it's like . . . just take a room full of people, and no one should have a feeling that everything's going to be fine tomorrow. And yet, we all, until something's happened, we all operate under this false sense of security. But once something has happened, like this, it's kind of like, the bubble's been burst. We realize that something could happen, because it has. So we always have that element of fear, where (others) don't have that. Not because they shouldn't have it, but because they've never had to deal with it.

For Ana, the loss was experienced as a lack of closure, a feeling of emotions not tended to, of losses not grieved.

I suppose if I was going to talk about educating the family and educating the patients, I would go beyond the transplant and try to educate them as well on how to bring closure. I don't think anybody does that. I don't think there's anybody that gives you any information or helps you or works with you through closure. Closure appears to be an individual, independent, whatever you do with it, and if you don't do anything with it, then I guess you don't have closure. Nobody seems to address it.

The trust in one's body is also lost. Following cancer, the body is no longer viewed as being sheltered from disease or even death. Eileen discussed her shifted view of her body—once trusted, now emphatically distrusted.

I don't trust my body, no. I am really a positive person, but it's failed me once, you know? It's like I don't have control. I always felt like I had my control and I think that control, once you face this, you've lost control, I mean, it's taken away from you. And so, I don't think I'll ever really trust (my body) again. I trust in my mind that I can kind of, you know, calm myself down, this kind of thing. But as far as the body, I've kind of lost that confidence.

DISCUSSION AND IMPLICATIONS

These patients illustrate that fear, a predominate reality when undergoing autologous BMT, is balanced with hope for survival. The overarching fear, fear of death, often was related to the unknown, including cancer recurrence. The fear of the unknown also came from being unprepared or inappropriately prepared physically and emotionally. Losses were intertwined with these fears and included loss of both control and trust in one's body. Patients discussed fear of leaving the hospital and not having someone "constantly looking at you to make sure that the cancer isn't back." These fears and losses changed their view of life and led to a need for help in bringing closure to the experience.

Fear in cancer survivors has been discussed extensively. Other researchers have found that cancer survivors fear recurrence (Fredette, 1995; Wong & Bramwell, 1992; Wyatt, Kurtz, & Liken, 1993). Northouse (1981) found that patients who had fewer significant others with whom they could discuss mastectomy-related apprehensions had higher levels of recurrence anxieties. In addition, patients who felt that their concerns were understood by significant others had less fear of recurrence. These fears underscore the value in assessing, eliciting, listening to, and understanding the concerns of autologous BMT patients.

Fear and anxiety associated with being discharged also have received continuing attention. Steeves (1992) and Gorzynski and Holland (1979) found patients with cancer feared leaving the protection of the hospital. Thomas, Glynne-Jones, Chait, and Marks (1997) found that 31% of a sample of 65 long-term cancer survivors attending an outpatient oncology clinic in the United Kingdom suffered from anxiety, a percentage level no different from anxiety levels of patients with active cancer. In Thomas et al.'s sample, 28% of the patients refused to be discharged from the clinic because they feared cancer recurrence would go undetected if they were discharged.

The losses these participants described also have been discussed. Nurses have identified nausea as a source of patient suffering because it is a precursor to vomiting and the act of vomiting in the presence of others was considered a humiliating act (Kahn & Steeves, 1995). These informants also discussed embarrassment about loss of physical control.

These patients talked about fear of the unknown, lack of preparation, and the need for accurate information about feelings, both physical and emotional. Whereas the primary intervention for nurses to use with patients when fears are discussed is active listening, the fear of the unknown calls for different interventions.

Johnson, Fieler, Jones, Wlasowicz, and Mitchell's (1997) research and self-regulation theory may provide direction for selecting the type of information that may be most useful to patients undergoing autologous BMT. Nursing interventions derived from self-regulation theory have shown that preparatory information that is concrete and objective assists patients. Concrete objective information includes physical sensations and symptoms, temporal characteristics, environmental features, and causes of sensation, symptoms, and experience (Johnson et al.). What is smelled, heard, tasted, felt, and seen encompasses the physical sensations and symptoms experienced. The duration and sequence of events are temporal characteristics. These can include how long pain is expected to last and when side effects begin, both of which are issues discussed by participants in this research. The characteristics of the treatment room and the people in the patient's surroundings are the environmental features. The cause of sensations, symptoms, and experiences needs to be explained so that no misunderstandings of the experience occur. Providing information that is concrete and objective enhances patients' understanding of what is happening to them. As patients in this study noted, fear of death from cancer recurrence was triggered by fear of the unknown. Although eliminating the fear of death is unlikely, concrete information could increase control. As Ana noted, "The more you know, the less control you will lose."

A complete description of an upcoming, stressful healthcare situation is not required to reduce psychological distress. And, indeed, participants in this study described terror from the details in the consent form. If the preparatory information provided to the patient contains some of the typical concrete, objective features, it will assist in guiding the patient to construct a realistic expectation of the experience (Johnson et al., 1997). As these informants noted, unique aspects exist in each autologous BMT experience. However, many commonalties also were noted, and accurate preparation for these commonalties may help reduce fear. Tarzian et al. (1999) discussed preparing patients for BMT and the need to individualize this preparation.

Research has supported the importance of adequately preparing BMT recipients for what to expect during and after BMT. Andrykowski et al. (1995) studied the psychosocial impact of BMT in adults, who, on average, were 42 months post-BMT. The study indicated that only a minority considered themselves to have "returned to normal." Less-than-normal physical, cognitive, occupational, sexual, and interpersonal functioning was reported. Those who reported the greatest level of psychological distress were those with the highest disparity between the actual and the expected level of functional status. This study's participants also noted feeling fear when symptoms lasted longer than they expected. Hengeveld, Houtman, and Zwann (1988) interviewed patients one to five years post-BMT concerning their emotional experiences and information and support given to them. All 17 patients reported severe emotional strain related to their illness, BMT, and consequences of both. Many patients felt they had been inadequately prepared for the emotional

and sexual problems they encountered following discharge.

Although patients in this study discussed many fears, they were quick to add their hope for survival. Hope among those with cancer has been discussed in some detail in the literature. Fear and hope were linked in a document published by the National Coalition for Cancer Survivors (Clark, 1995). Clark discussed fear of death and recurrence and hope. She noted the need for information and the importance of hope as a prerequisite for action. Hope, which she noted could never be false, is needed to transcend reality. Denial is different in that it avoids reality. She noted that hope changes as situations change and includes consideration of the future.

Professionals have discussed similar views. Morse and Doberneck (1995) discussed similarities and differences in hope among people in different situations. Those with breast cancer were constantly "hoping against hope," continuously battling to keep negative thoughts out. "Dealing with it" and "Keeping it in its place" were the two core categories identified in Ersek's grounded theory study (1992) that were used to describe the process of maintaining hope in adults undergoing BMT for leukemia. "Dealing with it" was defined as the process of facing and permitting the full range of emotions, behavior, and thoughts about the possible negative outcomes of the illness. "Keeping it in its place" was a process that occurred after the seriousness of the disease was recognized and entailed controlling the impact of the illness and the treatment through one's response to both.

Morse and Penrod (1999) also linked hope with the concepts of enduring, uncertainty, and suffering. One difference among these concepts is that hopeful people appreciate the effect of events on their past, present, and future and also have the goals and means, or routes, to move toward those goals. This requires a level of knowledge that is not limited in awareness and includes full comprehension and acceptance.

Bushkin (1993) described her personal battle with cancer. She wrote of the two roads those diagnosed with cancer travel: one is the road of hopelessness and the other is that of courage. One of the positive signposts on the road of courage is that of hope provided by supportive people. "Hope is the light in this land. It is any kind of light: an electric light, a candle, or the sun. It is also the light that comes from the supportive words of other travelers and guides. Without hope, the traveler will be without fuel or energy to walk. Hope and light create warmth and improved vision; but, even more importantly, with light, the traveler can see the road at night" (p. 873). Informants in this study support the idea that when nurses provide adequate preparation, fear of the unknown is reduced, and this promotes hope.

These informants described fears, losses, and hopes along with a sense that the BMT was a life-altering event or a liminal passage. A liminal passage is a transition. Liminal comes from the Latin word *limin,* meaning threshold (Brown, 1993). Birth, death, marriage, and other rites of passage have been described as liminal passages. Liminality is a time when growth and change are more possible because personal boundaries are more permeable (Floyd & Robbie, 1990; Gentry, Kennedy, Paul, & Hill, 1995; Stevens, 1991; Tarzian, 1998). Nurses caring for patients during liminal passages need to be aware that these are times when people are vulnerable, open to transformation, and need to be protected. As these informants demonstrated, how nurses responded to them created powerful memories.

CONCLUSION

Patients identified specific nursing actions as being helpful in allaying fear: provision of knowledge and information and preparation for each step in treatment and recovery. By understanding the relationship between hope and fear, nurses then can use specific strategies to decrease fear and increase hope in autologous BMT patients.

This research contributes to the body of nursing knowledge that supports the importance of patient preparation in reducing fears in patients with cancer. Information and opportunities to discuss fears and losses are important. Because

patients wonder whether they are doing "the same" as others, suggesting appropriate support groups or arranging meetings with someone who had an autologous BMT may be useful. Including family members in all these interventions, as appropriate, also may reduce their fears. Nursing education can emphasize these aspects of patient preparation. Further research is needed to explore the interplay between hope and fear in patients undergoing BMT, as well as in patients living with a life-threatening illness. In addition, research is needed to test the effectiveness of providing patients undergoing autologous BMT with the kind of information called for in self-regulation theory (Johnson et al., 1997).

The informants in this study clearly showed that nurses have a primary role in preparing patients to understand what to expect during this life-changing experience. Inadequate or inappropriate preparation clearly increased fears and interfered with hope. As one informant noted, "It's sort of like when you really want a drink of water, and someone gives you a cup of hot coffee. You know, yes, it's wet, but it's not quite what you need at the time." This underscores the importance of understanding patients' experiences and needs to provide the appropriate care. Stovall (1995) summarized these patients' experiences and provided guidance to nurses: "With communication comes understanding and clarity; with understanding, fear diminishes; in the absence of fear, hope emerges; and in the presence of hope, anything is possible" (p. 789).

The authors acknowledge the patients who participated in the interviews and gave generously of their time. The authors express their appreciation to Anita J. Tarzian, RN, PhD, for her thoughtful review of an earlier version of this article.

References

Andrykowski, M. (1994). Psychosocial factors in bone marrow transplantation: A review and recommendations for research. *Bone Marrow Transplantation, 13,* 357-375.

Andrykowski, M., Brady, M., Greiner, C., Altmaier, E., Burish, T., Antin, J., Gingrich, R., Mc-

Garigle, C., & Henslee-Downey, P. (1995). 'Returning to normal' following bone marrow transplantation: Outcomes, expectations, and informed consent. *Bone Marrow Transplantation, 15,* 573-581.

Brown, L. (Ed.). (1993). *The new shorter Oxford English dictionary.* Oxford, England: Clarendon Press.

Bushkin, E. (1993). Signposts of survivorship. *Oncology Nursing Forum, 20,* 869-875.

Clark, E. (1995). *You have the right to be hopeful.* Silver Spring, MD: National Coalition for Cancer Survivors.

Cohen, M.Z., Headley, J., & Sherwood, G. (in press). Spirituality in bone marrow transplantation: When faith is stronger than fear. *International Journal for Human Caring.*

Cohen, M.Z., Kahn, D., & Steeves, R. (in press). *Hermeneutic phenomenological research: A practical guide for nurse researchers.* Thousand Oaks, CA: Sage.

Ersek, M. (1992). The process of maintaining hope in adults undergoing bone marrow transplantation for leukemia. *Oncology Nursing Forum, 19,* 883-889.

Floyd, D., & Robbie, E. (1990). Obstetrical rituals and cultural anomaly: Part II. *Pre- and Peri-Natal Psychology Journal, 5*(1), 23-39.

Fredette, S. (1995). Breast cancer survivors: Concerns and coping. *Cancer Nursing, 18,* 35-46.

Gentry, J., Kennedy, P., Paul, C., & Hill, R. (1995). Family transitions during grief: Discontinuities in household consumption patterns. *Journal of Business Research, 34*(1), 67-79.

Gorzynski, J., & Holland, J. (1979). Psychological aspects of testicular cancer. *Seminars in Oncology, 6,* 125-129.

Hengeveld, M., Houtman, R., & Zwann, F. (1988). Psychological aspects of bone marrow transplantation: A retrospective study of 17 long-term survivors. *Bone Marrow Transplantation, 3,* 69-75.

Hjermstad, M.J., & Kaasa, S. (1995). Quality of life in adult cancer patients treated with bone marrow transplantation—A review of the literature. *European Journal of Cancer, 31A*(2), 163-173.

International Bone Marrow Transplant Registry. (1996). *IBMTR annual number of blood and marrow transplants worldwide, 1970-1995.* Retrieved from the World Wide Web: http://www.biostat.mcw.edu/IBMTR/

Johnson, J., Fieler, V., Jones, L., Wlasowicz, G., & Mitchell, M.L. (1997). *Self-regulation theory: Applying theory to your practice.* Pittsburgh: Oncology Nursing Press, Inc.

Kahn, D.L., & Steeves, R.H. (1995). The significance of suffering in cancer care. *Seminars in Oncology Nursing, 11,* 9-16.

Morse, J., & Doberneck, B. (1995). Delineating the concept of hope. *Image: Journal of Nursing Scholarship, 27,* 277-285.

Morse, J., & Penrod, J. (1999). Linking concept of enduring, uncertainty, suffering, and hope. *Image: Journal of Nursing Scholarship, 31,* 145-150.

Northouse, L. (1981). Mastectomy patients and the fear of cancer recurrence. *Cancer Nursing, 6,* 213-220.

Shuster, G., Steeves, R., Onega, L., & Richardson, B. (1996). Coping patterns among bone marrow transplant patients: A hermeneutical inquiry. *Cancer Nursing, 19,* 290-297.

Steeves, R. (1992). Patients who have undergone bone marrow transplantation: Their quest for meaning. *Oncology Nursing Forum, 19,* 899-905.

Stevens, P. (1991). Play and liminality in rites of passage: From elder to ancestor in West Africa. *Play and Culture, 4,* 119-123.

Stovall, E. (1995). Self-advocacy and cancer survivorship. *Illness, Crisis, and Loss, 5*(1), 199-203.

Tarzian, A.J. (1998). *Breathing lessons: An exploration of caregiver experiences with dying patients who have air hunger.* Unpublished doctoral dissertation. University of Maryland, Baltimore.

Tarzian, A.J., Iwata, P.A., & Cohen, M.Z. (1999). Autologous bone marrow transplantation: The patient's perspective of information needs. *Cancer Nursing, 22,* 103-110.

Thomas, S., Glynne-Jones, R., Chait, I., & Marks, D. (1997). Anxiety in long-term cancer survivors influences the acceptability of planned discharge from follow-up. *Psycho-Oncology, 6,* 190-196.

van Manen, M. (1994). *Researching lived experience: Human science for an action sensitive pedagogy.* Ontario, Canada: Althouse Press.

Whedon, M., & Ferrell, B.R. (1994). Quality of life in adult bone marrow transplant patients: Beyond the first year. *Seminars in Oncology Nursing, 10,* 42-57.

Wong, C., & Bramwell, L. (1992). Uncertainty and anxiety after mastectomy for breast cancer. *Cancer Nursing, 15,* 363-371.

Wyatt, G., Kurtz, M., & Liken, M. (1993). Breast cancer survivors: An exploration of quality of life issues. *Cancer Nursing, 16,* 440-448.

For More Information . . .

- American Bone Marrow Donor Registry
  http://www.abmdr.org/
- BMT Talk
  http://www.ai.mit.edu/people/laurel/Bmt-talk/bmt-talk.html
- Bone Marrow Donors
  http://www.bmdw.org/

These Web sites are provided for information only. The hosts are responsible for their own content and availability. Links can be found using ONS Online at www.ons.org.

Appendix C

From *Research in Nursing & Health* 23, 17-24, 2000.

POSITIVE AND NEGATIVE OUTCOMES OF ANGER IN EARLY ADOLESCENTS*

Noreen E. Mahon
Professor,
College of Nursing, Rutgers,
The State University of New Jersey,
Newark, NJ

Adela Yarcheski
Professor,
College of Nursing, Rutgers,
The State University of New Jersey,
Newark, NJ

Thomas J. Yarcheski
Associate Professor,
Department of Professional Management,
St. Thomas University,
Miami, FL

Abstract: *The purposes of this study were to examine symptom patterns and diminished general well-being as negative outcomes and vigor and change as positive outcomes of trait and state anger via two structural equation models. In a school auditorium, a convenience sample of 141 boys and girls, ages 12-14 years, responded to the Trait Anger Scale and the State Anger Scale and to instruments measuring general well-being, symptom patterns, vigor, and change. In the negative outcome model, results indicated that diminished general well-being and increased symptom patterns were outcomes of trait anger and state anger in early adolescents. In the positive outcome model, contrary to expectation, less vigor and less inclination to change were outcomes of trait anger in early adolescents, while state anger had no appreciable influence on the same variables. The findings suggest that anger, particularly trait anger, had a negative influence on the outcome variables studied.* (© 2000 John Wiley & Sons, Inc. *Res Nurs Health* 23:17-24, 2000)

Keywords: anger; well-being; symptoms; vigor; change; early adolescents

Theorists have described early adolescence as a developmental period of great stress, high vulnerability, mood changes, and emotional lability (Blos, 1962; Hamburg, 1974; Hartzell, 1984). More recently, theorists identified the emotion of anger as a major issue of concern during early adolescence (Pipher, 1994; Wilde, 1996). Yet, anger is underexamined in early adolescents, and study of either negative or positive outcomes of anger has been neglected in the empirical literature for this age group.

The negative outcomes of anger are clearly delineated in the theoretical literature. However, there is a paucity of research on the health outcomes of anger in early adolescents, such as diminished well-being and the manifestations of symptoms (Gaylin, 1984; Novaco, 1985, 1986), leaving open to question the risks of anger for this age group. The positive outcomes of anger, such as feelings of vigor and inclination to change (Freeberg, 1982; Gaylin, 1984; Izard, 1977, 1991; Lerner, 1975; Novaco, 1976), also are clearly delineated in the theoretical literature. Studies of the positive outcomes of anger in early adolescents are virtually nonexistent in the empirical literature, also leaving open to question the benefits of anger for this age group. Thus, the purposes of this study were to examine symptom patterns and diminished general well-being as negative outcomes of trait and state anger and to examine vigor and change as positive outcomes of trait and state anger in early adolescents.

A widely used conceptualization of anger is the one by Spielberger and colleagues (1983), which makes a distinction between state anger and trait anger. Trait anger is defined as the disposition of individuals to perceive a wide range of situations as frustrating or annoying, tending to respond to such situations with elevations in state anger. Spielberger (1996) defined state anger as "an emotional state marked by subjective feelings that vary in intensity from mild annoyance or irritation to intense fury and rage" (p. 1), which is generally accompanied by muscle tension and activation of the autonomic nervous system.

Spielberger (1972) has argued that personality traits and states, such as trait anger and state anger, reflect different types of psychological constructs. His theory points out the conceptual differences between traits and states as well as the relationship between them. According to Spielberger, personality traits are relatively enduring individual differences among people to perceive the world in a certain way or in dispositions to behave or react in a specified manner with predictable regularity. Personality traits also reflect individual differences in the frequency and intensity with which certain emotional states have been experienced in the past and differences in the probability that such states will be manifested in the future. Spielberger (1972) stated that "the stronger a particular personality trait, the more probable it is that an individual will experience the emotional state that corresponds to this trait ..." (p. 31). He added that the stronger the personality traits, the more likely that emotional states will be characterized by high levels of intensity. Spielberger suggested

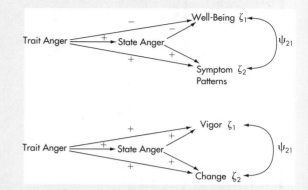

Figure 1. Proposed models for negative and positive outcomes of anger in early adolescents.

that when the state-trait theory is used in research both components should be included so that a fuller understanding of the relationship between the two variables and their relationship to other variables can be obtained. Thus, based on theory, it was hypothesized that trait anger contributes strongly and positively to state anger. In this study, the direct effects of both trait anger and state anger on the negative or positive outcomes and the indirect effects of trait anger through state anger on the same outcomes were estimated using bivariate regression models.

In the first model in the present study (see Figure 1) we examined the extent to which trait anger and state anger are related to diminished well-being and increased symptom patterns, two negative outcomes of anger. Several theorists have proposed an inverse relationship between anger and well-being (Gaylin, 1984; Novaco, 1985, 1986). As Gaylin (1984) indicated, anger is a complex psychophysical phenomenon with wide-ranging implications for physical, mental, and social well-being. Novaco (1985) proposed that many negative effects can result from anger, including impairments to psychological and physical well-being. In support of these theoretical statements, Schlosser (1990) reported an inverse correlation ($r = -.34$, $p < .01$) between trait anger and general well-being in a combined sample of 90 undergraduates, ages 17-19 years, and

87 undergraduates, ages 25-40 years. In the present study, adolescent general well-being was defined as a holistic, multidimensional construct incorporating mental/psychological, physical, and social dimensions (Columbo, 1986). Based on theory and research, it was hypothesized that trait anger and state anger each are inversely related to general well-being in early adolescents.

Perhaps because the biological system is implicated in the experience of anger, Averill (1982) postulated that anger may find an outlet in unusual ways, including psychosomatic disorders and bodily symptoms. Gaylin (1984) theorized that anger can be manifested psychosomatically through the expression of various symptoms. With reference to adolescents, Freeberg (1982) indicated that anger can result in such symptoms as weight loss, anorexia, sleep disturbances, withdrawal, and confusion. In support of these theoretical statements, Larson and Kasimatis (1991) reported positive correlations between anger and physical symptoms such as aches, pains, and gastrointestinal upsets in undergraduate students. Based on theory and research, it was hypothesized that trait anger and state anger each are positively related to symptom patterns. In this study, symptom patterns were defined as physical, psychological, and psychosomatic symptoms (Gurin, Veroff, & Feld, 1960).

Based on the theoretical relationships and empirical findings presented in the above model, it was hypothesized that trait anger has a direct effect on state anger, and that both trait anger and state anger have a direct effect on adolescent general well-being and symptom patterns. Further, it was hypothesized that trait anger has an indirect effect on both general well-being and symptom patterns through state anger (Figure 1).

Novaco (1975) has argued that the positive outcomes of anger often are overlooked due to our concerns about the negative behavioral implications of the concept. Later, Averill (1983) contended that anger is a common negative emotion that can have positive outcomes. In the second model in this study (see Figure 1) we examined the positive influence of trait anger and state anger on vigor and the inclination to change, two positive outcomes of anger.

In 1977, Izard theorized that anger imbues the individual with feelings of vigor, strength, and energy. More recently, Izard (1991) theorized that anger induces a sense of vigor, mobilizes energy for action, and that "we may never feel stronger or more invigorated than when we are really angry" (p. 248). Gaylin (1984) also suggested that anger invigorates the person, and Novaco (1976) proposed that anger increases the vigor with which one acts. The available literature indicates that these theoretical propositions have not been tested empirically in any population. In the present study, vigor was defined as a mood of vigorousness, ebullience, and high energy (McNair, Lorr, & Droppleman, 1992). As derived from theory, it was hypothesized that trait anger and state anger each are positively related to vigor in early adolescents.

A number of theorists have linked anger with the propensity to change. Novaco (1976) proposed that anger is a driving force for efforts at change. Gaylin (1984) suggested that anger has a powerful capacity to initiate internal change. Lerner (1985) argued that anger signals the necessity for change, and Tavris (1982) proposed that anger energizes change. Freeberg (1982) suggested that adolescents who have learned to express anger see themselves as being able to change their lives. An underlying theme in these aforementioned theoretical works is that the change resulting from anger is positive and constructive. The available literature indicates that these theoretical propositions have not been tested empirically in any population. In this study, the inclination to change was defined as seeking new and different experiences, readily changing opinions or values in different circumstances, and adapting readily to changes in the environment (Jackson, 1984). As derived from theory, it was hypothesized that trait anger and state anger each are positively related to change in early adolescents.

Based on the theoretical relationships posited in the above model, it was hypothesized that trait anger has a direct effect on state anger, and that both trait anger and state anger have a direct effect on vigor and inclination to change. Further, it was hypothesized that trait anger has an indirect effect on vigor and inclination to change through state anger (Figure 1).

METHOD

Sample

A sample size of 141 subjects was deemed adequate given the number of variables in each of the structural equation models tested in the present study (Tanaka, 1987). Using the guidelines by Elliott and Feldman (1990), the chronological ages of 12-14 years represented early adolescence in this study. As reported earlier (Yarcheski, Mahon, & Yarcheski, 1999), 180 students were approached to participate in the study; 156 voluntarily agreed to do so. Responses from 15 participants were excluded from the analyses due to incomplete data on some of the variables. The final sample consisted of 141 seventh and eighth graders who were between the ages of 12-14 years ($M = 12.8$; $SD = .61$); 78 were girls and 63 were boys. About 77% were White; the remaining 23% were African-American, Latino, or Asian-American.

Instruments

The State Anger and Trait Anger Scales of the State-Trait Anger Expression Inventory (STAXI) were used to measure state anger and trait anger (Spielberger, 1996). *State anger* is measured by 10 items using a 4-point summated rating scale that assesses the intensity of anger, or how angry one is feeling right now. *Trait anger* is measured by 10 items using a 4-point summated rating scale that assesses the frequency of anger, or how angry one generally feels. Higher scores on each of the measures indicate higher levels of either state anger or trait anger. Normative data on the STAXI is available for adolescents, ages 12-18 years (Spielberger, 1996).

The content validity for the State-Trait Anger Scale was determined by Spielberger et al. (1983) using the definitions of anger either as a person-ality trait or as an emotional state to develop items. Construct validity was assessed by Spielberger et al. (1983) using principal factor analysis with orthogonal rotation, which identified the state-trait anger scales. Fuqua et al. (1991) found a similar factor structure in 455 college students. Spielberger et al. (1983) also reported extensive evidence of concurrent, convergent, and discriminate validity for the scales with various samples. They reported the following alpha coefficient reliabilities for the State Anger Scale: .89 and .88 for female and male high school students, and .95 and .95 for female and male college students. In these same samples, coefficient alphas for the Trait Anger Scale were .82 and .84, and .91 and .89, respectively. In the present sample, the coefficient alphas were .97 for state anger and .89 for trait anger.

The short version of the Adolescent General Well-Being (AGWB) Questionnaire is a 39-item Likert-type scale that assesses the social, physical, and mental/psychological dimensions of well-being (Columbo, 1984). Scores on this 5-point scale can range from 39 to 195; higher scores reflect higher perceived general well-being. Examples of items are "I feel as happy as others" and "I like myself." To establish content validity for the AGWB Questionnaire, Columbo (1984) primarily generated items from his conceptual model of well-being in adolescents; secondarily, he selected items from existing reliable and valid well-being instruments for adolescents. Validity was assessed through multiple statistical analyses, such as item-to-total correlations and multiple factor analyses, all of which were conducted on data obtained from 940 adolescents, ages 14-18 years. Columbo (1984) reported a coefficient alpha of .92 for the 39-item questionnaire in 940 adolescents. Yarcheski, Scoloveno, and Mahon (1994) reported a coefficient alpha of .93 in 99 adolescents, ages 15-17 years. In the present sample, the coefficient alpha was .95.

The Symptom Pattern Scale measures physical, psychological, and psychosomatic manifestations of psychological distress (Gurin et al., 1960). The Symptom Pattern Scale is a 17-item,

5-point summated rating scale. Scores can range from 17 to 85; higher scores indicate the higher occurrence of symptom patterns. The instrument has content validity, and construct validity has been provided through factor analysis, the use of theoretically relevant variables, and the known-groups technique (Gurin et al., 1960). Yarcheski and Mahon (1986) reported a coefficient alpha of .77 for the Symptom Pattern Scale in 136 early adolescents; Yarcheski, Mahon, and Yarcheski (1992) reported a coefficient alpha of .78 for early adolescents; and, Mahon, Yarcheski, and Yarcheski (1993) reported .84 for 325 adolescents, ages 12-21 years. In the present sample, the coefficient alpha was .92.

The Vigor-Activity Subscale of the Profile of Mood States (POMS) is an 8-item adjective checklist that was used to measure vigor (McNair et al., 1992). The subscale is a 5-point summated rating scale. Scores can range from 0 to 32; higher scores indicate higher levels of vigor. McNair et al. (1992) provided evidence of concurrent, predictive, and construct validity, and factor analysis determined the six subscales on the POMS in a variety of healthy and clinical samples. In a study by Lubin et al. (1994), the Vigor-Activity subscale provided evidence of concurrent validity for the Depression Adjective Checklist with two adolescent samples. Internal consistency reliability coefficients for the Vigor-Activity Subscale were .89 and .87 in two studies of clinical samples (McNair et al., 1992). The POMS has been used with adolescents (Furst & Hardman, 1988; Lubin et al., 1994; McGowan, Miller, & Henschen, 1990), but reliabilities were not reported. In the present sample, the coefficient alpha was .80.

The Change Subscale of the Personality Research Form-E was used to measure inclination to change (Jackson, 1984). This subscale consists of 16 true-false items. Scores can range from 0 to 16; higher scores indicate higher levels of change. Examples of items are "When I find a good way to do something, I avoid trying new ways" and "Changes in routine bother me." Theories of personality were used to derive the subscales of the Personality Research Form, providing content validity for the instrument. Convergent validity for the Change Subscale was demonstrated in women and men by correlations of .24 or greater between change and the conceptually related subscales of complexity, innovation, breadth of interest, and tolerance on the Jackson Personality Inventory. Divergent validity was demonstrated by correlations of .12 or lower between change and the conceptually unrelated subscales of social participation and social adroitness. Reddon, Pope, Friel, and Sinha (1996) used the Jackson Personality Inventory with adolescents, ages 14-18 years, but they did not report reliabilities. Jackson (1984) reported a test-retest reliability for the Change Subscale of .69 in 135 subjects, a KR-20 reliability of .86 for 260 subjects, and an odd-even reliability of .65 for 84 college students. In the present sample, the KR-20 was .68.

Procedure

After approval to conduct the study was granted by the university Institutional Review Board, access was gained to an urban middle school. The principal and seventh and eighth grade teachers reviewed and approved the instrument packets for appropriateness of content and reading levels for seventh and eighth graders, except for those in special education classes.

One week prior to testing, all seventh and eighth graders who were not in special education classes received a packet containing an explanation about the study and a consent form for their parents. On the testing date one week later, students who had parental consent and gave informed consent as well participated in the study. Testing took place in the school auditorium where students responded to a demographic data sheet and the study instruments.

RESULTS

Descriptive statistics for the study variables are presented in Table 1. The correlations for the hypothesized relationships are presented in Table 2. Six of the ten relationships hypothesized across the two models were statistically significant. Correlations between trait anger and vigor, state

Table 1. Descriptive Statistics for Study Variables (N = 141)

Variable	M	SD	Range
State anger[a]	16.86	9.56	10-40
Trait anger[a]	22.43	7.70	10-40
Change	8.53	2.85	1-16
Vigor	19.39	7.09	2-32
Symptom patterns	39.44	13.87	17-83
Well-being	138.81	29.80	47-193

[a]From "An Empirical Test of Alternative Theories of Anger in Adolescents," by A. Yarcheski, N. E. Mahon, and T. J. Yarcheski, *Nursing Research*, 1999.

Table 2. Correlations for Hypothesized Relationships in Models 1 and 2 (N = 141)

Variable	State Anger	Trait Anger
Trait anger	.65[a]	—
Vigor	−.26*	−.34*
Change	−.12	−.25*
Symptom patterns	.58*	.61*
Well-being	−.58*	−.66*

[a]From "An Empirical Test of Alternative Theories of Anger in Adolescents," by A. Yarcheski, N. E. Mahon, and T. J. Yarcheski, *Nursing Research*, 1999.
*$p < .01$

anger and vigor, and trait anger and change were not in the direction hypothesized. The correlation between state anger and change was not statistically significant.

Each of the structural equation models was tested via the LISREL 7 program (Joreskog & Sorbom, 1989). To test the influence of trait anger and state anger on each of the outcome measures, as determined by the magnitude of the path coefficients, a bivariate regression analysis was done on a just-identified model, using a correlation between the error terms (correlated error term) for the two dependent variables to account for the relationship between them. The initial estimates (path coefficients) produced by the program are identical to maximum likelihood estimates because the model is just-identified with zero degrees of freedom and, thus, fits the data perfectly.

A path diagram of the model of negative outcomes of trait anger and state anger with its respective path coefficients and squared multiple correlations is presented in Figure 2. As hypothesized, trait anger had a direct effect on state anger. Relative to the negative outcomes, trait anger had a direct negative effect on well-being and a direct positive effect on symptom patterns. State anger had a direct negative effect on well-being and a direct positive effect on symptom patterns. As hypothesized, trait anger had statistically significant indirect effects on well-being (−.17) through state anger and on symptom patterns (.21) through state anger. The total effect of trait anger on well-being was −.66; the total effect of trait anger on symptom patterns was .61.

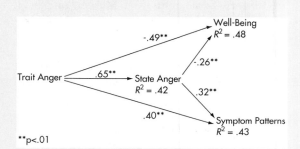

Figure 2. Results of testing negative outcomes of anger using bivariate regression analysis in early adolescents.

A path diagram of the model of positive outcomes of trait anger and state anger with its respective path coefficients and squared multiple correlations is presented in Figure 3. Again, as hypothesized, trait anger had a direct effect on state anger. Relative to the positive outcomes, the results were statistically significant for trait anger, but opposite to the direction predicted. Trait anger had direct negative effects on vigor and on change. State anger did not have a statistically significant direct effect on vigor or change. Contrary to expectations, trait anger did not have statistically significant indirect effects on vigor through state anger or on change through state anger. The total effect of trait anger on vigor was −.34; the total effect of trait anger on change was −.25.

In summary, trait anger had the greatest influence on diminishing general well-being, whereas state anger had the greatest influence on increasing symptom patterns. The influence of trait anger was greater in the model of negative out-

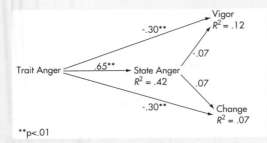

$$-.30^{**}$$

Vigor
$R^2 = .12$

$-.07$

Trait Anger $.65^{**}$ State Anger
$R^2 = .42$ $.07$

$-.30^{**}$

Change
$R^2 = .07$

$^{**}p<.01$

Figure 3. Results of testing positive outcomes of anger using bivariate regression analysis in early adolescents.

comes (symptom patterns and diminished well-being) than in the model of positive outcomes (vigor and change). State anger had a low to moderate influence in the model of negative outcomes (symptom patterns and diminished well-being). State anger had no significant influence on the positive outcomes (vigor and change).

DISCUSSION

As expected, based on Spielberger's (1972) state-trait theory, the path coefficient between trait anger and state anger was positive and strong. This finding gives credence to Spielberger's state-trait theory. According to this theory (Spielberger, 1996), trait anger is an acquired behavioral disposition that predisposes a person to perceive a wide range of situations as anger-provoking (i.e., annoying, frustrating, irritating), such as responding to questionnaires as the early adolescents did in the present study, and to react to such situations with elevations in state anger. Consistent with this theory, the higher the trait anger reported by the early adolescents in the present study, the higher the state anger reported by them.

In the model of negative outcomes, both trait anger and state anger diminished general well-being in early adolescents, and both findings are consistent with propositions by several anger theorists (Gaylin, 1984; Novaco, 1985, 1986) who posit that anger has harmful effects on well-being. Trait anger had a stronger negative influence on well-being in this sample than did state anger. Together trait anger and state anger explained 48% of the variance in general well-being (see Figure 2).

These findings add to the literature regarding the consequences of trait anger and state anger in early adolescents.

Because traits are relatively enduring characteristics of individuals, the negative influence of trait anger on general well-being is of concern in early adolescents. Spielberger (1966) stated that traits are developed during early childhood socialization and then tend to remain stable across the life span. In early adolescents, traits may not yet be fully developed and stabilized. Thus, interventions designed to modify trait anger might be effective and, in turn, increase the general well-being of early adolescents. Wilde (1996), who identified anger as a major problem during adolescence, recommends the use of rational-emotive behavior therapy to modify anger. To reduce anger, this therapy uses cognitive, emotive, and behavioral techniques to help adolescents find errors in their thinking and acting.

Both trait anger and state anger were related to increased symptom patterns in early adolescents, but trait anger had a somewhat stronger influence on symptom patterns than did state anger. Together, trait anger and state anger explained 43% of the variance in symptom patterns in this age group (see Figure 2), contributing to the knowledge base regarding the negative consequences of anger in early adolescents. The findings are consistent with propositions by several anger theorists (Averill, 1982; Freeberg, 1982; Gaylin, 1984) who posit that anger is manifested psychosomatically through the expression of various symptoms. Some of the symptoms, as measured in this study (Gurin et al., 1960), that were related to anger in the early adolescents were headaches, loss of appetite, upset stomach, difficulty getting up in the morning, and complaints of pains and ailments. Nurse practitioners working with early adolescents who present with such symptoms need to consider anger as a possible precursor of the symptomatology. When assessments reveal this to be the case, early adolescents may be helped by teaching them to express their anger in ways that do not compromise their health, as suggested by Freeberg (1982). It would be interesting to determine through longitudinal study whether trait anger and state anger predict psychosomatic disorders later in life in the same early adolescents who manifested high levels of symptom patterns due to trait anger and state anger earlier in life.

In the model of positive outcomes, contrary to expectation, the path coefficient indicated that trait anger was negatively related to vigor. This finding is surprising in that prominent theorists in the field of anger (Gaylin, 1984; Izard, 1977, 1991; Novaco, 1976) postulated a positive relationship between anger and vigor. Recently, Izard (1993) suggested that the vigor associated with anger is greater than that associated with any other emotion. However, the present findings indicate that trait anger is clearly enervating to early adolescents and reduces their vigor. In the absence of prior empirical work, replication of these findings in early adolescents and other age groups is indicated so that aforementioned theoretical statements can be further evaluated.

The correlation between state anger and vigor was statistically significant (see Table 1), but the path coefficient between the two variables was not (see Figure 3). These findings invite the following interpretation using Babbie's (1992) discussion of three-variable analysis. Trait anger is one determinant of state anger (Spielberger, 1972) and the two variables were related in the present study. When the influence of trait anger on state anger was controlled for in the statistical analysis of the structural equation model, the relationship between state anger and vigor vanished. Therefore, the correlation between state anger and vigor is spurious. In other words, because the path coefficient was of negligible magnitude in the model, there is no causal link between state anger and vigor. Their correlation is merely a product of the relationship found between trait anger and state anger and between trait anger and vigor in early adolescents. In addition, the negative correlation and path coefficient found between state anger and vigor was opposite to that hypothesized, which further challenges the positive direction postulated between anger and vigor by some theorists (Gaylin, 1984; Izard, 1977, 1991; Novaco, 1976).

Counter to the theorizing by Gaylin (1984) and Novaco (1976) who postulated that anger is a powerful motivator in promoting change, the higher the trait anger, the less inclined early adolescents were to seek new experiences, change opinions or values in different circumstances, and adapt to changes in the environment. From a methodological perspective, the personality characteristic of change, as measured in the present study, may not be wholly consistent with the action-oriented change suggested by these theorists. New instruments measuring the propensity for action-oriented change, and instruments that are more reliable than the one measuring personality-oriented change in the present study, are needed to pursue future research regarding the relationship between trait anger and change in early adolescents.

The correlation between state anger and change was not statistically significant (see Table 2), and the negative direction was opposite to that hypothesized. The path coefficient also was not statistically significant but the positive direction was consistent with that hypothesized. Given that neither the correlation nor path coefficient was significant, it is clear that state anger, a transitory emotional state, had little influence on the inclination to change in this sample of early adolescents.

In conclusion, in early adolescents, trait anger had a more powerful influence on both the negative and positive outcomes studied than did state anger. The negative outcomes of anger, both diminished well-being and increased symptom patterns, were clearly supported by the findings. The strongest relationship found was between trait anger and diminished general well-being, adding to the body of knowledge regarding the detrimental effects of anger. However, neither trait anger nor state anger contributed positively to the positive outcomes of vigor and inclination to change theorized in the literature. In fact, trait anger was found to de-energize and reduce vigor in early adolescents and to negatively influence their inclination to change. All findings considered, the experience of anger in early adolescents is ripe for continued study. Future analyses of anger should be done separately for boys and girls, and for early adolescents from different cultures so that a more comprehensive knowledge base can be developed.

References

Averill, J.R. (1982). Anger and aggression: An essay on emotion. New York: Springer-Verlag.

Averill, J.R. (1983). Studies on anger and aggression: Implications for theories of emotions. American Psychologist, 38, 1145-1160.

Babbie, E. (1992). The practice of social research (6th ed.). Belmont, CA: Wadsworth Publishing Company.

Blos, P. (1962). On adolescence. New York: The Free Press.

Columbo, S.A. (1984/1986). General well-being in adolescents: Its nature and measurement (Doctoral dissertation, Saint Louis University, 1984). Dissertation Abstracts International, 46, 2246B.

Elliott, G.R., & Feldman, S.S. (1990). Capturing the adolescent experience. In S.S. Feldman & G.R. Elliott (Eds.), At the threshold: The developing adolescent (pp. 1-53). Cambridge, MA: Harvard University Press.

Freeberg, S. (1982). Anger in adolescence. Journal of Psychosocial Nursing and Mental Health Services, 20, 29-31.

Fuqua, D.R., Leonard, E., Masters, M.A., Smith, R.J., Campbell, J.L., & Fisher, P.C. (1991). A structural analysis of the State-Trait Anger Expression Inventory. Educational and Psychological Measurement, 51, 439-446.

Furst, D.M., & Hardman, J.S. (1988). The iceberg profile in young competitive swimmers. Perceptual and Motor Skills, 67, 478.

Gaylin, W. (1984). The rage within. New York: Simon & Schuster.

Gurin, G., Veroff, J., & Feld, S. (1960). Americans view their mental health. New York: Basic Books.

Hamburg, B.A. (1974). Early adolescence: A specific and stressful stage of the life cycle. In G.V. Coehlo, D.A. Hamburg, & J.E. Adams (Eds.), Coping and adaptation (pp. 101-124). New York: Basic Books.

Hartzell, H.E. (1984). The challenge of adolescence. Topics in Language Disorders, 4, 1-9.

Izard, C.E. (1977). Human emotions. New York: Plenum Press.

Izard, C.E. (1991). The psychology of emotions. New York: Plenum Press.

Izard, C.E. (1993). Organizational and motivational functions of discrete emotions. In M. Lewis & J.M. Haviland (Eds.), Handbook of emotions (pp. 631-641). New York: Guilford Press.

Jackson, D.N. (1984). Personality research form manual (3rd ed.). Port Huron, MI: Research Psychologist Press.

Joreskog, K.G., & Sorbom, D. (1989). LISREL 7: A guide to the program and applications (2nd ed.). Chicago, IL: SPSS.

Larson, R.J., & Kasimatis, M. (1991). Day-to-day physical symptoms: Individual differences in the occurrence, duration, and emotion concomitants of minor daily illnesses. Journal of Personality, 59, 387-423.

Lerner, H.G. (1985). The dance of anger. New York: Harper and Row.

Lubin, B., Van Whitlock, R., McCollum, K.L., Thummel, H., Denman, N., & Powers, M. (1994). Measuring the short-term mood of adolescents: Reliability and validity of the state form of the Depression Adjective Checklists. Adolescence, 29, 591-604.

Mahon, N.E., Yarcheski, A., & Yarcheski, T.J. (1993). Health consequences of loneliness in adolescents. Research in Nursing & Health, 16, 23-31.

McGowan, R.W., Miller, M.J., & Henschen, K.P. (1990). Differences in mood states between belt ranks and karate tournament competitors. Perceptual and Motor Skills, 71, 147-150.

McNair, D.M., Lorr, M., & Droppleman, L.F. (1992). EDITS Manual for the Profile of Mood States. San Diego, CA: Educational and Industrial Testing Service.

Novaco, R.W. (1975). Anger control: The developmental evaluation of an experimental treatment. Lexington, MA: D.C. Heath and Company.

Novaco, R.W. (1976). The functions and regulations of the arousal of anger. American Journal of Psychiatry, 133, 1124-1127.

Novaco, R.W. (1985). Anger and its therapeutic regulation. In M.A. Chesney & R.H. Rosenman (Eds.), Anger and hostility in cardiovascular and behavioral disorders (pp. 203-226). New York: Hemisphere Publishing Corporation.

Novaco, R.W. (1986). Anger as a clinical and social problem. In R.J. Blanchard & D.C. Blanchard (Eds.). Advances in the study of aggression (Vol. 2, pp. 1-67) New York: Academic Press.

Pipher, M. (1994). Reviving Ophelia. New York: Ballantine Books.

Reddon, J.R., Pope, G.A., Friel, J.P., & Sinha, B.K. (1996). Leisure motivation in relation to psychosocial adjustment in young offender and high school samples. Journal of Clinical Psychology, 52, 679-685.

Schlosser, B. (1990). The assessment of subjective well-being and its relationship to the stress process. Journal of Personality Assessment, 54, 128-140.

Spielberger, C.D. (1966). Theory and research on anxiety. In C.D. Spielberger (Ed.), Anxiety and behavior (pp. 3-20). New York: Academic Press.

Spielberger, C.D. (1972). Anxiety as an emotional state. In C.D. Spielberger (Ed.), Anxiety: Current trends in theory and research. Vol. 1 (pp. 31-49). New York: Academic Press.

Spielberger, C.D. (1996). Manual for the State-Trait Anger Expression Scale. Port Huron, MI: Sigma Assessments Systems.

Spielberger, C.D., Jacobs, G., Russell, S., & Crane, R.S. (1983). Assessment of anger: The State-Trait Anger Scale. In J.N. Butcher & C.D. Spielberger (Eds.), Advances in personality assessment (pp. 161-189). Hillsdale, NJ: Lawrence Erlbaum.

Tanaka, J.S. (1987). "How big is big enough?": Sample size and goodness of fit in structural equation models with latent variables. Child Development, 58, 134-146.

Tavris, C. (1982). Anger: The misunderstood emotion. New York: Simon & Schuster.

Wilde, J. (1996). Treating anger, anxiety, and depression in children and adolescents. Washington, DC: Accelerated Development.

Yarcheski, A., & Mahon, N.E. (1986). Perceived stress and symptom patterns in early adolescents: The role of mediating variables. Research in Nursing & Health, 9, 289-297.

Yarcheski, A., Mahon, N.E., & Yarcheski, T.J. (1992). Validation of the PRQ85 Social Support Measure for adolescents. Nursing Research, 41, 332-337.

Yarcheski, A., Mahon, N.E., & Yarcheski, T.J. (1999). An empirical test of alternate theories of anger in early adolescents. Nursing Research, 48, 317-323.

Yarcheski, A., Scoloveno, M.A., & Mahon, N.E. (1994). Social support and well-being in adolescents: The role of hopefulness. Nursing Research, 43, 288-292.

Appendix D

From *Progress in Transplantation* 10(2): 81-87, 2000.

FAMILY ADAPTATION TO A CHILD'S TRANSPLANT: PRETRANSPLANT PHASE

Geri LoBiondo-Wood, PhD, RN
University of Texas,
Houston Health Science Center,
Houston, TX

Laurel Williams, MSN, RN
University of Nebraska Medical Center,
Omaha, NE

Kamiar Kouzekanani, PhD
University of Texas—Austin,
Austin, TX

Charles McGhee, PhD
University of Texas—San Antonio,
San Antonio, TX

The purpose of this study was to explore the relationship between family stress, family coping, social support, perception of stress, and family adaptation from the mother's perspective during the pretransplant period in the context of the Double ABC-X Model of Family Adaptation. The process of seeking a transplant for a child is very stressful, and before interventions can be developed, clinicians need to understand how aspects of family life are affected. Twenty-nine mothers whose children were being evaluated for a liver transplant constituted the sample for this exploratory study. Higher family strains, fewer coping skills, and higher perception of stress were related to more unhealthy family adaptation during the pretransplant phase. Data point to the need for close evaluation not only for the child's needs but for the family's needs as the family begins the process of seeking a transplant for the child. (Progress in Transplantation. 2000;10:81-87)

Transplantation is an accepted treatment for chronic liver disease in children. Seventy percent of all children who receive a liver transplant do so before they are 5 years old.[1] When parents are confronted by the reality that their child needs to be evaluated for an organ transplant, a whole set of issues, needs, and concerns arises. The issues of long waiting periods for scarce organs, financial burdens, chronic healthcare needs of the child, and stress on siblings and families related to the needs of a chronically ill child all weigh on the family and its resources.[2]

The literature also suggests that healthcare providers do not assess the needs of families well.[3-8] Providers need to know how to intervene with families in order to assist them in the transplant process. Before interventions can be developed, research needs to focus on how families are adapting to the reality of transplantation. This study begins the exploration of the relationship between family variables of stress, coping, social support, perception of stress, and family adaptation from the mother's perspective during the pretransplant period.

LITERATURE REVIEW

Transplantation is viewed as a process, with different phases that require the family to adapt. Each phase has the potential for crises and hardships. Throughout the life cycle, families are assumed to face hardships and crises and develop strengths and capabilities to deal with both minor and major disruptions. Some crises are short lived; others are more enduring and require not only adaptation but also change to meet new demands. Within the realm of healthcare, transplantation requires families to cope with both long-term adaptations and short-term crises.

Transplantation affects all aspects of individual and family life. No phase of the process has totally defined limits or costs in terms of time, physical and psychosocial factors, stress, and economics.[2,5-7] The research to date that is related to parents' responses prior to a child's transplantation has been scant.[5,7] Rodrigue et al,[5] in a study of 18 fathers whose children were evaluated for solid organ transplants, reported less parenting stress, more concern about family finances, and more limitations in family activities, compared to normative group data. Weichler[7] explored mothers' information needs at each stage of the liver transplant process and found that, prior to the child's transplant, the mother's information needs were related to the child's physical needs and status, as well as ways to emotionally support the child.

Prior to receiving a transplant, children and their families will have been in the healthcare system for varying lengths of time, dealing with multiple physical problems and therapies. Gold et al[8] reviewed descriptive information gathered over a 4-year period from parents who participated in a support group for parents whose children either had or were awaiting a heart or liver transplant. Parents in the preoperative stage described a sense of relief in knowing that their child was at a center that could offer treatment. On the other hand, parents felt a sense of loss of control of the care of their child. Parents also expressed a range of emotions, including guilt, depression, and anger.

Another study explored the impact of the child's liver transplant on the family from the mother's perspective during the posthospitalization period.[6] This study found that mothers felt that social support, better coping skills, and de-

creased levels of stress were significantly related to family adaptation in the first year after the child's transplant.

Unless a child has experienced an acute life-threatening illness involving the liver, most children arrive at the transplant center with a need for a transplant as a consequence of a progressive, chronic liver disease. As a result of liver disease, a child may have seen multiple care providers, undergone multiple tests and treatments, and developed multisystem complications, including hypersplenism, portal hypertension, and growth retardation.[9]

The initial step in becoming approved as a candidate for a transplant is generally a physical, psychosocial, and developmental evaluation of both the child and the family over the course of several days. Parents are also confronted with new staff and with the economic impact of the transplant, and they may have to travel to different states or cities to the transplant center. Once the child is accepted as a candidate for a transplant, there is a waiting period that may last weeks or years. During the waiting phase, families and children must cope with the chronic disease process; potential for the child's death; decisions about which parent should be the donor in the case of living-related transplantation; and the hope that a donor liver will become available. Transplantation, as a treatment for a chronic illness, is different from other chronic disease treatments in that children often can begin treatment as soon as the diagnosis is made. However, in end-stage liver disease, the sickest children are given transplants first because of the shortage of organs.[10] Parents are presented with a dilemma. Even though it is better to keep the child as well as possible preoperatively, the parents know that the sickest child receives an organ first.[8,11] Also, children and their families awaiting liver transplantation are waiting for another person, generally a child, to die. Parents have reported feelings of guilt related to awaiting another child's death.[7,8]

The process of seeking a transplant for a chronically ill child is a long-term process, with many challenges not only for the child, but for

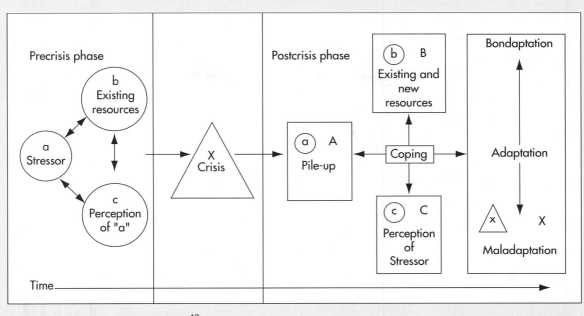

Double ABC-X Model of Family Adaptation[12]

the family as a whole. For this study, the factors that families confront were conceptualized using the Double ABC-X Model of Family Adaptation[12] (see figure). The concepts of the model are described within the context of the pretransplant period. The concept of pile-up (aA) reflects the idea that the family undergoes a pile-up of stressors and strains. These stressors and strains include usual family developmental demands, the stress related to waiting, financial burdens, and the feelings of loss of control. Family's existing and new resources—social support (bB)—are the family's ability to meet its demands and needs and include existing and expanded family support and resources. Within this framework, how families cope or manage is believed to be related to their adaptation. The family's perception of the stressor (cC) focuses on the family's view of the stressors and the meaning that family members give to the stressor. The diagnosis and treatment of liver disease in a child presents a host of uncertainties that the family confronts. Family adaptation (xX) is the component of the frame-work that denotes the continuum of outcomes toward which the family's efforts are directed.

The pretransplant phase of the process is the beginning of a journey that requires families to deal with multiple stressors and uncertainties. The postcrisis variables of the model were the focus of this study. The crisis events for families during the pretransplant period are the need for the child to be evaluated for a possible liver transplant, with incumbent stress, and the need to have and develop new resources, cope, and adapt.

METHODS

This study considers the postcrisis variables of the Double ABC-X Model.[12] Table 1 lists the postcrisis concepts of the model and the tools used to quantify each concept.

Sample

The subjects were 29 mothers, ranging in age from 19 to 44 years, whose children were being evaluated for a liver transplant (see Table 2). Because this was an exploratory study, no power analysis

Table 1. Family Concepts and Measures

Concept	Measure
Pile-up—Family strains (aA)	Family Inventory of Life Events and Changes
Existing and new resources (bB)	
Social support	Norbeck Social Support Questionnaire
Coping	Coping Health Inventory for Parents
Perception of stressor (cC)	Parent Perception of Uncertainty Scale Profile of Mood States
Family adaptation (xX)	McMaster's Family Assessment Device

Table 2. Sample Demographics (N = 29)

	Mean age	Range
Mother	28.8	19-44
Father	30.5	21-45
Child	3.3	.04-12.6
Marital status, no. (%)		
Single	4 (13.8)	
Married	22 (75.9)	
Divorced	3 (10.3)	

was performed. All mothers were able to read and understand English. The sample comprised 17 whites, 9 blacks, 1 American Indian, 1 Hispanic American, and 1 mother of unspecified ethnicity. Twenty (68.9%) of the mothers had attended or graduated from college. In the category of combined family income, 12 families (41.3%) earned below $20,000; 9 (31%) earned in the $20,001 to $30,000 range, and 5 earned above $30,001. The mean age of the children who were the transplant candidates was 3.3 years (SD, 4.3 years). Fifty-nine percent of the children were male.

Instruments

Six standardized tools were used to measure the concepts in the Double ABC-X model (see Table 1). The reliabilities for each of these instruments were calculated for this study and found to be .70 and above.

Family Inventory of Life Events and Changes (FILE).[13] The FILE is a 71-item tool used to measure family stress variables, with the added ability of measuring the pile-up of life events. A reliability coefficient of .81 for the total scale score (N = 2470) has been reported, indicating internal consistency.[13] Validity assessments of the instrument were made by correlating the FILE with the Family Environment Scale, another measure of family functioning.[14] The FILE was used in the current study to measure stress, with higher scores indicating higher stress levels.

Coping Health Inventory for Parents (CHIP).[15] The CHIP was devised to measure parents' coping responses in the management of family life when a child member is seriously and/or acutely ill. The CHIP is a 45-item tool with 3 scales: Family Integration, Cooperation, and an Optimistic Definition of the Situation; Maintaining Social Support, Self-Esteem, and Psychological Stability; and Understanding the Health Care Situation Through Communication with Other Parents and Consultation with the Health Care Team.[15] Coefficient alphas for the 3 scales are 0.79, 0.79, and 0.71, respectively, for the same sample. In a study of predictive validity, the parents' use of the 3 coping patterns was associated with improvement in the child's health status on 2 measures.[15] The CHIP was used in the current study to measure coping. Families with higher conflict record greater use (higher scores) of coping behaviors assessed by the CHIP, since this reflects an active effort on the part of families to manage conflict and adapt.[15]

Norbeck Social Support Questionnaire (NSSQ). The NSSQ is a 9-item, self-report questionnaire developed by Norbeck, Lindsey, and Carrieri[16] that measures multiple dimensions of social support. The NSSQ evaluates a person's total network, including number of support persons, frequency of contact, duration of relationship, total functional support, and total loss. Test-retest reliability yielded correlation coefficients ranging from .85 to .92 for functional and network items and .71 to .83 for number of persons and support loss, respectively.[16] Internal consistency ranges from .88 to .97.[17] Tests of concurrent and predictive validity have also been conducted.[16,18] The NSSQ was used in the current study to measure existing and new resources.

Parent Perception of Uncertainty Scale (PPUS). The PPUS was developed by Mishel[19] as an extension of her work on the construct of uncertainty in illness, specifically as it relates to parents' uncertainty experience concerning their child's illness. This 31-item instrument contains 4 subscales: Ambiguity, Lack of Clarity, Lack of Information, and Unpredictability. Reliability for the total scale is .91, and the subscales range from .72 to .87. The PPUS has also been evaluated for construct and predictive validity.[19] The PPUS was used in the current study to measure a parent's perception of uncertainty as a stressor. Higher scores reflect higher levels of uncertainty.

Profile of Mood States (POMS). The POMS is a 65-item adjective rating scale which measures 6 identifiable mood states: Tension-Anxiety, Depression-Dejection, Anger-Hostility, Vigor-Activity, Fatigue-Inertia, and Confusion-Bewilderment.[20] The POMS is a measure of an individual's level of mood and subjective affect. Internal consistency is reported to be .90 or above for all items within each factor. Validity has been established in multiple studies.[20] Although the current study researched how families adapt to a child's need for a transplant, the authors believe that an assessment of the individual's affect as an emotional response to the stressors of transplantation was important to study within the exploratory boundaries of the study.

McMaster Family Assessment Device (FAD). The FAD is a 60-item instrument designed as a multidimensional measure of family functioning and based on the McMaster Model of Family Functioning.[21] The FAD contains 6 subscales and a total scale score. The subscales are Problem Solving, Communication, Roles, Affective Responsiveness, Affective Involvement, and Behavior Control. The General Functioning score reflects an overall index of family functioning. Internal consistency using coefficient alpha from samples of psychiatric (N = 1138), medical (N = 298), and nonclinical (N = 627) samples ranges from 0.57 to .86. Test-retest reliability at a 1-week interval for the subscales and total scale ranged from .66 to .76.[22] Confirmatory factor analyses with the 3 samples provide support for the hypothesized structure of the instrument.[21] Scores on the scales have a possible range of from 1 (healthy) to 4 (unhealthy). In the current study, the FAD was used to measure the outcome variable of family adaptation.

Demographic information. Data gathered for purposes of sample description included characteristics of the children and parents, and medical factors related to end-stage liver disease.

Procedure

Following approval from the Institutional Review Board, the authors mailed a consent form to mothers whose children were scheduled for a transplant evaluation, explaining the study's aim and including a request for participation, directions, and the instruments. Mothers completed the instruments at the time of the evaluation and returned the completed forms at the end of the evaluation, or completed the instruments within 1 week of the evaluation and returned them by mail. Completion of the instruments was the condition of inclusion.

RESULTS

The reliability of each of the instruments used in this study was tested. Coefficients for all of the scales used were at least .70 and above. The Pearson Product Moment Correlation was used to test whether there were significant relationships between the independent variables of stress, coping, social support, perception of stressor, and mood state, and the dependent variable of family adaptation. Correlations that were found to be significant were generally moderate to strongly correlated. Table 3 presents the relationships among the subscales, total scores for each variable, and significance.

Stress

Overall family stress as measured by the FILE and family adaptation (on the FAD) were positively and

Table 3. Correlation Among Family Variables and Family Adaptation

	FAD subscales and general functioning						
	AI	AR	BC	C	PS	R	GF
Stress (FILE)							
Finance and business	.22	.06	.22	−.02	−.06	.37	.00
Marital strains	.62***	.62**	.07	.05**	.42**	.58**	.65***
Intrafamily strains	.06**	.73***	.17	.62**	.69***	.63***	.73***
Work-family transitions and strains	.05**	.48**	.27	.43**	.41*	.58**	.05**
Losses	.34	.43*	.23	.14	.29	.27	.36
Illness and family care strains	.36	.28	.03	.07	−.06	.28	.23
Pregnancy or childbearing strains	.19	.18	.04	.05	.14	.18	.07
Transition in and out	.54**	.20	−.03	.01	.06	.31	.25
Family legal violations	.47**	.01	−.13	.00	−.11	.23	.13
Total	.68***	.60**	.18	.41*	.40*	.64***	.58**
Resources (NSSQ)							
Affect	−.37	−.24	−.09	−.19	−.13	−.03	−.25
Affirm	−.34	−.19	−.12	−.16	−.01	−.03	−.02
Aid	−.32	−.21	−.01	−.16	−.12	−.29	−.21
Total network	−.31	−.16	−.01	−.12	.02	−.17	−.18
Total losses	.49*	.27	.08	.12	.04	.09	.22
Total functioning	−.35	−.21	−.01	−.17	−.12	−.03	−.22
Total	.02	.01	−.42*	−.07	−.04	−.19	.07
Coping (CHIP)							
Family	−.53**	−.79***	−.32	−.53**	−.6**	−.22	−.68***
Medical	−.07	−.52**	−.24	−.38	−.56**	−.08	−.45**
Support	−.18	−.49*	−.24	−.48*	−.48*	−.15	−.47**
Total	−.34	−.69***	−.31	−.54**	−.61**	−.19	−.62**
Stressors—Uncertainty (PPUS)							
Lack of clarity	.32	.11	.11	−.01	.14	.36	.01
Lack of information	.03	.13	−.05	−.13	.02	.37	.11
Unpredictability	.45*	.25	.37	.13	.17	.45*	.28
Ambiguousness	.51**	.36	.09	.34	.03	.39*	.28
Total	.58**	.34	.16	.21	.27	.53**	.26
Stressors (POMS)							
Tension-anxiety	.19	.19	.03	.28	.01	.36	.21
Depression-dejection	.05**	.05**	.12	.33	.25	.45*	.43*
Anger-hostility	.62***	.06**	−.06	.52**	.01	.39*	.57**
Vigor-activity	.02	−.16	−.52**	−.27	−.19	−.25	−.16
Confusion-bewilderment	.01	.15	.06	.19	.06	.45*	.16
Fatigue-inertia	−.02	−.11	−.12	−.03	−.16	.17	−.11
Total	.35	.40*	.13	.38**	.24	.47*	.37*

*$P < .05$; **$P < .01$; ***$P < .001$.

AI indicates affective involvement; *AR,* affective response; *BC,* behavior control; *C,* communications; *CHIP,* Coping Health Inventory for Parents; *FAD,* McMaster Family Assessment Device; *FILE,* Family Inventory of Life Events and Changes; *GF,* general functioning and total scale score; *NSSQ,* Norbeck Social Support Questionnaire; *POMS,* Profile of Mood States; *PPUS,* Parent Perception of Uncertainty Scale; *PS,* problem solving; *R,* roles.

significantly related (r = .58, P < .01). Testing of the subscales of the various instruments with the FAD subscales was also performed (see Table 3). The FAD subscales of affective involvement (r = .68, P < .001), affective response (r = .60, P < .01), coping (r = .41, P < .05), problem solving (r = .40, P < .05), roles (r = P < .001) and total family stress were significantly and positively related. The FILE subscales of marital strain, intrafamily, and work-family strains were significantly and positively related to all of the FAD subscales except behavior control.

Resources

Resources and social support as measured by the NSSQ demonstrated no significant relationships with family adaptation except for behavior control. Overall social support and behavior control were negatively and significantly related (r = −.42, P < .05).

Coping

Coping as measured by the CHIP was negatively and significantly related to family adaptation (r = −.62, P < .01). Significant negative relationships were found between the subscales of the CHIP, ie, family integration (r = −.68, P < .001), support (r = .47, P < .01), understanding of medical care (r = −.45, P < .01), and family adaptation. Also, the total score of the CHIP and the affective response and problem solving subscales of the FAD were all negatively and significantly correlated. There were no significant relationships among the FAD subscales of behavior control and roles and the CHIP, but there were mixed results among the remaining FAD subscales of affective involvement and communications.

Perception of Stressor

The relationship between the subscales of the PPUS and family adaptation demonstrated mixed results. Family adaptation was not significantly related to overall uncertainty. The subscales of affective involvement (r = .58, P < .001) and roles (r = .53, P < .01) were related significantly to uncertainty. Overall affective state of the mother was positively and significantly related

to family adaptation (POMS, r = .37, P < .05). When examining the various moods tested by the POMS, higher levels of depression and anger were significantly related to various aspects of poorer family adaptation.

DISCUSSION

Data from this study suggest that in this sample, for each subject both as the mother reporting family information and as an individual in the family, there is a relationship between increased family strains, fewer coping skills, and unhealthy family adaptation. In this sample, among the family stressors of marital strain, intrafamily strain, and work-family transitions, mothers with higher levels of these stressors related poorer family adaptation. This response may be caused by the chronic nature of the healthcare needs and child's disease process. Also, mothers who reported using fewer coping skills reported significantly more unhealthy family adaptation. The positive and significant relationship between unhealthy family adaptation and the mother's depression and anger is also important to note. These findings are significant because the evaluation is just the beginning step of the trajectory in the transplant process for the family. Each of the significant findings is the beginning of a picture that can lead to better understanding of how to assess and assist families who are beginning the path of seeking a transplant for a child.

This study has several limitations. The small sample size, limited to mothers, does not permit generalization to a larger population and does not include the father's perspective. Also, the data collection period and timing of the data collection were at a stressful time. It may have been too early in the process for the mothers to respond to the events; it might have been better to have queried the mothers several weeks after the evaluation.

The evaluation process is an important step in moving toward the actual transplant, and it should also be a beginning step in evaluating and working with the family in a larger context. Many services are offered to children who are evaluated for transplant. The study data suggest that care providers need to review and address the needs of both the child and the family during the evaluation. The child is closely assessed during the evaluation for potential needs and services. Services for evaluating the child and the family need to be available. Family services need to be timely and cost effective. In order to provide such services, healthcare providers need to know not only what services are most beneficial but also more information about the family's strengths and weaknesses.

Families are generally given a great deal of information about transplantation during the pretransplant evaluation. What information is integrated by the parents and how well the information is integrated are important elements to consider in light of expected stress and reported coping levels. Also, the form in which the information is delivered should be considered. If an individual is having difficulty coping and is very anxious, the amount of attention the individual can give to written or oral information is limited. It may be that an overview of the information should be given at first and details reinforced later.

It is not surprising that this study found high levels of stress, fewer coping skills, and some difficulty in family adaptation. The data reflect that the evaluation period is a stressful and critical period for the family. This study points to the need for further research. Family variables were measured at a single point in a process that extends over a long period. Fathers were not included, but fathers' responses to the stress of transplant evaluation need to be explored. Whether fathers share the same responses as do the mothers or have other responses needs to be understood in the light of care planning. Further research is needed to see how and if family adaptation changes over the process of transplantation in the light of other family variables in the model.

CONCLUSION AND RECOMMENDATIONS

As healthcare providers try to meet the needs of children who require transplant, they must re-

member that the children's parents and family members perform a critical role in total healthcare. Parents decide when to seek care, have to understand and use the vast amount of information given regarding the child's care, and provide the care needed by the child. Parents interact with the healthcare system on behalf of their child and thereby influence the child's care greatly. It is crucial for health providers to understand the way the child is perceived by the family before the transplant as well as after the transplant.

Variables of individual and family stress and of coping were found to correlate significantly with family adaptation prior to transplantation. The study data provide the basis for further research and evaluation of the impact of transplantation on the family as a whole. As healthcare providers move to cost containment and documentation of outcomes that affect the child's family and that family's ability to cope and care for a member with chronic healthcare needs, research needs to focus on what aspects of the child's care are compromised if the family's needs are not addressed. Based on the data from this study and the long-term healthcare needs, further explorations of the short-term and long-term impact of the child's transplant on the family are clearly needed to develop a picture of the child's and family's needs over time.

Acknowledgments

This research was funded by the National Institute of Nursing Research, National Institutes of Health, Washington, DC.

References

1. United Network for Organ Sharing. 1996 Annual Report of Transplant Recipients and the Organ Procurement and Transplant Network. Richmond, Va: United Network for Organ Sharing; 1997.
2. Suddaby EC. No simple answers: ethical conflicts in pediatric heart transplantation. *J Transplant Coord.* 1999;9:266-270.
3. Jacono J, Hicks G, Antonioni C. Comparison of perceived needs of family members of criti-

cally ill patients in intensive care and neonatal intensive care units. *Heart Lung.* 1990;19:33-38.

4. Martin SD. Coping with chronic illness. *Home Health Care Nurse.* 1995;13:50-54.

5. Rodrigue JR, MacNaughton K, Hoffman RG, et al. Perceptions of parenting stress and family relations by fathers of children evaluated for organ transplantation. *Psychol Rep.* 1996; 79:723-727.

6. LoBiondo-Wood G, Bernier-Henn M, Williams L. Impact of the child's transplant on the family: maternal perspective. *Ped Nurs.* 1992;18: 461-466.

7. Weichler, NK. Information needs of mothers of children who have had liver transplants. *J Ped Nurs.* 1990;5:88-96.

8. Gold LM, Kirkpatrick BS, Fricker FJ, Zittelli BJ. Psychosocial issues in pediatric organ transplantation: the parent's perception. *Pediatrics.* 1986;77:38-744.

9. Jurim O, Seu P, Busuttil R. Pediatric liver transplantation. In: Maddery WC, Sorrell MF, eds. *Transplantation of the Liver.* 2nd edition. Norwalk, Conn: Appleton & Lange; 1995.

10. United Network for Organ Sharing. *UNOS Update.* 1995;11:15-17, 40.

11. Heffron TG, Emond JC. Living-related donor liver transplantation. In: Maddery WC, Sorrell MF, eds. *Transplantation of the Liver.* 2nd edition. Norwalk, Conn: Appleton & Lange; 1995.

12. McCubbin HI, Patterson JM. In McCubbin HI, Sussman MB, Patterson JM, eds. *Social Stress and the Family Marriage: Marriage and Family Review.* New York, NY: Harcourt Brace; 1983:67-137.

13. McCubbin HI, Patterson JM, Wilson L. Family inventory of life events and changes. In: McCubbin HI, Thompson A, eds. *Family Assessment and Inventories for Research and Practice.* Madison, Wis: University of Wisconsin, Madison; 1987.

14. Moos R. *Family Environment Scales.* Palo Alto, Calif: Consulting Psychologists Press; 1974.

15. McCubbin HI, McCubbin M, Nevin R, Cauble AE. Coping health inventory for parents (CHIP). In: McCubbin HI, Thompson A, eds. *Family Assessment for Research and Practice.* Madison, Wis: University of Wisconsin, Madison; 1982.

16. Norbeck JS, Lindsey AM, Carrieri VL. Further development of the Norbeck social support questionnaire: normative data and validity testing. *Nurs Res.* 1983;32:4-9.

17. Norbeck JS, Lindsey AM, Carrieri VL. The development of an instrument to measure social support. *Nurs Res.* 1981;30:264-269.

18. Brandt PA. Clinical assessment of social support of families with handicapped children. *Compr Ped Nurs.* 1984;7:1189-1193.

19. Mishel M. Parent's perception of uncertainty concerning their hospitalized child. *Nurs Res.* 1983;32:324-330.

20. McNair DM, Lorr M, Doppleman LF. *POMS Manual for Profile of Mood States.* San Diego, Calif: Educational and Industrial Testing Service; 1971.

21. Epstein NB, Bishop DS, Baldwin LM. McMaster model of family functioning: A view of the normal family. In: Walsh A, ed. *Normal Family Processes.* New York, NY: Guilford Press; 1982.

22. Brown GB, Arpin K, Corey P, Fitch M, Gafni A. Prevalence and correlates of family dysfunction and poor adjustment to chronic illness in specialty clinics. *J Clin Epidemiol.* 1990;43:373-383.

Glossary

A

a priori From Latin: the former; before the study or analysis.

abstract A brief, comprehensive summary of a study.

accessible population A population that meets the population criteria and is available.

after-only design An experimental design with two randomly assigned groups—a treatment group and a control group. This design differs from the true experiment in that both groups are measured only after the experimental treatment.

after-only nonequivalent control group design A quasiexperimental design similar to the after-only experimental design, but subjects are not randomly assigned to the treatment or control groups.

alternate form reliability Two or more alternate forms of a measure are administered to the same subjects at different times. The scores of the two tests determine the degree of relationship between the measures.

analysis of covariance (ANCOVA) A statistic that measures differences among group means and uses a statistical technique to equate the groups under study in relation to an important variable.

analysis of variance (ANOVA) A statistic that tests whether group means differ from each other, rather than testing each pair of means separately, ANOVA considers the variation among all groups.

animal rights Guidelines used to protect the rights of animals in the conduct of research.

anonymity A research participant's protection in a study so that no one, not even the researcher, can link the subject with the information given.

antecedent variable A variable that affects the dependent variable but occurs before the introduction of the independent variable.

applied research Tests the practical limits of descriptive theories but does not examine the efficacy of actions taken by practitioners.

assent An aspect of informed consent that pertains to protecting the rights of children as research subjects.

assumption A basic principle assumed to be true without the need for scientific proof.

auditability The researcher's development of the research process in a qualitative study that allows a researcher or reader to follow the thinking or conclusions of the researcher.

axial coding A data-analysis strategy used the grounded theory method. It requires intense coding around a single theme.

B

basic research Theoretical or pure research that generates, tests, and expands theories that explain or predict a phenomenon.

beneficence An obligation to do harm and to maximize possible benefits.

benefit Potential positive outcomes of participation in research study.

bias A distortion in the data-analysis results.

bracketed A process during which the researcher identifies personal biases about the phenomenon of interest to clarify how personal experience and beliefs may color what is heard and reported.

C

case studies The study of a selected phenomenon that provides an in-depth description of its dimensions and processes.

case study method The study of selected contemporary phenomenon over time to provide an in-depth description of essential dimensions and processes of the phenomenon.

chance error Attributable to fluctuations in subject characteristics that occur at a specific point in time and are often beyond the awareness and control of the examiner. Also called random error.

chi-square (x^2) A nonparametric statistic that is used to determine whether the frequency found in each category is different from the frequency that would be expected by chance.

close-ended item Question that the respondent may answer with only one of a fixed number of choices.

cluster sampling A probability sampling strategy that involves a successive random sampling of units. The units sampled progress from large to small. Also known as *multistage sampling*.

cohort The subjects of a specific group that are being studied.

computer database Print database that is put on software programs that can be accessed on-line or on CD-ROM via the computer.

concealment Refers to whether the subjects know that they are being observed.

concept An image or symbolic representation of an abstract idea.

conceptual definition General meaning of a concept.

conceptual framework A structure of concepts and/or theories pulled together as a map for the study.

conceptual literature Published and unpublished non–data-based material, such as reports of theories, concepts, synthesis of research on concepts, or professional issues, some of which underlie reported research, as well as other nonresearch material.

conceptual model A set of interrelated concepts that symbolically represents a phenomenon.

concurrent validity The degree of correlation of two measures of the same concept that are administered at the same time.

conduct of research The analysis of data collected from a homogenous group of subjects who meet study inclusion and exclusion criteria for the purpose of answering specific research questions or testing specified hypotheses.

confidence interval Quantifies the uncertainty of a statistic or the probably value range within which a population parameter is expected to lie.

confidentiality Assurance that a research participant's identity cannot be linked to the information that was provided to the researcher.

consent See *informed consent*.

consistency Data are collected from each subject in the study in exactly the same way or as close to the same way as possible.

constancy Methods and procedures of data collection are the same for all subjects.

constant comparative method A process of continuously comparing data as they are acquired during research with the grounded theory method.

construct An abstraction that is adapted for scientific purpose.

construct replication The use of original methods, such as sampling techniques, instruments, or research design, to study a problem that has been investigated previously.

construct validity The extent to which an instrument is said to measure a theoretical construct or trait.

consumer One who actively uses and applies research findings in nursing practice.

content analysis A technique for the objective, systematic, and quantitative description of communications and documentary evidence.

content validity The degree to which the content of the measure represents the universe of content, or the domain of a given behavior.

context Environment where event(s) occurs.

contrasted-group approach A method used to assess construct validity. A researcher identifies two groups of individuals who are suspected to have an extremely high or low score on a characteristic. Scores from the groups are obtained and examined for sensitivity to the differences. Also called known-group approaches.

uniform or

control Measures used to ... constant the condition ... investigation occurs ... experimental

control group The ... eceive an ... investigation that ... comparison group. **nonprobability**

intervention o ... ses the most readily

convenience ... bjects as subjects in **sampling**

access ... trategy for assessing ... hich two or more tools

a stu ... asure the same construct

conv ... subjects. If the measures ... dated, convergent validity ... orted.

... gree of association between

...y A type of nonexperimental ... that examines the ... tween two or more variables. ... s in qualitative research to ensure ... validity, or soundness of data.

...-related validity Indicates the degree ... elationship between performance on the ... measure and actual behavior either in the present (concurrent) or in the future (predictive).

critical reading An active interpretation and objective assessment of an article during which the reader is looking for key concepts, ideas, and justifications.

critical thinking The rational examination of ideas, inferences, principles, and conclusions.

critique The process of objectivity and critically evaluating a research report's content for scientific merit and application to practice, theory, or education.

critiquing criteria The criteria used for objectively and critically evaluating a research article.

Cronbach's alpha Test of internal consistency that simultaneously compares each item in a scale to all others.

cross-sectional study A nonexperimental research design that looks at data at one point in time, that is, in the immediate present.

culture The system of knowledge and linguistic expressions used by social groups that allows the researcher to interpret or make sense of the world.

Cumulative Index to Nursing and Allied Health Literature (CINAHL) A print or computerized database; computerized CINAHL is available on CD-ROM and on-line.

D

data Information systematically collected in the course of a study; the plural of datum.

database A compilation of information about a topic organized in a systematic way.

data-based literature Reports of completed research.

data saturation A point when data collection can cease. It occurs when the information being shared with the researcher becomes repetitive. Ideas conveyed by the participant have been shared before by other participants; inclusion of additional participants does not result in new ideas.

debriefing The opportunity for researchers to discuss the study with the participants and for participants to refuse to have their data included in the study.

deductive reasoning A logical thought process in which hypotheses are derived from theory; reasoning moves from the general to the particular.

degrees of freedom The number of quantities that are unknown minus the number of independent equations linking these unknowns; a function of the number in the sample.

delimitations Those characteristics that restrict the population to a homogeneous group of subjects.

Delphi technique The technique of gaining expert opinion on a subject. It uses rounds or multiple stages of data collection, with each round using data from the previous round.

dependent variable In experimental studies, the presumed effect of the independent or experimental variable on the outcome.

descriptive/exploratory survey A type of nonexperimental research design that collects descriptions of existing phenomena for the purpose of using the data to justify or assess current conditions or to make plans for improvement of conditions.

descriptive statistics Statistical methods used to describe and summarize sample data.

design The plan or blueprint for conduct of a study.

developmental study A type of nonexperimental research design that is concerned not only with the existing status and interrelationship of phenomena but also with changes that take place as a function of time.

diffusion The strategy for promoting adoption of evidence-based practices.

direct observation A method for measuring psychological and physiological behaviors for purposes of evaluating change and facilitating recovery.

directional hypothesis Hypothesis that specifies the expected direction of the relationship between the independent and dependent variables.

dissemination The communication of research findings.

divergent validity A strategy for assessing construct validity in which two or more tools that theoretically measure the opposite of the construct are administered to subjects. If the measures are negatively correlated, divergent validity is said to be supported.

domains Symbolic categories that include the smaller categories of an ethnographic study.

downlink A receiver for programs beamed from other agencies that allows a person to participate in telecommunications conferences.

E

electronic database The electronic means by which journal sources (periodicals) of data-based and conceptual articles on a variety of topics (e.g., doctoral dissertations) are found, as well as the publications of professional organizations and various governmental agencies.

element The most _unit about which_ information is colle

eligibility criteria Th restrict the populatio _teristics that_ group of subjects. _ogeneous_

emic view The natives' o world.

empirical analytical A gen quantitative research appro _of the_ hypotheses.

empirical The obtaining of evid objective data.

empirical literature A synonym fo literature; see _data-based literature_

Epistemology The theory of knowle branch of philosophy that concerns people know what they know.

equivalence Consistency or agreement a observers using the same measurement or agreement among alternate forms of a t

error variance The extent to which the variance in test scores is attributable to error rather than a true measure of the behaviors.

ethics The theory or discipline dealing with principles of moral values and moral conduct.

ethnographic method A method that scientifically describes cultural groups. The goal of the ethnographer is to understand the natives' view of their world.

ethnographic research See _ethnography._

ethnography A qualitative research approach designed to produce cultural theory.

etic view An outsider's view of another's world.

evaluation research The use of scientific research methods and procedures to evaluate a program, treatment, practice, or policy outcomes; analytical means are used to document the worth of an activity.

evaluative research The use of scientific research methods and procedures for the purpose of making an evaluation.

evidence-based practice The conscious and judicious use of the current "best" evidence in the care of patients and delivery of health care services.

evidence-based guidelines A set of guidelines that allow the researcher to better understand the evidence base of certain practices.

ex post facto study A type of nonexperimental research design that examines the relationships among the variables after the variations have occurred.

experiment A scientific investigation in which observations are made and data are collected by means of the characteristics of control, randomization, and manipulation.

experimental design A research design that has the following properties: randomization, control, and manipulation.

experimental group The group in an experimental investigation that receives an intervention or treatment.

external criticism A process used to judge the authenticity of historical data.

external validity The degree to which findings of a study can be generalized to other populations or environments.

extraneous variable Variable that interferes with the operations of the phenomena being studied. Also called *mediating variable.*

F

face validity A type of content validity that uses an expert's opinion to judge the accuracy of an instrument.

factor analysis A type of validity that uses a statistical procedure for determining the underlying dimensions or components of a variable.

findings Statistical results of a study.

Fisher's exact probability test A test used to compare frequencies when samples are small and expected frequencies are less than six in each cell.

fittingness Answers the questions: Are the findings applicable outside the study situation? Are the results meaningful to the individuals not involved in the research?

frequency distribution Descriptive statistical method for summarizing the occurrences of events under study.

G

generalizability (generalize) The inferences that the data are representative of similar phenomena in a population beyond the studied sample.

grand theory All-inclusive conceptual structures that tend to include views on person, health, and environment to create a perspective of nursing.

grounded theory Theory that is constructed inductively from a base of observations of the world as it is lived by a selected group of people.

grounded theory method An inductive approach that uses a systematic set of procedures to arrive at theory about basic social processes.

H

historical research method The systematic compilation of data resulting from evaluation and interpretation of facts regarding people, events, and occurrences of the past.

history The internal validity threat that refers to events outside of the experimental setting that may affect the dependent variable.

homogeneity Similarity of conditions. Also called internal consistency.

hypothesis A prediction about the relationship between two or more variables.

hypothesis-testing validity A strategy for assessing construct validity in which the theory or concept underlying a measurement instrument's design is used to develop hypotheses that are tested. Inferences are made based on the findings about whether the rationale underlying the instrument's construction is adequate to explain the findings.

I

independent variable The antecedent or the variable that has the presumed effect on the dependent variable.

inductive reasoning A logical thought process in which generalizations are developed from specific observations; reasoning moves from particular to the general.

inferential statistics Procedures that combine mathematical processes and logic to test hypotheses about a population with the help of sample data.

informed consent An ethical principle that requires a researcher to obtain the voluntary participation of subjects after informing them of potential benefits and risks.

innovation diffusion Process by which an innovation or research findings are communicated through various channels over time among the members of a profession.

institutional review boards (IRBs) Boards established in agencies to review biomedical and behavioral research involving human subjects within the agency or in programs sponsored by the agency.

instrumental case study Research that is done when the researcher pursues insight into an issue or wants to challenge a generalization.

instrumentation Changes in the measurement of the variables that may account for changes in the obtained measurement.

integrative research review Synthesis review of the literature on a specific concept or topic.

internal consistency The extent to which items within a scale reflect or measure the same concept.

internal criticism A process of judging the reliability or consistency of information within an historical document.

internal validity The degree to which it can be inferred that the experimental treatment, rather than an uncontrolled condition, resulted in the observed effects.

internet The global electronic network that links a cadre of participating networks (e.g., commercial, educational, and governmental agencies).

interrater reliability The consistency of observations between two or more observers; often expressed as a percentage of agreement between raters or observers or a coefficient of agreement that takes into account the element of chance. This usually is used with the direct observation method.

interrelationship/difference studies The classification of a nonexperimental research design that attempts to trace relationships among variables. The four types are correlational, ex post facto, prediction, and developmental.

interval The level of measurement that provides different levels or gradations in response. The differences or intervals between responses are assumed to be approximately equal.

interval measurement Level used to show rankings of events or objects on a scale with equal intervals between numbers but with an arbitrary zero (e.g., centigrade temperature).

intervening variable A variable that occurs during an experimental or quasiexperimental study that affects the dependent variable.

intervention Deals with whether or not the observer provokes actions from those who are being observed.

interviews A method of data collection in which a data collector questions a subject verbally. Interviews may be face-to-face or performed over the telephone, and they may consist of open-ended or close-ended questions.

intrinsic case study Research that is undertaken to have a better understanding of the essential nature of the case.

item to total correlation The relationship between each of the items on a scale and the total scale.

J

justice Human subjects should be treated fairly.

K

key informants Individuals who have special knowledge, status, or communication skills and who are willing to teach the ethnographer about the phenomenon.

knowledge-focused triggers Ideas that are generated when staff read research, listen to scientific papers at research conferences, or encounter evidence-based practice guidelines published by federal agencies or specialty organizations.

Kuder-Richardson (KR-20) coefficient The estimate of homogeneity used for instruments that use a dichotomous response pattern.

kurtosis The relative peakness or flatness of a distribution.

L

level of significance (alpha level) The risk of making a type I error, set by the researcher before the study begins.

levels of measurement Categorization of the precision with which an event can be measured (nominal, ordinal, interval, and ratio).

life context The matrix of human-human-environment relationships emerging over the course of one's life.

Likert-type scales Lists of statements on which respondents indicate whether they "strongly agree," "agree," "disagree," or "strongly disagree."

limitation Weakness of a study.

linear structural relationships (LISREL) A computer program developed to analyze covariance and the testing of complex causal models.

literature Print and non-print sources such as books, chapters of books, journal articles, critique reviews, abstracts published in conference proceedings, professional and governmental reports, and unpublished doctoral dissertations.

lived experience In phenomenological research a term used to refer to the focus on living through events and circumstances (prelingual) rather than thinking about these events and circumstances (conceptualized experience).

longitudinal study A nonexperimental research design in which a researcher collects data from the same group at different points in time.

M

manipulation The provision of some experimental treatment, in one or varying degrees, to some of the subjects in the study.

matching A special sampling strategy used to construct an equivalent comparison sample group by filling it with subjects who are similar to each subject in another sample group in relation to preestablished variables, such as age and gender.

maturation Developmental, biological, or psychological processes that operate within an individual as a function of time and are external to the events of the investigation.

mean A measure of central tendency; the arithmetic average of all scores.

measurement The assignment of numbers to objects or events according to rules.

measurement effects Administration of a pretest in a study that affects the generalizability of the findings to other populations.

measures of central tendency Descriptive statistical procedure that describes the average member of a sample (mean, median, and mode).

measures of variability Descriptive statistical procedure that describes how much dispersion there is in sample data.

median A measure of central tendency; the middle score.

mediating variable A variable that is between or occurs between an independent and dependent variable and can produce an indirect effect of the independent variable on the dependent variable. Also called *extraneous variable*.

MEDLINE The print or computerized database of standard medical literature analysis and retrieval system on-line; it is also available on CD-ROM.

metaanalysis A research method that takes the results of multiple studies in a specific area and synthesizes the findings to make conclusions regarding the area of focus.

methodological research The controlled investigation and measurement of the means of gathering and analyzing data.

microrange theory The linking of concrete concepts into a statement that can be examined in practice and research.

midrange theory A focused conceptual structure that synthesizes practice-research into ideas central to the discipline.

modal percentage A measure of variability; percent of cases in the mode.

modality The number of peaks in a frequency distribution.

mode A measure of central tendency; most frequent score or result.

model A symbolic representation of a set of concepts that is created to depict relationships.

mortality The loss of subject from time 1 data collection to time 2 data collection.

multiple analysis of variance (MANOVA) A test used to determine differences in group means; used when there is more than one dependent variable.

multiple regression Measure of the relationship between one interval level dependent variable and several independent variables. Canonical correlation is used when there is more than one dependent variable.

multistage sampling (cluster sampling) Involves a successive random sampling or units (clusters) that programs from large to small and meets sample eligibility criteria.

multitrait-multimethod approach A type of validity that uses more than one method to assess the accuracy of an instrument (e.g., observation and interview of anxiety).

N

naturalistic research A general label for qualitative research methods that involve the researcher going to a natural setting, that is, to where the phenomena being studied is taking place.

network sampling (snowball effect sample) A strategy used for locating samples that are difficult to locate. It uses social networks and the fact that friends tend to have characteristics in common; subjects who meet the eligibility criteria are asked for assistance in getting in touch with others who meet the same criteria.

nominal The level of measurement that simply assigns data into categories that are mutually exclusive.

nominal measurement Level used to classify objects or events into categories without any relative ranking (e.g., gender, hair color).

nondirectional hypothesis One that indicates the existence of a relationship between the variables but does not specify the anticipated direction of the relationship.

nonequivalent control group design A quasiexperimental design that is similar to the true experiment, but subjects are not randomly assigned to the treatment or control groups.

nonexperimental research design Research design in which an investigator observes a phenomenon without manipulating the independent variable(s).

nonparametric statistics Statistics that are usually utilized when variables are measured at the nominal or ordinal level because they do not estimate population parameters and involve less restrictive assumptions about the underlying distribution.

nonparametric tests of significance Inferential statistics that make no assumptions about the population distribution.

nonprobability sampling A procedure in which elements are chosen by nonrandom methods.

normal curve A curve that is symmetrical about the mean and unimodal.

null hypothesis A statement that there is no relationship between the variables and that any relationship observed is a function of chance or fluctuations in sampling.

O

objective Data that are not influenced by anyone who collects the information.

objectivity The use of facts without distortion by personal feelings or bias.

observed score The actual score obtained in a measure.

ontology The study of being, of existence, and its relationship to non-existence.

open-ended item Question that the respondent may answer in his or her own words.

operational definition The measurements used to observe or measure a variable; delineates the procedures or operations required to measure a concept.

operationalization The process of translating concepts into observable, measurable phenomena.

ordinal The level of measurement that systematically categorizes data in an ordered or ranked manner. Ordinal measures do not permit a high level of differentiation among subjects.

ordinal measurement Level used to show rankings of events or objects; numbers are not equidistant, and zero is arbitrary (class ranking).

P

paradigm From the Greek word meaning "pattern," it has been applied to science to describe the way people in society think about the world.

parallel form reliability See *alternate form reliability.*

parameter A characteristic of a population.

parametric statistics Inferential statistics that involve the estimation of at least one parameter, require measurement at the interval level or above, and involve assumptions about the variables being studied. These assumptions usually include the fact that the variable is normally distributed.

path analysis A statistical technique in which the researcher hypothesizes how variables are related and in what order and then tests how strong those relationships or paths are.

Pearson correlation coefficient (Pearson r) A statistic that is calculated to reflect the degree of relationship between two interval level variables. Also called Pearson product moment correlation coefficient.

percentile A measure of rank; percentage of cases a given score exceeds.

phenomenological method A process of learning and constructing the meaning of human experience through intensive dialogue with persons who are living the experience.

phenomenological research Phenomenological research is based on phenomenological philosophy and is research aimed at obtaining a description of an experience as it is lived in order to understand the meaning of that experience for those who have it.

phenomenology A qualitative research approach that aims to describe experience as it is lived through, before it is conceptualized.

philosophical beliefs The system of motivating values, concepts, principles, and the nature of human knowledge of an individual, group, or culture.

philosophical research Based on the investigation of the truths and principles of existence, knowledge, and conduct.

physiological measurement The use of specialized equipment to determine physical and biological status of subjects.

pilot study A small, simple study conducted as a prelude to a larger-scale study that is often called the "parent study."

population A well-defined set that has certain specified properties.

population validity Generalization of results to other populations.

prediction study A type of nonexperimental research design that attempts to make a forecast or prediction derived from particular phenomena.

predictive validity The degree of correlation between the measure of the concept and some future measure of the same concept.

primary source Scholarly literature that is written by a person(s) who developed the theory or conducted the research. Primary sources include eyewitness accounts of historic events, provided by original documents, films, letters, diaries, records, artifacts, periodicals, or tapes.

print databases Indexes, card catalogues, and abstract reviews. Print indexes are used to find journal sources (periodicals) of data-based and conceptual articles on a variety of topics, as well as publications of professional organizations and various governmental agencies.

print index See *print databases.*

probability The probability of an event is the event's long-run relative frequency in repeated trials under similar conditions.

probability sampling A procedure that uses some form of random selection when the sample units are chosen.

problem statement An interrogative sentence or statement about the relationship between two or more variables.

problem-focused triggers Those that are identified by staff through quality improvement, risk surveillance, benchmarking data, financial data, or recurrent clinical problems.

process consent In qualitative research the ongoing negotiation with subjects for their participation in a study.

product testing Testing of medical devices.

program A list of instructions in a machine-readable language written so that a computer's hardware can carry out an operation; software.

propositions The linkage of concepts that lays a foundation for the development of methods that test relationships.

prospective study Nonexperimental study that begins with an exploration of assumed causes and then moves forward in time to the presumed effect.

psychometrics The theory and development of measurement instruments.

purposive sampling A nonprobability sampling strategy in which the researcher selects subjects who are considered to be typical of the population.

Q

qualitative measurement The items or observed behaviors are assigned to mutually exclusive categories that are representative of the kinds of behavior exhibited by the subjects.

qualitative research The study of research questions about human experiences. It is often conducted in natural settings, and uses data that are words or text rather than numerical in order to describe the experiences that are being studied.

quantitative measurement The assignment of items or behaviors to categories that represent the amount of a possessed characteristic.

quantitative research The process of testing relationships, differences, and cause and effect interactions among and between variables. These processes are tested with either hypotheses and/or research questions.

quasiexperiment Research designs in which the researcher initiates an experimental treatment but some characteristic of a true experiment is lacking.

quasiexperimental design A study design in which random assignment is not used but the independent variable is manipulated and certain mechanisms of control are used.

questionnaires Paper and pencil instruments designed to gather data from individuals.

quota sampling A nonprobability sampling strategy that identifies the strata of the population and proportionately represents the strata in the sample.

R

random access memory (RAM) A computer's memory that the user can read or change.

random selection A selection process in which each element of the population has an equal and independent chance of being included in the sample.

randomization A sampling selection procedure in which each person or element in a population has an equal chance of being selected to either the experimental group or the control group.

range A measure of variability; difference between the highest and lowest scores in a set of sample data.

ratio The highest level of measurement that possesses the characteristics of categorizing, ordering, and ranking and also has an absolute or natural zero that has empirical meaning.

ratio measurement Level that ranks the order of events or objects and that has equal intervals and an absolute zero (e.g., height, weight).

reactivity The distortion created when those who are being observed change their behavior because they know that they are being observed.

recommendation Application of a study to practice, theory, and future research.

records or available data Information that is collected from existing materials, such as hospital records, historical documents, or videotapes.

refereed journal or peer-reviewed journal A scholarly journal that has a panel of external and internal reviewers or editors; the panel reviews submitted manuscripts for possible publication. The review panels use the same set of scholarly criteria to judge if the manuscripts are worthy of publication.

relationship/difference studies Studies that trace the relationships or differences between variables that can provide a deeper insight into a phenomenon.

reliability The consistency or constancy of a measuring instrument.

reliability coefficient A number between 0 and 1 that expresses the relationship between the error variance, true variance, and the observed score. A 0 correlation indicates no relationship. The closer to 1 the coefficient is, the more reliable the tool.

replication The repetition of a study that uses different samples and is conducted in different settings.

representative sample A sample whose key characteristics closely approximate those of the population.

research The systematic, logical, and empirical inquiry into the possible relationships among particular phenomena to produce verifiable knowledge.

research base The accumulated knowledge gained from several studies that investigate a similar problem.

research-based practice Nursing practice that is based on research studies; that is, supported by research findings.

research-based protocols Practice standards that are formulated from findings of several studies.

research hypothesis A statement about the expected relationship between the variables; also known as a scientific hypothesis.

research literature A synonym for data-based literature.

research problem Presents the question that is to be asked in a research study.

research question A key preliminary step wherein the foundation for a study is developed from the research problem and results in the research hypothesis.

research utilization A systematic method of implementing sound research-based innovations in clinical practice, evaluating the outcome, and sharing the knowledge through the process of research dissemination.

respect for persons People have the right to self-determination and to treatment as autonomous agents; that is, they have the freedom to participate or not participate in research.

retrospective data Data that have been manifested, such as scores on a standard examination.

retrospective study A nonexperimental research design that begins with the phenomenon of interest (dependent variable) in the present and examines its relationship to another variable (independent variable) in the past.

review of the literature An extensive, systematic, and critical review of the most important published scholarly literature on a particular topic. In most cases it is not considered exhaustive.

risk Potential negative outcome(s) of participation in research study.

risk-benefit ratio The extent to which the benefits of the study are maximized and the risks are minimized such that the subjects are protected from harm during the study.

S

sample A subset of sampling units from a population.

sampling A process in which representative units of a population are selected for study in a research investigation.

sampling error The tendency for statistics to fluctuate from one sample to another.

sampling frame A list of all units of the population.

sampling interval The standard distance between the elements chosen for the sample.

sampling unit The element or set of elements used for selecting the sample.

saturation See *data saturation.*

scale A self-report inventory that provides a set of response symbols for each item. A rating or score is assigned to each response.

scholarly literature Refers to published and unpublished data-based and conceptual literature materials found in print and nonprint forms.

scientific approach A logical, orderly, and objective means of generating and testing ideas.

scientific hypothesis The researcher's expectation about the outcome of a study; also known as the research hypothesis.

scientific literature A synonym for data-based literature; see *data-based literature.*

scientific merit The degree of validity of a study or group of studies.

scientific observation Collecting data about the environment and subjects. Data collection has specific objectives to guide it, is systematically planned and recorded, is checked and controlled, and is related to scientific concepts and theories.

secondary analysis A form of research in which the researcher takes previously collected and analyzed data from one study and reanalyzes the data for a secondary purpose.

secondary source Scholarly material written by person(s) other than the individual who developed the theory or conducted the research. Most are usually published. Often a secondary source represents a response to or a summary and critique of a theorist's or researcher's work. Examples are documents, films, letters, diaries, records, artifacts, periodicals, or tapes that provide a view of the phenomenon from another's perspective.

selection The generalizability of the results to other populations.

selection bias The internal validity threat that arises when pretreatment differences between the experimental group and the control group are present.

semiquartile range A measure of variability; range of the middle 50% of the scores. Also known as semiinterquartile range.

simple random sampling A probability sampling strategy in which the population is defined, a sampling frame is listed, and a subset from which the sample will be chosen is selected; members randomly selected.

skew Measure of the asymmetry of a set of scores.

snowball effect sampling (network sampling) A strategy used for locating samples difficult to locate. It uses social network and the fact that friends tend to have characteristics in common; subjects who meet the eligibility criteria are asked for assistance in getting in touch with others who meet the same criteria.

social desirability The occasion when a subject responds in a manner that he or she believes will please the researcher rather than in an honest manner.

Solomon four-group design An experimental design with four randomly assigned groups—the pretest-posttest intervention group, the pretest-posttest control group, a treatment or intervention group with only posttest measurement, and a control group with only posttest measurement.

split-half reliability An index of the comparison between the scores on one half of a test with those on the other half to determine the consistency in response to items that reflect specific content.

stability An instrument's ability to produce the same results with repeated testing.

standard deviation (SD) A measure of variability; measure of average deviation of scores from the mean.

standard error of the mean The standard deviation of a theoretical distribution of sample means. It indicates the average error in the estimation of the population mean.

statistical hypothesis States that there is no relationship between the independent and dependent variables. The statistical hypothesis also is known as the null hypothesis.

statistical reliability An index of the interval consistency of responses to all items of a single form of measure that is administered at one time.

stratified random sampling A probability sampling strategy in which the population is divided into strata or subgroups. An appropriate number of elements from each subgroup are randomly selected based on their proportion in the population.

survey studies Descriptive, exploratory, or comparative studies that collect detailed descriptions of existing variables and use the data to justify and assess current conditions and practices, or to make more plans for improving health care practices.

symbolic interaction A theoretical perspective that holds that the relationship between self and society is an ongoing process of symbolic communication whereby individuals create a social reality.

systematic Data collection carried out in the same manner with all subjects.

systematic error Attributable to lasting characteristics of the subject that do not tend to fluctuate from one time to another. Also called constant error.

systematic sampling A probability sampling strategy that involves the selection of subjects randomly drawn from a population list at fixed intervals.

T

t statistic Commonly used in nursing research; it tests whether two group means are more different than would be expected by chance. Groups may be related or independent.

target population A population or group of individuals that meet the sampling criteria.

test A self-report inventory that provides for one response to each item that the examiner assigns a rating or score. Inferences are made from the total score about the degree to which a subject possess whatever trait, emotion, attitude, or behavior the test is supposed to measure.

testable Variables of proposed study that lend themselves to observation, measurement, and analysis.

testing The effects of taking a pretest on the scores of a posttest.

test-retest reliability Administration of the same instrument twice to the same subjects under the same conditions within a prescribed time interval, with a comparison of the paired scores to determine the stability of the measure.

text Data in a contextual form, that is narrative or words that are written and transcribed.

theoretical framework Theoretical rationale for the development of hypotheses.

theoretical literature A synonym for conceptual literature; see conceptual literature.

theoretical sampling Used to select experiences that will help the researcher test ideas and gather complete information about developing concepts when using the grounded theory method.

theory Set of interrelated concepts, definitions, and propositions that present a systematic view of phenomena for the purpose of explaining and making predictions about those phenomena.

time series design A quasiexperimental design used to determine trends before and after an experimental treatment. Measurements are taken several times before the introduction of the experimental treatment, the treatment is introduced, and measurements are taken again at specified times afterward.

time-sharing Several users working on one mainframe via terminals at the same time.

triangulation The expansion of research methods in a single study or multiple studies to enhance diversity, enrich understanding, and accomplish specific goals.

true experiment Also known as the pretest-posttest control group design. In this design, subjects are randomly assigned to an experimental or control group, pretest measurements are performed, an intervention or treatment occurs in the experimental group, and posttest measurements are performed.

type I error The rejection of a null hypothesis that is actually true.

type II error The acceptance of a null hypothesis that is actually false.

U

uplink The ability to broadcast conferences so that they can be attended from a distance.

V

validation sample The sample that provides the initial data for determining the reliability and validity of a measurement tool.

validity Determination of whether a measurement instrument actually measures what it is purported to measure.

variable A defined concept.

W

web browser Software program used to connect or "read" the World Wide Web (www).

world wide web (www) A conceptual group of servers on the internet. The web is multiple hypertext linked together in an internet network that criss-crosses the whole internet like a spider web.

worldview Another label for paradigm, see above, the way people in society think about the world.

Z

Z score Used to compare measurements in standard units; examines the relative distance of the scores from the mean.

Index

A

A priori, 214
Abstract, 37, 44
Abstract reviews, 91*b*
Accessible population, 242
Accuracy
  interviews and questionnaires and, 303
  research design and, 189-190
Advanced statistics, 359-360
After-only experimental design, 207*f*, 208-209
After-only nonequivalent control group design, 212*f*, 213
Agency for Health Research and Quality, 91*t*, 93*t*, 420, 421*b*
Aims of inquiry, 128, 128*t*
Alpha level, 352-353
Alternate form reliability, 324, 327
American Association of Critical Care Nurses website, 420
American Nurses Association human rights guidelines, 271-272, 272*b*
American Pain Society website, 420
American Thoracic Society website, 421
Analysis of covariance, 228, 230, 357
Analysis of variance, 356
Analysis understanding, 40-41
Anecdotes, 300
Animal rights, 284-285, 286*b*
Anonymity, 273*t*, 274*t*, 276
  questionnaires and, 304
Antecedent variable, 206, 212
AORN Online, 92*t*
Assent, 282
Associate level nurse
  literature review by, 81*t*
  role in research process, 10
Associated causal analysis techniques, 230
Association for Women's Health website, 420-421
Assumptions, critical reading and, 36
Audit and feedback, 432
Auditability, 157, 158*t*, 168*b*
Authenticity of records, 305
Available data, 304-305

B

Baccalaureate level nurse
  literature review by, 81*t*
  role in research process, 10-11

Page numbers followed by f [the "f" is in ital] indicate figures; t, [the "t," in ital] tables; b, [the "b," in ital] boxes.

Backward solution, 359
Bakas Caregiving Outcomes Scale, 314
Beneficence, 267, 270*b*
Benefits, 270
Best Evidence website, 421
Best Practices Network website, 421
Bias
  bracketing and, 145
  consistency in data collection and, 296
  in convenience sampling, 244
  in purposive sampling, 246-247
  in systematic sampling, 252
  interviewer, 304
  records and available data and, 305
  sampling procedures and, 257
  selection, 195*t*, 197
Bimodal distribution, 338, 339*f*
Biobehavioral interface, 297
Biological measurements, 296-298
Bracketing, 134, 145
Braden Scale, 315-316
Brainstorming, 52, 55*f*

C

Cabinet and Council on Nursing Research, 7
Card catalog, 90, 91*b*
Care Continuity Instrument, 318-319
Caregiver Reciprocity Scale, 317*t*, 317-318
Case report, 152
Case study, 126, 132-133, 152-154
Causal modeling, 230
Causal relationship, 62
Causal-comparative study, 228*t*, 228-229
Causality issue in nonexperimental research, 229-231
Center for Advanced Nursing Practice, 415-417
Centers for Health Evidence website, 421
Chance error, 313
Change champion, 431, 431*b*
Charmaz' guidelines for ethnographical writing, 162
Child involvement in research, 282
Chi-square, 357
Chronic illness, research opportunities in, 25
Classic experiment, 207*f*, 207-209
Clinical Evidence website, 93*t*
Close-ended items, 301, 302*f*
Cluster sampling, 244*t*, 250-251
Cochrane Library website, 91*t*, 93*t*, 421
Code of ethics, 266